Invasive Investigation of the Heart

A GUIDE TO
CARDIAC CATHETERISATION AND
RELATED PROCEDURES

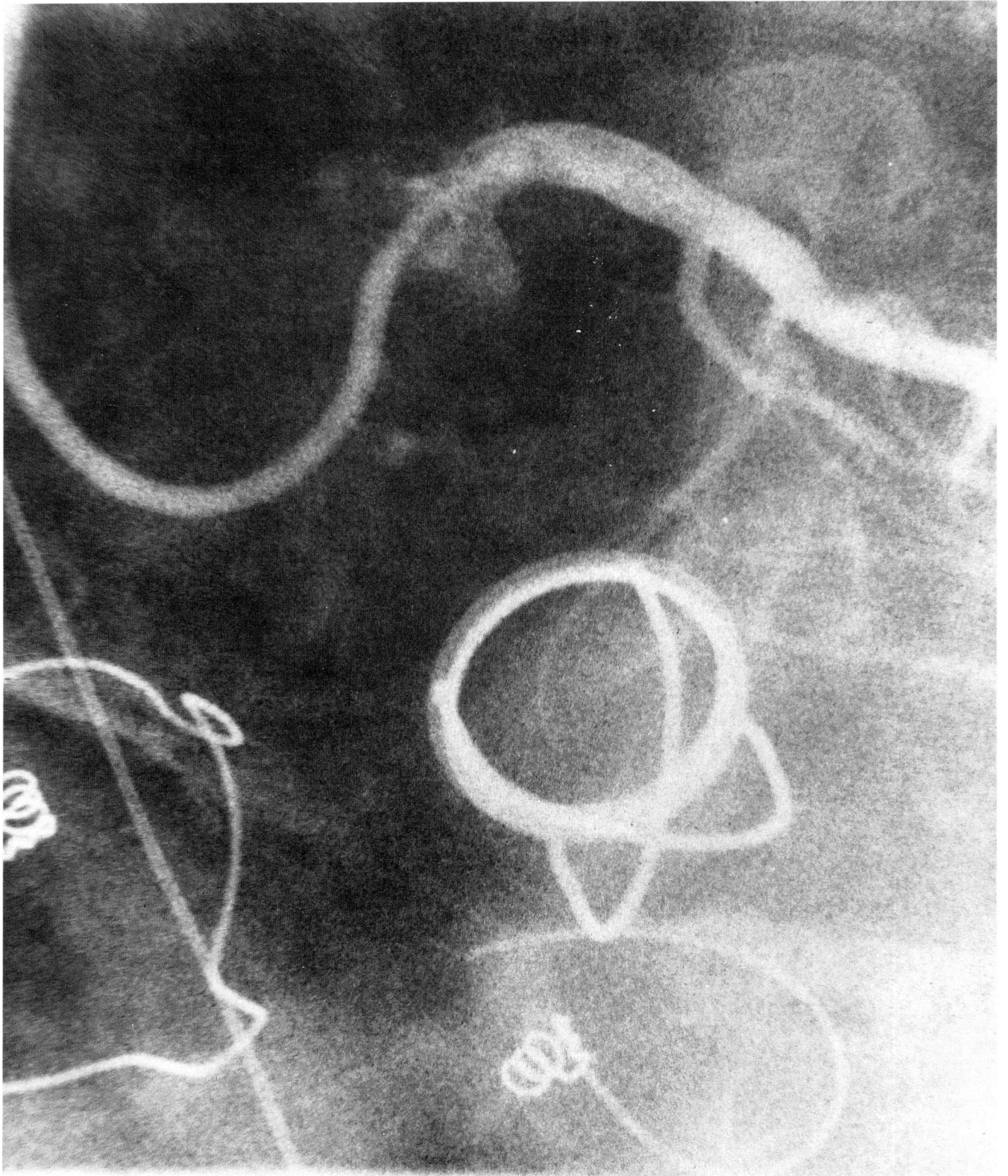

Hardware!

Invasive Investigation of the Heart

A GUIDE TO

CARDIAC CATHETERISATION AND

RELATED PROCEDURES

GRAHAM MILLER

MA, BSc, DM, FRCP
Consultant Cardiologist and Director
Cardiac Laboratories
Brompton Hospital
London

BLACKWELL SCIENTIFIC PUBLICATIONS
OXFORD LONDON EDINBURGH BOSTON MELBOURNE

Dedicated to
The Cardiac Technicians and Nurses of
the Brompton Hospital — without whose skills
it would not be possible and without whose
friendship it would not have been
so much fun

© 1989 by
Blackwell Scientific Publications
Editorial offices:
Osney Mead, Oxford OX2 0EL
  (*Orders*: Tel: 0865−240201)
8 John Street, London WC1N 2ES
23 Ainslie Place, Edinburgh EH3 6AJ
3 Cambridge Center, Suite 208
  Cambridge, Massachusetts 02142, USA
107 Barry Street, Carlton
  Victoria 3053, Australia

First published 1989

Set in Palatino and Helvetica
by Setrite Typesetters, Hong Kong
Printed and bound in Great Britain
by William Clowes Limited, Beccles and London

DISTRIBUTORS

USA
  Year Book Medical Publishers
  200 North LaSalle Street
  Chicago, Illinois 60601
  (*Orders*: Tel: (312) 726−9733)

Canada
  The C.V. Mosby Company
  5240 Finch Avenue East
  Scarborough, Ontario
  (*Orders*: Tel: (416) 298−1588)

Australia
  Blackwell Scientific Publications
  (Australia) Pty Ltd
  107 Barry Street
  Carlton, Victoria 3053
  (*Orders*: Tel: (03) 347−0300)

British Library
Cataloguing in Publication Data
Miller, Graham A.H. (Graham Austin Herrock)
  Invasive investigation of the heart.
  1. Man. Heart. Diagnosis. Catheterisation
  I. Title
  616.1'20754

ISBN 0−632−02027−X

Contents

PART 1   TECHNIQUES

PART 2   CATHETERISATION IN SPECIFIC DISORDERS

APPENDICES

Additional Contributors

R. BALCON MD FRCP FACC
Consultant Cardiologist
London Chest Hospital
Bonner Road
London

M.A. BRANTHWAITE MD FRCP FFARCS
Consultant Physician and Anaesthetist
Brompton Hospital
Fulham Road
London

K. DAWKINS BSc MD MRCP
Consultant Cardiologist
Wessex Cardiothoracic Centre
Southampton General Hospital
Tremona Road
Southampton
formerly *Clinical Fellow in Transplantation*
  Cardiology
Stanford University Medical Centre
Stanford
USA

D. DENISON PhD FRCP
Consultant in Respiratory Physiology
Brompton Hospital
Fulham Road
London
Professor of Clinical Physiology
National Heart and Lung Institute
London

I.H. KERR MB FRCP FRCR
Consultant Radiologist
Brompton Hospital
Fulham Road
London

C. MORGAN BM FFARCS
Consultant in Intensive Care and Anaesthesia
Departments of Intensive Care and Anaesthesia
Brompton Hospital
Fulham Road
London

E. ROWLAND MB BS
Lecturer Cardiothoracic Institute
Cardiac Department
Brompton Hospital
London

L.D.R. SMITH BSc MBBS MRCP
formerly *Research Fellow*
presently *Visiting Scientist*
IBM Scientific Centre
2 St Clement Street
Winchester
Locum Snr Registrar
Cardiac Department
St Thomas's Hospital
Lambeth Palace Road
London

Preface

Much of the appeal of the discipline of Cardiology lies in its use of practical procedures, pre-eminently the techniques of cardiac catheterisation. There is great satisfaction to be gained when a procedure has been completed speedily, safely and without discomfort to the patient and, as a result, the outstanding questions have been answered and future management made clear. This book is addressed to cardiologists undertaking catheterisation procedures in the hope that a description of the various procedures will be of use in helping them to develop the necessary skills.

Since the aim of catheterisation is to reach a diagnosis it seemed important to devote a major portion of the book to a description of the findings that enable one to reach a specific diagnosis and to exclude alternatives. This section, profiles of acquired and congenital heart disease, forms the second part of the book. The problem here was what to put in — and what to leave out. Clearly it is impossible to describe all the possible variations of congenital heart disease in a general text. Yet the haemodynamic and angiographic characteristics of congenital lesions provide such insight into cardiac function in general that I was unable to resist temptation — and congenital heart disease is covered in some detail for this reason.

No attempt is made to provide a general textbook of cardiology — physical signs, electrocardiographic findings and treatment are not discussed. More controversially I have not attempted an exhaustive description of the various ways in which cardiac function may be studied under conditions of stress — exercise, pacing, the infusion of drugs. Here I plead bias: questioning how far the many derived indices truly affect the management of the individual patient and whether the information could not have been obtained in simpler ways. The interests of the patient, not the doctor, are paramount. The patient is ill served by a long and uncomfortable study the results of which will make no difference to his treatment. The questions which should be asked, before anyone is subjected to catheterisation, are 'What is the purpose of the study?', 'What is the information required — and will it make any difference to his management?' and 'Can this information be obtained in other, simpler, ways?'

But catheterisation can often provide the answer more quickly and more definitively than a battery of other tests. 'Invasion' must not be seen as inherently wrong while 'non-invasive' investigation, like cleanliness, is next to Godliness. What is bad is an invasive investigation that is badly performed or designed. I have devoted considerable space to the risks of catheterisation, and their avoidance — and make no apology for doing so.

Finally I acknowledge a great debt to the friends and colleagues who have contributed to this text. Believing that you can only write well about a subject if you are an expert, I have sought out such experts to write those sections in which I was less than expert — or frankly ignorant. All are, or have been, colleagues at the National Heart and Chest Hospitals and all have given their time to what is often a thankless task — I thank them now.

My thanks too to the staff of Blackwell Scientific Publications: to Peter Saugman for his cheerful encouragement and, in particular, to Karen Anthony for creating order out of chaos.

Graham Miller 1988

Introduction

The history of cardiac catheterisation begins in 1929 when Werner Forssmann first demonstrated that it was possible to introduce a catheter into the human heart — his own — without complications [1], but it was not until the 1940s that cardiac catheterisation started to develop into the technique that, today, is part of the routine investigation of cardiac disease. Initially right heart catheterisation was used to provide information about cardiac physiology — by Cournand and his associates in the US [2] and by McMichael and Sharpey-Schafer in England [3]. Catheterisation was first used for *diagnostic* purposes in 1945 [4] and left heart catheterisation was first performed by Zimmerman in 1950 [5]. The impact of cardiac catheterisation cannot be overstated: for the first time it was possible to check, in the living patient, the validity of clinical diagnosis by a technique that provided unequivocal, quantifiable information. With the development of selective angiography, pictorial information was added and the heart was no longer inaccessible; on the contrary it became one of the most accessible organs and yielded more and more of its secrets. The discipline of Cardiology had a dual appeal; fact had replaced speculation and there was a place for those who enjoyed developing technical skills.

However, the demise of cardiac catheterisation has been predicted at many times in the past 25 years. As rheumatic fever became a rare disease in the post-antibiotic era and as each new 'non-invasive' technique was developed it was predicted that there would be a diminishing need for the skills of the 'invasive cardiologist'. The reverse has turned out to be the case; the number of catheterisation laboratories and the number of patients studied by invasive techniques have increased dramatically. The need for cardiologists and others trained in the techniques of cardiac catheterisation has increased rather than diminished.

Is it true, however, that the 'case mix' has changed over the years. Rheumatic fever and its cardiac sequelae are seen less frequently — at least in the affluent societies of the West — and the catheterisation laboratory is less often called upon to study patients with rheumatic valve disease. There are reasons for this other than the decreasing frequency of rheumatic fever. Firstly, advances in surgical technique have made unnecessary the assessment of the relative degrees of mitral stenosis and regurgitation; valve replacement is an option which was not available in the era of closed mitral valvotomy. Secondly, echocardiography provides answers to many of the questions that formerly could only be answered by cardiac catheterisation. But it is important to remember that the reliability of echocardiographic signs had, initially, to be checked against the findings at catheterisation. In this regard echocardiographic diagnosis is no different from clinical diagnosis; the reliability of physical signs had also, initially, to be determined by catheterisation. Thus cardiac catheterisation is the 'gold standard'. We may dispense with catheterisation when alternative diagnostic tests are reliable or when additional information will not affect management and it is right that we should; catheterisation has a small risk but not a zero-risk. The first questions that the physician should ask are: 'Is catheterisation necessary in this case? Will the information obtained materially affect the management of the patient?' There is still controversy about the need for catheterisation in, for example, mitral valve disease [6–8] but we must not allow vested interests to affect our judgement — and this applies to both the enthusiasts for non-invasive techniques and to the 'invasivists'.

That catheterisation provides the 'gold standard' is one reason why patients may still need to be studied in the laboratory; if there is doubt and if the findings can influence management then catheterisation is indicated.

It is advancing surgical technique that has resulted in the continuing growth of cardiac catheterisation; in particular the development of surgical techniques for the management of coronary artery disease has led to the explosive growth of selective coronary arteriography — first developed by Mason Sones at the Cleveland Clinic [9].

The surgery of congenital heart disease has made such enormous strides that it is sometimes hard to remember that the surgical treatment of congenital cardiac defects has a history little longer than that of postwar cardiac catheterisation. These advances would not have been possible without an increasing precision of diagnosis provided by cardiac catheterisation; the catheterisation of neonates and infants with congenital heart disease has been another growth area, one demanding considerable technical and intellectual skills (see Chapter 17). Here, too, echocardiography can substitute for catheterisation in a growing number of cases and the indications for catheterisation in congenital heart disease are continually changing. While non-invasive techniques can provide a detailed description of the abnormal anatomy they can only provide indirect information about the resulting physiological disturbance. Accurate determination of pulmonary flow and resistance is one such physiological measurement and the measurement of pulmonary arteriolar resistance remains an indication for catheterisation in patients with congenital heart disease. This important subject is discussed in Chapter 9.

The success of surgery in the field of congenital cardiac disease is providing a new group of patients in whom catheterisation is required — those who would not, formerly, have survived into adulthood but who are now presenting, in increasing numbers, with late complications. Such patients pose problems which are unfamiliar to both adult and paediatric cardiologists and for this reason a separate chapter is devoted to congenital heart disease in adult life (Chapter 18).

Cardiac transplantation has an established clinical role and the ways in which the catheterisation laboratory contributes to the preoperative assessment and postoperative management of patients undergoing transplantation is discussed in Chapter 23. Unfortunately the application of new surgical techniques produces problems of its own; we may need to study fewer patients with untreated rheumatic valve disease but we have to learn how to study more and more of the problems that can follow cardiac surgery. Prosthetic valve malfunction and dehiscence, graft occlusion and myocardial dysfunction are but some of the penalties to be paid for surgical advance.

A new field of activity — interventional cardiology — has sprung up to provide a new challenge. Percutaneous transluminal coronary angioplasty is the most obvious example and is described in Chapter 14; other techniques already established include balloon valvuloplasty and therapeutic embolisation (Chapter 5). The clinical application of laser techniques is on the horizon and there is no doubt that many other techniques will be developed. All make heavy demands on the time and skill of laboratory-based physicians.

If the case mix has changed, and is continually changing, so too is the way that cases are managed. Studies which needed an hour or more to complete are now completed in a dozen minutes. And there is ample evidence to show that the mortality and morbidity associated with cardiac catheterisation has also fallen significantly [10]. To a large extent these improvements are the result of technical developments; in particular the very great improvement in X-ray equipment which has made catheterisation easier, quicker and safer.

While there is no doubt that studies are now completed more rapidly than used to be the case it is not possible to demonstrate that this, by itself, has contributed to the reduced mortality and morbidity. From the patient's point of view, though, the less time the study takes the better. The more that catheterisation can be seen by the patients as a simple, routine, procedure with little associated discomfort and anxiety the better. We owe it to our patients to strive towards this ideal.

The implications are clear; catheterisation is a skill which requires training and which, to be retained, requires constant practice. The days when a cardiologist thought of himself as equally competent by the bedside and in the catheterisation laboratory — on the basis of performing one or two studies a week — are past. Today the cardiologist (or radiologist) who specialises in invasive studies — the laboratory-based cardiologist — is a sub-specialist in his own right. It is to those who are developing the skills that make for good, safe catheterisation that this book is addressed. The skills, technical and manipulative, that are needed for diagnostic catheterisation are the same skills that are needed for performing other, therapeutic, procedures in cardiology. The aspiration of a pericardial effusion, pacemaker wire insertion, percutaneous intra-aortic balloon pumping and cardiopulmonary resuscitation are examples of such procedures which are not part of diagnostic catheterisation. Because learning to perform these invasive procedures is part of the training of a cardiologist they, too, are described here.

Finally, in learning how to perform cardiac catheterisation, the cardiologist has to learn *balance*. The patient is entitled to expect a quick, safe, 'diagnostic' study. The investigator may wish to satisfy his curiosity by extending the study to provide information that is not directly relevant to the management of the particular patient being studied. 'Research' studies are of the second type. There is no real problem when a study is clearly recognised as having a 'research' content; the protocol must have been approved by the local ethics committee and the patient must give his informed consent. Such studies should be in two parts: the initial study should be directed towards obtaining the information that is needed for patient management; the second part of the study, the research component, can follow and can be abandoned, without losing diagnostic information, at any time that the risk or discomfort to the patient becomes significant. 'Balance' is more difficult to achieve in what appear to be straightforward diagnostic studies. A speedily completed study that fails to provide a vital piece of information is a disservice to the patient and puts him in double jeopardy; either the study has to be repeated or surgery may be embarked on without adequate preoperative information. On the other hand, seeking information — the coronary anatomy, for example, or detailed evaluation of ventricular performance during stress — in a patient in whom management is unaffected by the findings also increases risk and discomfort unjustifiably. Often such extended studies are performed 'because they are laboratory practice'. The patient's interests, not those of the laboratory, are paramount and the good operator *knows when to stop*. This book is intended to be a *practical* guide and concentrates on conventional diagnostic procedures. Those who wish to explore the many additional techniques that can be used to provide more detailed assessment of cardiac physiology and performance must look elsewhere. It is possible to derive a multitude of 'indices' and to calculate them to several decimal places; whether or not such indices and calculations have any real meaning is another matter.

Except in cases where only limited information is sought the end-result of a catheterisation study is to provide a definitive diagnosis. The operator assembles the haemodynamic and angiographic data and produces a report which summarises the anatomical and physiological abnormalities that are present. This can only be done if the significance of the findings is recognised. A description of the invasive investigation of the heart must, therefore, include both 'how to do it' and 'what does it mean?' Section 2, 'Catheterisation in Specific Disorders', attempts to illustrate the haemodynamic and angiographic findings in most of the conditions encountered in the catheterisation laboratory. Inevitably some selection is involved; illustrating all known varieties of congenital cardiac defects would require a book several times larger than this one. But if, at the end of a study, the operators can find a description here that matches the findings in the study they have just completed and if they can do so at least nine times out of ten then this book will have achieved its purpose.

REFERENCES

1 Forssmann W. Die Sondierung des rechten Herzens. *Klin Wochenschr* 1929;**8**:2085.
2 Cournand AF, Ranges HS. Catheterisation of the right auricle in man. *Proc Soc Exp Biol Med* 1941;**46**:462.
3 McMichael J, Sharpey-Schafer EP. The action of intravenous digoxin in man. *Q J Med* 1944;**13**:1123.
4 Brannon ES, Weens HS, Warren JW. Atrial septal defect: study of haemodynamics by the technique of right heart catheterisation. *Am J Med Sci* 1945;**210**:480.
5 Zimmerman HA, Scott RW, Becker NO. Catheterization of the left side of the heart in man. *Circulation* 1950;**1**:357.
6 St John Sutton MG *et al.* Valve replacement without preoperative cardiac catheterization. *New Engl J Med* 1981;**305**:1233.
7 Roberts WC. Reasons for cardiac catheterization before cardiac valve replacement. *New Engl J Med* 1982;**306**:1291.
8 Rahimtoola SH. The need for cardiac catheterization and angiography in valvular heart disease is not disproven. *Ann Int Med* 1982;**97**:433.
9 Sones FM *et al.* Cine coronary arteriography. *Circulation* 1959;**20**:773(abs).
10 Adams DF, Abrams HL. Complications of coronary arteriography: a follow-up report. *Cardiovasc Radiol* 1979;**2**:89.

PART 1
Techniques

The catheterisation laboratory

The successful installation and operation of a cardiac catheterisation laboratory involves the cooperation of cardiologists, radiologists, equipment manufacturers, physiological measurement technicians and many more. Before a laboratory can be commissioned a number of questions have to be answered of which the most important are:

1 Does the setting justify the installation of a catheterisation laboratory?

2 What are the rooms that are needed and how big should they be?

3 Is the laboratory to be concerned with the study of coronary artery disease only, of all forms of acquired heart disease, of congenital heart disease or of all three?

4 Depending on the answer to **3** above what X-ray and other equipment is most suitable?

5 What staff are required and how, and by whom, is their work to be organised?

IS A CATHETERISATION LABORATORY JUSTIFIED?

Two factors are of concern here: the relationship with a cardiac surgical unit and the anticipated case-load. Firstly, there can be no doubt that, ideally, catheterisation laboratories should only exist in centres with a cardiac surgical unit. Complications requiring immediate surgical intervention are rare but they do occur and cannot be predicted. It is naive to imagine that it is possible to preselect 'simple' cases that will never pose problems. The need for on-site surgical back-up is greater today than in the past as a result of an increasing interventional role of the catheterisation laboratory — coronary angioplasty, intracoronary thrombolysis and so on. A second reason for a close relationship

with a cardiac surgical centre is that the laboratory staff need to be familiar with the individual requirements of the surgical team — what specific information the surgeon requires in his particular practice. Much time and expense is wasted and discomfort caused to the patient by performing, in referring hospitals, studies which have to be repeated to the satisfaction of the surgical centre. If studies are to be performed in a centre without a cardiac surgical unit there must be close liaison with the surgical centre so that studies need not be repeated. Paediatric cases should only be catheterised in centres with an active paediatric cardiology unit and paediatric cardiac surgical programme. There is no justification for the occasional paediatric study in a centre normally concerned exclusively with adult cardiac disease.

The second consideration in deciding if a laboratory is justified is the projected case-load. Laboratories performing a small number of studies each year are unlikely to develop the sort of expertise which is the only way to keep the complication rate down to acceptable levels. In one, multicentre, study of the complications of coronary arteriography laboratories performing less than 100 studies each year had a complication rate which was eight times higher than that experienced by laboratories undertaking 400 or more studies per year [1]. Not only is the complication rate higher but the cost per case rises exponentially as the case-load diminishes. The capital cost of the X-ray and other equipment needed in a catheterisation laboratory is very high — and the equipment has a limited life which is unlikely to be more than 10 years. If we assume the cost of equipping a catheterisation laboratory to be, for example, £500 000 and the life of the equipment to be 10 years (an optimistic estimate) then we have to write down the value of the equipment by £50 000/year. Inspection of Fig. 1.1 shows how, for a

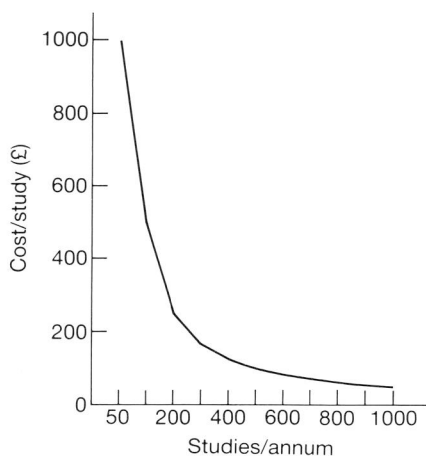

Fig. 1.1 Cost per case related to case-load.

laboratory performing 300 studies each year this represents an additional cost/study of just over £166. Were the laboratory to perform 1000 studies each year the additional cost/study would be only £50. The curve relating cost to case-load begins to flatten at about 300 studies/year and it is, perhaps, for this reason that the Inter-Society Commission for Heart Disease Resources recommended a minimum case-load of 300/year [2]. But it is perfectly possible for a single laboratory to perform 1000 to 1500 studies/year, more if the majority are coronary arteriograms, less if the work is primarily paediatric. An optimal case-load should, therefore, be something in this region and alternative options should be considered if the case-load is likely to be significantly less.

THE ROOMS NEEDED FOR A CATHETERISATION LABORATORY

The rooms that will be needed for a catheterisation laboratory complex consist of (1) a 'core' of rooms linked to the procedure room, and (2) the surrounding supporting facility.

1 *The 'core'*. This consists of (a) the procedure room, (b) the X-ray equipment room, (c) one or two control rooms for the radiographic controls and physiological recording equipment, (d) a 'clean' preparation room for assembling the instrument trolleys, and (e) a 'dirty' room for dis-assembling and initial cleaning of the instruments, catheters, etc. It is also

desirable to have an additional room for catheter storage and preparation. Sterilisation is likely to be a central, hospital, facility but the initial cleaning, labelling and preparation of re-usable catheters and instruments is best done by those who are directly responsible for their use.

2 *The surrounding support facility*. This will include a large room for data analysis and computer-based storage and retrieval, several rooms for viewing and reporting cine films and offices for professional, technical and secretarial staff. Considerable space will be needed for storage of equipment and of records. The services of an electronics department will be needed.

The procedure room. A minimum of some $47\,m^2$ has been suggested [2] but is unlikely to accommodate the additional equipment and personnel that will be needed for interventional and emergency work; 60 to $65\,m^2$ is a more desirable figure. In order to accommodate the X-ray tube/intensifier suspension a minimum ceiling height of 3 m (10 ft) is required. A rectangular shape with length slightly greater than breadth is suitable; the long axis of the patient support table being parallel with the long axis of the room. The building structure must be capable of bearing a considerable weight and the walls must incorporate a suitable shielding material for X-ray protection. Air-conditioning is essential as the equipment generates considerable heat and neither the equipment nor the staff work well at high temperatures. Lighting must be good but dark-room capability is not needed and staff satisfaction is improved if natural lighting is available when cases are not being studied. With today's high quality image intensifier/television systems there is no need to darken the room during fluoroscopy but some dimming of the lights is desirable; this is best achieved automatically by linking the dim/bright lighting controls to the operation of the fluoroscopy foot switch. Finally the floor need not be antistatic but must be washable. A false ceiling will allow equipment cables to be altered without major disturbance.

The X-ray equipment room. Ideally the X-ray generator(s) and cine pulse unit should not be inside the procedure room where they take up valuable space but should be separately housed. This room must be closely adjacent as the maximum permissible length for the high voltage cables is 18 m and for cables to constant potential equipment is 12 m. A floor area of about 9 m² will be needed.

Monitoring room(s). In order to shield staff from radiation it is desirable that the radiographic and video-tape controls and the physiological monitoring and recording equipment and their operators are housed in a separate 'cockpit'. This monitoring room is shielded from the procedure room and the partition must include a large area of lead-containing glass up to a minimum of some 2 m from the floor. The shielding must not impose a significant 'communication barrier' as complete understanding between the operator and the technical staff is essential. Hence the large area of glass and, if necessary, an intercommunication system between the two rooms. The same information must be available to the recording and X-ray technicians and to the operator in the procedure room. Thus the fluoroscopic image should be displayed on a second television monitor in front of the recording technician and an oscilloscope showing the ECG and pressure tracings should be positioned alongside the fluoroscopic display in front of the operator. In the US a single technician may operate both the physiological monitoring and recording equipment and the radiographic controls. In the UK regulations require that X-ray equipment be operated by a qualified radiographer — hence two technicians and two consoles or two monitoring rooms. If possible the monitoring room should have a 'computer floor' to allow for installation of new equipment and wiring without the need for structural alterations.

THE CASE 'MIX' AND APPROPRIATE EQUIPMENT

Although the work load of many laboratories consists almost entirely of the study of coronary artery disease it seems unwise to design the equipment with only these studies in mind. Some patients with coronary artery disease may have large, poorly functioning, ventricles requiring a larger X-ray field size than is ideal for visualising the coronary anatomy suggesting that, even for a dedicated 'coronary laboratory', there should be a choice of field size. Fortunately such dual mode intensifiers exist with the facility for instant switching between a small field size of 12 to 17 cm (5 to 7 in), which is ideal for visualising the coronaries, to a larger field of 22 to 25 cm (9 to 10 in) suitable for ventriculography. For routine, diagnostic studies a single plane system will suffice for all forms of acquired heart disease.

An essential component of all systems designed for cardiac investigation is a suspension which can be angulated in both the coronal and sagittal plane. All the major manufacturers provide such suspensions which allow the angiographer to obtain combinations of both oblique and cranially or caudally angulated views. The ideal format of such suspensions is of the 'U' or parallellogram type; apart from other disadvantages the C-arm configuration does not readily allow visualisation of the area of the iliac artery — essential if there is difficulty in advancing a catheter in this region.

The imaging system which is almost universally employed is 35 mm cine film. Serial film has the advantage over cine film in providing better definition but has a maximum filming rate of 6 f.p.s and a limited number of exposures. In the perfect laboratory, serial filming would be provided as an alternative to cine filming and is undoubtedly superior for a few applications — notably for pulmonary arteriography and peripheral arteriography. Unfortunately there are penalties; apart from the added expense the addition of a serial film changer usually involves the complexity of adding a second X-ray tube and generator. Combined systems which use a single tube in either serial or cine mode involve extra bulk attached to the image intensifier with resulting loss of manoeuvrability.

If the laboratory is to study paediatric patients then a biplane system is needed. Such systems will incorporate the same suspension, with its facility for obtaining angulated views, together with a second X-ray tube and intensifier mounted on a similar suspension and providing simultaneous filming in a second plane (not necessarily at right angles to the first). The main advantage of biplane systems is that they provide two views of the (often complex) anatomy for a single injection of radio-opaque contrast medium. Since the maximum permissible amount of contrast medium that can be given during a study is about 4 ml/kg it is obvious that the availability of biplane filming can be crucial in allowing completion of a study in, for example, a 2.0 kg neonate in whom a maximum of 8 ml of contrast can be given.

Equally it is obvious that such considerations do not apply in adult work in which injection volumes seldom exceed 30 ml/angiogram and seldom more than twice that for the whole study. It is possible that, with recently developed non-ionic media and with digital subtraction techniques, paediatric work will be possible with lower volumes per injection than are needed at present; if so then there may be a diminished need for biplane systems even in the study of congenital heart disease.

Biplane systems have other advantages, however; in particular the ability instantly to change from anteroposterior to lateral fluoroscopy can be very helpful in determining the orientation of the catheter during exploration of the heart or during procedures such as balloon atrial septostomy and coronary angioplasty.

With the exception of biplane X-ray equipment a dedicated paediatric laboratory will differ little from one designed for the study of adults though a separate anaesthetic room is desirable as is an on-line system for measuring oxygen consumption.

The patient support table is integral with the X-ray tube suspension. Both floor and ceiling mounted supports are available, the latter having the advantage of leaving a clear floor area but tending to be less rigid if external cardiac massage is needed in an emergency. U-arm or parallellogram tube suspensions require a clear area beneath much of the patient's body so that the table top has to be both strong and radiolucent; carbon fibre is the material of choice. The table top should be 'floating'; that is capable of being moved freely in all directions in the horizontal plane. The table should be considerably longer, at the foot end, than is needed to accommodate the patient; this extra length is needed as a 'work bench' to support catheters, guide wires and so on during coronary angioplasty and other 'interventional' procedures. It should be possible for the operator to lock and unlock the table at a touch.

A television monitor, positioned at a comfortable height and distance, provides the fluoroscopic image and should be flanked by a second monitor on which is displayed the currently recorded pressure signal(s) and electrocardiogram. The operator should only have to look in one direction to obtain all the essential information. A second video monitor is needed for displaying a previously recorded (analogue or digital) image for comparison ('road map') with the real-time image during coronary angioplasty.

An audio signal ('bleep') triggered by the QRS complex of the electrocardiogram provides warning of any untoward arrhythmias even when the operator's attention is elsewhere. It should not be necessary for the recording technician to draw his attention to ECG abnormalities or to changes in waveform; minimising conversation maximises concentration. Finally a video tape (or disc) recording system coupled to the television chain allows immediate play back of the angiocardiograms.

Other equipment in the catheterisation laboratory

As well as functioning as an X-ray room a catheterisation laboratory fulfils some of the functions of an operating theatre and those of a physiological laboratory. As a specialised theatre there is a need for full anaesthetic equipment with gases and suction available. Full operating-theatre sterility is neither possible nor desirable and infection almost unknown though a higher level of sterility is needed if the laboratory is to be used for permanent pacemaker implantation. Nonetheless sterile discipline is needed and imposes disciplined behaviour on the laboratory staff. Scrub-up is best done in the procedure room so that the operator can keep in touch while the patient is being prepared or, in the case of some infants and children, being anaesthetised. Resuscitation equipment will include external defibrillation and a full range of emergency drugs. The laboratory is an unusually safe environment since pressure, ECG and fluoroscopic monitoring is more constantly available than is often the case in emergency situations.

As a physiological measurement laboratory the essential measuring and recording equipment will include:

1 Strain-gauge pressure transducers with an hydraulic calibration/flush system. At least three, equi-sensitive, transducers will be needed. The measurement of valve gradients requires simultaneous records from two sites and a third pressure channel is needed as a 'spare'.

2 ECG channel and electrodes. For most studies a single channel is all that is needed but a second channel provides a spare and may, sometimes, be used for intracardiac recording, etc. A multiple (12-lead) display is desirable during coronary angioplasty.

3 Reflection oximeter. For most purposes reflection

oximetry is the ideal technique for the measurement of oxygen saturation of blood samples. Although slightly less accurate than some other techniques it has the advantage of providing a read-out in no more than 15 s, and of using small (0.4 ml) amounts of blood. Reflection oximetry is inaccurate at very low saturations and at high saturations when the patient is breathing high concentrations of oxygen. An alternative technique for measuring oxygen content should be available therefore — blood gas (Po_2) analysis or fuel cell. If neonatal and infant studies are to be done then blood gas analysis must be available.

4 Cardiac output determination. The accurate measurement of cardiac output by the Fick method will require some method of measuring oxygen consumption. Alternatives include expired air collection and analysis using a Tissot spirometer or mass spectrometry. Alternatively a thermodilution technique with appropriate computer read-out provides a quick, simple method of determining output in most cases.

5 Amplifiers and recording system. The recording system must be capable of superimposing the traces. This may be done by obtaining a photographic recording from the tube face of an oscilloscope or by using either a light-beam or ink-jet system. A permanent record may be obtained by using light sensitive (photographic) paper or ultraviolet sensitive paper while the ink-jet system employs conventional paper. Each system has its advantages and disadvantages but whichever is chosen it is essential that the information displayed on the monitor in the procedure room reflects exactly the true situation as being recorded in the monitoring room. On-line computer assisted analysis of pressure records is available and a digital read-out can be provided for the operator though too much information display can be confusing. The recorder must have a minimum of four channels; six or eight channel recorders are more usual.

6 Many other techniques are employed, indicator dilution techniques and catheter-tip manometry for example, but the choice of these will depend on the particular interests of the laboratory.

7 If paediatric cases are to be studied a radiolucent warming pad will be needed to prevent hypothermia in neonates.

8 Emergency equipment. A D/C cardioverter capable of delivering synchronised countershock must be available and checked for proper functioning each day. Appropriate, small-sized, paddles must be connected during paediatric studies. A standby external pacemaker and pacing catheter must be readily available though it will only be needed on very rare occasions. The anaesthetic equipment will include laryngoscopes and endotracheal tubes for emergency ventilation and a full range of emergency drugs.

PERSONNEL

In addition to the operator a minimum of three (four in the UK) other people will be needed for performing a study. These are: (1) a scrub nurse or physician in training to assist the operator, (2) a circulating nurse or technician to provide extra items of equipment, catheters, etc., to load and operate the angiographic injector syringe to analyse blood samples and to comfort the patient. In practice two such circulating nurses or technicians are usually needed. Monitoring and recording of the physiological signals will require (3) a technician stationed in the monitoring cubicle and (in the UK) the X-ray controls will be the responsibility of (4) a radiographer.

Overall direction of the catheterisation laboratory or laboratories should be the responsibility of a physician acting as laboratory director. The probability is that this individual will be a cardiologist; what is certain is that he must be fully trained in all those aspects of cardiology which bear on the functioning of the laboratory. He must be familiar with the management — surgical and medical — of cardiac patients so that he can ensure that the laboratory provides the information needed for management decisions.

REFERENCES

1 Adams DF, Fraser DB, Abrams HL. The complications of coronary arteriography. *Circulation* 1973;**48**:609.
2 Friesinger GC *et al.* Optimal resources for examination of the heart and lungs: cardiac catheterization and radiographic facilities. *Circulation* 1983;**68**:893A.

The tools of catheterisation

The tools of catheterisation are the catheters themselves, guide wires, sheath introducers, needles, manometer tubing and various stopcocks and adaptors for connecting the catheter to the pressure transducer.

CATHETERS

The construction of cardiac catheters is more complex than appears at first sight. The ideal catheter needs to have a number of characteristics; it must be flexible, especially at the tip, but not so flexible that it is impossible to manipulate. It must be smooth internally and externally and resist platelet adherence and thrombus formation. It must withstand high pressures without rupturing during angiography. It must be radio-opaque and easily visible during fluoroscopy. It should have a small external diameter so that it can be introduced easily and yet have the largest possible internal diameter for ease of sampling and to permit a high rate of flow during angiography. No single catheter combines all the characteristics that may be needed for a particular purpose and, as a result, catheters are available in a multitude of forms.

Catheter construction

Cardiac catheters may be made of woven Dacron, of polyurethane, of polyethylene, of polyvinylchloride (PVC) or of Teflon.

Woven Dacron catheters consist of an inner framework of Dacron fibres woven in tubular form and covered with a smooth, radio-opaque, outer coating of polyurethane. Such catheters have superb manipulability and are ideal for 'exploring' the heart with very little risk of damaging the vessels or myocardium. Some woven Dacron angiographic catheters incorporate a reinforcing nylon core which allows a higher injection pressure to be used and increases the flow rate of contrast medium during angiography. These, and other, catheters may incorporate a stainless-steel wire mesh within the body of the catheter. The purpose of the wire mesh is to improve 'torque control' so that a given degree of twist imparted to the proximal part of the catheter is transmitted, without loss, to the catheter tip. Woven Dacron catheters can be 'heat-moulded' by immersing the tip in boiling water, reshaping the curve and then cooling in cold water; however, they do not retain the new shape for long after being re-introduced as they soften, markedly, in the body after being re-introduced. Woven Dacron catheters manufactured by the United States Catheter and Instrument Company (USCI) incorporate a metallic tin filler to provide radio-opacity and all have the same grey colour imparted by this filler.

Polyurethane catheters have the valuable characteristic of retaining their preformed shape when introduced into the circulation. Many preformed catheters have to be straightened (e.g. by a guide wire) before they can be introduced but the original shape is recovered when the guide wire is removed. Whereas woven Dacron catheters tend to be of 'simple' shape — that is straight except for a gentle bend at the distal end — the family of extruded polyurethane catheters includes many that are preshaped for special purposes. The shape of these catheters can be modified by heat-moulding and the new shape is well retained within the circulation. Polyurethane catheters have a limited shelf-life; polymer ageing may lead to fracture and these catheters should not be used after the printed expiry date — usually 3 years [1].

Polyethylene catheters are similar to polyurethane catheters but may be slightly stiffer and more thrombogenic; this latter disadvantage is overcome by routine heparinisation of the patient at the beginning of the study. Polyethylene catheters also retain a preformed shape and can be heat-moulded.

Polyvinylchloride (PVC) catheters are the softest and least traumatic but have poor memory and poor manoeuvrability; they are ideal for flow-directed (e.g. Swan−Ganz), balloon-tipped catheters.

Teflon catheters are designed to permit high flow rates for angiography when a large bolus injection is required — as for aortography. They are less flexible than other catheters and for this reason should not be used for exploring the heart since there is a real danger of perforating the myocardium. This characteristic, together with their low coefficient of surface friction (0.04 as compared with 0.21 for polyethylene and 1.35 for polyurethane), can be an advantage in some special applications when a catheter is required to penetrate the subcutaneous tissues. For example, they can be used for percutaneous, trans-apical, left ventriculography or for draining pericardial effusions by the apical or sub-xiphoid routes.

Catheter sizes

Three dimensions are important when choosing a catheter for a particular purpose: the external and internal diameters, and the usable length. Diameters may be given in millimetres or in fractions of an inch but for convenience are usually referred to by their 'French gauge' (F). *The external diameter in millimetres can be obtained by dividing the French gauge by 3 (e.g. 6F = 2 mm OD).* Woven Dacron catheters made by the USCI are colour coded for French gauge at the butt end. The diameters of the most frequently used catheters are given in Table 2.1.

Catheters made by the Cordis Corporation have a 'key' printed on the hub:
1 Thin-wall, unbraided — blue hub with white lettering (max. pressure 500 p.s.i. (3450 kPa)).
2 Standard, braided — white hub with black lettering (max. pressure 1000 p.s.i. (6900 kPa)).
3 High flow, braided — white hub with red lettering (max. pressure 1000 p.s.i. (6900 kPa)).
4 'Super flow', unbraided — white hub with blue lettering (max. pressure 800 p.s.i. (5520 kPa)).

Table 2.1   Diameters of the most frequently used catheters.

French gauge	Colour code	OD (mm)	OD (in.)
4.0F	Red	1.33	0.052
5.0F	Silver	1.67	0.065
6.0F	Green	2.00	0.078
7.0F	Brown	2.33	0.091
8.0F	Blue	2.67	0.104
9.0F	Black	3.00	0.118

OD = external (outside) diameter.

Three numbers are printed on the hub: the French gauge (external diameter), the length of the catheter and the guide wire size that the catheter will accept. For example 7 80 038 indicates that the catheter is 7F, 80 cm long and will accept a 0.038″ guide wire.

In some cases the colour of the catheter provides the key to its construction; for example, braided catheters made by William Cook (incorporating a wire mesh for torque control) are coloured green (or blue — 'superior' torque control).

The internal diameter will depend on the type of construction: those which are designed to give high flow rates will have a larger internal diameter for a given French gauge at the expense, usually, of some torque control and features such as a wire mesh within the wall. They are referred to as 'thin-wall' catheters. The internal diameters of standard and thin-wall catheters are given in Table 2.2.

Table 2.2.   Internal diameters (ID) of standard and thin-wall catheters.

Size (French gauge)	Standard		Thin-wall	
	ID (in.)	ID (mm)	ID (in.)	ID (mm)
4	0.018	0.46	0.023	0.58
5	0.026	0.66	0.034	0.86
6	0.036	0.91	0.046	1.17
7	0.046	1.17	0.058	1.47
8	0.056	1.42	0.068	1.73
9	0.064	1.63	0.078	1.98

The length of a catheter should be little more than is needed to reach all parts of the heart from the chosen entry site. This is particularly important when the catheter is to be used for angiography since the maximum obtainable flow rate is dependent on the length of the catheter. The longer the catheter the greater the resistance to flow and the slower the rate of injection. It follows that the smaller catheters (4.0, 5.0 and 6.0F) which are designed for paediatric use tend to be available in 50 or 80 cm lengths and larger catheters only in longer lengths — 100 or 125 cm.

Catheter design

The simplest type of catheter consists of no more than a hollow tube with a single hole at its distal end and a Luer-lock fitting at the proximal end. The 'Cournand' catheter [2] is of this type (Fig. 2.1). Such catheters have a number of disadvantages; in particular they are unsuitable for angiography since the high-pressure jet of contrast medium emerging from the end-hole will cause the catheter to recoil violently in the opposite direction and the jet may also penetrate the myocardium ('intramyocardial injection'). To overcome this problem catheters which are intended for angiography have multiple side-holes from which the contrast emerges and, often, a closed end [3]. Thus cardiac catheters may be divided into two broad categories: those designed for 'exploring' the heart (by pressure measurement and taking blood samples) and angiographic catheters.

CATHETERS DESIGNED PRIMARILY FOR
EXPLORING THE HEART

'Exploring catheters' should be flexible to minimise the possibility of damaging the myocardium, and should have no more than two side-holes. With the possible exception of 'balloon catheters' (see below) all 'exploring' catheters must have a curve of about 30° a few centimetres from the end. It is obvious that it would be impossible to steer a completely straight catheter; by adding a curve towards the tip, rotational movements are converted into left/right or anterior/posterior movements of the catheter tip. In addition the curve makes it possible to abut the tip against the myocardium so that further advance of the catheter results in a loop being formed (see Chapter 4 on 'catheter manipulation'). Exploring catheters need not be of large diameter or particularly short; 5 or 6F are adequate for neonates and infants and 7 or 8F adequate for children and adults. 4.0F catheters may be used in desperation if no other catheter can be introduced through a very small vessel but the lumen is so small that it is difficult to

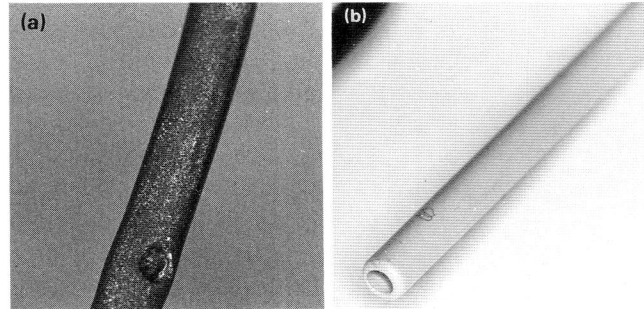

Fig. 2.1 'Exploring catheters': (a) Goodale–Lubin. Note the 'birds-eye' side-holes in addition to the end-hole. (b) Cournand. There is an end-hole only.

obtain an 'undamped' pressure, particularly if there is any thrombus formation. A satisfactory angiogram is almost impossible to obtain through a standard 4F catheter though a special, 'ultra-thin-wall', 4F pigtail catheter has been shown to give satisfactory results (see under 'Pigtail angiographic catheters' below). There must be an end-hole so that the indirect left atrial ('wedge') pressure can be obtained. There must be no more than two side-holes as multiple side-holes would make it impossible to assess valve gradients — some side-holes might be below and some above the valve giving a false impression of the severity and site of a stenosis. The original *Cournand* catheter (Fig. 2.1b) has an end-hole and no side-holes and is ideal for obtaining a record of the 'wedge' pressure. However, it has the serious disadvantage that the end-hole may be partially or completely obstructed by impinging against the myocardium; attempts to sample through the catheter are thus frustrated and the suction against the myocardium generates ectopic beats. The catheter has then to be moved and the sequence is repeated so that a carefully sought position within the heart is lost and the catheter has to be repositioned. The ideal exploring catheter has an end-hole and two 'birds-eye' side-holes very close to the tip; this is the *Goodale–Lubin* catheter (Fig. 2.1a) [4]. The side-holes, being close to the tip, do not, as a rule, prevent a 'wedge' pressure being obtained.

Flow-guided catheters. These are flexible PVC catheters with a balloon at the tip. The original Swan–Ganz balloon catheter [5] was designed for bedside catheterisation of the pulmonary artery without the need for fluoroscopy (Fig. 2.2). A separate lumen

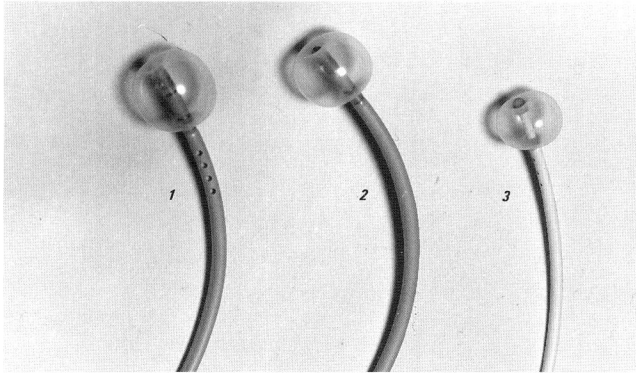

Fig. 2.2 Flow-guided, balloon-tipped, catheters (Swan−Ganz):
(1) 7F flow-guided angiographic catheter; closed-end and
multiple side-holes proximal to the balloon. (2) 7F 'monitoring'
catheter. There is a single end-hole; the inflated balloon extends,
slightly, beyond the tip of the catheter. (3) 5F flow-guided,
angiographic catheter for paediatric work.

allows the balloon to be inflated with air (or carbon dioxide if there is a possibility of right-to-left shunting) and acts as a 'sail' helping to carry the catheter with the blood flow. When the inflated balloon occludes a pulmonary artery the distal lumen will record the indirect left atrial (wedge) pressure. These catheters also find many uses in the catheterisation laboratory. Their tendency to be carried with the blood flow may enable the operator to reach a site which cannot be reached by conventional catheter manipulation [6]. For this reason balloon-tipped catheters are particularly useful in the study of congenitally malformed hearts. A further advantage is that the inflated balloon projects a short distance beyond the catheter tip, thus spreading the forces when the tip impinges against the myocardium and reducing the incidence of ectopic beats and the risk of perforating the heart. Many modifications of the original catheter exist; there are versions with multiple side-holes for angiography and the balloon allows 'balloon occlusion angiography' to be performed (see Chapter 7). There are triple lumen versions in which the distal opening allows recording of pulmonary artery or wedge pressures while a proximal opening allows recording of right atrial pressure or, since a thermistor can be incorporated, the injection of cold saline for determination of (thermodilution) cardiac output. Another version incorporates a pacing electrode. The incorporation of optical fibres in a recently introduced version allows continuous recording of oxygen saturation of

mixed venous blood when the catheter is attached to an external microprocessor.

In some balloon-tipped catheters (e.g. the *Berman* angiographic catheter) the balloon is recessed so that the catheter may be introduced through a sheath of the same French gauge. Others require a sheath introducer 1F larger than the catheter size in order to accommodate the additional thickness of the deflated balloon.

The only other 'exploring catheters' that need to be mentioned are *double-lumen catheters*. These, as their name indicates, have two fine lumens and are designed to permit the simultaneous recording of two pressures; for example, the pressures proximal and distal to a stenotic valve so as to allow accurate measurement of a valve gradient. In many cases valve gradients which are of importance are adequately measured by sequential records (e.g. as the catheter is withdrawn from the left ventricle to the aorta) but small gradients may be significant across the tricuspid valve and may require a double-lumen catheter for proper display. Caution must be exercised when interpreting the results obtained with these catheters as the fine lumen may give a 'damped' pressure recording unless great care is taken to flush the lumens and keep them free of thrombus.

Transducer-tip catheters. These catheters (Millar, Gaeltech; Fig. 2.3b) have miniature pressure transducers mounted at the tip. Since the pressure record does not involve transmission via a column of fluid (as in conventional catheter−manometer systems) the problems of damping and resonance are eliminated and high-fidelity, artefact-free pressure records can be obtained. These high-fidelity records are essential if the first derivative of the pressure (dp/dt) is to be recorded. Some versions have a lumen and side-holes allowing sampling or angiography to be performed through the same catheter. Transducer-tip catheters are expensive and difficult to manipulate within the heart and blood vessels; to some extent the latter problem can be overcome by using a long sheath, positioned using a conventional catheter which is then replaced by the transducer-tip catheter.

Camino Laboratories catheters. These are transducer-tip catheters in which fibre-optics are used to transmit the pressure signal to an external microprocessor. The catheters are cheaper than the Millar and Gaeltech

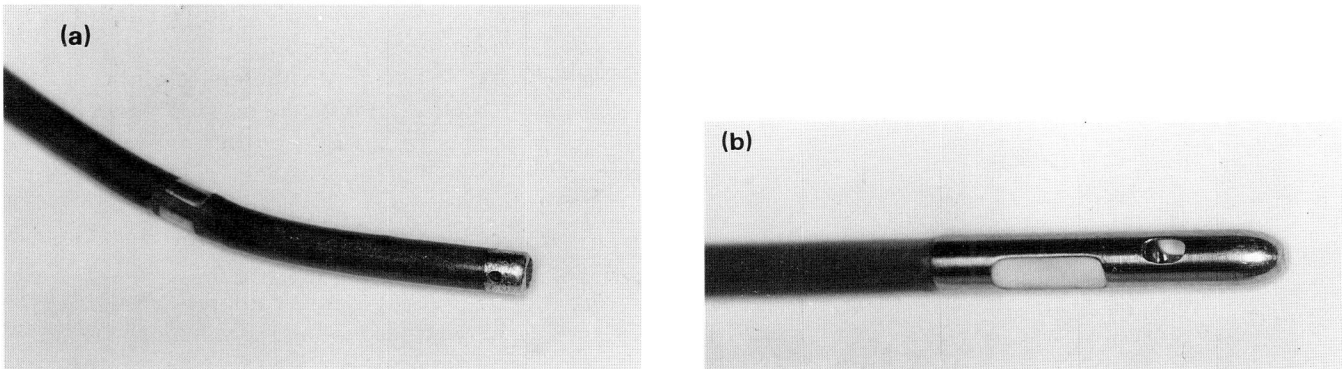

Fig. 2.3 (a) Zucker multipurpose bipolar electrode catheter. There are two side-holes (in the distal electrode) and an end-hole. The two platinum electrodes are situated 1.5 cm apart. This catheter can be used as an 'exploring' catheter for pressure measurements and oximetry and allows recording of intracardiac electrocardiograms. The catheter is often used as a standby pacemaking catheter in situations where there is a possibility of a serious arrhythmia being precipitated during the study. (b) Catheter-tip manometer (Gaeltech) — micromanometer mounted at the end of a catheter for high-fidelity recording of intracardial pressures.

transducer-tip catheters but share the disadvantage that zeroing is impossible after the catheter has been inserted.

ANGIOGRAPHIC CATHETERS

Most general purpose angiographic catheters have multiple side-holes, each with a matching hole opposed to it at 180° or spirally arranged so that the recoil force is counteracted by an equal and opposite force. Ideally the end of the catheter should be closed so that there is no backward recoil. However, many angiographic catheters do have an end-hole though this is a small one designed to accept a guide wire and nothing more. Originally this was to enable the catheter to be introduced percutaneously over a guide wire by the 'Seldinger' technique [7]. Today we have 'sheath' introducers [8] which make possible the percutaneous insertion of closed-end catheters; nonetheless it is often useful to be able to pass a guide wire through a catheter in order to facilitate entry to an otherwise inaccessible site and most angiographic catheters have a small end-hole for this reason. The ideal angiographic catheter permits the injection of a large volume of (viscous) contrast medium in a short time and at low pressure. The longer and narrower a catheter is the more the resistance to the passage of contrast medium. Thus the ideal catheter is no longer than is necessary to reach all parts of the patient's heart and is of the largest possible bore compatible with entry through

the artery or vein being used and compatible with safe manipulation within the heart.

The following list of angiographic catheters includes those which are in common use.

Ventriculography and general purpose angiographic catheters. Eppendorf and National Institutes of Health (NIH) catheters (Figs 2.4 and 2.5). These general purpose, angiographic catheters are very similar. They have a closed end and cannot, therefore, be used with a guide wire. They can be used for right and left ventriculography, for aortography and pulmonary arteriography or for angiography of the great veins or right atrium. Both are of thin-wall construction, have six side-holes and a nylon inner core reinforcement. The NIH catheter is rather stiff and should not be used for exploring the heart as there is an increased risk of perforating the myocardium. The Eppendorf catheter differs from the NIH in that the nylon reinforcing core only extends 20 cm from the hub so that the tip is more flexible than is that of the NIH catheter. The NIH catheter is available in woven Dacron and polyethylene versions. The Eppendorf is of woven Dacron construction.

Catheterisation of the right ventricle and pulmonary artery can be difficult when the approach is from the leg. An angled version of the pigtail ventriculography catheter, the *Grollman* catheter (Fig. 2.9b) [9], passes easily through the right ventricle when this approach is used; in many centres this is the prefered catheter for selective pulmonary arteriography.

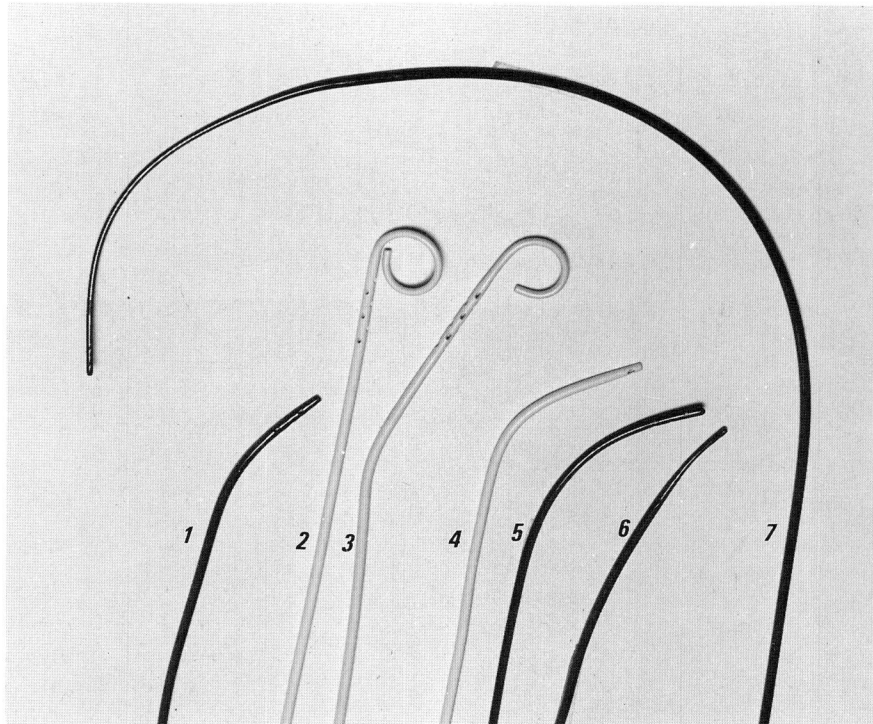

Fig. 2.4 A selection of angiographic catheters. (1) Gensini, (2) pigtail, (3) angled pigtail (Van Tassel technique for stenotic aortic valves), (4) multipurpose, (5) NIH, (6) Lehman ventriculographic, and (7) Shirey (note the long, 5F, tapered distal 7.5 cm. The proximal shaft is 8F).

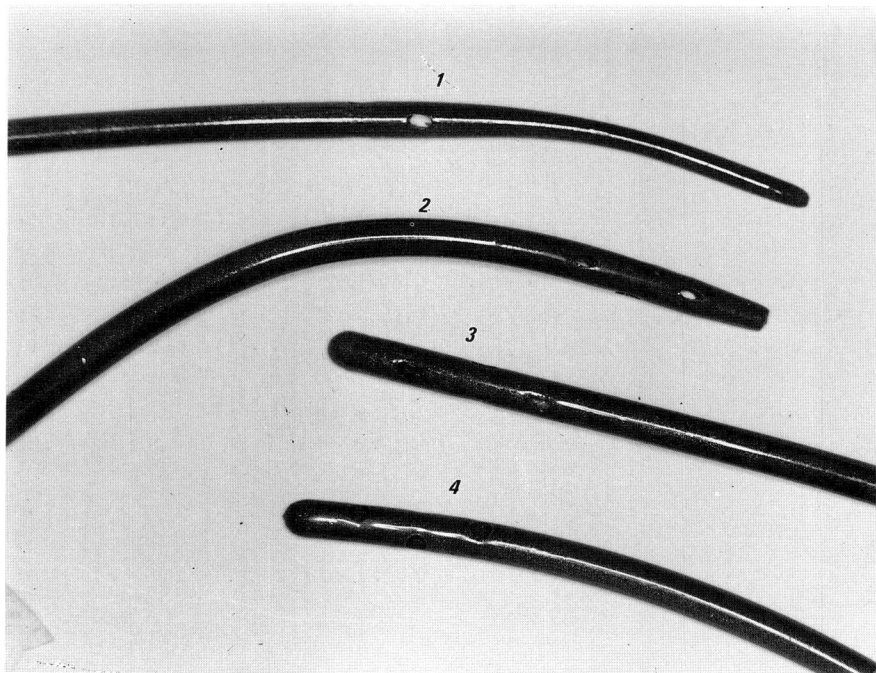

Fig. 2.5 Close-up views of angiographic catheters. (1) Lehman ventriculography, (2) Gensini, (3) Eppendorf, and (4) NIH.

Lehman ventriculography catheter (Figs 2.4 and 2.5). (Note that there is also a 'Lehman' exploring catheter which is a thin-wall version of the Cournand catheter.) This thin-wall catheter also has a closed end but differs in that it has only four side-holes and the last centimetre or so is much narrower (4.0 or 5.0F) than the shaft of the catheter, thus forming a short tapered tip. It is designed to facilitate the negotiation of stenotic (aortic) valves or tortuous vessels. Great care should be used if this catheter is introduced from the arm as the relatively rigid shaft and fine pointed tip makes it possible to perforate the vessel wall — particularly at the junction between the subclavian and innominate artery. It is better to use an open-tip catheter that will accept a guide wire and use the guide wire to lead the catheter around tortuosities or through stenotic valves.

Shirey angiography catheter (Fig. 2.4). This catheter is similar to the Lehman catheter but the thin tapered tip (5.0F or 6.0F) is 7.5 cm long and has its side-holes at the end of the thin tip section rather than in the wide shaft as does the Lehman. The catheter was designed to allow the tip to be looped within the left ventricle for retrograde catheterisation of the left atrium through the mitral valve — an excellent and neglected technique [10]. It is also a good catheter for negotiating tortuous vessels and may sometimes traverse a stenotic aortic valve when all other catheters have failed (when used for this purpose it must be used without looping). It is of woven Dacron construction.

'Pigtail' ventriculography catheter (Fig. 2.4). This is the ideal catheter for left ventriculography. As its name suggests the catheter terminates in a loop resembling a pig's tail; there is an open end to accept a guide wire and there are 12 non-opposed side-holes. The pigtail configuration means that the tip impinges against the myocardium not as a point but as a small loop and as a result is less liable to provoke ventricular ectopic beats. This same feature also means that it can be advanced through a great vessel with less danger of becoming lodged under an atheromatous plaque and causing a dissection. The catheter may be introduced percutaneously over a guide wire (Seldinger technique) or, more usually, through a sheath introducer fitted with a haemostatic valve. It may also be introduced via an arteriotomy (e.g. from the brachial artery), in which case the pigtail tip must, initially, be straightened by leading with a guide wire. Introduced from the arm in this way the pigtail catheter and guide wire will readily traverse the often tortuous subclavian/innominate junction. The catheter will readily cross a normal aortic valve but has to be straightened with a guide wire if the valve is stenotic.

There are several variants of the pigtail catheter. An angled variant (Van Tassel technique; Fig. 2.4) is designed to aid in crossing stenotic valves [11], but these catheters are still less likely to achieve the object than are catheters without a pigtail configuration.

Pigtail catheters with three radio-opaque markers 2 cm apart (Cordis 'Quanticor', USCI 'Cardiomarker') allow calculation of X-ray magnification factor [12] for measurement of ventricular volumes.

For neonatal use a 50-cm-long, Teflon, 'ultra-thin-wall' catheter (UMI) has been designed [13] which has a 4.0F external diameter but an internal diameter of 0.92 mm (equivalent to a standard 6.0F catheter) instead of 0.58 mm as in conventional thin-wall 4.0F catheters. Excellent flow rates can be achieved with this catheter but it must be manipulated with a 0.025″ guide wire in place to prevent buckling at the side-holes.

Gensini angiographic catheter (Figs 2.4 and 2.5). This catheter is designed for percutaneous insertion and has an end-hole, to take a guide wire, and six side-holes. It is a thin-wall catheter with a slightly tapered tip to facilitate passage through the subcutaneous tissues and the vessel wall. With the arrival of sheath introducers equipped with haemostatic valves the traditional Seldinger technique of percutaneous entry is largely a thing of the past. However, Gensini catheters are still of use as they can be used with a guide wire when this is needed to pass awkward or tortuous sites. Since the end of the catheter has only the usual gentle curve and not the pigtail configuration this is one of the best catheters for crossing stenotic aortic valves; when used for this purpose catheterisation should be from the arm via a brachial arteriotomy.

Brockenbrough transseptal catheter (Fig. 2.6). The transseptal technique [14] involves the transfemoral (vein) insertion of a preshaped Teflon catheter within which is a (sheathed) needle 69 cm long. When the end of the catheter has engaged the limbus of the

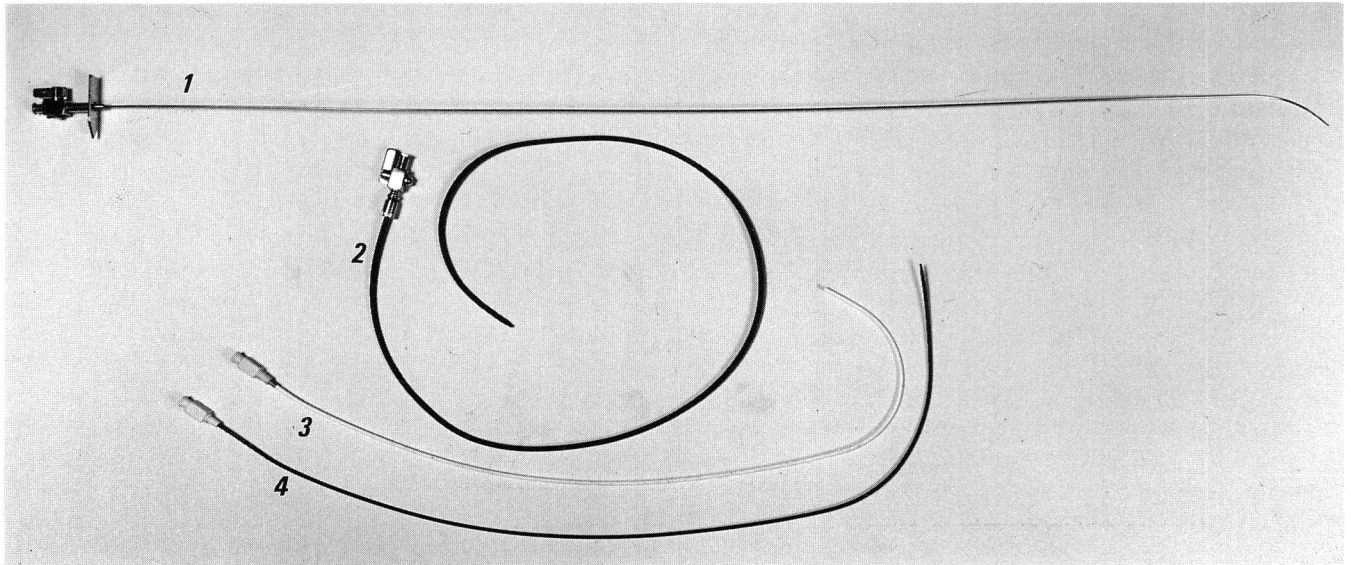

Fig. 2.6 Transseptal catheterisation. (1) Brockenbrough transseptal needle, (2) Teflon Brockenbrough transseptal catheter, (3 and 4) USCI Mullins transseptal set: (3) long sheath, (4) catheter.

foramen ovale the needle is advanced (unsheathed) to puncture the interatrial septum and the catheter then advanced over the needle to enter the left atrium. The technique is described in detail in Chapter 3. The Brockenborough catheter has a curved end (2.0–3.5 cm in diameter) to facilitate passage across the mitral valve to the left ventricle, and six side-holes in addition to the end-hole. A smaller version is produced for paediatric work and a modification of the technique (USCI Mullins transseptal introducer) is also available which permits the transseptal introduction of a long sheath so that closed-end and other catheters or bioptomes may be introduced to the left heart by the transseptal technique [15]. A similar 'long-sheath modification' of the transseptal technique using a modified pigtail catheter has been described for use in adult patients [16].

CORONARY ARTERIOGRAPHY CATHETERS

Most catheters for coronary arteriography are pre-shaped but the catheter first developed for selective coronary arteriography, the *Sones* catheter [17], is a conventional catheter with a long tapered tip, an open end and four side-holes; it is inserted via a brachial arteriotomy. This catheter has the merit of being safe to use and can be used for cannulating both the left and the right coronary arteries; however, it requires more manipulative skill than do the various preshaped coronary arteriography catheters. Many operators use the Sones catheter for left ventriculography (with a low flow rate) so that one catheter will suffice for the whole of a 'coronary study'. This is bad practice as the Sones catheter is more liable to produce intramyocardial injections of contrast medium than do true ventriculography catheters such as the pigtail, NIH or Gensini. The Sones catheter is produced with both long and short tapered tips to allow for different sized aortic roots. Finally, this, and similar catheters such as the 'multipurpose' catheter in Fig. 2.4, may sometimes enable one to cross a difficult (stenotic) aortic valve.

Judkins femoral-coronary catheters (Fig. 2.7b) [18]. These were the first of the preshaped coronary arteriography catheters. They are designed for percutaneous insertion via the femoral artery and should be inserted over a guide wire even if an introducing sheath is being used. Separate, and differently shaped, right and left coronary catheters have to be used and a third catheter used for ventriculography. Different radius curves are available to allow for differing configurations of the aortic root: the 4 cm curve is generally the most useful (Fig. 2.8) a 3.5 cm curve may be needed when the aortic root is small, and 5 and 6 cm curves are available for use when the aortic root is dilated. The catheters have an end-hole but no side-holes. Coronary cannulation is very easy with these catheters as they are designed to 'seek out' the coronary ostia and need a minimum of manipulation. The chief disadvantages of the Judkins technique are those attendant on any percutaneous arterial approach — the possibility of bleeding and haematoma formation which may be of concern if patients are to be discharged the same day. Thin-wall, high-flow Judkins catheters of small gauge (nos. 5 or 6F) have been developed with the aim of reducing the risk of bleeding, since there is a smaller entry hole, while retaining an adequate rate of delivery of contrast medium.

Amplatz coronary catheter (Fig. 2.7b) [19, 20]. This is a preshaped, end-hole catheter originally designed for coronary cannulation by the percutaneous transfemoral approach though the catheter can be used

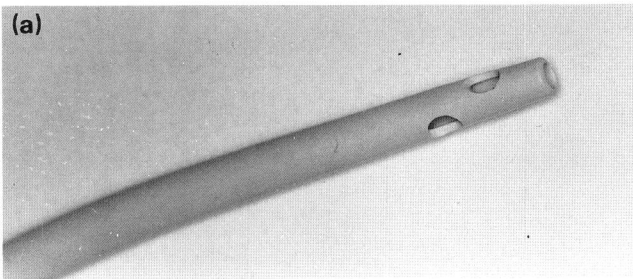

Fig. 2.7 (a) The tip of the Sones coronary arteriographic catheter showing the end-hole and four side-holes.

from the brachial artery. The catheter is shaped so as to sit in the sinus of Valsalva and thence enter the coronary ostia. It has two distinct configurations designed for left (L) and right (R) coronary cannulation and is available in a number of curve sizes: L 1—4 and R 1—3 for use in different sized aortic roots. The chief advantage of the Amplatz coronary catheter is that it provides an alternative to the Judkins technique when the transfemoral approach has been used but when it has not been possible to cannulate the coronary arteries with the Judkins catheters.

Castillo coronary catheter (Fig. 2.7b) [21]. This, in the author's opinion, is the ideal coronary arteriography catheter. The Castillo technique [22] combines the advantages of easy coronary cannulation resulting from the preset curve with the advantage of the brachial arteriotomy — haemostasis by direct suture rather than by pressure and thrombus formation. The same catheter can be used for cannulation of both the left and right coronary ostia and of vein grafts; a separate ventriculography (pigtail) catheter must be used to obtain a left ventriculogram. Insertion from the brachial arteriotomy is achieved without the need for a straightening guide wire though a guide wire will be needed to straighten the pigtail ventriculography catheter. In their standard form these catheters have no side-holes. In the author's opinion, side-holes add to the safety of coronary arteriography. When a catheter has only an end-hole it is possible for the tip to be inserted beneath an atheromatous plaque and the emergent jet of contrast

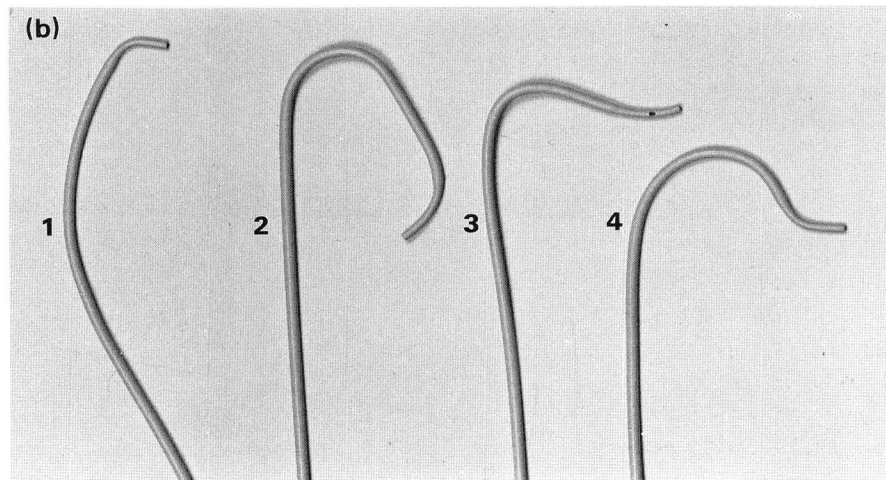

(b) A selection of catheters used for coronary arteriography: (1) femoral right coronary (Judkins technique), (2) femoral left coronary (Judkins), (3) brachial coronary (Castillo technique) — modified by the addition of four side-holes, (4) femoral left coronary (Amplatz technique).

(a)

*Primary curve

Secondary curve

(b)

*

Primary curve

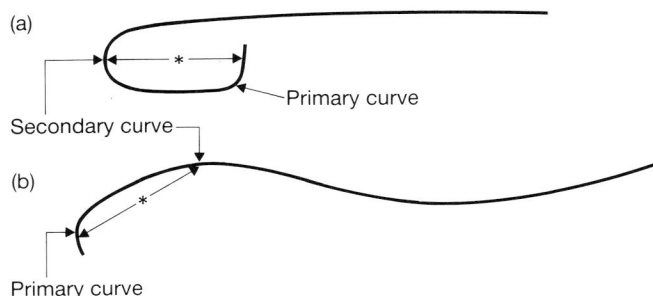

Fig. 2.8 Judkins coronary arteriography catheter: (a) femoral left coronary, (b) femoral right coronary (end-hole; no side-holes). Catheter are designated by the length between the primary and secondary curves* e.g.:

No.	Length(cm)	Description/use
I	3·5	Small aorta
II	4·0	Standard
III	5·0	Dilated aorta
IV	6·0	Poststenotic dilatation

medium may cause dissection of the coronary artery. When there are side-holes the contrast medium has an alternative exit even when the tip is against the vessel wall or an atheromatous plaque. In addition it is possible for some coronary blood flow to continue via the side-holes even when the catheter is occluding the coronary ostium. Finally spill-over of contrast medium results in better opacification of the coronary ostia and less danger of missing ostial stenosis than when a single jet of contrast medium emerges from a deeply engaged, single-end-hole catheter. Fortunately a variant of the Castillo catheter is available to order which has four side-holes in addition to the end-hole. Castillo catheters are available with three sizes of curve: I for small aortic roots, II for most purposes, and III for patients with a dilated aortic root or high take-off of the left coronary.

Soft-tip catheters (Angiomedics, Inc.). These polyurethane catheters are unusual in that there is a deformable, bulb-like tip designed to reduce intimal trauma or plaque dissection and thus increase the safety of coronary cannulation. A wire mesh is incorporated for torque control and there are soft-tip versions of several of the standard coronary and ventriculography catheters [23].

The 'multipurpose catheter' (Fig. 2.4) is similar to the

Sones catheter and designed to allow coronary arteriography and left ventriculography to be performed with a single catheter using a percutaneous transfemoral approach [24].

Coronary bypass catheters (Fig. 2.9). These pre-shaped, polyurethane catheters are designed for selective cannulation of coronary bypass grafts by the percutaneous, transfemoral approach. Versions are available for cannulating left and right coronary bypass grafts but often a 'right Judkins' catheter will do the job equally well. Another version with two oppositely directed curves (Greenburg, Fig. 2.9 [25]) has been designed for cannulating grafts which have been inserted high on the aortic arch. The 'Sidewinder' IV catheter, originally designed for cerebral arteriography [26], is an excellent graft-seeking catheter for transfemoral use [27]; it is also an excellent catheter for bronchial (collateral) cannulation.

When the brachial approach is used it will be found that the Castillo coronary arteriography catheter is very suitable for cannulating aortocoronary (saphenous vein) bypass grafts. Internal mammary artery grafts pose a difficult problem and a transfemoral approach using a catheter with a backward pointing tip (Fig. 2.9) is needed to cannulate this vessel though a special catheter is available which is designed to allow internal mammary cannulation from a right transbrachial approach [28] (Fig. 2.9b).

INTERVENTION CATHETERS

Atrial septostomy (Rashkind) catheter (Fig. 2.10). This, the first of the widely used 'intervention catheters' has a single purpose: to create a tear in the interatrial septum so as to allow mixing of systemic venous and pulmonary venous blood across the resulting 'septostomy'. Its first, and still most important, use was in complete transposition of the great arteries [29]. Since it is in neonates that septostomy is required, the catheter is small (usually no. 5F) and contains a single lumen through which it is possible to inflate the balloon with dilute contrast medium. The balloon is mounted at the tip of the catheter and has a maximum volume of 2.0—4.0 ml. The septostomy catheter produced by Edwards Laboratories has a preset angle proximal to the balloon allowing easy passage across the foramen ovale; it is the catheter of choice for balloon atrial septostomy.

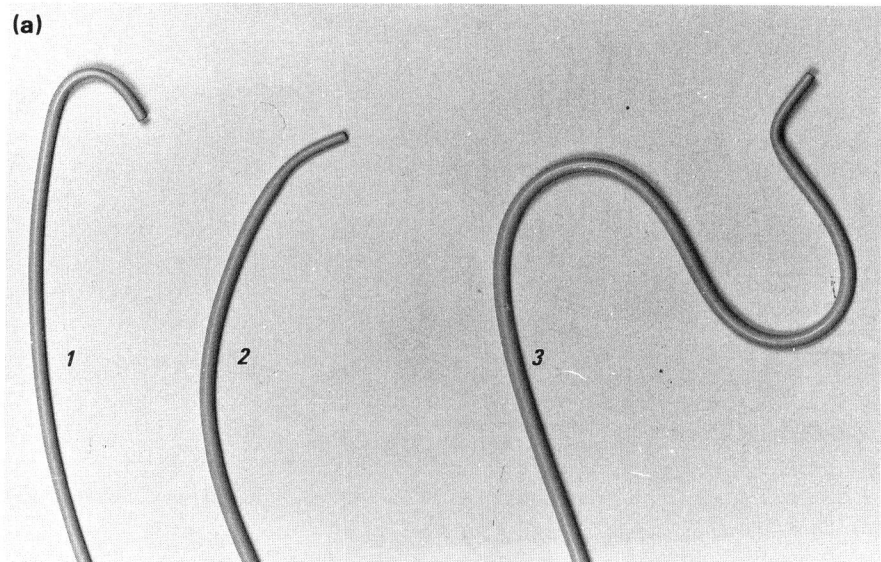

Fig. 2.9 (a) A selection of graft-seeking catheters. (1) Femoral internal mammary artery, (2) femoral right coronary bypass and (3) femoral coronary bypass (Greenburg technique).

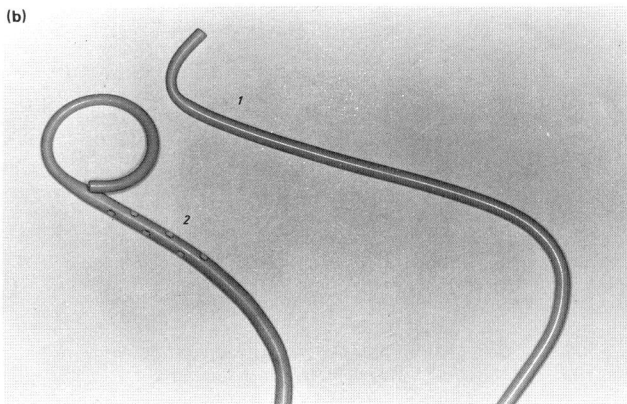

(b) Two more preshaped catheters. (1) Brachial internal mammary — for cannulating the left internal mammary artery from the right brachial artery. (2) 'Grollman' version of the pigtail catheter for pulmonary arteriography.

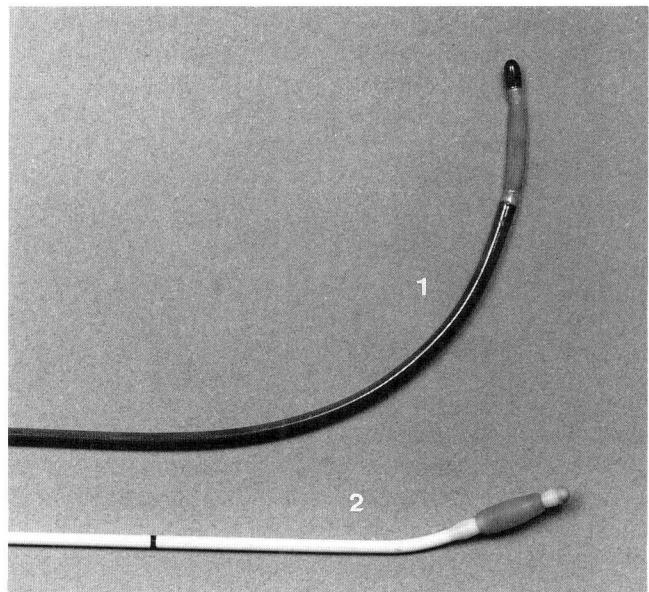

Fig. 2.10 Atrial septostomy catheters. (1) 'Rashkind' recessed-balloon septostomy catheter (USCI), (2) American Edwards Laboratories 'Miller' atrioseptostomy catheter.

After 1 month of age the interatrial septum may be too thick to tear by balloon septostomy and a *blade septostomy catheter* (Fig. 2.11) is available at the end of which a knife blade may be unsheathed in order to incise the atrial septum as the catheter is withdrawn across it [30, 31].

Balloon valvuloplasty catheters (Fig. 2.12). These catheters are designed to allow a stenotic valve (e.g. pulmonary valve) to be split by inflating a relatively large, sausage-shaped balloon which is positioned across the valve. The catheters contain two lumens, one of which allows the catheter to be threaded over a guide wire while the other allows the balloon to be inflated, at high pressure, with dilute contrast medium. The balloon is non-distensible; that is to

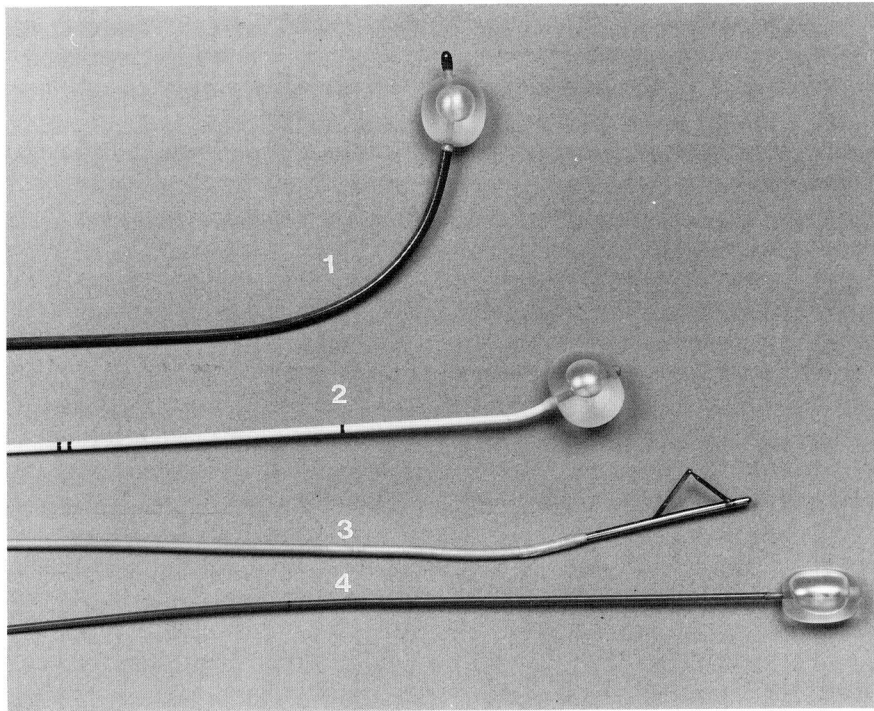

Fig. 2.11 Atrial septostomy (1) USCI recessed balloon, (2) Edwards Laboratories septostomy catheter, (3) Park blade septostomy catheter (William Cook Incorporated), and (4) Embolectomy, 4F Fogarty embolectomy catheter.

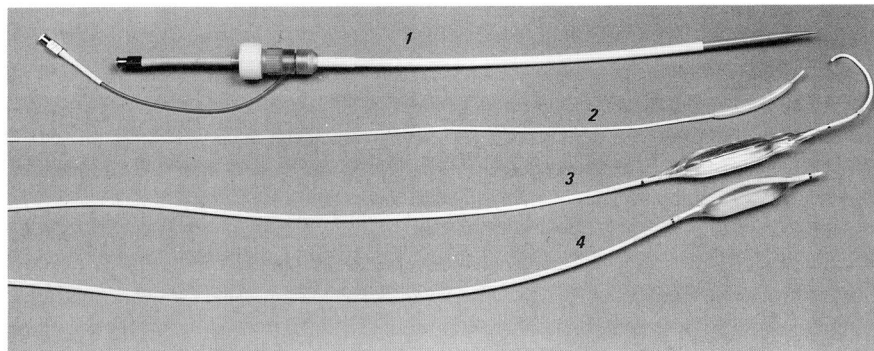

Fig. 2.12 Valvuloplasty. (1) 14F sheath dilator/introducer with Touhy—Borst adjustable haemostatic valve and side-arm, (2) Olbert, (3) Cribier—Letac dual-diameter balloon for aortic valvuloplasty — note the pigtail end, and (4) monofoil balloon (Mansfield Scientific).

say it will enlarge only to the predetermined maximum diameter. Excessive pressure thereafter will only rupture the balloon. There are a number of sizes available (8—25 mm diameter) appropriate to the diameter of the valve ring or vessel to be dilated.

A 'trefoil' valvuloplasty catheter has been developed [32] for aortic valvuloplasty; the single balloon is replaced by three, radially distributed, balloons. This catheter allows forward flow of blood during inflation via the interstices between the balloons. As a result there is no loss of consciousness and the balloon maintains a more stable position across the valve ring. Balloon valvuloplasty catheters used for

aortic valvuloplasty should have a pigtail tip. The, often violent, to-and-fro movement that occurs as balloon inflation obstructs left ventricular outflow could result in myocardial perforation by the tip of a straight catheter. The 'Cribier—Letac' aortic valvuloplasty catheter is of pigtail configuration and is available with a 'stepped' balloon allowing progressive dilatation of the valve. Balloon stability can be improved by the use of a long sheath which extends around the aortic arch and butresses the valvuloplasty catheter.

Coronary angioplasty (PTCA) catheters. A number of

special introducing and dilating catheter systems are available for dilating atherosclerotic lesions of the coronary arteries. The important subject of coronary angioplasty and the catheters required is discussed in Chapter 14.

Embolisation catheters (Figs 2.13 and 2.14). A number of devices have been developed for occluding pathological vessels such as those supplying arteriovenous fistulae. *Spring coils* can be ejected through a simple delivery catheter; the coils incorporate Dacron fibres and occlusion of the vessel results from thrombus formation around the coil. The technique is simple and the coils are cheap but occlusion is somewhat less precise than with the alternative technique of balloon occlusion. The *Debrun* technique of balloon occlusion employs miniature balloons which are tied to the end of the central catheter of a coaxial delivery system. When in position the balloon is filled with a rapidly hardening silicone gel and detached by withdrawing the fine, central catheter into the tip of the coaxial delivery catheter. A more convenient system (Becton–Dickinson) uses a mechanically detachable valved balloon filled with contrast medium. The use of these catheters is discussed in Chapter 5.

Pacing catheters. These catheters are described in the chapter devoted to pacemaking and electrophysiological studies (Chapter 22).

Fogarty embolectomy catheter (Fig. 2.11). This catheter is used to remove thrombus from vessels [33]. In the catherisation laboratory it is occasionally needed to remove thrombus from the brachial artery when poor technique has resulted in loss of the radial pulse. The catheter has a single lumen and a distal balloon which can be inflated with saline or dextrose. It is available in several sizes; 4F is suitable for brachial 'embolectomy'. The catheter is inserted by a cut-down and arteriotomy and advanced through the thrombus, with or without the aid of a stiffening stylet. The balloon is then inflated and the catheter slowly withdrawn so as to deliver the thrombus through the arteriotomy. It is best to allow the balloon diameter to adjust, slightly, to the calibre of the vessel by keeping gentle pressure on the inflating syringe rather than fixing the volume of fluid within the balloon.

The list of catheters given above, long though it is, includes only those catheters which are in common

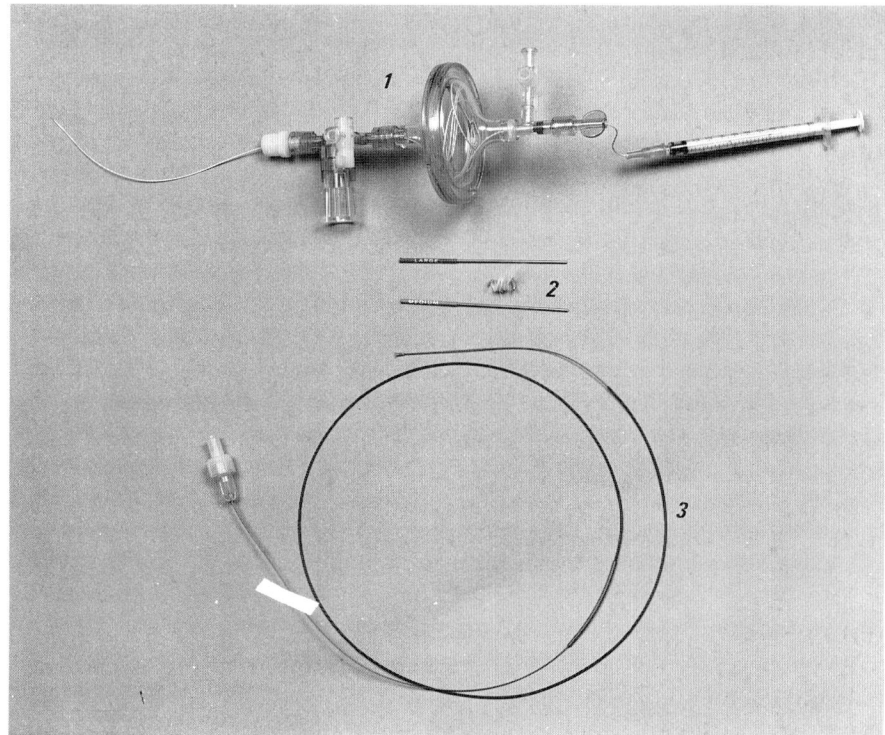

Fig. 2.13 Embolisation. (1) Delivery chamber for Becton–Dickenson mini-balloon embolisation catheter, (2) Gianturco spring coil and cartridges, and (3) Debrun coaxial balloon embolisation catheter.

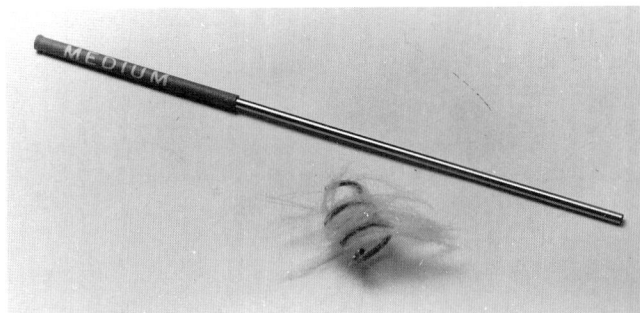

Fig. 2.14 Gianturco spring coil and cartridge.

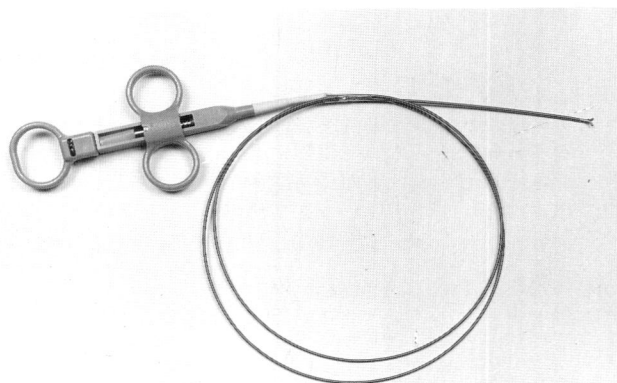

Fig. 2.15 King's endomyocardial bioptome (disposable — Cordis Corporation).

use or which are used in our laboratory. Nonetheless the physician coming to cardiac catheterisation for the first time or early in his experience will find that the list includes all those catheters which will be needed for routine diagnostic catheterisation as well as some which are needed for techniques which are other than routine. New developments which have not yet found general clinical use include laser catheters, plaque-removing catheters and angioscopy catheters [34].

The details of the way in which the catheters are used will be found in Chapters 3 and 4 and in those chapters dealing with catheterisation of specific lesions.

Catheters are the most obvious items which are employed during cardiac catheterisation but they are not the only ones. The remainder of this chapter will deal with other tools of catheterisation which make cardiac catheterisation safe and slick and as atraumatic as possible: bioptomes, introducing devices, guide wires, needles and the like.

BIOPTOMES

Two types of endomyocardial bioptomes (biopsy forceps) are in general use. The Scholten bioptome, which has one fixed and one movable cutting jaw, and the King's College Hospital bioptome in which both jaws move. The King's bioptome (Fig. 2.15) is available in two lengths, 104 and 50 cm and 6F. This bioptome is flexible and easy to use and is available as a disposable item (Cordis Corporation). The bioptome is introduced through a long sheath which is positioned with the aid of a pigtail ventriculography catheter. The jaws are operated by a three-ring handle and are kept closed by a spring until the central ring is pulled backwards.

SHEATH INTRODUCERS (Fig. 2.16)

The introduction of the Hoffman–Desilets type of sheath introducer [8] was an important advance as this device allowed the percutaneous, transfemoral introduction of all types of catheter (closed or open-ended) without the need for repeated exchange over a guide wire. As a result, saphenous or femoral vein cut-down is now only employed in neonates and infants in whom femoral vein puncture has proved impossible. The device consists of an assembly of (1) a short guide wire — straight or J-tipped, (2) a tapered 'dilator', and (3) a snug-fitting mylar sheath which is slightly shorter than the dilator. This basic pattern, which is used for transvenous catheter insertion, is adapted for transarterial (and transvenous) use by the addition of a one-way haemostatic valve and side-port in the hub. The haemostatic valve reduces blood loss and prevents the entry of air during exchange of a transvenous catheter. The side-port, with attached tubing and stopcock, allows the arterial pressure to be recorded or fluids to be infused during catheterisation. As a rule the sheath should be of the same French gauge as the catheter that is to be used. However, the haemostatic valve allows smaller catheters to be inserted without blood loss. If the side-port is to be used for arterial pressure measurement a sheath is needed which is 1F larger than the catheter. The technique of vessel entry using these devices is described in Chapter 3.

Fig. 2.16 Percutaneous entry. (1) Dilator/sheath assembly with haemostatic valve and side-arm for arterial catheterisation, (2) no. 19 'butterfly' needle (see text), (3) short-bevel vascular needle (and syringe), (4) short guide wire as used with (1), and (3) J-tipped versions are available, (5) Hoffman—Desilets dilator and sheath (dis-assembled) without haemostatic valve for transvenous entry.

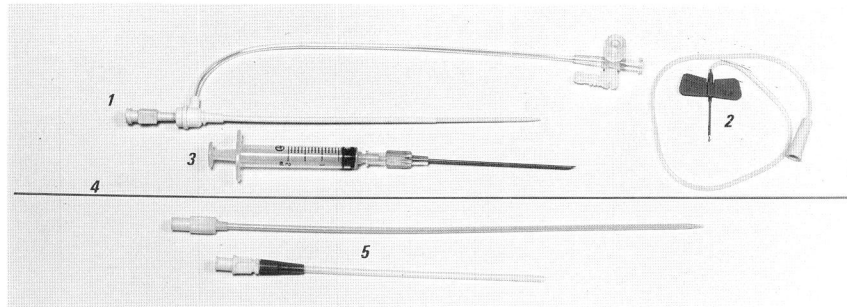

Long sheaths. Sheaths of considerably greater length are available. When introduced together with a pig-tail ventriculography catheter they allow the pigtail catheter to be replaced by a bioptome (for endomyo-cardial biopsy) or by a transducer-tip catheter (for high-fidelity pressure recording). Somewhat shorter sheaths can be positioned in a tortuous or ather-omatous iliac and femoral artery so that subsequent catheter insertion and exchange is facilitated and the danger of subintimal dissection is avoided.

Split sheaths. These are designed to split along their length so that they can be removed with the catheter in place. They are of use for multiple catheter inser-tion through the same puncture site (see Chapter 22). They also facilitate the introduction of large balloon valvuloplasty catheters. The balloon splits the sheath but its passage through the subcutaneous tissues is eased. The sheath is removed once the balloon has entered the vessel. Some split sheaths have no hub; great care must be taken to ensure that the sheath is not carried in with the catheter and 'lost' within the vessel. It is our practice to guard against this happening by attaching a haemostat to the proximal end of the split sheath.

GUIDE WIRES

Guide wires have a number of important uses. They form an essential part of the technique of percu-taneous vessel entry; the vessel is entered with a needle, a guide wire is advanced through the needle, the needle is removed and the catheter or dilator/sheath assembly advanced over the guide wire. Guide wires are used to lead an end-hole catheter through a tortuous vessel or across a stenotic valve.

Guide wires are needed to straighten preshaped catheters as they are advanced to the aortic root. They may help in reaching a site that cannot be reached by catheter manipulation alone and they can be used to stiffen a catheter which is tending to form a loop instead of advancing. Most guide wires consist of a spirally wound wire surrounding a central core and incorporate an inner safety wire attached to the tip. This safety wire prevents detachment of the flexible tip and its loss within the circulation should it fracture and separate from the rest of the wire. The central core tapers towards its distal end and stops short of the end of the spirally wound outer wire. As a result the leading tip is flexible. Guide wires are available with varying lengths of flexible tip, the most commonly used length being 3 cm. It is essential to check that the flexible end is about to be inserted first — careless insertion of the rigid end could result in vessel damage or perforation. The most commonly used guide wires are Teflon coated with resulting in-creased smoothness and ease of use. It is impossible to clean guide wires which are, therefore, for single use only and discarded at the end of the procedure.

J-guide wires

Guides with a curved tip are known as 'J-guides' and among other uses allow the guide to be passed up tortuous or atheromatous vessels without the risk of becoming lodged against the intima or beneath an atheromatous plaque. Curves of varying radii (15, 7.5, 3 or 1.5 mm) are available. J-guides with small radii cannot be inserted through the hub of a needle or catheter and are supplied with a small plastic introducing sleeve to straighten the tip before insertion. Straight guide wires can be given a curved tip if they are drawn firmly across the edge of a metal instrument while being held against the instrument by firm finger pressure.

Movable-core guide wires. In these wires the central (straight) core is attached to the butt of the wire but not to the distal (floppy) end. The first few centimetres of the butt separate from the rest of the outer coil and pulling on the butt withdraws the central core and increases the length of the floppy tip. The tip may be straight or of a 'J' configuration. This, last, type is of considerable usefulness as the wire is straight-tipped when the core is advanced (and easily inserted, therefore) but assumes the 'J' form when the core is retracted. Such wires approach the ideal of a 'universal guide wire'. Teflon-coated central cores move more freely than uncoated ones.

Exchange guide wires. Guide wires are available in various lengths — 125 or 150 cm are the most generally useful lengths. Exchange guides are 260 or 300 cm long and are designed to allow the original catheter to be removed and a new one threaded over the wire without disturbing the position of the tip of the wire within the heart. For example, a stenotic aortic valve may have been crossed with a catheter which is unsuitable for ventriculography. By using an exchange guide it is then possible to place a pigtail catheter in the left ventricle though this catheter would not, initially, cross the aortic valve.

Sizes of guide wires. Guide wires are available in a number of thicknesses varying from 0.025″ to 0.045″ (finer wires are used for coronary angioplasty — see Chapter 14). It is best to confine the routinely used guides to two thicknesses, say 0.025″ for paediatric and 0.035″ for adult work, in order to avoid possible confusion. Table 2.3 shows the minimum catheter and needle sizes which will accept two standard guide wire sizes. No 7F balloon flotation catheters will accept a 0.025 guide wire but a no. 5F catheter will only accept a 0.014″ and a no. 6F a 0.018″ guide wire — guides which are usually used for coronary angioplasty.

VESSEL DILATORS

When a vein (or artery) has been exposed by a cut-down some device is needed which will hold the vessel open so that the catheter can be

Table 2.3 Minimum catheter and needle sizes which will accept three standard guide wire sizes.

Guide wire diameter		Thin-wall needle gauge	Catheter FG	
In.	mm		Standard	Thin-wall
0.025	0.6	19	5	5
0.035	0.9	18	6	6
0.038	1.0	17	7	6

FG = French gauge.

introduced — as with a shoe-horn. Angled forceps are sometimes used but these 'tent' the opening so that a triangular opening is expected to accept a circular catheter. It is best to use an introducer which is a half circle in cross-section and has a pointed tip. Such introducers are easily made from thin-wall stainless-steel tubing (Fig. 3.1). Although it may seem unnecessary to dwell on such trivial accessories the possession of a suitable introducer may, especially in neonatal work, make the difference between success and failure.

NEEDLES

Needles designed for entering vessels (vascular needles) are thin-wall needles and must have a short bevel. The inside of the hub must be gently tapered to allow the introduction of a guide wire. Traditionally two-part, re-usable needles with a central trochar and outer cannula (e.g. Cournand, 'Seldinger' needles) were used in catheterisation laboratories. Today disposable needles are used and most prefer one-part needles designed to puncture one wall of the vessel only and not to transfix it. The vessel is punctured with the bevel uppermost; for this reason vascular needles should have some indication of the orientation of the needle incorporated in the hub. For percutaneous entry in neonates and infants a no. 19 gauge 'butterfly' cannula (Fig. 2.16) is ideal and will accept a 0.025″ guide wire. Correct vessel entry is signalled by free flow of blood along the clear plastic tubing attached to the needle — this tubing has to be cut off close to the hub before a guide wire can be inserted.

Left ventricular puncture needles for the transapical measurement of left ventricular pressure can be 19 gauge but must be at least 10 cm long. An 18 gauge needle will be needed if a guide wire and catheter are to be inserted (e.g. for pericardial aspiration or transapical left ventriculography).

OTHER ACCESSORIES

These include manometer tubing, rotating adaptors, stopcocks and manifolds, all of which are important as they help to make catheterisation as simple as possible; where technology can help full advantage should be taken of it. We owe it to the patient (and ourselves) to make catheterisation as easy, slick and atraumatic as possible. Almost all of these items are available as disposable equipment. Manometer tubing should be as short as possible to avoid degrading the frequency response of the fluid-filled catheter-manometer system. Three-way stopcocks allow blood sampling without breaking the integrity of the fluid-filled system. Manifolds are needed for coronary arteriography (Fig. 2.17). They consist of a rotating, Luer-lock connection for the catheter and a port for pressure measurement/flush, a port for the supply of contrast medium and a port for the injecting syringe.

CARE AND STERILISATION OF CATHETERS

Today virtually all cardiac catheters are packaged ready sterilised and labelled 'For single use only'.

This instruction, though deriving from the American Federal Drugs Administration regulations and medicolegal considerations obtaining in the USA, is also of great benefit in reducing the risks of infection and ensuring that the catheter is in perfect condition, but cardiac catheters are not cheap and it is still common practice to re-use at least the more expensive varieties. Some catheters cannot be re-used, notably balloon-tipped catheters, and neither can guide wires.

If catheters are to be re-used the dangers and disadvantages involved are (1) that repeated sterilisation may alter the characteristics of the catheter making it less easy to manipulate or making it brittle so that it may actually fracture; (2) if any blood clot remains in the lumen it may enter the bloodstream of the next patient and cause a 'pyrogenic reaction'; (3) the 'anti-thrombogenic' coating applied to some catheters will be lost with a danger of causing micro-embolisation; and finally (4) unless sterilisation is complete there is a danger of infection. Preparing catheters for re-use thus involves, firstly, a cleaning process which will remove all traces of thrombus from the lumen and, secondly, sterilisation of the catheter.

To clean a catheter the following steps should be followed:

1 Manually flush and clean the outside of the catheter with tap water — as soon as possible after use.
2 The catheter is then connected to a pressure flushing system and flushed with water for 30 minutes to 1 hour.
3 Soak the catheter in Detergicide (USCI) solution for at least 30 minutes.

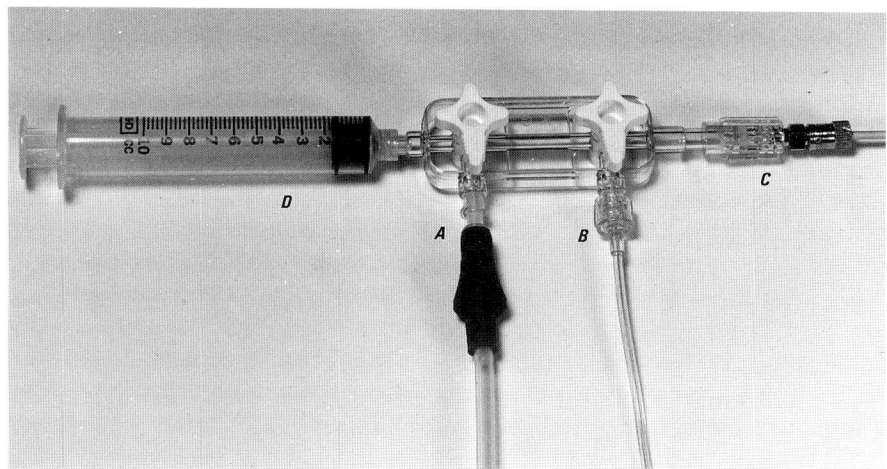

Fig. 2.17 Disposable manifold for coronary arteriography: (A) connection to reservoir of contrast medium, (B) connection to pressure transducer, (C) rotating Luer-lock connector to catheter, and (D) 10 ml syringe (Luer-lock) for injection of contrast medium.

4 Flush the lumen of the catheter with 1000 ml of Detergicide solution by gravity drip.

5 Finally rinse with 1000 ml of distilled water using a similar gravity drip system.

The catheter is then wrapped for sterilisation by ethylene oxide. When wrapping the catheter the diameter of the coils should be as large as possible to avoid fracturing at a sharp bend and to make it easy to manipulate in subsequent use. Woven Dacron catheters (virtually the only type that are still re-used) may be given the correct tip configuration by inserting a wire mandrel or, in the case of closed-end catheters, by enclosing the tip in a correctly shaped external stainless-steel sleeve.

REFERENCES

1 Schneider RM *et al.* Fracture of a polyurethane catheter in the aortic arch. A complication related to polymer aging. *Cathet Cardiovasc Diagn* 1983;**9**:197.

2 Cournand A, Ranges HA. Catheterization of the right auricle in man. *Proc Soc Exp Biol Med* 1941;**46**:462.

3 Rodriguez-Alvarez A, Martinez de Rodriguez G. Studies in angiocardiography: the problems involved in the rapid, selective and safe injections of radiopaque materials. Development of a special catheter for selective angiography. *Am Heart J* 1947;**53**:841.

4 Goodale WT, Lubin M, Banfield WG, Hackel DB. Catheterization of the coronary sinus, right heart and other viscera with a modified venous catheter. *Science* 1949;**109**:117.

5 Swan HJC, Ganz W *et al.* Catheterization of the heart in man with use of a flow-directed balloon-tipped catheter. *New Engl J Med* 1970;**283**:447.

6 Jones SM, Miller GAH. Catheterisation of the pulmonary artery in complete transposition of the great arteries using the Swan−Ganz flow-directed catheter, *Br Heart J* 1973;**35**:298.

7 Seldinger SI. Catheter replacement of the needle in percutaneous arteriography, a new technique. *Acta Radiol* 1953;**39**:368.

8 Desilets DJ, Hoffman R. A new method of percutaneous catheterization. *Radiology* 1965;**85**:147.

9 Grollman JH, Renner JW. Transfemoral pulmonary angiography: update on technique. *AJR* 1981;**136**:624.

10 Shirey EK, Sones FM. Retrograde transaortic and mitral valve catheterization. Physiologic and morphologic evaluation of aortic and mitral valve lesions. *Am J Cardiol* 1966;**18**:745.

11 Baur HR, Mruz GL, Erickson DL, Van Tassel RA. New technique for retrograde left heart catheterization in aortic stenosis. *Cathet Cardiovasc Diagn* 1982;**8**:299.

12 Se Do Cha, Incarvito J, Maranhao V, New method: calculation of magnification factor from an intracardiac marker. *Cathet Cardiovasc Diagn* 1983;**9**:79.

13 Keane JF, Freed MD, Fellows KE, Fyler DC. Pediatric cardiac angiography using a 4 French catheter. *Cathet Cardiovasc Diagn* 1977;**3**:313.

14 Brockenbrough EC, Braunwald E. New technique for left ventricular angiocardiography and transseptal left heart catheterization. *Am J Cardiol* 1960;**6**:1062.

15 Mullins CE. New catheter and technique for transseptal left heart catheterization in infants and children. *Circulation* 1979;**251**(suppl II):59−60.

16 Laskey WK, Kusiak V, Untereker WJ, Hirshfeld JW. Transseptal left heart catheterization: utility of a sheath technique. *Cathet Cardiovasc Diagn* 1982;**8**:535.

17 Sones FM, Shirey EK. Cine coronary artriography. *Mod Concepts Cardiovasc Dis* 1962;**31**:735.

18 Judkins MP. Selective coronary arteriography. 1. Percutaneous transfemoral technique. *Radiology* 1967;**89**:815.

19 Amplatz K, Formamek G, Stranger P, Wilson W. Mechanics of selective coronary catheterization via femoral approach. *Radiology* 1967;**89**:1040.

20 White RI, French RS, Amplatz K. An improved technique for right coronary artery catheterization. *Am J Radiol Roentgen Ther* 1971;**13**:562.

21 Wells E *et al.* A simplified method for left heart catheterization including coronary arteriography. *Chest* 1973;**63**:959.

22 Zir LM, Dinsmore RE, Goss C, Harthorne JW. Experience with preformed catheters for coronary arteriography by the brachial approach. *Cathet Cardiovasc Diagn* 1975;**1**:303.

23 Van Tassel RA. *et al.* A less traumatic catheter for coronary arteriography. *Cathet Cardiovasc Diagn* 1985;**11**:187.

24 Schoonmaker FW, King SB. Coronary arteriography by the single catheter percutaneous femoral technique: experience with 6800 cases. *Circulation* 1974;**50**:735.

25 Greenburg BH *et al.* Arteriographic findings in patients with aortocoronary saphenous vein bypass grafts and associated manual core endarterectomy. *Circulation* 1974;**50**:735.

26 Arani DT. A time saving technique in angiography of aorto-coronary bypass grafts. *Cathet Cardiovasc Diagn* 1981;**7**:301.

27 Simmons CR, Tsao EC, Thompson JR. Angiographic approach to the difficult aortic arch: a new technique for transfemoral cerebral angiography in the aged. *Am J Radiol Roentgen Ther* 1973;**119**:605.

28 Singh RN. Internal mammary arteriography: a new catheter technique by right brachial approach. *Cathet Cardiovasc Diagn* 1980;**6**:439.

29 Rashkind WJ, Miller WW. Creation of an atrial septal defect without thoracotomy: palliative approach to complete transposition of the great arteries. *JAMA* 1966;**196**:991.

30 Park SC *et al.* A new atrial septostomy technique. *Cathet Cardiovasc Diagn* 1975;**1**:195.

31 Park SC *et al.* Clinical use of blade septostomy. *Circulation* 1978;**58**:600.

32 Van den Berg EJM *et al.* New triple lumen balloon catheter for percutaneous (pulmonary) valvuloplasty. *Cathet Cardiovasc Diagn* 1986;**12**:352.

33 Fogarty TJ *et al.* Method for extraction of arterial emboli and thrombi. *Surg Gynecol Obstet* 1963;**116**:241.

34 Cortis BS *et al.* Angioscopy *in vivo. Cathet Cardiovasc Diagn* 1984;**10**:493.

CHAPTER 3

Techniques of catheterisation — access to the left and right heart

This chapter will describe the various techniques available for catheter insertion and access to the cardiac chambers and great vessels. 'Special' techniques such as transseptal and left ventricular puncture will be described but descriptions of how to manipulate the catheter within the heart are left to Chapter 4. 'Interventional' techniques such as valvuloplasty and embolisation therapy are discussed in Chapter 5.

PREPARATION OF THE PATIENT

Adult patients should regard the forthcoming catheterisation study as a minor, routine procedure which is almost (but not completely) free from risk and discomfort and which will only take a short time to complete. Needless to say they seldom do. Nonetheless much can be done to encourage this desirable attitude. Whenever possible patients should be shown the laboratory and receive a simple explanation of the function of the various items of equipment and a simple explanation of what is involved in the procedure. This is best done by a nurse — perhaps on the evening before the study is scheduled. They should be told that the only discomfort involved will be the injection of local anaesthetic at the entry site and a 'warm flush' lasting 30 seconds at the time of angiography. They will not feel the catheter within the heart though they may feel the odd 'extra heart beat'. If there are other patients who have experienced the procedure their reassurance is likely to be even more valuable. If this is done adult patients seldom need any premedication though the exceptionally nervous patient

may need premedication with 10 mg diazepam (valium) by mouth 1 hour before the study. Antibiotic cover is not needed. Anticoagulants need not be discontinued unless direct left ventricular puncture is planned. Atropine should not be given as a routine premedication; it should, however, be given at the first sign of an impending vasovagal reaction. The patient appears uncomfortable, his face is pale and the pulse rate falls. Atropine sulphate, 0.6 to 1.2 mg, can then be given by whatever route is immediately available — intravenous or intra-arterial. In practice this is an uncommon event; it occurs in patients who are anxious or following painful stimuli — both should be avoided by sensible preparation and good technique.

Patients scheduled for catheterisation should not have eaten or drunk anything for 4 hours prior to the study. This precaution is more to prevent vomiting at the time of angiography than as a precaution in case general anaesthesia is required. This instruction is often applied over-enthusiastically; the patient coming to the laboratory as the last case in the afternoon is often found to have had nothing to eat or drink since the previous night! We allow a light early breakfast for patients due for study in the morning and full meals up to, and including morning coffee for those scheduled for a study in the afternoon.

As far as possible everything should be done to make the procedure seem a minor one; thus we have most patients walk the short distance to the laboratory rather than transporting them on a trolley; by analogy patients walk to a minor procedure such as an X-ray but are wheeled to a major one such as an operation.

Although efforts such as these are designed to make the procedure seem trivial preparation should not, in fact, be casual. Informed, signed and witnessed consent must be obtained. The HBsAg (Australia antigen) status must be known as special precautions have to be taken if the patient is HBsAg positive. Any known allergies must be recorded. It is assumed that the clinical state will be as good as can be achieved by medical therapy and that the results of all relevant investigations are known. Drug treatment should not be altered with the exception of appropriate adjustment of insulin dosage in diabetics. It is unwise — and, for obvious reasons, distressing for the patient — to give a powerful diuretic shortly before the study.

Many, perhaps most, studies can be performed on a 'day case' (out-patient) basis. The main reason that they are not, other than logistic reasons, is fear of bleeding at the site of percutaneous, transarterial, entry; this objection does not apply if a brachial arteriotomy is used and there is, therefore, a powerful economic argument in favour of this approach.

CHOOSING THE SITE OF ENTRY

Anyone who sets out to catheterise the heart should be equally adept at all the standard techniques of catheterisation. He is then free to choose whichever approach is most likely to provide a solution to the problems posed by each individual patient. The first question that the operator must ask is 'What is the primary object of the study in this patient?' It may be that the aortic valve gradient must be obtained in which case an approach from the arm provides the greatest chance of success. It may be that there is thought to be an atrial septal defect in which case the defect will most easily be crossed if the approach is from the leg. Of course it is to be hoped that all relevant information will flow smoothly and rapidly from the study but unfortunately this does not always happen. One reason why it does not always happen is that the operator has chosen an approach which is less than optimal for solving the problem posed by a particular patient. This is most easily understood if we look at the advantages and disadvantages of each approach.

Catheterisation from the arm

RIGHT HEART CATHETERISATION FROM THE ARM

1 *Advantages.* This is the best approach for reaching the pulmonary artery and 'wedge' position. It is usually easy to enter an overriding aorta via the ventricular septal defect (VSD) (e.g. in tetralogy of Fallot). There is a better chance of reaching the right heart than from the leg if an absent inferior vena cava (IVC) with azygos continuation is suspected (e.g. in laevo-isomerism).

2 *Disadvantages.* The arm gets in the way for lateral angiocardiography and will have to be moved. In congenital heart disease it is difficult or impossible to cross an atrial septal defect (ASD) or patent foramen ovale and hence a left heart study which might have been obtained by a transvenous approach may require an arterial cut-down or puncture. Percutaneous catheterisation of an antecubital vein may be impossible and of the axillary vein is dangerous so that a cut-down is needed. It may be impossible to catheterise the IVC if Mustard's operation has been performed (in complete transposition). Balloon atrial septostomy is impossible.

LEFT HEART CATHETERISATION FROM THE ARM

1 *Advantages.* This approach offers the best chance of crossing (retrogradely) a stenotic aortic valve. In aortic dissection there is probably less danger of entering the false lumen than if the approach was from the leg. In congenital heart disease an ascending aortogram can be obtained in cases of aortic interruption or severe coarctation where this would be impossible, or difficult, from the leg.

2 *Disadvantages.* A retrograde arterial approach from the arm requires an arteriotomy; from the leg a percutaneous approach is required. Thus the decision 'arm or leg?' is often in reality 'cut-down or percutaneous?'. The merits and demerits of an arteriotomy or percutaneous arterial approach are discussed below but there are, in addition, some special situations in which the arterial approach is best made from the leg. The brachial artery may be small in the young patient or the patient of slender build (particularly in the female). Because of the

position of the X-ray tube or intensifier it is impossible to obtain a true lateral angiocardiogram without repositioning the arm. It is difficult, when the approach is from the arm, to engage the catheter tip in the left subclavian for studying a left Blalock anastomosis or a left internal mammary-coronary artery graft. It may be difficult to engage systemic-to-pulmonary collaterals or bronchial arteries. Finally there are always some patients in whom the anatomy is such that one approach may fail while another may succeed. Thus an aberrant right subclavian artery (from descending aorta), tortuous vessels or a greatly dilated aortic root may all frustrate attempts to reach the left heart from the arm.

Catheterisation from the leg

RIGHT HEART CATHETERISATION FROM THE LEG

1 *Advantages.* Most of the advantages and disadvantages of an approach from the leg are simply the reverse of those discussed in relation to the approach from the arm. In particular the simplicity of both the transvenous and transarterial percutaneous (sheath introducer) technique makes an approach from the leg attractive. Some manoeuvres may only be possible from the leg; these include crossing an ASD or foramen ovale and transseptal puncture to reach the left heart, atrial septostomy and balloon valvuloplasty for pulmonary or mitral valve stenosis. It is usually possible to reach the SVC from the IVC when Mustard's operation has been performed.

2 *Disadvantages.* It is marginally more difficult to reach the pulmonary artery and obtain a 'wedge' pressure from the leg than from the arm — particularly if the right atrium is enlarged or if there is tricuspid regurgitation . If pulmonary embolism is suspected there is a danger of dislodging more thrombus. In congenital malformations, especially those with atrial isomerism, an absent intrahepatic segment of IVC with azygos continuation makes it very difficult to reach the right ventricle.

LEFT HEART CATHETERISATION FROM THE LEG

1 *Advantages.* An approach from the femoral artery is required for the Judkins technique of coronary arteriography and this is the usual approach for percutaneous transluminal coronary angioplasty (PTCA) and for left ventricular biopsy. Bronchial arteries and collateral vessels are more easily engaged and embolised.

2 *Disadvantages.* The major practical disadvantage of the approach from the leg is the difficulty that may be experienced in crossing a stenotic aortic valve. Other situation which can cause problems are aortic dissection (when the catheter may enter the false lumen) and, in congenital heart disease, difficult or impossible studies in cases of aortic interruption and coarctation. Retrograde, percutaneous, catheterisation of the femoral artery should be avoided in the obese patient and in patients with suspected aorto-iliac arterial disease.

TECHNIQUES FOR ENTERING VESSELS

In order to spare the patient unnecessary discomfort it is desirable to enter both artery and vein (if both are required) from the same site. Thus in this section both entry to artery and vein will be discussed under 'site of entry'. Three sites are commonly used: (1) the antecubital fossa (median cubital or basilic vein and brachial artery), (2) the inguinal region (saphenous vein and femoral artery and vein), and (3) the axilla (axillary artery and vein). Other sites are the supra- and subclavicular approach to the subclavian vein (and, rarely, artery), the internal jugular vein, the umbilical artery and vein (in the neonate), and the direct percutaneous transapical approach to the left ventricle.

The antecubital fossa

As with all approaches the skin and subcutaneous tissues should first be cleaned with an antiseptic preparation such as povidone-iodine (Betadine) or chlorhexidine (Hibitane). The skin and subcutaneous tissues are anaesthetised with 5−10 ml of a 1% or 0.5% solution of lidocaine hydrochloride (Xylocaine) which acts, within 1−2 minutes and is effective for about 1 hour 15 minutes. The local anaesthetic must not contain added adrenaline (epinephrine). Care should be taken to avoid puncturing the vessel (especially the artery during the injection of local anaesthetic and to avoid intravascular injections.

VENOUS ACCESS

In many patients the median cubital vein will be visible through the skin and if right heart catheterisation is all that is required a very short (0.5 cm), transverse, incision will be all that is needed before the vein can be exposed by blunt dissection with a haemostat. Ties (e.g. catgut) are placed around the vein above and below the point of entry. The use of a blunt-pointed introducer ('dilator') of semi-circular cross-section will facilitate the introduction of the catheters (Fig. 3.1). It is important that a *medial* vein is chosen, a large lateral (cephalic) vein may tempt the unwary but this vein joins the axillary vein at a sharp angle which may be difficult or impossible, to negotiate. If both a left and right heart study are to be performed then it is best to make the incision over the brachial artery at the point of maximal pulsation. Even though there may not be an obvious superficial vein at this point the chances are that an adequate vein will be discovered during the isolation of the artery or lying close beside it.

ARTERIAL ACCESS

A short, transverse incision is made in the antecubital fossa over the point of maximal pulsation of the brachial artery. Blunt dissection is used to expose a 1 to 1.5 cm length of the brachial artery while an assistant retracts the tissues and the biceps tendon laterally. Tapes are passed above and below the artery and a small transverse incision made in the artery using fine scissors or the point of a no. 11 blade with the sharp side uppermost.

Hints

1 Remember that vessels lie in a 'conduit' surrounded by fatty tissue, if the dissection is exposing muscle it is in the wrong place.
2 The median nerve lies medial to the brachial artery. If the nerve is touched during the dissection (the patient will complain of parasthesiae) the dissection is too medial.
3 Although often very superficial the brachial artery lies beneath the biceps tendon which will usually have to be retracted laterally to expose the artery.
4 An artery which is unusually superficial and smaller than expected is probably the ulnar artery ('early bifurcation'). Avoid using this small artery; if

challenged by a large catheter there will be pain followed by spasm of the artery and loss of confidence by the patient. A little further dissection will expose a larger (radial) artery lying a little deeper and more laterally.
5 If the artery cannot be found quickly (and the whole dissection should take no more than 2 or 3 minutes) remove the retractors and relocate the artery by palpation. Quite often it will be found that the assistant has been retracting the artery along with the biceps tendon.

When the vessels have been isolated a small incision with fine pointed scissors or scalpel blade allows the catheter or guide wire to be inserted. If the incision is small it will usually be found that the catheter 'seals' the hole in the artery and no further haemostasis is required; if not the tapes will have to be tightened around the artery and catheter. Never tighten the tapes so much that it is difficult to advance the catheter; if so the slight resistance that is felt if a catheter impinges against the vessel wall or a branch or an atheromatous plaque will be obscured and disaster may follow as the catheter is advanced further. A delicate sense of touch is very important in catheterisation. If an end-hole catheter (e.g. 'pigtail') is used for the arterial study then the catheter should be lead into the artery by 10 cm or so of the guide wire — flexible tip first. *Never* advance a guide wire (or catheter) against resistance, this is how intimal dissections are caused followed by possible occlusion of the artery.

REPAIRING THE ARTERIOTOMY: AVOIDING COMPLICATIONS

The major potential complication of a brachial arteriotomy is loss of the radial pulse; it is the reason why many operators shun this approach in favour of the percutaneous, transfemoral, approach. Local arterial complications should occur in less than 1% of cases and are usually the result of poor technique. Three such errors of technique can lead to problems: (1) poor arterial repair, (2) damage to the artery proximal to the entry point and, possibly, (3) inadequate heparinisation.

Arterial repair

The artery should be repaired with interrupted transverse sutures. A 'purse-string' suture allows rapid closure of the artery at the end of the procedure and is satisfactory in most instances; but it narrows the vessel. It is best, therefore, to get into the habit of using interrupted sutures and a transverse repair in all cases. The suture material need be no thicker than 6/0 (8/0 in neonatal and infant work). Thicker suture material obscures the repair and makes it difficult to do a neat job; as in most craftmanship a neat job of work is also a sound one. If a double throw is used initially the first tie will not slip while a further two ties are added. The needle should be 'atraumatic' and the suture material of a non-slip type such as braided polyester (Ethibond). Four interrupted sutures are usually all that are required. Great care must be taken not to pick up the posterior wall with a suture during a repair; the use of a (reversed) straight, semi-circular introducer (Fig. 3.1) to guard the posterior wall during placement of the first two lateral stay sutures helps to avoid this complication. Angled arterial clamps (e.g. paediatric vascular occlusion clamp GU 3662 (Fig. 3.2) GU Manufacturing Company: see Appendix 2 for address) are used to obtain haemostasis during the repair without tension on the artery. Often one sees haemostasis being obtained by traction on the tapes while the operator is attempting to pull the edges of the fragile artery together with fine suture material— against the tension applied by his assistant! There is no sense in making such difficulties for oneself or in using thick 'bulldog' clamps or any instruments that do not make the repair easy and quick. At the end of the repair the artery is allowed to fall back into its bed with the clamps off but at least one loose tape still around it in case the radial pulse is poor and the repair has to be redone. The patient should not be allowed to leave the laboratory unless the radial pulse is easily palpable; 'spasm' as a cause of an absent pulse is more an excuse for poor technique than a genuine physiological phenomenon.

If the repair is good and the radial pulse still not present the probable reason is that clumsy catheter or guide wire manipulation has caused an intimal dissection somewhere between the subclavian and the site of entry. It has already been stressed that this can result if the catheter or guide wire is advanced against resistance. This may also happen if the catheter is introduced at too sharp an angle; the artery should be allowed to resume its straight course by slackening the upper tape as the catheter or guide wire is inserted at a shallow angle.

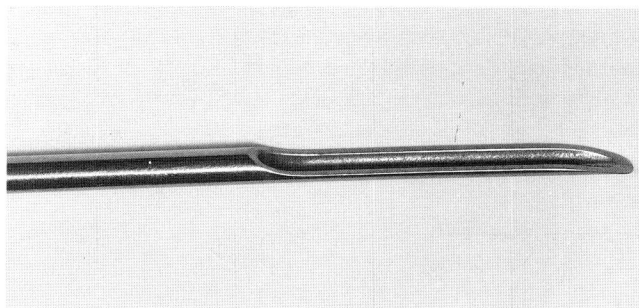

Fig. 3.1 Introducer made from thin-wall stainless-steel tubing. May also be used (open-side uppermost) during arterial repair to guard the posterior wall of the brachial artery during insertion of the first two stay sutures.

The complication is difficult to deal with though gently withdrawing a no.4F Fogarty embolectomy catheter through the artery in the upper arm may 'iron out' the intimal flap and remove associated thrombus. Thrombus formation as the immediate cause of an absent radial pulse is very rare since all patients having an arteriotomy should be heparinised; it is our practice to administer 1.0 mg/kg body weight of heparin intra-arterially through the catheter when it has reached the ascending aorta. This single bolus will provide adequate anticoagulation for 40 minutes [1] but only about 40% of patients will remain adequately heparinised if the study lasts for more than 90 minutes — few studies do, or should. Giving heparin by local infusion distal to the arteriotomy is useless (the dose is too small for whole-body heparinisation and is rapidly washed out by collateral flow) and painful for the patient.

The femoral approach

CUT-DOWN IN NEONATES AND INFANTS

Before the development of sheath introducers the only way that closed-end catheters could be introduced from the leg was by a cut-down. Today a cut-down is only likely to be employed in neonates or infants when a percutaneous technique has failed or is judged to be beyond the operator's skill. Following local anaesthesia an incision is made parallel to the inguinal ligament and 1.0 to 1.5 cm below it. The lateral extremity of the incision should be in line with the femoral artery (located by palpation) and

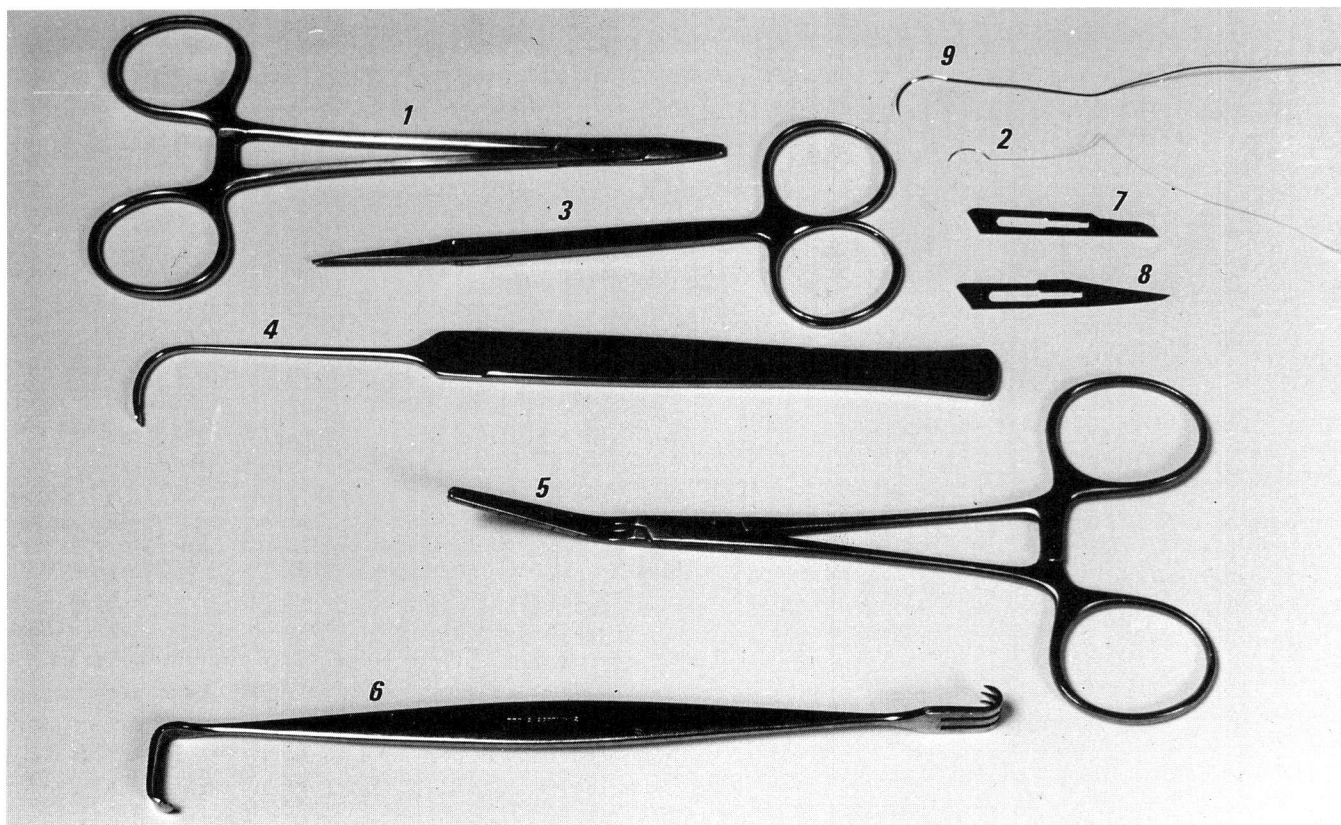

Fig. 3.2 Cut-down. Arteriotomy. Some of the instruments used for arterial cut-down. (1) Small, non-toothed, needle holders for arterial repair. (2) 6/0, atraumatic curved needle and braided polyester suture for repair of arteriotomy. (3) Fine, pointed scissors. (4) Aneurysm needle — used in conjunction with curved 'mosquito' haemostat for retraction and blunt dissection of tissues during exposure of the brachial artery. (5) Angled paediatric vascular occlusion clamp (two needed) used for haemostasis during arterial repair. (6) Retractor (two needed) used by assistant during exposure of the brachial artery. (7) No. 15 scalpel blade (skin incision). (8) No. 11 scalpel blade — may be used instead of scissors for arteriotomy. (9) Curved cutting needle and 3/0 silk for skin suture.

its length about 1.0 to 1.5 cm. Blunt dissection should expose the saphenous vein. If the vein is too small to accept the catheter there is no option but to explore the vein towards the inguinal ligament; the saphenofemoral junction provides the next possible entry site; failing that the femoral vein will have to be exposed. Unfortunately an incision distal enough to uncover the saphenous vein is too distal to be ideal for the femoral vein so that this dissection becomes progressively more difficult. An alternative that may be chosen is to seek the femoral vein from the beginning. This requires, in the neonate, an incision which is just below the inguinal ligament. The femoral vein lies immediately medial to the artery and somewhat 'deep' to it. Ligatures must be placed above and below the entry site but despite these it is often difficult to avoid some blood loss as

the catheter is being introduced. The rather difficult dissection in a neonate, the problem of blood loss and the need to repair the femoral vein at the end of the procedure are strong arguments for the percutaneous (sheath) technique or, failing this, for using the saphenous vein if at all possible.

Hints

1 Even if it has proved impossible to introduce a sheath percutaneously it is a good idea to tie a sheath into the femoral vein if it has been isolated by cut-down. This will make it easy to change catheters without the problem of blood loss each time.
2 Be very sure that it is the vein, and not the artery, before opening the vessel. The femoral artery of a neonate is small and thin-walled and, if there is

arterial desaturation, may look very like a vein. Naturally if the artery has been incised, intentionally or by mistake, it must be repaired using 8/0 interrupted sutures as described for the repair of a brachial arteriotomy above — as must the vein.

PERCUTANEOUS TECHNIQUE

This is the ideal way to enter femoral vessels. The basic technique is easily described: following local anaesthesia the vessel is located by palpation and punctured by a short-bevel needle. A guide wire is passed through the needle to lie some distance up the vessel before the needle is removed and replaced by a tapered-tip catheter or introducer/sheath assembly [2, 3] which is advanced over the guide wire. The guide wire and introducer are then withdrawn leaving the sheath in the vessel. The catheter(s) can be introduced and exchanged through the sheath, and catheterisation commenced.

VENOUS ACCESS

The femoral vein lies immediately medial to the artery. In the adult, imagine each to be about the same thickness as a finger. Locate the artery below the inguinal ligament by palpation and thoroughly anaesthetise the skin and subcutaneous tissues with 1.0 or 0.5% lignocaine. Take plenty of time about making sure exactly where the artery lies, when you think the exploring finger is directly above the artery move the finger slightly to the left and right and confirm that the arterial pulsations are now felt first to one and then the other side of the finger tip. Make a 2—3 mm incision in the skin over the vein (and artery if an arterial study is to be performed as well) with the point of a no. 15 blade (a no. 11 blade is often used but there is a danger of penetrating too far with this dagger-like blade; even of entering the artery. A no. 15 blade will only penetrate a few millimetres). Using a short-bevel needle attached to a 2 ml syringe advance the needle at about a 45° angle to where you think the vein should be; keeping suction on the plunger of the syringe all the time. The moment the needle enters the vein the plunger can move back and blood will enter the syringe. The reason for advocating the use of a small volume syringe is that this moment, when the plunger can move and blood be aspirated, is more

immediately noticeable than would be the case if a larger syringe were used. Provided blood enters the syringe easily the needle can be detached, lowered to a more horizontal position and the guide wire inserted through it and advanced some distance up the vein. As always, *never* advance the guide wire against resistance. If the guide wire will not pass readily, remove it and check that there is free flow of blood; moving the needle slightly if necessary. When the guide wire is in place, remove the needle and pass the assembly of vessel dilator and sheath over the wire and into the vein twisting the assembly as it is advanced. Finally remove the dilator and introduce the catheter through the sheath. Sheath introducers (e.g. Hoffman—Desilets) designed for entering veins have no haemostatic valve. In some situations (especially when studying congenital heart disease) it may be anticipated that several catheters of different sizes will be needed to complete the study. For example a no. 5F balloon-tipped catheter may be needed to obtain the pulmonary artery pressure in a case of complete transposition but a no. 7F angiographic catheter needed to obtain good ventriculograms. If this is so it is wise to use an introducer equipped with a haemostatic valve and side-arm of a size adequate to take the largest catheter you envisage using. This way blood loss due to a catheter in an overlarge sheath will be avoided. The sheath must always be purged of air by opening the stopcock of the side-arm before introducing the catheter.

In the neonate or infant, the standard needles supplied by the manufacturers for use with sheath introducers are too large and have too long a bevel to allow clean puncture of the 1 to 2 mm diameter femoral vein. A helpful trick is to use a short-bevel no. 19 'butterfly' needle. This has a short length of clear plastic tubing attached and if used without a syringe it will be found that the moment of entry is signalled by blood appearing in this clear tubing. The rate and steadiness with which blood advances up the plastic tubing gives an excellent indication of whether or not the needle tip is free within the lumen of the femoral vein. When free backflow has been obtained the plastic tubing is cut off and the butt of the needle and a 0.025″ guide wire inserted through the needle and into the vein.

If a cut-down is used to isolate the saphenous vein in an adult (due to non-availability of a sheath introducer) the incision will need to be 4 to 5 cm below the inguinal ligament. The saphenous vein is most easily isolated by feel; a finger in the incision will discover the vein as a firm cord which can be rolled beneath the finger tip. A haemostat can be guided 'blind' by the exploring finger and used to elevate the vein. The vein is secured by passing the haemostat and a ligature beneath it.

ARTERIAL ACCESS

The traditional 'Seldinger' technique of arterial puncture [4] employed a trochar and cannula and entry was signalled by blood spurting from the end of the cannula. Puncture involved transfixing the artery before the trochar was removed and then slowly withdrawing the cannula at a more horizontal angle until this jet of blood was observed. Although this technique is still employed it is more sensible to make use of the facility, available in all catheterisation laboratories, of monitoring pressure at the needle tip to signal entry to the femoral (or any other) artery. To do this a standard short-bevel needle, which will accept a guide wire, is attached to a strain-gauge pressure transducer via a length of plastic 'manometer tubing'. The needle is advanced with the pressure at its tip displayed on an oscilloscope. An undamped arterial pressure signals vessel entry and there is no need to puncture both walls of the artery. Damped oscillations signal the point at which the needle is very near to puncturing the artery or, more importantly, that the needle tip is not quite free within the lumen. A sudden fall in tissue pressure to near zero indicates that the needle has missed the artery and is now too deep. Slight adjustments of the needle position until there is an 'undamped' arterial pressure ensure that the subsequent insertion of the guide wire and catheter will be 'clean' with no damage to the artery other than the essential single entry hole.

Catheter insertion can be over the guide wire (e.g. with Gensini-type catheters) but it is more usual to use a dilator/sheath assembly fitted with a haemostatic valve [3]. These 'valved sheaths' allow multiple catheter changes without the need for repeated guide wire insertions and with minimal damage to the vessel wall. The side-arm of the sheath should be purged with blood before the catheter is inserted to avoid the introduction of (a small amount) of air.

At the end of the procedure, the sheath/catheter is removed and finger pressure applied to the puncture site for at least 10 minutes until a haemostatic plug has formed and there is no visible bleeding.

The disadvantage of the percutaneous, transfemoral (arterial), approach is that there may be delayed bleeding or haematoma formation at the puncture site. For this reason patients have to remain in bed for some hours after the procedure (overnight in some institutions). Haematoma formation, as a complication of the technique, is almost certainly under-reported. Out-patient catheterisation becomes a questionable procedure. Our preference, for these reasons, is to use a brachial arteriotomy in the majority of cases.

It may be difficult, or impossible, to traverse a tortuous, atheromatous iliac artery from the leg and the transfemoral approach should be avoided in patients with suspected aorto-iliac disease. In obese patients it may be difficult to localise the femoral artery by palpation and difficult to obtain haemostasis by manual compression. Haemostasis may also be difficult to obtain in patients with a wide pulse pressure due to aortic regurgitation or an aortopulmonary shunt. In all such patients the alternative brachial approach should be considered.

The axilla

This approach is not widely known or practised but can be invaluable in many cases of congenital heart disease. The approach requires a cut-down in the right axilla. A percutaneous approach has been employed but anyone who has cut-down on the axilla will be struck by the way in which the cords of the brachial plexus surround the axillary artery and vein and not, therefore, surprised that brachial palsies have been reported as a complication of the percutaneous approach. Local anaesthetic should be injected into the loose subcutaneous tissue and not deeply around the brachial plexus. There are usually three skin creases in the infant's axilla and the incision should be at the level of the middle one of these. If the incision is made too near to the chest wall the dissection reveals numerous, small chest-wall veins but not the main axillary vein. Too far along the upper arm and again the main axillary artery and vein fail to appear. A semi-transparent aponeurosis will be found immediately beneath the skin and subcutaneous fat and the brachial plexus and axillary vein will be visible through this. The aponeurosis is divided by blunt dissection and the axillary vein found among the nerve cords in an inferomedial position. Further gentle separation of the nerves will reveal the axillary artery in a more superior (lateral) position. The hunt for the artery is guided by looking for its pulsations. The operator must be able to distinguish the different appearance of nerve trunks and arteries.

Although this dissection sounds frightening it is, in fact, remarkably easy — easier, thanks to the superficial position of the structures, than the dissection of the femoral artery and vein. The chief difficulty with this approach in the neonate is negotiating the sharp downward bend needed to enter the superior vena cava (SVC) from the subclavian vein. The axillary vein and artery are as large as the femoral vessels. Familiarity with this approach may allow access to the heart when other approaches have failed as well as providing a solution to specific problems such as access to the ascending aorta in cases of aortic interruption. As always entry to small vessels is facilitated by using a semi-circular introducer. As always the artery and vein must be repaired with meticulous technique — using 8/0 suture material.

Transapical left ventricular puncture [5]

This technique has two uses: (1) to measure the gradient between the left ventricle and aorta or wedge, and (2) to obtain a left ventricular angiocardiogram. In both cases it is used only when the left ventricle cannot be entered by more conventional techniques. In the first case it is only necessary to enter the ventricle with a fine (19 gauge) 10 cm long, needle in order to measure left ventricular pressure. Complications are rare and it is probable that left ventricular puncture is less hazardous than the alternative of transseptal puncture. The technique will, of course, only be needed when retrograde passage through the aortic valve is impossible, in severe aortic stenosis for example.

The second use for the technique, to obtain a left ventriculogram [6, 7], is needed when it is impossible to enter the left ventricle either antegradely through the mitral valve (following transseptal puncture) or retrogradely through the aortic valve — typically when both valves have been replaced by tilting disc prostheses.

The first step, following sterilisation of the skin, is to locate the left ventricular apex by palpation. Then

place the tip of some metal implement — a scalpel handle for example — at what appears to be the apex as located by palpation. Fluoroscopy will now reveal how accurate this was. If the point chosen and marked with the radio-opaque implement turns out not to be the radiological apex the implement is moved until it appears to be just lateral to the true apex and this is the point selected for puncture. The skin, deep tissues and pleura are anaesthetised and the hypodermic needle replaced by a fine, 10 cm long needle attached to a pressure transducer by a length of manometer tubing for continuous monitoring of pressure at the needle tip. The needle is advanced upwards, backwards and to the right; aiming at the back of the right shoulder. The orientation of the needle can be checked by fluoroscopy. The point at which the needle tip touches the cardiac apex can be felt as cardiac movement is transmitted through it; there are often one or two ventricular ectopic beats at this time. Advancing the needle a centimetre or so further should produce a distinct 'puncturing' sensation and the continuously monitored pressure should change to an undamped ventricular waveform. It is important to ensure that the pressure IS undamped and that a clear a-wave and end-diastolic pressure are being obtained. If not, the needle tip is not free within the cavity of the ventricle and a false pressure may be recorded.

Possible complications include haemopericardium with tamponade and pneumothorax; they are rare but the patient should be closely monitored for some hours after return to the ward and should have a portable chest X-ray performed an hour or so later.

The technique of transapical left ventriculography (Fig. 3.3) is identical in the first stages except that a larger bore needle must be used; one that will accept an 0.035″ or 0.038″ guide wire. When a good ventricular pressure has been obtained and recorded the manometer tubing is disconnected and a guide wire advanced to lie freely within the cavity of the left ventricle. The needle is removed and replaced with a short, Teflon, Gensini catheter. To minimise the size of the puncture hole a small diameter (Fig. 3.4) (no. 6F) catheter can be used; to obtain a satisfactory angiogram through such a fine catheter it should be as short as possible — say 15 to 20 cm long. Such catheters are available to special order. Teflon is the preferred material as it is relatively rigid with a low coefficient of friction and will force its way through the tissues following the track of the guide wire. It

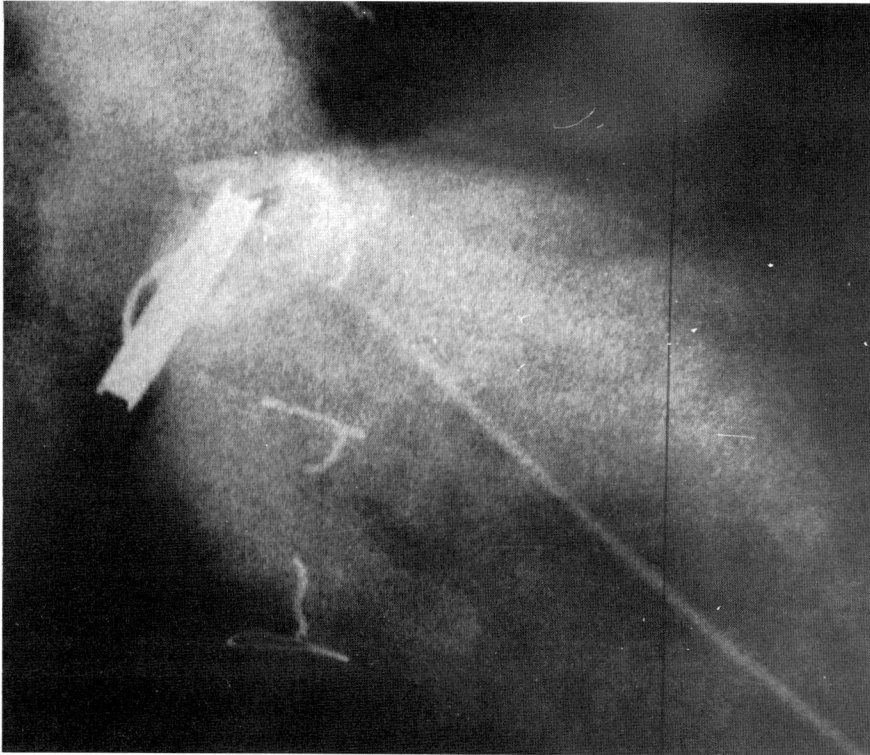

Fig. 3.3 Percutaneous transapical left
ventriculography. Antegrade entry to the
left ventricle is guarded by a Bjork–Shiley
tilting disc mitral prosthesis and
retrograde entry by an Omniscience aortic
prosthesis.

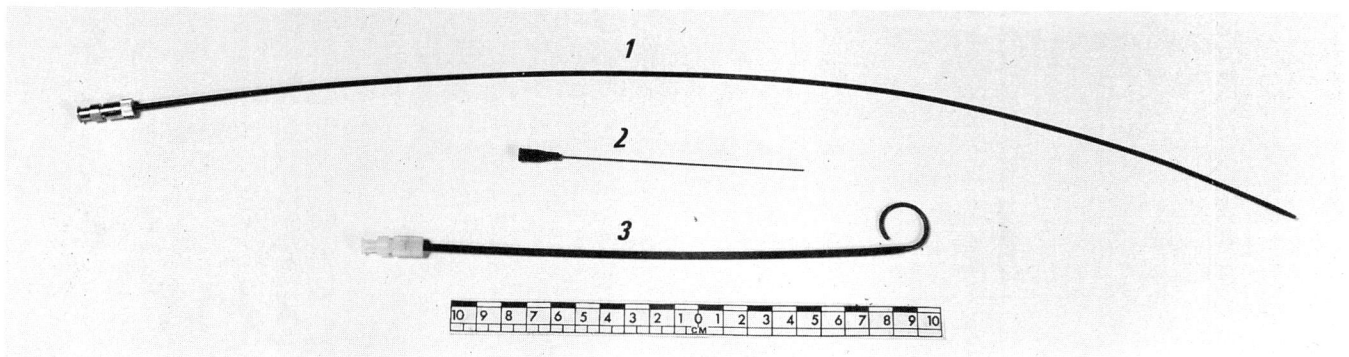

Fig. 3.4 Transthoracic left ventricular puncture. Pericardial drainage. (1) 50 cm long, 6F, Teflon Gensini catheter for transapical left
ventriculography. (2) 10 cm no. 19 needle for transapical left ventricular puncture and pressure measurement. (3) 20 cm Teflon pigtail
catheter for pericardial drainage.

is possible to advance the guide wire and then the
catheter further so as to enter the left atrium or the
aorta from the left ventricle [8].

Brockenbrough transseptal puncture

This technique [9–11] was in common use some
years ago but is less often practised today. It is

however, an essential part of balloon mitral valvuloplasty. The technique allows access to the left atrium
and left ventricle for both pressure measurement
and angiography and thus permits detailed assessment of mitral valve function. This was important
when mitral valvotomy was the only operation that
was available but is less important in the era of
open valve surgery and valve replacement.

The technique involves percutaneous puncture of the right femoral vein as described above. A guide wire is used to lead the special Teflon transseptal catheter through the IVC and right atrium until the tip of the catheter lies in the SVC. The guide wire is then replaced by 71 cm long transseptal needle (Fig. 2.6) connected, by manometer tubing, to a pressure transducer. This needle is advanced through the lumen of the catheter until its sharp point is just sheathed within the Teflon catheter. It is wise to follow the progress of the needle tip up the catheter by fluoroscopy since it has been known for the needle to perforate the catheter wall. The last few centimetres of the needle have a gentle curve; as the needle traverses the catheter it will tend to rotate this way and that as the curved tip follows the course of the catheter through the iliac vein and IVC — allow it to do so freely. The catheter is 2 cm shorter than the needle so that, to remain safely sheathed, 3 cm of the butt of the needle must remain unsheathed at the groin. This should be checked before the procedure starts so that the operator is familiar with the appearances of the assembly both when the needle is sheathed and when it is un-sheathed. As soon as the catheter tip is withdrawn from the SVC to a high right atrial position the curve of the needle within the catheter will cause the catheter to adopt the same curve. A pointer attached to the butt of the needle allows the operator to determine the orientation of the catheter tip and enclosed needle. The sheathed needle should point medially and 45° posteriorly as the catheter tip is slowly drawn down the interatrial septum. The upper part of the septum is related to the aortic root and the catheter may be seen to move slightly to the left as it is withdrawn to below the bulge of the aortic root. This is not the point for atrial puncture; puncture here results in a recognised complication of the technique — aortic puncture. With further downwards withdrawal of the catheter/needle assembly the tip is felt to move slightly to the left as it engages beneath the limbus of the foramen ovale. At this point the needle is advanced so that it protrudes beyond the catheter tip and punctures the atrial septum. The pressure record should now change to show a higher (left atrial) pressure. If the aortic root has, inadvertently, been punctured an aortic waveform will be displayed; provided that puncture was with the fine needle tip only this is unlikely to result in a serious complication. Acci-

dental aortic root puncture is most likely when the root is dilated [12]. The position should be checked by sampling through the needle; fully saturated blood confirms a left atrial position for the needle tip. Finally the Teflon catheter is advanced over the needle to the left atrium and the needle can then be withdrawn. Advancing the catheter still further should result in it entering the left ventricle through the mitral valve; the catheter has a preformed curve to assist in this manoeuvre. Counter-clockwise rotation at the hub will cause the tip to point anteriorly in the direction of the mitral orifice.

A variant of this technique employs an assembly consisting of a Teflon dilator within a long sheath. The dilator has no side-holes and is used over a Brockenbrough transseptal needle in just the same way as described for the Brockenbrough catheter. When the dilator and sheath have entered the left atrium the long dilator is withdrawn leaving the curved end of the sheath positioned in the left atrium ready to accept a variety of catheters. Both this device the USCI Mullins transseptal catheter introducer set (Fig. 2.6) [13] and the conventional Brockenbrough catheter and needle are available in adult and paediatric sizes.

The subclavian vein

The percutaneous approach to the right heart via the subclavian vein is more often used for the insertion of pacemaker wires than for diagnostic catheterisation but may occasionally be needed when all other routes are barred. The subclavian vein lies directly behind the clavicle in its middle third and joins the internal jugular vein behind the sternoclavicular joint to form the innominate vein. The subclavian artery lies a few millimetres behind the vein and the apex of the pleura a few millimetres behind the artery. The subclavian vein may be punctured from above or below the clavicle though the infraclavicular approach is the one most frequently used. The site of entry is immediately below the clavicle at the junction of its medial and middle third. A small tubercle may be palpated beneath the clavicle at this point. Following lidocaine anaesthesia of the skin a small incision is made with the tip of a no. 15 scalpel blade. Using a no. 21 needle the subcutaneous tissue is anaesthetised and the needle simultaneously advanced beneath the clavicle aiming at a point 2 cm above the suprasternal notch and keeping the needle at an angle of about 30° to the chest wall. Intermittent suction on the attached syringe will result in the aspiration of blood as soon as the vein is entered. The fine needle can then be changed for one that will accept a guide wire (e.g. 18 gauge) and the vein entered along the same track. The short bevel should be directed inferomedially so as to direct a guide wire towards the innominate vein rather than towards the internal jugular vein. A sheath introducer is then inserted over the guide wire in the usual way. As with all venous entry from the upper body (subclavian and internal and external jugular veins) there is a danger of air aspiration when the patient inspires. For this reason the sheath introducers used must incorporate a haemostatic valve. The side-port and tubing must be purged before the catheter is introduced. When a syringe is detached from a needle in the vein (e.g. prior to guide wire insertion) the patient should be asked to hold his breath or breathe out and the hub of the needle immediately closed with a finger or thumb. Subclavian vein puncture is facilitated if a pad (e.g. a rolled towel) is placed between the patients shoulder-blades; the patient should be asked to turn his head towards the opposite side — to the left for puncture of the right subclavian vein.

Complications of subclavian vein puncture include pneumothorax, haemothorax and inadvertent puncture of the subclavian artery; this last complication being of importance because of the difficulty in controlling bleeding since manual compression is impossible. The approach may have a higher complication rate than do alternative routes of venous access [14].

The internal jugular vein

This (percutaneous) approach [15—17] is also used more frequently for pacemaker wire insertion or central venous pressure monitoring than for diagnostic catheterisation. To cannulate the vein the patient's neck is extended by placing a pad beneath his shoulders and his head turned to the opposite side. The internal jugular vein lies laterally to the carotid artery in the centre of a triangle formed by the medial end of the clavicle, the lateral border of the sternal head of the sternocleidomastoid and the medial border of the sternal head of the same muscle. Puncture of the vein and insertion of a sheath introducer is accomplished in the usual way

after the vein has been punctured with a no. 18 gauge needle. The introducer sheath must be equipped with a haemostatic valve to guard against air embolism. After anaesthesia with lidocaine a small skin incision is made in the centre of this triangle (3—4 cm above the sternoclavicular joint and 1—2 cm lateral to the sternal head of the sternocleidomastoid). The needle should be directed caudally and posteriorly at an angle of about 30° to the frontal plane — aiming at the nipple on the same side. If the vein is not entered at the first attempt a steeper angle and/or a slightly more lateral direction may be tried. The needle should not be directed more medially as the carotid artery lies medial to the vein at this point and could be punctured.

Ventricular biopsy [18]

Left ventricular endomyocardial biopsy using the King's bioptome [19—21] — obtainable as a disposable item from the Cordis Corporation (see Appendix 2 for address) is most easily performed from percutaneous puncture of the femoral artery. The left ventricle is entered retrogradely using a pigtail catheter contained within a long sheath which covers all but the last few centimetres of the catheter. The catheter is then withdrawn leaving the sheath in position to guide the biopsy forceps into the left ventricle and towards the apex or lateral wall. When the tip of the bioptome is clear of the sheath its jaws can be opened, the bioptome is advanced further so that the open jaws impinge against the myocardium when they are closed (firmly) and the bioptome removed with a small piece of myocardium held within the two cup-shaped jaws. Slight resistance as the bioptome is withdrawn signals the successful removal of tissue. Advancing the bioptome with the jaws open probably reduces the (very small) risk of perforating the heart.

Although the technique is simple there are some problems that may be encountered.
1 Even with high quality fluoroscopy it may be difficult to see exactly where the end of the sheath is lying within the ventricle. The jaws cannot be opened until they are clear of the sheath which should be a centimetre or so away from the myocardium to allow the jaws to impinge against the myocardium in a fully open position. It takes some practice to position the end of the sheath correctly;

one guide to its position is provided as the pigtail catheter is withdrawn since the curled end of the catheter will be straightened as it enters the sheath; the point at which this happens can be observed and noted.

2 The sheath has no side-holes and will be occluded if the open end lies against the myocardium. The sheath is thin and will kink easily. If either of these things happen there will be no back-flow of blood to purge the sheath as the bioptome is withdrawn. Air is drawn into the sheath as the bioptome is withdrawn and the next time the bioptome is inserted it acts as a piston and forces air into the ventricle with a very real danger of causing air embolism. Air embolism by this mechanism is the major potential complication of the technique. It is vitally important to purge the sheath each time; adjusting its position if necessary. Thrombus forming within the sheath can result in embolism by the same mechanism and heparinisation is advisable to prevent this happening.

3 The reverse effect — excessive blood loss through the sheath — can be overcome by inserting a haemostatic valve into the butt of the sheath; if this is done it is doubly important to open the stopcock of the side-arm of the haemostatic valve to purge all air before inserting the bioptome.

4 If the arch of the aorta forms a tight curve it is possible that the stiff bioptome will not follow the sheath but will penetrate it. This, potentially dangerous, complication must be watched for — always use fluoroscopy to follow the passage of the bioptome through the sheath.

Left ventricular biopsy using the King's bioptome and long sheath technique can also be performed from a brachial arteriotomy.

Right ventricular endomyocardial biopsy is performed in similar fashion. The catheter and long sheath are introduced percutaneously into the femoral vein. The catheter is advanced to the apex of the right ventricle and the sheath advanced a little so that it too lies in the right ventricle. The catheter is then removed and the sheath purged of air and connected to the pressure transducer to check that a right ventricular pressure is still being recorded. The bioptome is advanced through the sheath and clockwise rotation of the bioptome and sheath should ensure that it is pointing towards the ventricular septum. This is most easily appreciated by

fluoroscopy in the left oblique projection; the bioptome should be directed inferiorly and *posteriorly*.

The bioptome is now advanced until the jaws are free of the sheath and can be opened; further advance will cause the open jaws to impinge against the septum. The jaws are closed and a firm tug on the bioptome should produce a biopsy sample.

Right ventricular biopsy using the Scholten bioptome [22, 23] from the internal jugular vein is described in the chapter devoted to the management of cardiac transplantation (Chapter 23). Left ventricular endomyocardial biopsy can be performed in children using the transseptal, long sheath technique [24]. The various techniques of endomyocardial biopsy have been reviewed by Mason [23].

Other 'long sheath' techniques

The ability to introduce a long sheath over a guiding catheter allows the introduction of special catheters, such as catheter-tip manometers or velocity probes, which are too rigid or too delicate to be manipulated into the heart in the usual way. A long sheath can also be used to overcome problems with tortuous and atheromatous iliac arteries. Following initial negotiation of the tortuous segment with the aid of a J-guide a long sheath can be left in place so that further catheter changes are guided through the sheath and the risk of subintimal dissection is minimised.

The umbilicus

There are two umbilical arteries and an umbilical vein. An umbilical artery is often catheterised, during the first week of life, for monitoring arterial pressure and blood gases. The umbilical vein can be cannulated for the first few days of life. Both routes have been used for diagnostic catheterisation though the technique has not found widespread acceptance.

The technique involves thorough cleaning of the umbilicus (sepsis is a potential complication) and the insertion of two stay sutures. The vessels are probed and thrombus extracted. A catheter inserted into the umbilical artery will pass caudally to the iliac artery and can then be advanced cephalad to the aortic arch where it may traverse the ductus and enter the pulmonary artery [26, 27].

If the umbilical vein is cannulated it may, in about half the attempts, be possible to traverse the ductus venosus and enter the inferior vena cava and right heart. Damage to hepatic structures is a possible complication.

REFERENCES

1 Dehmer GJ, Haagen D, Malloy CR, Schmitz JM. Anticoagulation with heparin during cardiac catheterisation and its reversal by protamine. *Cathet Cardiovasc Diagn* 1987;**13**:16.
2 Desilets DJ, Hoffman R. A new method of percutaneous catheterization. *Radiology* 1965;**85**:147.
3 Hillis LD. Percutaneous left heart catheterization and coronary arteriography using a femoral artery sheath. *Cathet Cardiovasc Diagn* 1979;**5**:393.
4 Seldinger SI. Catheter replacement of the needle in percutaneous arteriography, a new technique. *Acta Radiol* 1953;**39**:368.
5 Brock R, Milstein BB, Ross DN. Percutaneous left ventricular puncture in the assessment of aortic stenosis. *Thorax* 1956;**11**:163.
6 Semple T, McGuinness JB, Gardner H. Left heart catheterisation by direct left ventricular puncture, *Br Heart J* 1968;**30**:402.
7 Wong CM, Wong PHC, Miller GAH. Percutaneous left ventricular angiography. *Cathet Cardiovasc Diagn* 1981;**7**:425.
8 Wong PHC, Chow JSF, Chen WWC, Miller GAH, Aortic catheterisation via percutaneous left ventricular puncture. *Cathet Cardiovasc Diagn* 1983;**9**:421.
9 Brockenborough EC, Braunwald E. A new technique for left ventricular angiocardiography and transseptal left heart catheterization. *Am J Cardiol* 1960;**6**:1062.
10 Ross J. Transseptal left heart catheterization: a new method of left atrial puncture. *Ann Surg* 1959;**149**:395.
11 Ross J, Braunwald E, Morrow AG. Transseptal left atrial puncture: new technique for the measurement of left atrial pressure in man. *Am J Cardiol* 1959;**3**:653.
12 Lew AS *et al.* Recent experience with transseptal catheterization. *Cathet Cardiovasc Diagn* 1983;**9**:601.
13 Mullins CE. New catheter and technique for transseptal left heart catheterization in infants and children. *Circulation* 1979;(suppl II) **251**:59—60.
14 Chokshi DS, Hildner FJ. Subclavian vein catheterization: a reassessment. *Cathet Cardiovasc Diagn* 1976;**2**:1.
15 Belani KG, Buckley JJ, Gordon JR, Castaneda W. Percutaneous cervical central venous line placement; a comparison of the internal and external jugular vein routes. *Anesth Analg* 1980;**59**:40.
16 Rao TL, Wong AY, Salem MR. A new approach to percutaneous catheterization of the internal jugular vein (lateral approach). *Anaesthesiology* 1977;**46**:362.
17 Latson LA *et al.* Percutaneous cardiac catheterization via the internal jugular vein in infants and children. *Cathet Cardiovasc Diagn* 1986;**12**:198.
18 Sakakibara S, Konno S. Endomyocardial biopsy, *Jpn Heart J* 1962;**3**:537.
19 Richardson PJ. Kings endomyocardial bioptome. *Lancet* 1974;**1**:660.
20 Brooksby IAB, Swanton RH, Jenkins BS, Webb-Peploe MM. Long sheath technique for introduction of catheter tip manometer or endomyocardial bioptome into left or right heart. *Br Heart J* 1974;**36**:908.
21 Brooksby IAB *et al.* Left ventricular endomyocardial biopsy, 1. Description and evaluation of the technique. *Cathet Cardiovasc Diagn* 1977;**3**:115.
22 Caves PK, Stinson EB, Billingham ME, Shumway NE. Percutaneous transvenous endomyocardial biopsy in human heart recipients (experience with a new technique) *Ann Thorac Surg* 1973;**16**:325.
23 Mason JW. Techniques for right and left ventricular endomyocardial biopsy. *Am J Cardiol* 1978;**41**:887.
24 Rios B, Nihill MR, Mullins CE. Left ventricular endomyocardial biopsy in children with the transseptal long sheath technique. *Cathet Cardiovasc Diagn* 1984;**10**:417.
25 Bloomfield DA. Overcoming the problem of tortuous vessel negotiation. *Cathet Cardiovasc Diagn* 1984;**10**:303.
26 Linde LM *et al.* Umbilical vessel cardiac catheterization and angiocardiography. *Circulation* 1966;**34**:984.
27 Sapin SO, Linde LM, Emmanouilides GC. Umbilical vessel angiocardiography in the newborn infant. *Pediatrics* 1963;**31**:946.

CHAPTER 4

Techniques of catheterisation — catheter manipulation

Successful catheterisation depends on choosing the appropriate catheter, described in Chapter 2, and the appropriate approach, described in Chapter 3. This chapter will describe the ways in which 'conventional' catheters are manipulated within the heart in order to reach the desired site. Manipulations needed for catheterising cases of both acquired and congenital heart disease are described. 'Special' techniques such as transseptal catheterisation and transapical puncture have been described in Chapter 3; interventional techniques are described in Chapter 5 and the techniques of coronary arteriography in Chapter 13.

Some general principles apply to all catheter manipulation.

1 Most 'conventional' catheters have a gentle curve towards the tip; if the curve is pointing to the left then clockwise rotation of the hub will cause the catheter tip to point more posteriorly — and vice versa. If the tip points to the right, clockwise rotation has the opposite effect — the tip points more anteriorly. In practice this becomes automatic so that the experienced operator may not be conciously aware of the movements that he makes in order to advance the catheter. If there is doubt, changing to lateral fluoroscopy (if available) or rotating the tube/intensifier suspension to an oblique position will allow one to check that the desired anterior or posterior orientation has been achieved.

2 Movements of the catheter should be gentle but *positive*. A mark of the inexperienced operator is that the catheter position remains unchanged during prolonged fluoroscopy (and prolonged radiation exposure to both operator and patient). Catheters and guide wires should *never* be advanced against unexpected resistance.

3 The pressure waveform transmitted from the catheter tip should always be continuously displayed during catheter manipulation. In this way entry to a new chamber will be instantly recognisable. Errors such as advancing the catheter through the coronary sinus in mistake for the right ventricle will be avoided; in the former instance the position may suggest that the catheter is in the right ventricle but a low, 'atrial' pressure is displayed revealing the true situation.

4 Guide wires are often used to assist in advancing a catheter. Merely advancing the catheter over a guide wire is not always successful; the catheter forms a loop and the tip may actually retract as a result. Success with a guide wire often depends on simultaneously advancing the catheter while *withdrawing* the stiff part of the guide wire through it.

RIGHT HEART CATHETERISATION FROM THE ARM

The techniques that will be described under this heading are those that are needed to reach the superior and inferior vena cavae, the right atrium and ventricle and the pulmonary artery and pulmonary arterial 'wedge' positions.

Superior vena cava (SVC) and right atrium

As a rule entry to these sites poses no problems; the catheter is advanced from an arm vein (median cubital, basilic or axillary) and passes smoothly through the axillary and subclavian veins before turning caudally to reach the superior vena cava and right atrium. In the neonate, and occasionally in the adult, there may be difficulty in negotiating the sharp angle between the horizontally directed sub-clavian vein and the vertically directed SVC. This difficulty may be overcome (1) by 'heat-moulding' a sharper terminal curve on the catheter or by chang-ing the catheter to one with a sharper curve, (2) by asking the patient to inspire deeply as the catheter is advanced (or asking the anaesthetist to provide a deep inspiration), or (3) by advancing the catheter horizontally across the left innominate vein until it impinges against the junction with the left internal jugular vein when further advance may cause a down-wards loop to form at the right subclavian/SVC junction (Fig. 4.1). This loop can then be advanced into the right atrium taking the catheter tip into the atrium; if the tip of the catheter can be fixed against some part of the atrial wall withdrawing the catheter will now straighten the loop allowing catheterisation to proceed normally. Unfortunately this manoeuvre often fails as the catheter tip merely passes up the left internal jugular vein. (4) It may help if the patient's arm is extended above his head. (5) If an end-hole catheter is being used it may be possible to use a J-guide wire to negotiate the difficult angle and then to advance the catheter over the guide into the right atrium. (6) A balloon-tipped catheter can be used; inflation of the balloon at the subclavian/SVC junction may allow the bloodstream to carry it into the right atrium.

Heat moulding is achieved by placing the distal few centimetres in boiling water for a few seconds and then moulding the desired curve by hand before placing the catheter tip in cold water to fix the new curve. All these manoeuvres have a general appli-cation and may be used in any situation where access is difficult.

Entering the inferior vena cava (IVC)

The key to entering the IVC from the arm is to avoid the formation of a loop. This happens when the catheter tip impinges against the floor of the right atrium; the catheter must be withdrawn and re-advanced without allowing such a loop to form. The inferior (and superior) cava enter the *posterior* aspect of the right atrium. Often an oblique course of the catheter below the diaphragm indicates entry to an hepatic vein; again a slight withdrawal and rotation followed by re-advancing the catheter will allow entry to the IVC.

Entering the right ventricle: traversing the tricuspid valve (Fig. 4.2)

This is the key manoeuvre in right heart catheter-isation. The technique is as follows: (1) Rotate the catheter so that its tip points laterally within the right atrium. (2) Advance the catheter so that its tip impinges the lateral wall of the right atrium and a loop is formed. (3) Rotate the catheter through 180° so that the distal limb of the loop lies against the interatrial septum with the tip superior to the opening of the tricuspid valve. (4) *Slowly* withdraw the cath-eter a centimetre or so until the catheter tip comes level with the tricuspid orifice when the tip will suddenly move to the left as it traverses the valve and enters the right ventricle. If the manoeuvre is carried out in this way the catheter tip will be pointing towards the outflow tract of the right ventricle and further advance will result in the catheter entering the pulmonary artery. It is possible to enter the right ventricle simply by advancing a catheter whose tip is pointing inferiorly and medially but the catheter tip will then be in the apex of the right ventricle. This position is desirable for pacemaker wire inser-tion but it is not possible to enter the pulmonary artery from this position.

Problems which may be encountered with this manoeuvre are: (1) it may be difficult to engage the tip of the catheter against the wall of the atrium — especially when the atrium is dilated, (2) if there is tricuspid regurgitation, the catheter tip may not stay in the ventricle long enough for it to be advanced to the pulmonary artery, and (3) if there is a dilated coronary sinus (as occurs when a left SVC drains to coronary sinus) the catheter will persist in entering this channel rather than the tricuspid valve. The solution to the first of these problems is to realise that the vital loop formation can be achieved provided that the catheter tip can be persuaded to impinge against the myocardium *somewhere* — anywhere — it does not have to be the lateral wall of the atrium. The problem of tricuspid regurgitation may be overcome by selecting a larger (and, therefore, stiffer) catheter or by stiffening the catheter by in-serting a guide wire, flexible end first, to within a few centimetres of the catheter tip. A balloon catheter is unlikely to provide the answer, useful though it can be in most other difficult situations. When the catheter persists in entering the coronary sinus the operator should remember that the opening of the

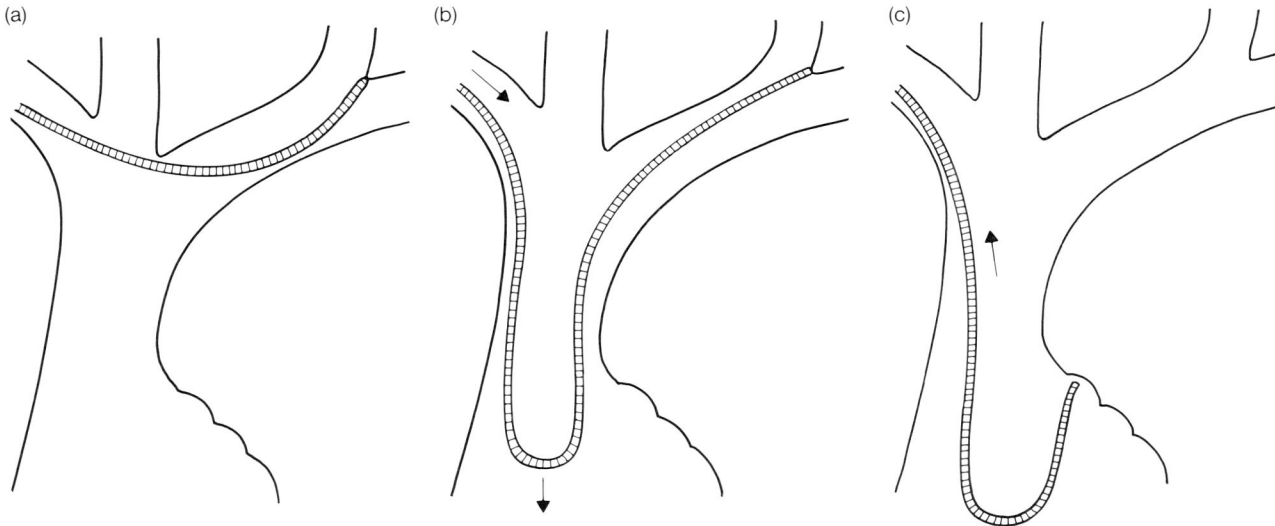

Fig. 4.1 The 'reverse loop' technique for difficult entry to the SVC. (a) Abut the catheter against the left innominate/internal jugular or subclavian junction. (b) Advance the catheter so that it forms a downward loop in SVC. (c) Straighten the loop after it has entered the right atrium by abutting the tip against the atrial wall and withdrawing the catheter (a guide wire may be needed to help remove the loop).

coronary sinus is *posterior* to the tricuspid orifice. Attempts should be made to rotate the catheter tip to a more anterior position before allowing it to move inferiorly and engage the tricuspid valve.

Pulmonary artery and 'wedge'

Provided that the catheter has crossed the tricuspid valve as described above, so that the tip is pointing towards the outflow tract, onward advance to the pulmonary artery should be a simple matter. Problems arise when the catheter tip is pointing towards the apex or lies *medially* within the ventricle. The pulmonary artery arises to the *left* of the aorta; a medial position of the catheter tip often means that it is entangled in the subvalve apparatus of the tricuspid valve. In this case the catheter should be withdrawn to the right atrium and the 'loop and rotate' manoeuvre repeated so as to recross the tricuspid valve finishing with a leftward and superior direction of the catheter tip.

The pulmonary artery 'wedge' position is obtained by further advancing the catheter out into the lung fields until it will go no further and the pressure trace changes from an arterial to an atrial waveform. The distal few centimetres of the catheter are often seen to become somewhat straightened at this time.

Confirmation that the wedge position has been obtained may sometimes be gained by sampling fully saturated blood but this is not always possible; nor is it often needed. Obtaining a good 'wedge' may be difficult when (1) there is pulmonary vascular disease, or (2) when there is a dilated right atrium allowing the catheter to loop in the atrium instead of advancing to a distal pulmonary artery. The use of a guide wire to stiffen the catheter or a larger and stiffer catheter may overcome these problems. It is often helpful to get the patient to take a deep inspiration while advancing the catheter to the wedge position. If all else fails a balloon catheter of the Swan−Ganz type will usually provide the solution; the balloon *must* be inflated *before* allowing it to pass outward to the wedge position. Inflation of the balloon while in a small pulmonary artery can lead to rupture of the artery and fatal intrapulmonary haemorrhage has occurred as a result [1, 2]. The balloon should not remain inflated in the wedge position for more than a minute or so.

RIGHT HEART CATHETERISATION FROM THE ARM IN CONGENITAL HEART DISEASE

It is impossible to cover all situations that may be

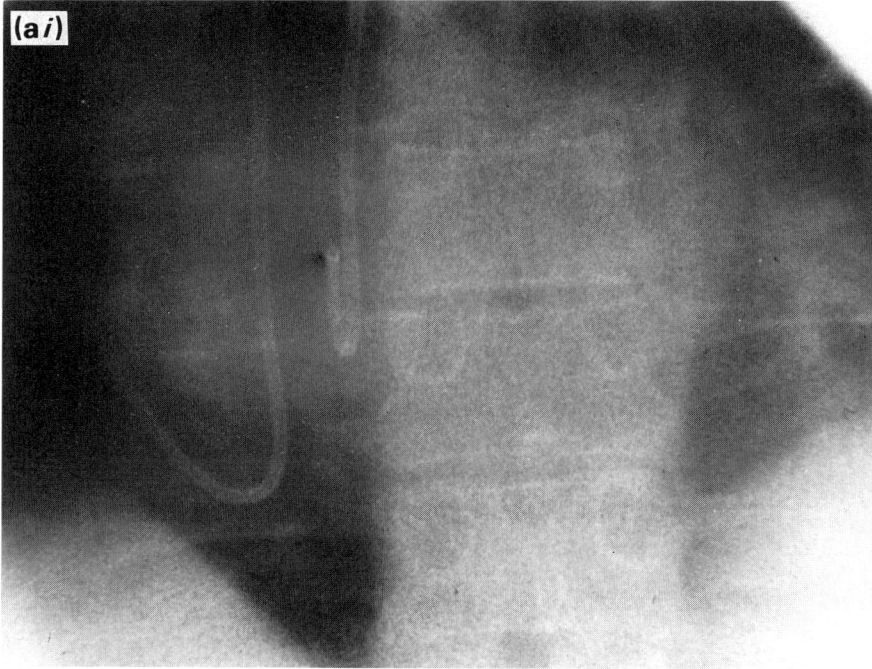

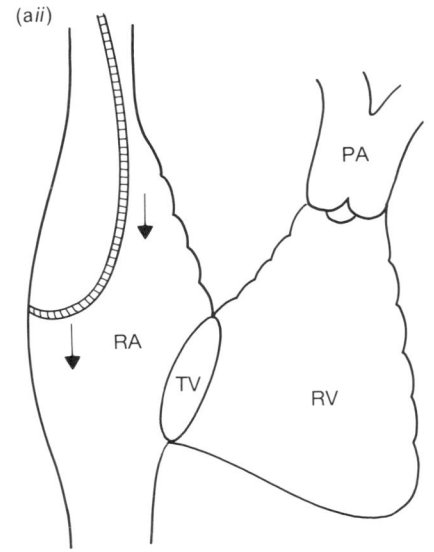

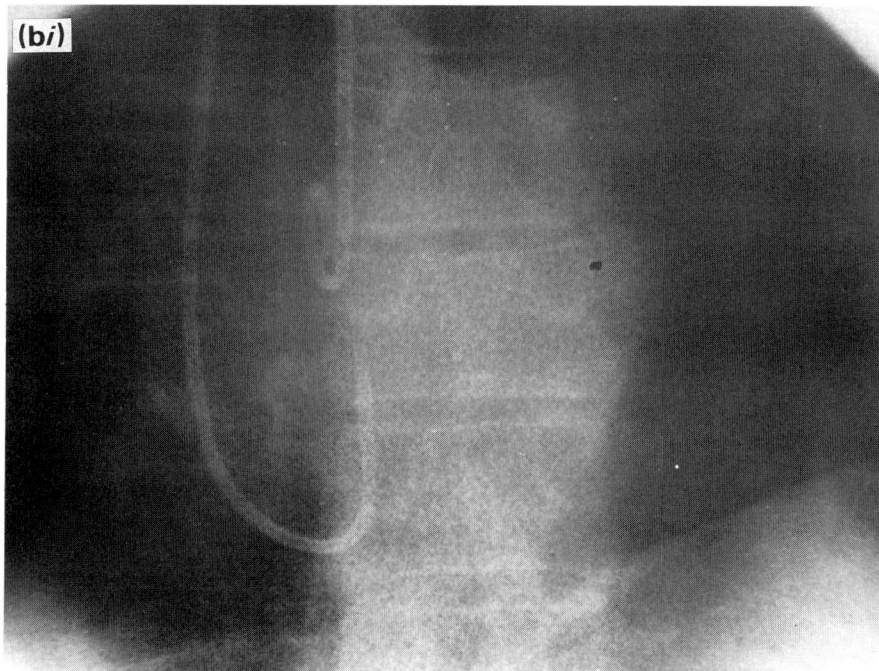

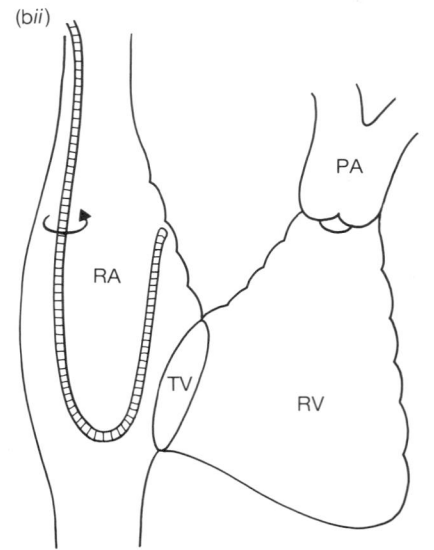

(ci)

(cii)

(d)

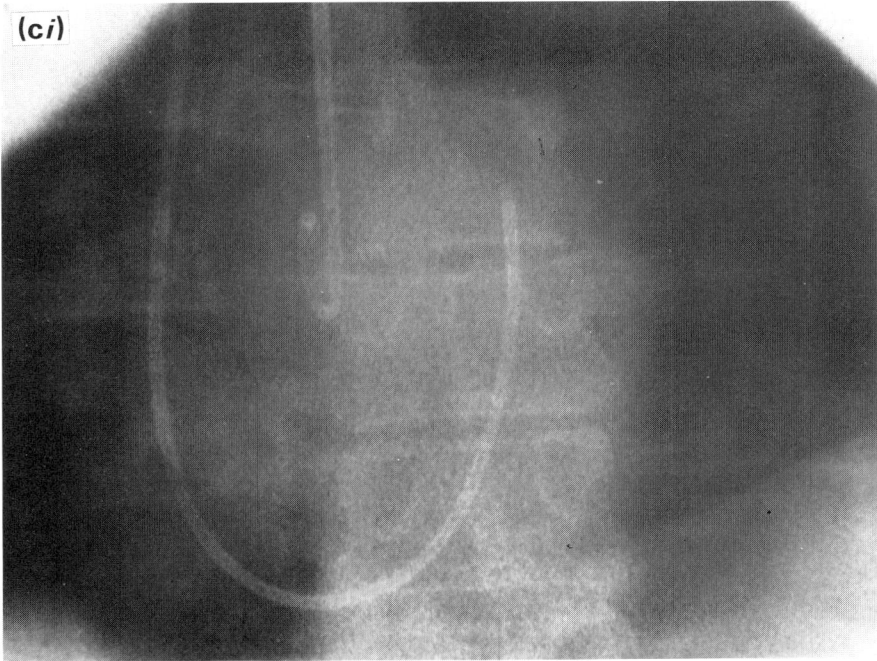

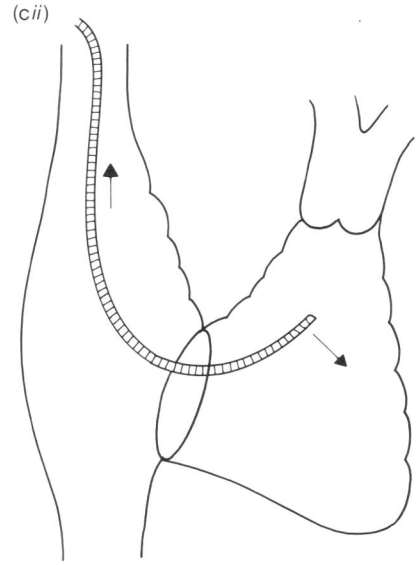

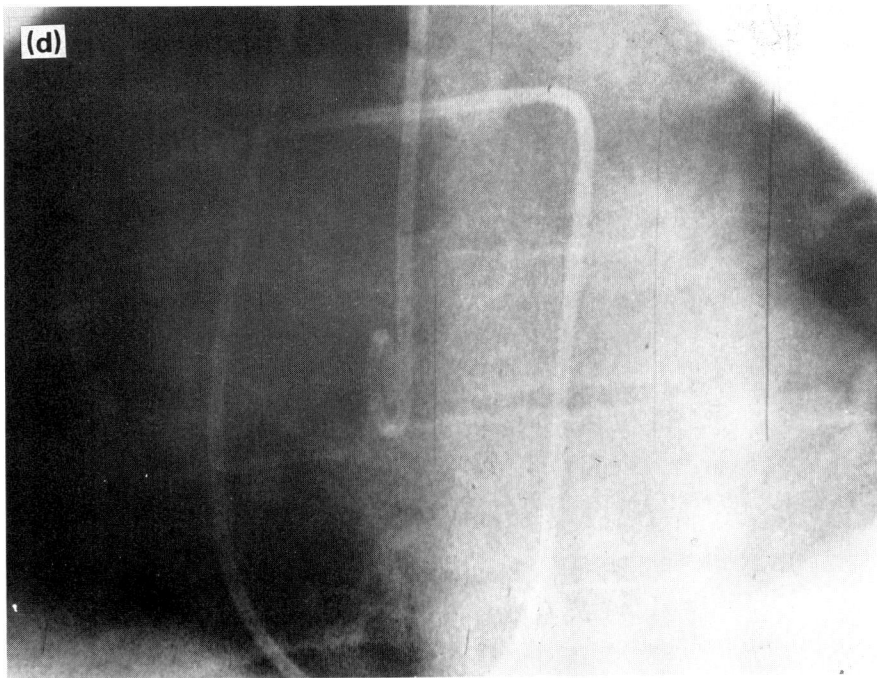

Fig. 4.2 Entering the right ventricle (and pulmonary artery) from the right atrium. (ai and ii) Abut catheter against lateral wall of right atrium to form a loop. (bi and ii) Rotate the loop so that the loop is directed medially with the catheter tip against the interatrial septum. (ci and ii) Withdraw the catheter so that the tip travels down the atrial septum and then 'flips' through the tricuspid valve pointing towards the right ventricular outflow tract. (d) Finally advance the catheter to enter the right and left pulmonary artery.

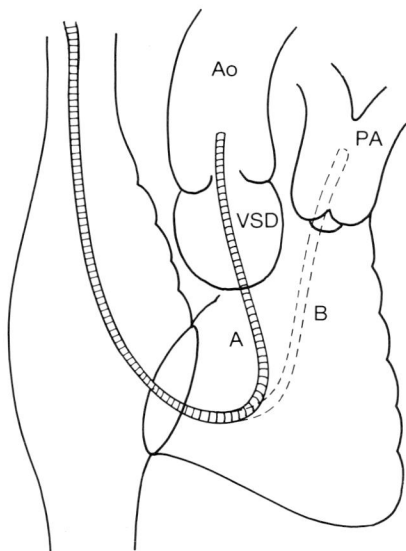

Fig. 4.3 Entry to aorta via VSD (e.g. tetralogy of Fallot) — the catheter must be kept in a *medial* position. If allowed to move to the left (laterally) as in position B, it may be possible to enter the pulmonary artery.

met with but some common abnormalities can be described as they may modify the above manoeuvres.

Entry to aorta via a ventricular septal defect (VSD) or when the aorta arises from the right ventricle. When the aortic valve lies to the right of the pulmonary valve (the usual situation) it is often possible to enter it from the right ventricle by crossing a VSD *provided* the catheter tip is kept in a medial position (Fig. 4.3) within the ventricle while being advanced towards the outflow tract — the reverse of the usual lateral position needed to enter the pulmonary artery. This manoeuvre is particularly likely to be successful when there is an overriding aorta, as in the tetralogy of Fallot. It will also be successful when the aorta arises from the right ventricle (e.g. in transposition, double outlet right ventricle).

Crossing a ventricular septal defect. If the aorta has been entered as described above it is often possible to manipulate the catheter into the left ventricle. While screening in the lateral or left oblique projection (so that anterior and posterior directions can be appreciated — they cannot with anteroposterior screening) the catheter is *slowly* withdrawn from the aorta until the moment at which the pressure changes

to a ventricular waveform. At this moment an attempt should be made to point the catheter tip posteriorly and advance it to the left ventricle (Fig. 4.4).

Entering the pulmonary artery in tetralogy and pulmonary stenosis. In tetralogy of Fallot the catheter often enters the aorta (as described above); if the catheter is withdrawn to the right ventricle and allowed to move to the left it may now be possible to advance it to the pulmonary artery (Fig. 4.3). Caution is needed when attempting pulmonary artery catheterisation in tetralogy as there is a danger of provoking infundibular 'shut-down'. Propranolol (0.1 mg/kg) may be given prophylactically in tetralogy to guard against infundibular shut-down. The catheter should not be left in the pulmonary artery any longer than is necessary to obtain the desired information since its presence may compromise flow through the narrow outflow tract.

In pulmonary valve stenosis the use of a guide wire may help in traversing the valve.

Entering the pulmonary artery in 'corrected transposition'. 'Corrected transposition' is a convenient term to describe the combination of atrioventricular and ventriculo-arterial discordance in which the aorta usually arises to the *left* of the pulmonary artery. Entering the pulmonary artery in this situation can be difficult (1) because the catheter tip must be kept in a *medial* position within the right ventricle in order to be directed towards the medially placed pulmonary artery, and (2) because the pulmonary valve arises more posteriorly than usual and there is a blind-ending 'pouch' of the outflow tract of the venous ventricle (morphologic *left* ventricle). The simplest answer to these problems is to use a balloon-tipped catheter.

Crossing a patent arterial duct. In all but a small minority of cases the duct communicates with the *left* pulmonary artery. To cross a duct it is therefore necessary to direct the catheter tip superiorly, posteriorly and to the left (i.e. towards the left pulmonary artery) when it will cross the duct and enter the descending aorta. Success is signalled by a change from pulmonary artery to aortic pressure and by the fact that the catheter can be advanced to below the diaphragm as it traverses the descending aorta. When the duct is small it may only be possible to cross it with a small (no. 5 or 6F) catheter and on occasion a

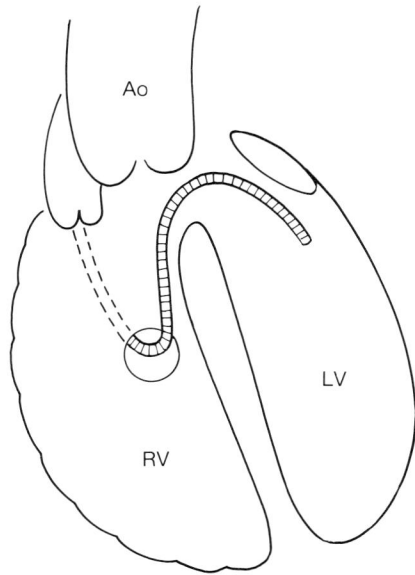

Fig. 4.4 Left oblique projection. Crossing the VSD to enter the left ventricle. If the catheter is slowly withdrawn from the aorta (Fig. 4.3) and pointed posteriorly as soon as the ventricular pressure is recorded, it may be possible to enter the left ventricle.

guide wire will be needed to assist in the manoeuvre. If a guide wire is used it should not be advanced beyond the catheter tip until the catheter has been directed towards the opening of the duct at the junction between the main and left pulmonary artery.

Aortopulmonary septal defect ('window') is a rare anomaly; from the point of view of catheter manipulation it is distinguished from a patent duct by the fact that the catheter crossing the defect from the pulmonary artery will enter the *ascending* aorta and not the descending thoracic aorta as it does when a duct is crossed.

Crossing an atrial septal defect (ASD). This is a difficult manoeuvre to perform when catheterisation is performed from the arm (and very easy when performed from the leg). Perhaps the best hope lies in forming the usual loop with the distal arm of the loop positioned high on the interatrial septum and orientated posteriorly and to the left. As the catheter is withdrawn the tip may move to the left while an atrial pressure is still being recorded — indicating that the tip of the catheter is now in the left atrium. Frequently, however, the catheter will only enter the right ventricle during this manoeuvre. An alternative is to direct the catheter tip to the left and inferiorly

in the hope that it will cross the defect instead of entering the apex of the right ventricle. In *atrioventricular defects* (septum primum ASD, AV canal) the problem is not that the catheter will not enter the left atrium but that it immediately enters the left ventricle and it may be difficult to manipulate the catheter to the right ventricle and pulmonary artery; a balloon-tipped catheter may be needed.

RIGHT HEART CATHETERISATION FROM THE LEG (Fig. 4.5)

When the femoral or saphenous veins are used for right heart catheterisation it will be found that entry to the right ventricle and pulmonary artery are slightly more difficult than when the approach is from the arm but that it is easy to cross an atrial septal defect or patent foramen ovale.

The cavae and right ventricle. There is seldom any difficulty in traversing the IVC to reach the right atrium though the catheter tip may engage in renal or hepatic veins as it is advanced. Any resistance to its smooth passage is an indication for fluoroscopy and slight withdrawal and re-orientation of the catheter tip. When the catheter tip is in the right atrium and pointing to the right, counter-clockwise rotation will cause the tip to point posteriorly and further advance will cause it to enter the SVC. Clockwise rotation would cause the tip to sweep anteriorly and become trapped in the right atrial appendage. Entry to the SVC is largely a matter of avoiding the catheter tip impinging against the atrial wall and forming a loop. It is precisely this manoeuvre, however, which is the key to entering the right ventricle. The loop which will form against the lateral wall of the atrium is, of course, the reverse of that formed when the approach is from the arm; the loop is convex *above*. Clockwise rotation causes the tip to sweep anteriorly and come to point medially and *inferiorly*. At this point the tip of the catheter should move to the left as it traverses the tricuspid valve and enters the right ventricle.

Pulmonary artery. Entering the pulmonary artery from the right ventricle is the difficult part of right heart catheterisation from the leg. Having entered the right ventricle, as described above, the catheter tip will be directed inferiorly and to the left; further clockwise

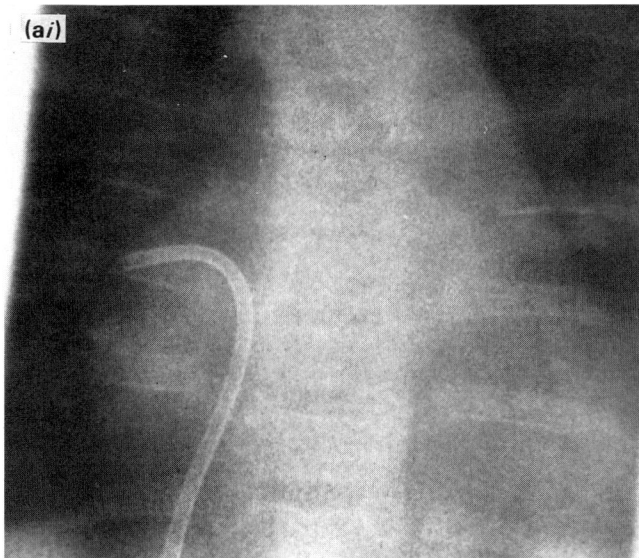
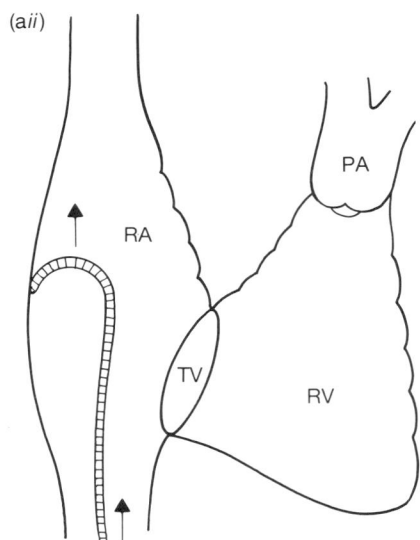

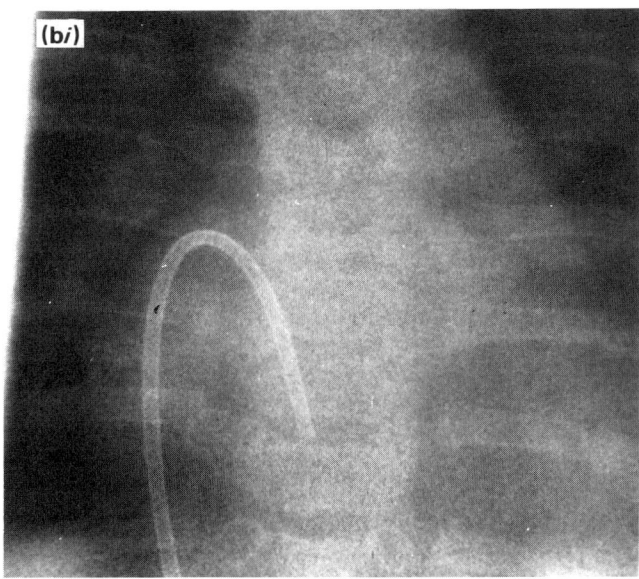
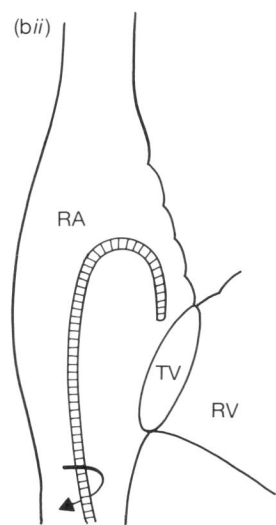

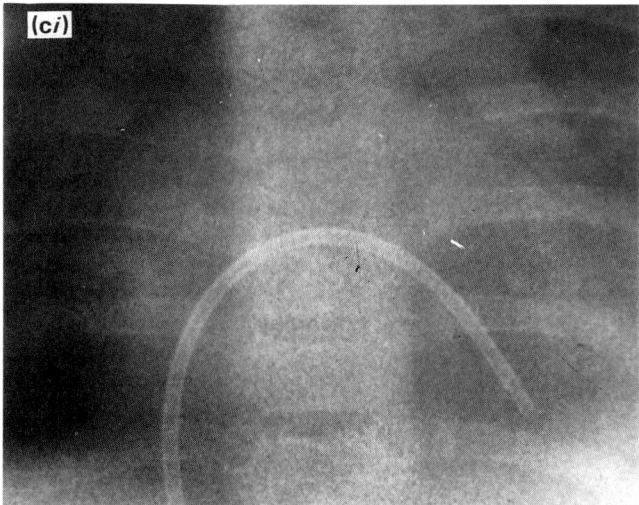
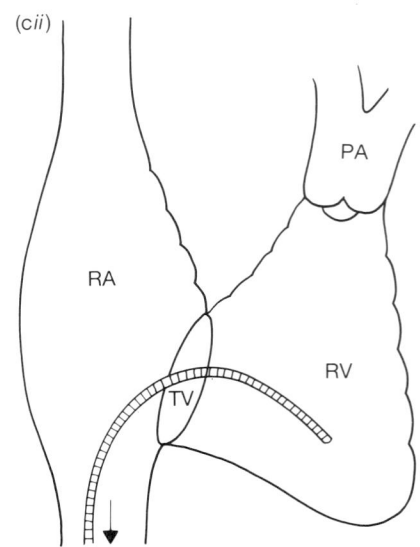

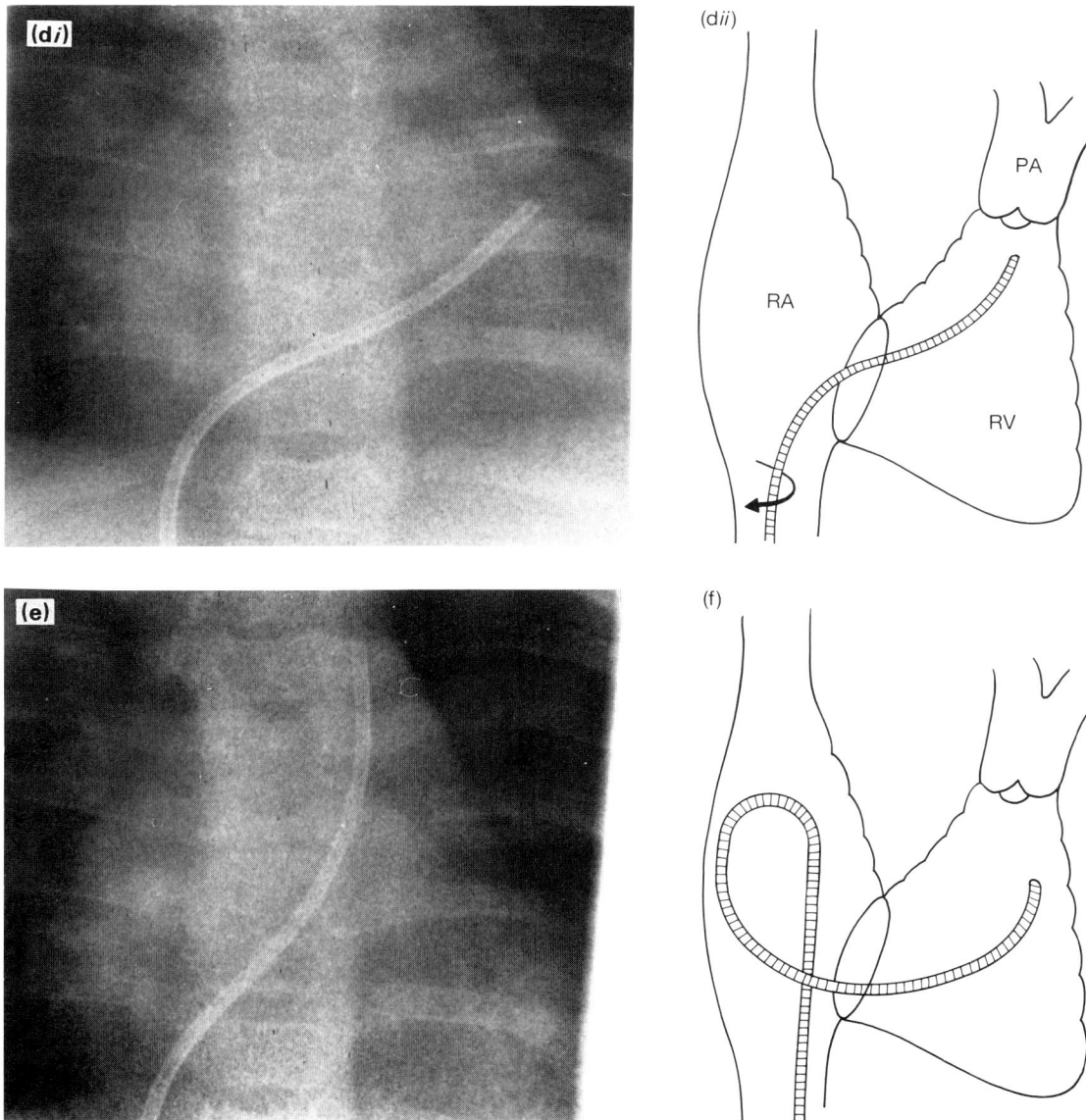

Fig. 4.5 Entering the right ventricle and pulmonary artery when the approach is from the leg. (a*i* and *ii*) Form a loop by abutting the catheter tip against the atrial wall. (b*i* and *ii*) Rotate the loop clockwise (or anti-clockwise) until it points medially. (c*i* and *ii*) Withdraw the catheter (slightly) until the tip enters the right ventricle. (d*i* and *ii*) *Slowly* rotate the catheter *clockwise* to coax the catheter tip to point towards the outflow tract. (e) Finally advance the catheter to the pulmonary artery. (f) An alternative, 'reverse-loop' technique which aims the catheter tip towards the outflow tract.

rotation should cause the tip to point superiorly (and to the left). It is often quite difficult to hold this position so as to advance the catheter further and enter the pulmonary artery. If a pulmonary arterioiogram is all that is required the preshaped 'Grollman' pigtail catheter will be found to traverse the right ventricle with ease [3]. If a wedge pressure is sought then an end-hole catheter must used; guide wires or a balloon catheter may be needed in difficult cases.

RIGHT HEART CATHETERISATION FROM THE LEG IN CONGENITAL HEART DISEASE

Entering the left atrium and ventricle (Fig. 4.6)

The ease with which an ASD or foramen ovale can be crossed to allow access to the left heart is the reason why this approach is usually the preferred one in cases of congenital heart disease. The catheter tip is directed medially (to the left) superiorly and *posteriorly* when further advance will result in it crossing the interatrial septum to reach the left atrium. Further advance will cause the catheter to enter left sided pulmonary veins; rotating the catheter in a clockwise fashion until the tip points to the right will allow entry to the right sided pulmonary veins. Difficulty arises when attempting to traverse the mitral valve to gain entry to the left ventricle. The gentle curve of the catheter, which is ideal for crossing the atrial septum, tends to lead the tip of the catheter into the left atrial appendage. What is needed now is a much sharper curve which will direct the catheter tip *inferiorly*. This is recognised in the technique of transseptal puncture in which the Brockenbrough needle maintains a gentle curve for septal puncture but the catheter has a much sharper inbuilt curve which it adopts as soon as the needle is removed. Success with a conventional catheter is achieved if the operator remembers (1) that the mitral valve is relatively medial within the cardiac silhouette, and (2) that the catheter tip must be rotated *anteriorly* (counter-clockwise rotation) in order to cross the mitral valve. Often an inexperienced operator persists in trying to cross the mitral valve with the catheter tip in too lateral a position so that it never becomes free of the left atrial appendage. If there is persisting

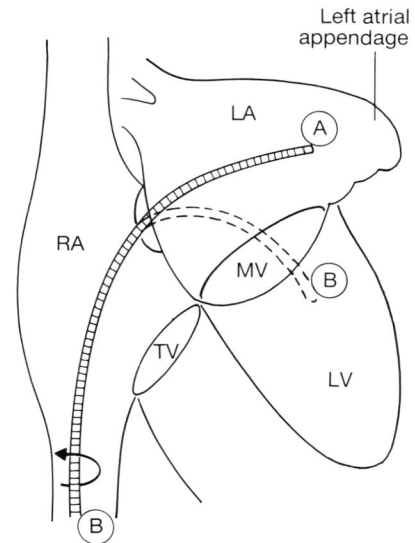

Fig. 4.6 (A) The position adopted by a catheter which has crossed an ASD or foramen ovale. (B) The mitral valve lies *medially* and a sharp anterior , downward turn of the catheter is needed to transverse the mitral valve and enter the ventricle. This will require an anti-clockwise rotation to bring the catheter tip anteriorly.

difficulty in crossing the mitral valve then heat-moulding a sharper curve, changing the catheter to one with a sharper curve or forming a loop in the left atrium to encourage it to adopt (temporarily) a sharper curve are all manoeuvres that have to be tried. Alternatively a balloon-tipped (angiographic) catheter can be used. Whatever happens the operator must not persist in advancing a catheter which is in the left atrial appendage; perforation of the appendage will be the only result.

Azygos continuation of the IVC

This anomaly occurs most commonly in association with laevo-isomerism but can occur in other examples of congenital heart disease. When present, right heart catheterisation from the leg can be difficult or impossible; a balloon catheter may be needed in order to reach the right ventricle and pulmonary artery. The operator should be alerted when the catheter, apparently lying in the right atrium, adopts a straight course and cannot be made to form a loop. A small injection of contrast medium will show the catheter lying in an azygos vein which courses superiorly to join the SVC.

LEFT HEART CATHETERISATION FROM THE ARM

Under this heading will be described the manipulations that are needed to enter ascending and descending aorta, the left ventricle, the left atrium and major branches and collaterals arising from the aorta. The techniques of coronary artery catheterisation are described in Chapter 13.

Ascending and descending aorta

There is seldom any difficulty in reaching the aortic arch from a retrograde arterial approach from the arm (branchial or axillary arteries). Sometimes the catheter will enter branches of the subclavian and axillary arteries around the shoulder girdle; since the catheter should be advanced under fluoroscopic control this should be appreciated and the catheter withdrawn and redirected.

Difficulty may also be experienced in traversing the junction between the subclavian and innominate arteries. This is a 'danger point' at which intimal dissection can occur during attempts to advance the catheter; the use of a J-guide wire or a pigtail catheter is indicated if there is any difficulty at this point. The combination of a pigtail catheter and guide wire is a very good one for traversing difficult angles or tortuous vessels. By allowing the tip of the catheter to adopt part of its inbuilt curve and by alternating the lead between catheter and guide wire most awkward bends can be negotiated safely. The last point of potential difficulty is at the aortic arch where a 'late take-off' of the subclavian artery may lead the catheter across the aortic arch and into the descending, rather than the ascending, aorta. Manipulation here is aided by using a left oblique projection so that the difference between a posterior course and the desired anterior one can be appreciated. Again the use of guide wires may help, as may a deep inspiration from the patient. On occasion, origin of the right subclavian from the descending aorta will frustrate all attempts to reach the left ventricle from the arm. This anomaly is not infrequent in infants and children with congenital heart disease but is very rare in adults with acquired heart disease.

Crossing the aortic valve: retrograde catheterisation of the left ventricle

There is seldom any difficulty in traversing a normal aortic valve; problems arise when the valve is stenosed and even minor degrees of aortic stenosis can make this a difficult manoeuvre. If a pigtail catheter is used it is usually sufficient merely to advance the catheter against the valve when it will enter the left ventricle without further effort. If this does not happen there are three steps that may be tried. (1) Advance the catheter so that it begins to form a loop above the valve, as the catheter is then withdrawn the end of the catheter may straighten and cross the valve (Fig. 4.7). (2) Make repeated advances of the catheter with different degrees of rotation resulting in different orientations of the curled end of the catheter in relation to the valve orifice. (3) Try the effect of a guide wire either to alter the curve of the catheter or to lead the catheter through the valve. Pigtail catheters are available with a 145 and 155° angulation of the distal 7 cm to aid in crossing the aortic valve in patients with aortic stenosis and a dilated aortic root. While more likely to succeed than the conventional, straight, variety no pigtail catheter is as suitable for crossing a 'difficult' valve as are ones without the curled pigtail-tip.

It is helpful to remember that normal aortic valve cusps are so widely open in systole that there is an uninterrupted channel into the left ventricle with the sinuses of Valsalva hidden away behind the open cusps. As a result success is dependent on the forward movement of the catheter coinciding with ventricular systole and is not the result of skilful direction of the catheter. Conversely, failure is due to having engaged the sinus of Valsalva by advancing the catheter during diastole. It is not suggested that deliberate timing of the catheter movement is necessary (if the valve is normal) but that the operator must withdraw the catheter fully so as to disengage from the sinus before re-advancing it for another attempt at crossing the valve. This is not the case when there is aortic stenosis and success here *does* depend on directing the catheter towards the valve orifice and timing the advance to coincide with ventricular systole. The secret of crossing a stenotic aortic valve is to be able to direct the catheter tip towards the orifice; as a rule this means that the catheter has to be directed away from the right sinus of Valsalva and towards the left. A plethora of

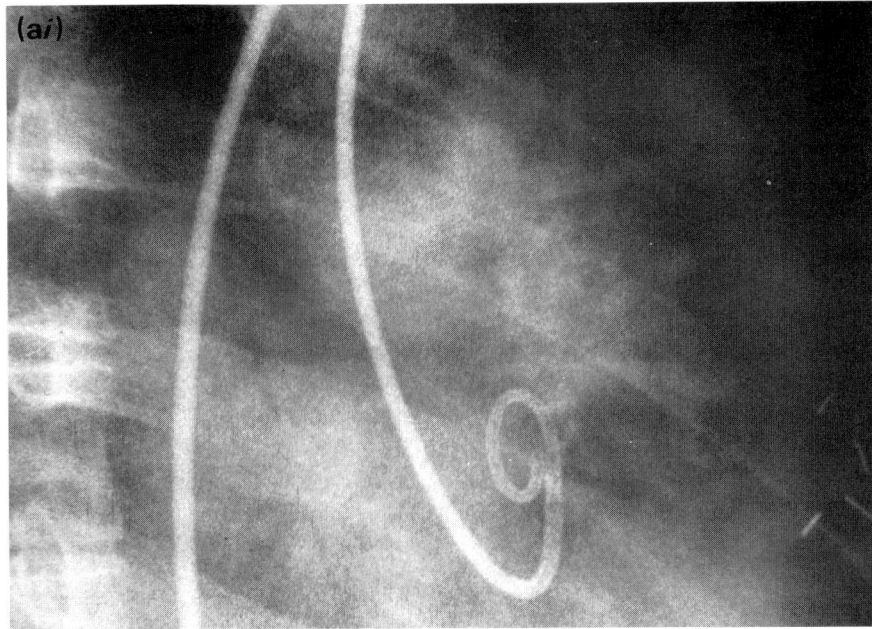

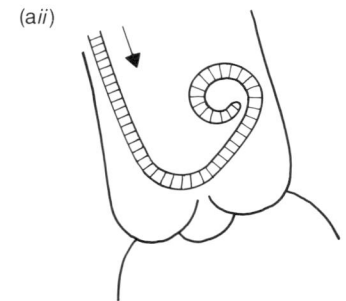

Fig. 4.7 Crossing the aortic valve retrogradely with a pigtail catheter. (a*i* and *ii*) Advance the catheter until it straddles the valve.

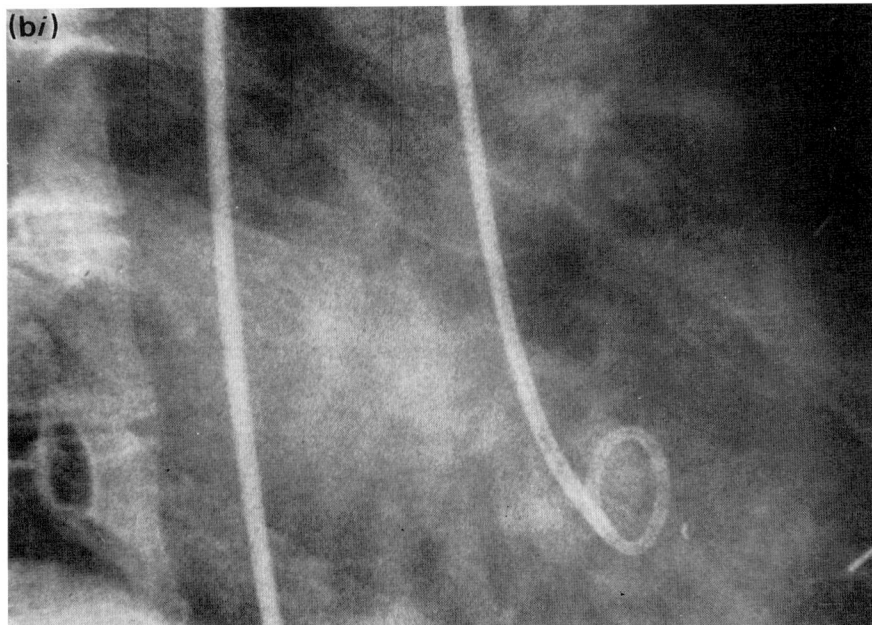

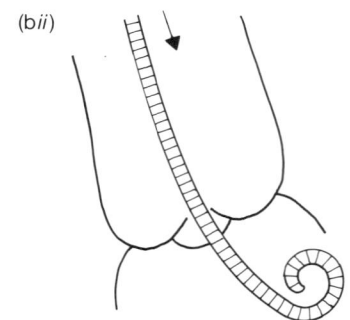

(b*i* and *ii*) Slowly withdraw the catheter — as the tip crosses the valve it may prolapse into the left ventricle.

reports describing a 'new' method of crossing stenotic aortic valves (particularly when the approach is from the leg) attest to the difficulty of this manoeuvre [4–7]. Almost without exception it will be found that the method advocated involves the use of a catheter with good torque control (e.g. 'positrol', 'torque control' incorporating a wire mesh) or using a catheter with an inbuilt distal curve that will direct the tip, or a guide wire, towards the left and allow the whole plane of the valve to be explored. Thus a right Judkins or a Castillo coronary catheter can be used to direct a guide wire to the left. The combination of a pigtail catheter and guide wire allows different angulations of the emerging guide; a short protruding length allows the curved tip of the catheter to direct the wire to the left, more protrusion of the wire straightens the curve and directs the wire more towards the right. Catheters such as torque control versions of the Sones, Multipurpose or Gensini are particularly suitable for crossing stenotic aortic valves. The various techniques that have been used for crossing stenotic aortic valves have been reviewed by Laskey [8].

The valve orifice may be eccentric; the problem here is to identify its position. It may be found by trial and error but the position of a powerful jet emerging from the orifice is often helpful. The catheter tip will be seen (and often felt) to vibrate when it is in this jet and attempts should be made to advance the catheter while maintaining the tip in this jet. Loss of vibration indicates that the catheter tip is no longer in line with the valve orifice. A small injection of contrast medium can be used to display the position of the valve orifice. Alternatively attempts at crossing the valve can be abandoned until aortography has been performed; review of the video record will reveal the position of the valve orifice and provide a map for subsequent attempts to cross the valve.

When the purpose of the study includes coronary arteriography it is sensible to abandon abortive attempts to cross the valve and proceed with coronary arteriography. There is a chance that the catheter will enter the ventricle during manipulation for coronary cannulation; the operator can then take both the advantage and the credit! Thus the Castillo catheter can be used to direct a guide wire through the valve; an 'exchange' guide must then be used to change to a catheter which is suitable for ventriculography (e.g. pigtail).

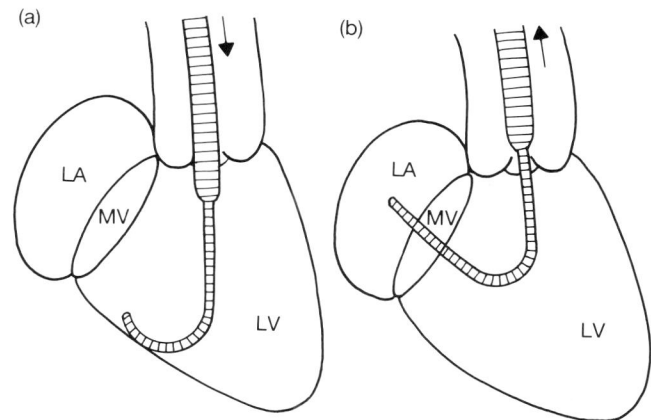

Fig. 4.8 Retrograde catheterisation of the left atrium using a Shirey catheter. (a) Form a posteriorly directed loop in the left ventricle. (b) (Right oblique projection.) Withdraw the catheter with the tip pointed superiorly and to the right until it crosses the mitral valve.

Most investigators base their estimate of the severity of aortic stenosis on the gradient obtained as the catheter is withdrawn from the ventricle to the aorta. If simultaneous records of ventricular and systemic pressure are demanded the alternatives are to use two arterial catheters inserted from different sites, to use femoral pressure recorded from the side-arm of a valved introducing sheath (after 'calibrating' for phase shift and peripheral amplification) or to use a double-lumen catheter. A double-lumen pigtail catheter which permits ventriculography and simultaneous recording of left ventricular and aortic pressures has been described [9].

Retrograde left atrial catheterisation (Fig. 4.8)

This manoeuvre is accomplished using a 'Shirey' catheter which has a long, flexible, tip (no. 5F). A right oblique projection is used for fluoroscopy since it profiles the mitral orifice and makes it easy to distinguish between the rightward and superior position of the left atrium and the leftward and inferior position of the ventricle. A loop is formed within the ventricle so that the flexible tip of the catheter is directed towards the mitral orifice. Entry to the left atrium is achieved either by further advance of the catheter or by withdrawing the catheter so as to pull the upward-pointing tip into the left atrium. Ventricular ectopic beats are to be expected during the formation of the loop but the soft and flexible tip makes this a safe technique deserving of wider application [10].

LEFT HEART CATHETERISATION FROM THE ARM IN CONGENITAL HEART DISEASE

In most cases of congenital heart disease a transvenous approach will provide all the required information since entry to the left heart is often achieved via septal defects or a foramen ovale. It follows that when a retrograde arterial approach is needed it is to solve specific problems or needs. The most obvious of these is when a transvenous approach has *not* allowed access to the left heart or aorta. Other situations which may demand a retrograde arterial approach include: (1) the need for an aortogram in instances of aortopulmonary communications (persistent ductus, aortopulmonary window, persistent arterial trunk, aortopulmonary collaterals and shunts). (2) Aortic anomalies when the aorta has not been reached (or cannot be reached) transvenously (coarctation, aortic atresia, aortic interruption, ruptured sinus of Valsalva, aortic insufficiency). (3) To record aortic valve, subvalve and supravalve gradients. (4) To obtain a coronary arteriogram (anomalous origin of left coronary from the pulmonary artery or anomalous origin of the left or arterior descending branch from the right coronary in tetralogy of Fallot). (5) To obtain a ventriculogram when the chamber (left, right or outflow chamber) cannot be reached transvenously.

Much of what has been discussed in relation to a retrograde arterial approach in acquired heart disease applies equally when the approach is used in congenital heart disease. Crossing a stenotic aortic valve is often surprisingly easy in neonates and infants — perhaps because the small diameter of the aorta relative to the catheter helps to guide the catheter tip to the centre of the stenosed valve. In aortic atresia the minute lumen of the ascending aorta may be occluded by the catheter and bradycardia results as coronary flow ceases — the catheter must be withdrawn to the aortic arch. The same complication can occur when a catheter crosses the duct in aortic atresia since all systemic and coronary flow is duct-dependent in this condition [11].

Coronary arteriography is seldom required in neonates and preshaped catheters of a suitably small size are not available; however the coronaries can often be cannulated using a no. 5F catheter of the Goodale—Lubin type. Indeed it is common for such catheters to enter the coronaries during attempts to cross the aortic valve; the operator should be aware of this possibility since the position adopted by the catheter resembles that adopted when it is in the left ventricle — and a large injection of contrast medium would be fatal.

Retrograde arterial catheterisation from the arm may be needed for selective cannulation of systemic-to-pulmonary collaterals which cannot be entered from the leg; the catheter will have to be manipulated across the aortic arch so as to enter the descending thoracic aorta.

Retrograde arterial catheterisation may allow access to the right heart — as when it crosses a VSD — the salvation of many a study in patients with no remaining venous access!

Finally, an alternative to retrograde arterial catheterisation in neonates and infants is to use a flow-directed (Swan—Ganz or Berman) angiographic catheter which has been introduced transvenously. After the catheter has crossed the atrial septum inflation of the balloon (using carbon dioxide) will allow the catheter to be carried through the left ventricle and into the aorta [12]. Similarly the aorta may be reached from the right ventricle in conditions with abnormal ventriculo-arterial connection (discordant or double outlet).

LEFT HEART CATHETERISATION FROM THE LEG

There is little to add to what has been discussed in regard to the retrograde arterial approach from the arm. Tortuous and atheromatous iliac arteries can cause problems and a J-guide should be used if there is the slightest difficulty in traversing these vessels. Intimal dissections are easily created and retroperitoneal haematoma is a possible complication. When such tortuous vessels have been traversed and subsequent catheter changes are anticipated (e.g. for coronary arteriography) a long sheath can be passed over an exchange guide wire and this long sheath used to guide subsequent catheters safely past the tortuosities and atheromatous plaques [13]. The technique of crossing the aortic valve is much the same as when the approach is from the arm but the operator has much less control over the position of the catheter tip. For this reason it is advisable to use an approach from the arm when a stenotic aortic valve has to be crossed. Techniques for crossing stenotic aortic valves when the approach is from the leg have been referred to already [4−8].

The retrograde transfemoral approach is used for cannulating aortopulmonary collaterals, bronchial arteries and systemic-to-pulmonary shunts of the Blalock type. Engaging bronchial arteries is often difficult; a catheter of the 'side-winder' type [14] may overcome this problem. The transfemoral approach is the technique of choice for cannulating left internal mammary-coronary grafts though techniques are described which allow internal mammary cannulation from the contralateral arm [15, 16]. The technique of transfemoral coronary arteriography is discussed in Chapter 13.

REFERENCES

1 Lapin ES, Murray JA. Hemoptysis with flow directed cardiac catheterisation. *JAMA* 1972;29:1246.
2 Kelly TF *et al*. Perforation of the pulmonary artery with Swan−Ganz catheters. Diagnosis and surgical management. *Ann Surg* 1981;193:686.
3 Grollman JH, Renner JW. Transfemoral pulmonary angiography: update on technique. *AJR* 1981;136:624.
4 Laskey WK *et al*. A safe and rapid technique for retrograde catheterization of the left ventricle in aortic stenosis. *Cathet Cardiovasc Diagn* 1982;8:429.
5 Crochet D, de Laguerenne J, Petitier H. New pre-shaped catheter for investigation of aortic stenosis by femoral approach: a study of 100 cases. *Cathet Cardiovasc Diagn* 1980;6:337.
6 Agarwal JB, Klein LW. A new catheter design for use in patients with critical aortic stenosis. *Cathet Cardiovasc Diagn* 1986;12:139.
7 Arnold JR, Fraser DJ, Nocero MA. New technique for retrograde catheterization of stenosed aortic valve. *Am Heart J* 1974;88:128.
8 Laskey WK. Editorial: (Percutaneous) retrograde left ventricular catheterization in aortic valve stenosis. *Cathet Cardiovasc Diagn* 1986;12:75.
9 Stoebe T, Adicoff A, Weir EK, Chesler E. Simultaneous measurement of aortic and left ventricular pressures in aortic stenosis using a double lumen pigtail catheter. *Cathet Cardiovasc Diagn* 1984;10:515.
10 Shirey EK, Sones FM. Retrograde transaortic and mitral valve catheterization. Physiologic and morphologic evaluation of aortic and mitral valve lesions. *Am J Cardiol* 1966;18:745.
11 Miller GAH. Aortic atresia. Diagnostic cardiac catheterisation in the first week of life. *Br Heart J* 1971;33:367.
12 Waldman JD, Pappelbaum JS, Turner SW. Antegrade left heart catheterisation. *Cathet Cardiovasc Diagn* 1977;3:321.
13 Bloomfield DA. Overcoming the problem of tortuous vessel negotiation. *Cathet Cardiovasc Diagn* 1984;10:303.
14 Simmons CR, Tsao EC, Thompson JR. Angiographic approach to the difficult aortic arch: a new technique for transfemoral cerebral angiography in the aged. *Am J Radiol Roentgen Ther* 1973;119:605.
15 Singh RN. Internal mammary arteriography: a new catheter technique by the right brachial approach. *Cathet Cardiovasc Diagn* 1980;6:439.
16 Dorros G, Lewin RF. Angiography of the internal mammary artery via the contralateral brachial artery. *Cathet Cardiovasc Diagn* 1987;13:138.

Interventional techniques

In recent years the catheterisation laboratory has undergone a transformation as a number of techniques have been developed for the *treatment* of heart disease using catheter-transportable devices. Pacemaking and percutaneous transluminal coronary angioplasty (PTCA) are the most obvious examples and are so important that separate chapters are devoted to these techniques. Pacemaking and His bundle ablation are discussed in Chapter 22 and PTCA in Chapter 14. Percutaneous intra-aortic balloon counter-pulsation is described in the chapter on cardiac intensive care (Chapter 21). Of the other therapeutic catheter techniques balloon atrial septostomy was the first to be developed but technological advances now allow the catheterising physician to treat pulmonary, aortic and mitral stenosis, coarctation of the aorta, pulmonary arteriovenous fistula and many more conditions. Balloon valvuloplasty is now the treatment of choice for 'classical' valvar pulmonary stenosis and balloon angioplasty the treatment of choice for recoarctation, branch pulmonary stenosis and stenoses of intracardiac baffles.

The status of other interventional techniques has still to be defined. Balloon valvuloplasty can certainly reduce transvalvargradients in mitral and aortic stenosis but there is no reason to suppose that the long-term results will be any better than those that can be obtained surgically. Restenosis is likely to be at least as common as it is following closed (surgical) valvotomy and valve replacement has a track record that will be hard to beat. As a result patient selection is of prime importance and attention is being focussed on those patients said to be at high risk for open heart surgery. It is important that enthusiasm for a new technique, one that puts the power of the surgeon into the hands of the cardiologist, is not allowed to pre-empt a careful assessment of the risks and benefits of the two, competing, treatment options.

No attempt will be made here to discuss the question of patient selection. Instead the presently available techniques will be described in the knowledge that not all may pass the test of time and that the next few years will see other developments in interventional techniques.

BALLOON ATRIAL SEPTOSTOMY

Balloon atrial septostomy, developed by Rashkind and Miller in 1966 [1] for the palliation of complete transposition of the great arteries, is still an essential, life-saving, part of the management of many patients with this condition.

The technique involves passing a special, balloon-tipped catheter (Figs 2.10 and 2.11) from the saphenous or femoral vein to the left atrium via the foramen ovale. The balloon is then inflated with approximately 2 cc of dilute contrast medium and the catheter is withdrawn until it presses against the atrial septum (Fig. 5.1). A sharp tug on the shaft of the catheter will then cause the inflated balloon to rupture the atrial septum as it passes through it before impacting in the inferior vena cava. The catheter should be re-advanced, immediately, to place the balloon in the mid-right atrium where it can be deflated.

The atrial septal defect (septostomy) so created allows mixing of pulmonary and systemic venous blood at atrial level with a consequent increase in arterial saturation. In almost all cases this increased mixing will permit survival until surgical correction is undertaken.

Hints

1 The Edwards Laboratories septostomy catheter has a 35° bend 2 cm from the tip which allows easy entry to the left atrium. It is our preferred catheter.

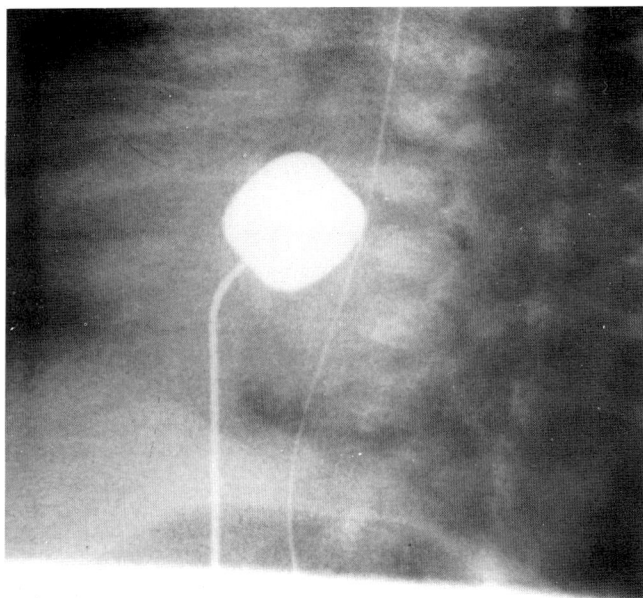

Fig. 5.1 Atrial septostomy. The septostomy catheter has been passed to the left atrium via the foramen ovale and the balloon inflated with 1−2 ml of dilute contrast medium. Prior to inflation the catheter position in the left atrium is confirmed by lateral fluoroscopy showing it to be posteriorly positioned. The inflated balloon has been positioned against the atrial septum; a sharp pull on the catheter will now cause it to tear the septum as it is pulled through and into the right atrial/inferior caval junction.

2 Because of the relatively small size of the neonatal saphenous or, more usually, femoral vein a single-lumen atrial septostomy catheter is used; the lumen provides for balloon inflation but there is no second lumen to provide a pressure record as a guide to the position of the catheter tip. In the anteroposterior projection it is difficult to distinguish between the appearance when the catheter tip is in the right ventricular outflow tract and when it is correctly positioned in the left atrium. If an inflated balloon were to be withdrawn from the right ventricle it might avulse the tricuspid valve. Fluoroscopy in the lateral projection is the simplest way of distinguishing between the two positions. If the catheter tip is in the left atrium it will lie posteriorly, it will be anterior if in the right ventricle. A left atrial position is confirmed if further advance leads the tip of the catheter outside the cardiac shadow into a pulmonary vein. The balloon must not be inflated while the catheter tip is in a pulmonary vein or the left atrial appendage. Finally if the catheter tip impinges on

myocardium it may stimulate ectopic beats — atrial if correctly positioned, ventricular if not.

3 If the septostomy catheter is introduced percutaneously a no. 7 sheath will be needed; the shaft of the catheter is 5F but the added thickness of the balloon requires a larger sheath. A haemostatic valve on the sheath will prevent blood loss.

4 The balloon will accept 1.8 ml of dilute contrast medium providing an inflated balloon 15 mm in diameter. Further inflation to provide a larger balloon has been advocated but the left atrium may well be little larger than the size of a balloon inflated with this amount of contrast medium; 1−2 ml of contrast medium is probably a safe quantity.

PARK BLADE ATRIAL SEPTOSTOMY

Severe arterial desaturation is present from birth in neonates with complete transposition so that septostomy is likely to be performed within the first week or so of life. At this time the atrial septum is thin and easily torn. Occasionally, presentation may be delayed and the atrial septum found to be too tough to be torn by a balloon. A catheter-mounted knife technique (blade septostomy) has been used to perform atrial septostomy in such patients [2−4]. A small surgical blade lies within a longitudinal slit at the end of a 65 cm long, 5F polyethylene catheter (see catheter 3, Fig. 2.11, William Cook, see Appendix 2 for address). The proximal end of the blade is attached to a guide wire within the lumen of the catheter. The distal end of the blade is linked to one end of a lever the other end of which is pivoted within the catheter tip. Advancing the guide wire causes the blade to protrude through the slit in the wall of the catheter. A side-port at the hub of the catheter allows the catheter to be flushed. This side-port provides a guide to blade orientation since the orientation of the side-port is the same as that of the blade. The catheter is rotated so that the blade is orientated inferiorly, anteriorly and to the left. The catheter is then slowly withdrawn, with the blade extended, thus incising the atrial septum. The blade is sheathed after it has entered the right atrium.

Although transposition of the great arteries is the commonest indication for atrial septostomy it has been useful in some other conditions where egress from the left or right atrium is critically restricted; tricuspid and pulmonary atresia, total anomalous pulmonary venous connection and mitral stenosis or hypoplasia are examples.

BALLOON VALVULOPLASTY AND ANGIOPLASTY

Pulmonary valve stenosis (Fig. 5.2)

Balloon valvuloplasty [5] has replaced surgical valvotomy for the treatment of 'typical' pulmonary valve stenosis. The ideal subject is a patient aged 6 months or more in whom there is moderate to severe valvar stenosis with a thin, mobile valve which 'domes' in systole. Younger patients and even neonates have been treated successfully but the need to introduce a relatively large catheter makes the technique technically difficult in such patients. Balloon pulmonary valvuloplasty has been used successfully in adults [6] in whom two balloons may be needed to provide the necessary combined diameter [7]. Patients with thickened, dysplastic valves such as are commonly found in Noonan syndrome, are not suitable candidates for balloon pulmonary valvuloplasty [8].

Balloon valvuloplasty is performed via a percutaneous puncture of the femoral vein. Following right ventricular angiography the position of the pulmonary valve as seen in the lateral projection is noted and may be marked on the face of the monitor screen. An end-hole catheter (e.g. no 6 Goodale–Lubin) is positioned in the distal left or right pulmonary artery and a long ('exchange') guide wire advanced through it to the same position. The end-hole catheter is then removed leaving the guide wire in place. The skin incision in the groin is enlarged slightly and the special balloon catheter advanced percutaneously over the guide wire until the sausage-shaped balloon is centred on the pulmonary valve. Passage of the large balloon catheter through the subcutaneous tissues is facilitated by prior dilatation with a no. 8–10F dilator or by using a 'split sheath'.

Hints

1 Passing the large catheter through the subcutaneous tissues is accomplished with rotation in the direction (usually counter-clockwise) which keeps the balloon furled against the shaft of the catheter. To avoid needless damage to the vein it should be rotated in the same direction during withdrawal.

2 There may be difficulty in traversing the right ventricle with the stiff valvuloplasty catheter. As with any difficult manipulation, using a guide wire success often depends on withdrawing the guide wire slightly as the catheter is advanced ('counter-traction'). The guide wire can then be re-advanced on its own and the procedure repeated. Simply pushing the catheter over a static guide wire is likely to result in buckling of the wire and loss of its position in the distal pulmonary artery. A relatively stiff guide wire will help and a 6F thin wall Goodale–Lubin catheter will accept a 0.038″ guide wire. The balloon is wetted before insertion but not inflated. Air can be withdrawn and replaced by dilute contrast medium when the balloon is safely within the inferior vena cava (IVC).

3 Thrombus forms very readily among the folds of the balloon; we heparinise the patient before performing balloon valvuloplasty.

4 It is important to position the balloon with its mid-point at the pulmonary valve. In the anteroposterior projection the right ventricular outflow tract and main pulmonary artery are angled away from the viewer so that the exact position of the pulmonary valve is difficult to define. As the balloon is inflated with dilute contrast medium it may, if incorrectly centred, advance or retract itself beyond, or proximal to, the valve without rupturing it. It is for this reason that the use of lateral fluoroscopy is recommended with the position of the valve marked on the monitor face (Fig. 5.2d). As the balloon is inflated, with as much force as the operator can manage, an indentation will be seen which disappears suddenly as the valve commissures split. The balloon is non-distensible; that is it will expand to its preset maximum diameter and no further. Excessive pressure beyond this point may cause the balloon to rupture longitudinally but will not damage the valve ring.

5 A balloon size (diameter) should be chosen which is up to 25% larger than the valve ring [7]. The two most common causes of failure are using too small a balloon and positioning the balloon too proximally or too distally. The diameter of the valve ring may be obtained from the angiogram (allowing for X-ray magnification) or by echocardiography. In practice an 18 mm balloon seems ideal for children over 1 year of age. During the initial inflation a waist will be seen in the balloon at the level of the pulmonary valve. Excessive waisting indicates that the balloon

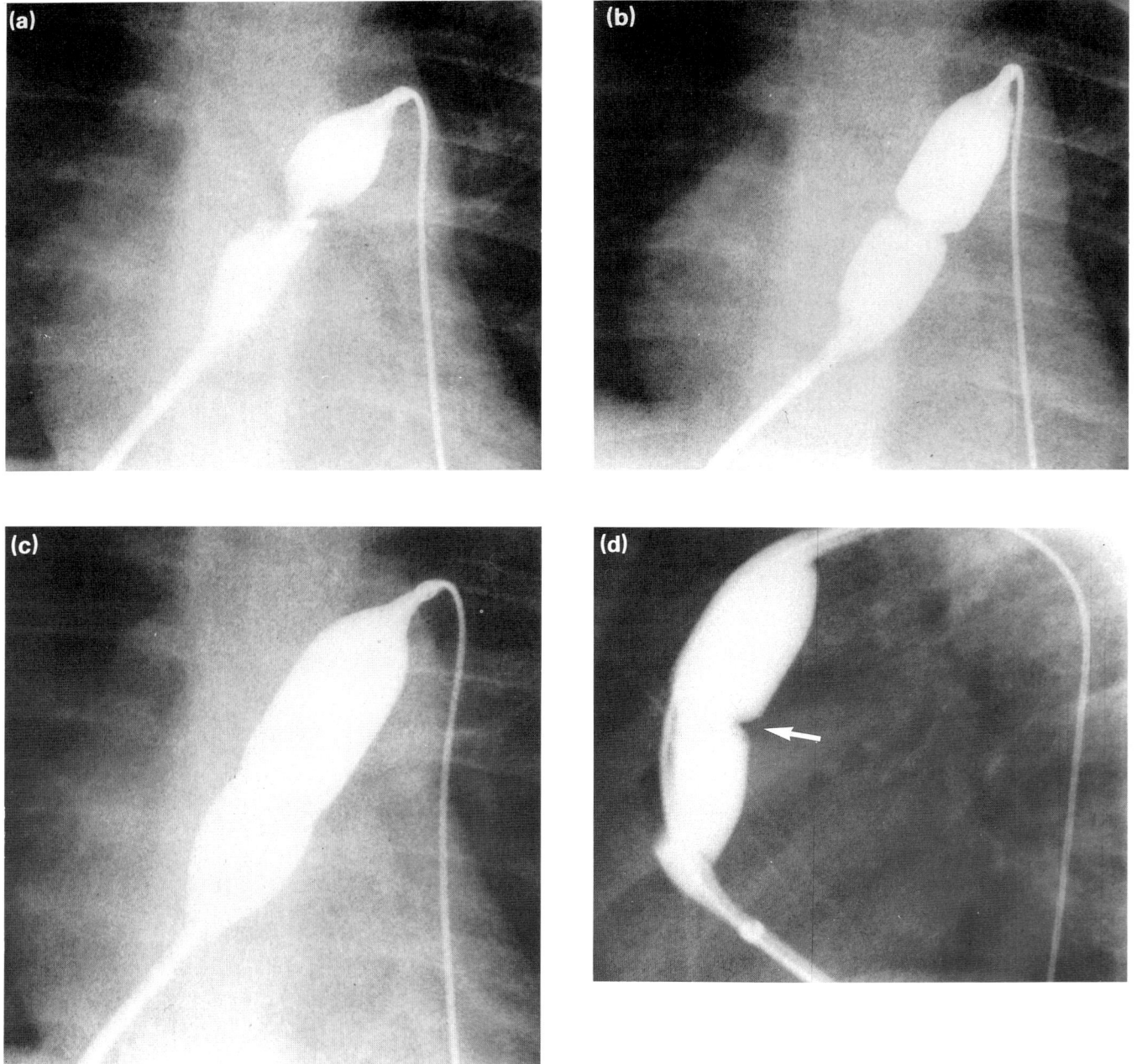

Fig. 5.2 Balloon pulmonary valvuloplasty. (a) Guide wire positioned in the distal left pulmonary artery. Balloon correctly centred on the stenotic pulmonary valve. Waisting of the balloon is seen as balloon inflation begins. (b) Balloon almost fully inflated but waisting still present. (c) Waisting has suddenly disappeared as the valve splits. Balloon valvuloplasty completed. (d) Balloon pulmonary valvuloplasty for pulmonary valve stenosis. Lateral projection showing the balloon correctly centred on the stenotic pulmonary valve which is causing a posterior indentation (arrow) — though a single indentation of this type may be due to flexing of the balloon.

is too large while minimal waisting suggests that a larger balloon will be needed. During full inflation this waisting will be seen to disappear, suddenly, as the valve tears; a sign of successful valvuloplasty.

The results of balloon pulmonary valvuloplasty are very satisfactory; in patients with moderately severe stenosis gradients are significantly reduced or abolished with (so far) no evidence of restenosis. In those with severe pulmonary stenosis there is usually some residual gradient but some, at least, of this residual gradient may be due to infundibular hypertrophy. As is the case following surgical valvotomy such residual gradients diminish over the next few months as right ventricular hypertrophy regresses.

Important complications have not, so far, been reported and clinically detectable pulmonary regurgitation is rare following balloon valvuloplasty.

Aortic stenosis

Balloon valvuloplasty for aortic stenosis (Fig. 5.3) has been employed in two groups of patients. In children with congenital aortic stenosis [9] balloon valvuloplasty may allow surgical valvotomy to be postponed — hopefully for some years. In adults balloon aortic valvuloplasty has been employed in patients who are not suitable candidates for surgical treatment. Such patients include those with 'end-stage', calcific, aortic stenosis and poor left ventricular function in whom even mild relief of stenosis might allow clinical improvement and safer surgical treatment at a later date. Others who have been treated include the aged and patients in whom there is a contraindication to bypass surgery, who have refused surgery or in whom surgery would, for some reason, be at a very high risk [10—12].

Balloon valvuloplasty for aortic stenosis poses a number of problems — not all of which have yet been solved:

1 There is a high incidence of (femoral) arterial complications due to damage to the vessel wall and intima by the large catheter and balloon [11]. The catheter is (usually) too large to be introduced from the brachial artery and most operators have employed a percutaneous, transfemoral, approach. An alternative approach that we have tried is by arteriotomy from the axillary artery. This approach provides a

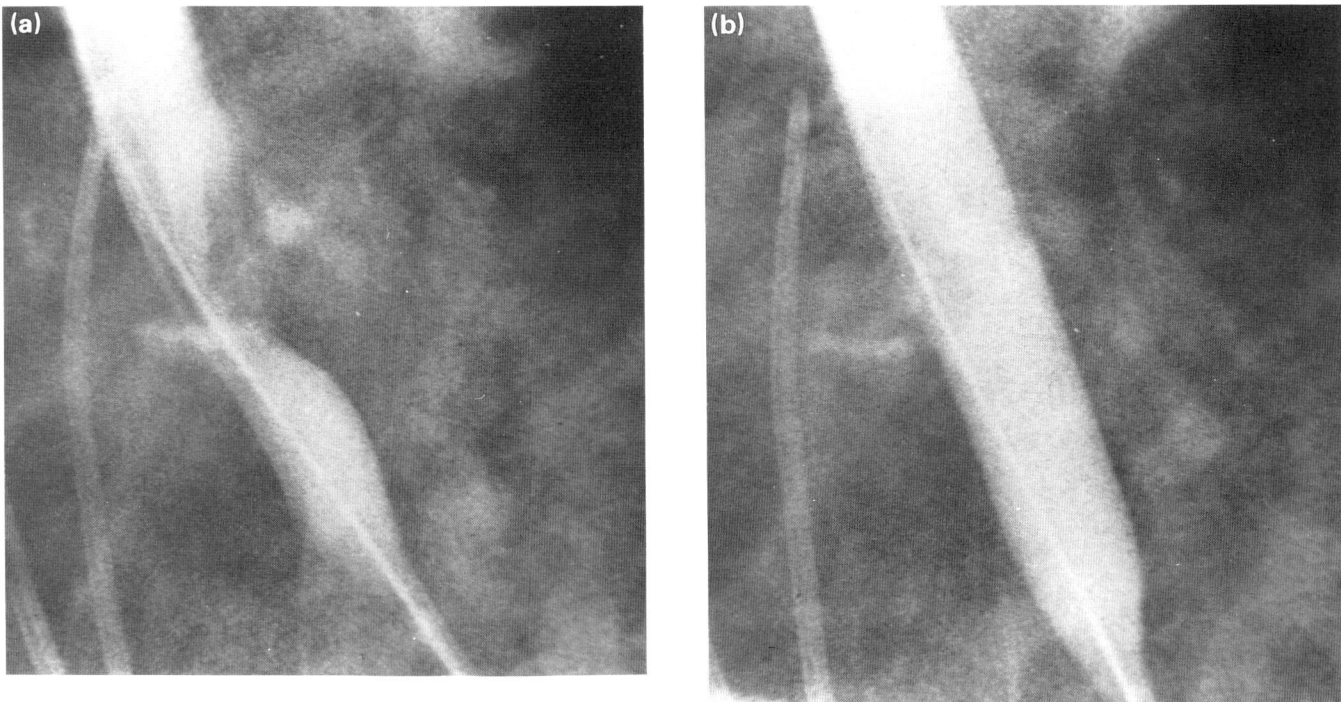

Fig. 5.3 Balloon aortic valvuloplasty for calcific aortic stenosis. (a) Indentation of the partially inflated balloon is seen at the level of the calcified aortic valve. (b) In the same patient the balloon is now fully inflated and waisting has disappeared with relief of the stenosis.

large artery: it is easier to cross the stenotic aortic valve from the arm and haemostasis is achieved by direct suture. However intimal damage is still a problem and can be difficult to repair. An antegrade, transvenous, approach (transseptal) has been employed in order to avoid the problem of arterial damage but this technique has not been widely adopted.

Balloon catheters are too large to be inserted through conventional introducer sheaths but valvuloplasty sheaths are now available up to 16F (Schneider–Medintag). For balloons up to 23 mm diameter use a 14F introducer, 16F is needed for a 25 mm balloon. These sheaths incorporate an adjustable haemostatic valve and a side-arm (Fig. 2.12). Despite their large size they have proved easy to use and have greatly simplified the transfemoral insertion of valvuloplasty balloons.

Dorros and associates [13] have described a double-balloon technique, one balloon 10 mm in diameter being inserted percutaneously from the femoral artery (using a 12F side-arm sheath) and the other via a brachial arteriotomy. In this way the size of each balloon can be reduced, thus minimising arterial trauma, while the combined diameters of the balloons across the aortic valve are equivalent to that of a much larger single balloon. Two 0.038″ exchange guide wires are first positioned in the left ventricle and the balloons advanced, simultaneously, over these guides.

2 It is difficult to maintain a stable position with the balloon centred on the valve; the inflated balloon tends to be ejected into the aorta during systole and to-and-fro movement of the catheter has resulted in the pointed tip of the (stiff) catheter perforating the myocardium with resulting tamponade. To guard against this complication it is essential that several centimetres of guide wire should be allowed to extend beyond the end of the catheter; a large diameter J-curve should be hand-moulded at the end of the guide wires so as to allow excess wire to be accommodated within the ventricle and ensure that the stiff part of the wire is guiding the balloon(s) across the valve (Fig. 5.4). A special guide wire is available with a long flexible tip and an unusually stiff proximal portion to provide support for the balloon. Finally, valvuloplasty catheters incorporating a pigtail tip will reduce the risk of myocardial damage during the procedure.

The trefoil-balloon valvuloplasty catheter

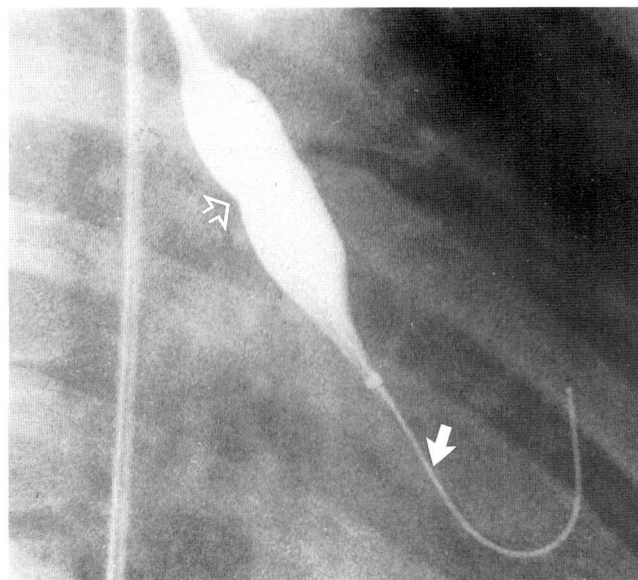

Fig. 5.4 Balloon aortic valvuloplasty. A single balloon is being used and has been advanced over a guide wire whose tip has been formed into a large radius J-shaped curve which lies within the cavity of the left ventricle (solid arrow). This curved wire serves to protect the myocardium from damage caused by the tip of the catheter as it moved to-and-fro during balloon inflation. The indentation caused by the stenotic aortic valve is seen (open arrow).

(Schneider–Medintag) shown in Fig. 5.5 may be more stable than a single balloon since it allows some forward flow between the radially mounted balloons during inflation. Yet another design, the Cribier–Letac valvuloplasty catheter (Fig. 5.6), has a single balloon the diameter of which increases at the mid-point to allow progressive dilatation without the need for a catheter change. This catheter also incorporates a pigtail tip and distal and proximal lumens allowing the valve gradient to be measured before and after valve dilatation.

3 In the unanaesthetised patient the profound hypotension that inevitably accompanies balloon inflation can be distressing. The balloon should be deflated as soon as the patient's level of consciousness begins to be impaired — 10 seconds of inflation is probably enough. The bradycardia and hypotension that accompanies balloon inflation may be partly of reflex origin; premedication with atropine is recommended. Death has been reported resulting from cerebral damage occurring during prolonged hypotension and bradycardia following balloon inflation.

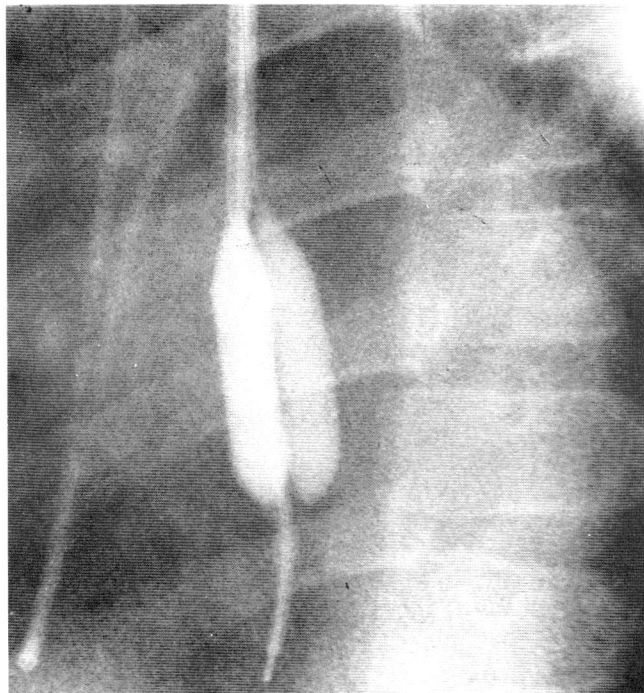

Fig. 5.5 Balloon aortic valvuloplasty — a 'trefoil' balloon is being used in this example.

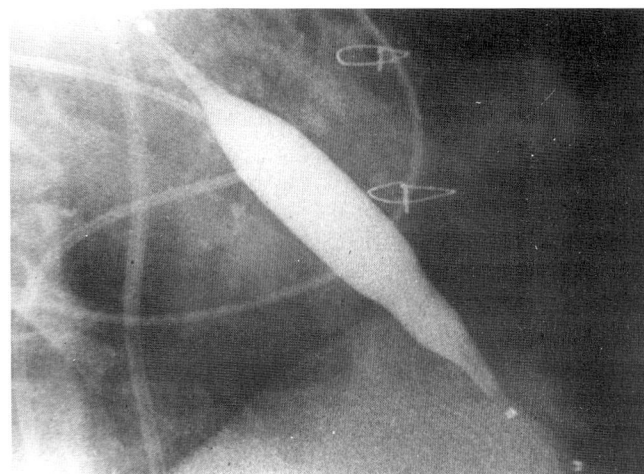

Fig. 5.6 Balloon aortic valvuloplasty. Cribier–Letac valvuloplasty catheter. The balloon has two, different, diameters; it also has a pigtail tip (not seen in this illustration).

4 In children transverse tears of the aorta have resulted from rupture of a balloon larger than the aortic diameter [14]. Inflation of a long balloon which is traversing the aortic arch will deform the arch as it straightens during inflation [14] and this is another possible cause of aortic wall rupture. A short balloon should be chosen the diameter of which is no more than 110% of the annulus or aortic diameter [15]. It is probable that relief of calcific aortic stenosis results from fracture of calcified nodules and/or separation of fused commissures [16] and that this can be achieved with balloons no larger than the annulus diameter. Larger balloons can cause avulsion of leaflets and severe aortic regurgitation. The situation is therefore unlike that in pulmonary valvuloplasty where over-sized balloons give the best results. Cribier and associates, with a large experience of valvuloplasty in calcific aortic stenosis, have recommended progressive dilatation starting with a 15 mm balloon and progressing to an 18 and, if necessary, 20 mm balloon [11].

5 Attempted aortic valvuloplasty is sometimes frustrated by inability to cross the valve and by tortuosity of the iliac arteries in a group of elderly, arteriosclerotic, patients.

6 Finally, whole-body heparinisation is indicated and it may be wise to flush the balloon with carbon dioxide and then dilute contrast medium to guard against air embolism should the balloon rupture.

Although aortic valve gradients can be reduced and calculated valve area increased by balloon valvuloplasty, the place of balloon valvuloplasty in calcific aortic stenosis remains controversial [46]. Inspection of such valves following valvuloplasty often reveals little change. Stenosis is due to rigidity of the calcified cusps and it seems unlikely that mere balloon inflation will do much to alter the morphology of such valves. The situation is different in children with non-calcified, mobile, congenitally stenotic aortic valves. Such valves respond well to balloon valvuloplasty.

Coarctation of the aorta (Fig. 5.7)

Although successes have been reported [17, 18] balloon angioplasty has not found general acceptance as primary treatment for uncomplicated native aortic coarctation. Aneurysm formation [47] and aortic rupture [19] have occurred and early recurrence has been common [17, 20]. The procedure may have a place in the palliation of individual cases where surgery is contraindicated or at high risk due to other conditions.

On the other hand balloon angioplasty is ideal

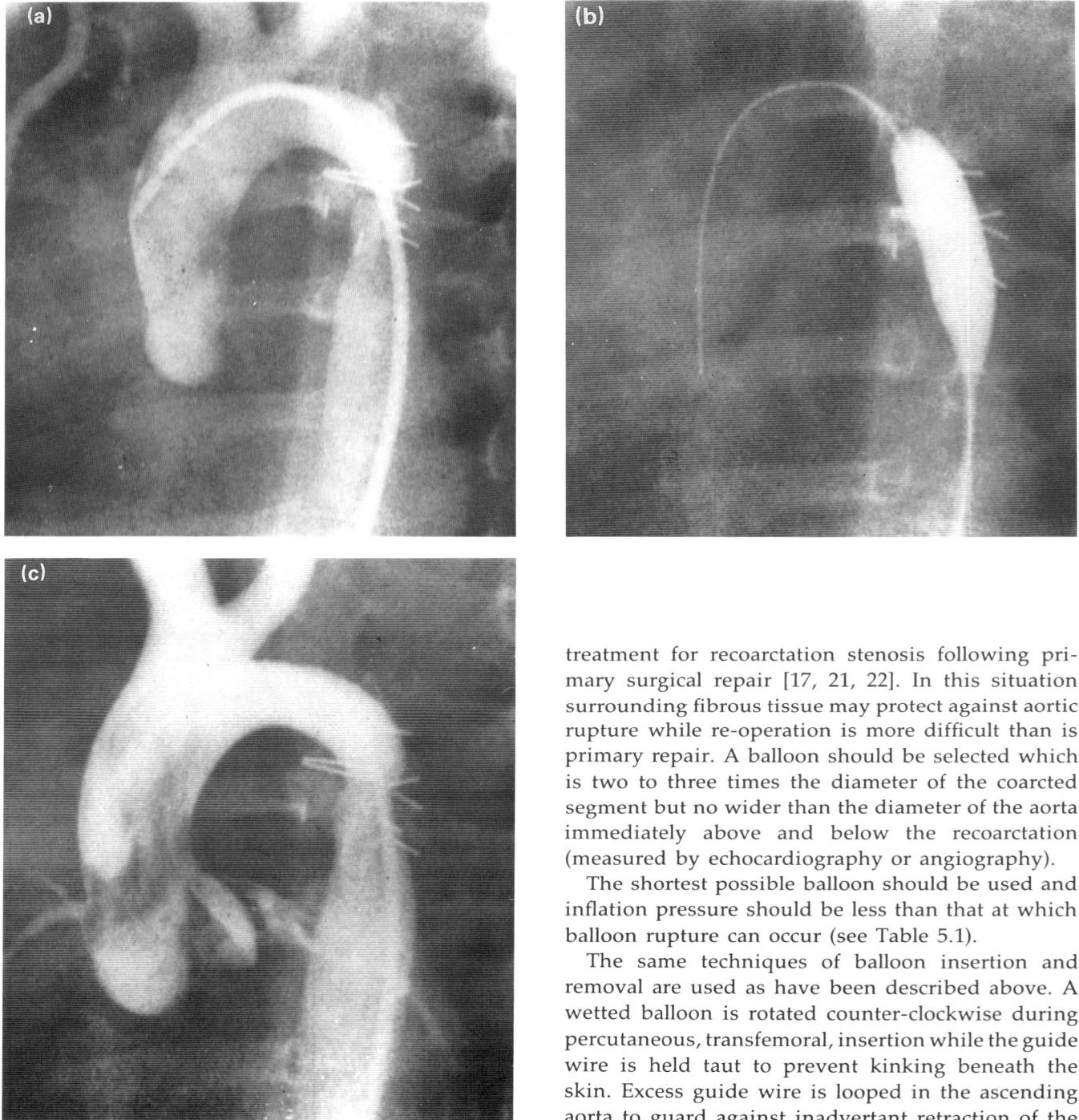

Fig. 5.7 Balloon angioplasty for aortic recoarctation. Before (a). during (b) and after (c) balloon angioplasty.

treatment for recoarctation stenosis following primary surgical repair [17, 21, 22]. In this situation surrounding fibrous tissue may protect against aortic rupture while re-operation is more difficult than is primary repair. A balloon should be selected which is two to three times the diameter of the coarcted segment but no wider than the diameter of the aorta immediately above and below the recoarctation (measured by echocardiography or angiography).

The shortest possible balloon should be used and inflation pressure should be less than that at which balloon rupture can occur (see Table 5.1).

The same techniques of balloon insertion and removal are used as have been described above. A wetted balloon is rotated counter-clockwise during percutaneous, transfemoral, insertion while the guide wire is held taut to prevent kinking beneath the skin. Excess guide wire is looped in the ascending aorta to guard against inadvertant retraction of the guide during balloon insertion.

Because of the risk of perforating the aorta, the dilated segment must not be recrossed by an unguarded catheter; any subsequent catheter exchange (e.g. for repeat angiography) must be made over the guide wire which is left in position in the arch or

Table 5.1 Manufacturers specifications for balloon catheters.

OD (mm)	Balloon length (cm)	Guide (")	Shaft (F)	Max. pressure (kPa)
Mansfield Scientific (Meditech)				
4	2	0.018	4.5	616.1 (6.1 atm)
12−23	3	0.038	9−10	313.1−353.5 (3.1−3.5 atm)
Schneider−Medintag				
19	4	0.035	8	252.5 (2.5 atm)
Trefoil (3×10)	4	0.035	9	505 (5 atm)
Trefoil (3×12)	4	0.035	9	404 (4 atm)
Schneider−Medintag (paediatric)				
4.2−5.0	1.0	0.014	4.3	707−808 (7−8 atm)
6.0−8.0	1.5	0.020	5	707−808 (7−8 atm)
8.0−10.0	2.0	0.035	7	505−707 (5−7 atm)
13−19	3.0	0.035	8	202−404 (2−4 atm)

ascending aorta. A Gensini catheter, which is straight and has both an end- and side-holes, is ideal for postangioplasty studies.

Mitral stenosis

Balloon valvuloplasty has been used to treat rheumatic and congenital mitral stenosis [23−25]. A transseptal technique is used employing a long sheath. A balloon-tipped catheter is advanced to the left atrium and the balloon inflated with carbon dioxide so as to carry the catheter through the mitral valve and left ventricle to the aorta. An exchange guide wire is then advanced through this catheter until its tip lies in the descending aorta at the level of the diaphragm. The sheath and balloon-tipped catheter are removed (leaving only the guide wire in place) and an 8 mm balloon angioplasty catheter advanced over this wire and used to enlarge the opening in the atrial septum. Finally this catheter is replaced by a larger (e.g. 25 mm) balloon catheter which is inflated when correctly positioned across the mitral valve. Alternatively a 'bifoil' (Schneider−Medintag) catheter or two monofoil [25] catheters can be used. If two balloons are used it will be necessary to position two guide wires in the descending aorta — a double-lumen flow-guided catheter has been used to achieve this. A large diameter, long introducer (dilator) set is available (Schneider−Medintag) to allow balloon mitral valvuloplasty by a long sheath technique.

Balloon mitral valvuloplasty is contraindicated if echocardiography reveals thrombus in the left atrium. Since a large opening has to be created in the atrial septum to accommodate the angioplasty balloon there is a possibility that a left-to-right interatrial shunt will result. Most, but not all, such shunts have been small [25]; if the valvuloplasty balloon is too long or too proximally positioned, a significant atrial defect can be created by inflation of the large valvuloplasty balloon across the atrial septum. A left-to-right shunt, by 'decompressing' the left atrium, may contribute to gradient reduction. The true situation can only be evaluated by recalculating valve area; thermodilution cannot be used to estimate mitral valve flow if the thermistor is in the pulmonary artery and there is a significant left-to-right shunt at atrial level.

A two-balloon technique, has been used to treat rheumatic tricuspid stenosis [26].

Other applications of balloon angioplasty

Balloon angioplasty has a major part to play in the remodelling of stenotic or hypoplastic pulmonary arteries [27, 28]. Balloon diameters three to four times the diameter of the stenoses are needed. Using a balloon-tipped catheter a 0.038" guide wire is positioned as far distally as possible in a large branch pulmonary artery. The balloon catheter is threaded over the guide wire in the usual way until it straddles the lesion. The balloon is inflated until the indentation disappears or the maximum safe inflation pressure has been reached. Inflation times of up to 30 seconds may be needed. As with coarctation angioplasty, and for the same reasons, subsequent catheter exchanges must be performed over the exchange guide wire and a non-pigtail catheter used for postdilatation angiography.

Stenosed anastomoses (e.g. at the end of a systemic-to-pulmonary shunt) also respond to balloon dilatation. Where pulmonary flow is largely shunt-dependent the inflation time must be short.

Stenoses at the upper and lower limbs of atrial baffles (Mustard's operation) are difficult to treat surgically but respond well to balloon dilatation [29, 30]. These lesions are very compliant and balloons five to ten times the diameter of the stenosis are recommended (Fig. 5.8).

Stenoses of individual pulmonary veins have not responded to attempted balloon dilatation [31].

It is probable that many other applications will be found for the technique but it is too early to say which will be found to survive the test of time.

TRANSCATHETER OCCLUSIVE PROCEDURES

Transcatheter occlusion has been used to treat systemic and pulmonary arteriovenous fistulae [32, 33], to occlude unwanted surgical (systemic-to-pulmonary) shunts [34, 35] and congenital systemic-to-pulmonary collaterals [36] and to occlude the blood supply to a source of bleeding (e.g. bronchial arteries). A number of different systems have been employed:
1 Gelfoam particles.
2 Ivalon sponge particles.
3 Gianturco (spring) coils.
4 Detachable, silicone-gel-filled, balloons (Debrun system).
5 Detachable, contrast-filled, balloons (Bard−Parker).

Gelfoam. Ivalon

Embolisation with gelfoam particles requires only that the vessel to be embolised is selectively catheterised with a suitable (end-hole) catheter. Gelfoam is supplied in sheets 1 mm thick and must be

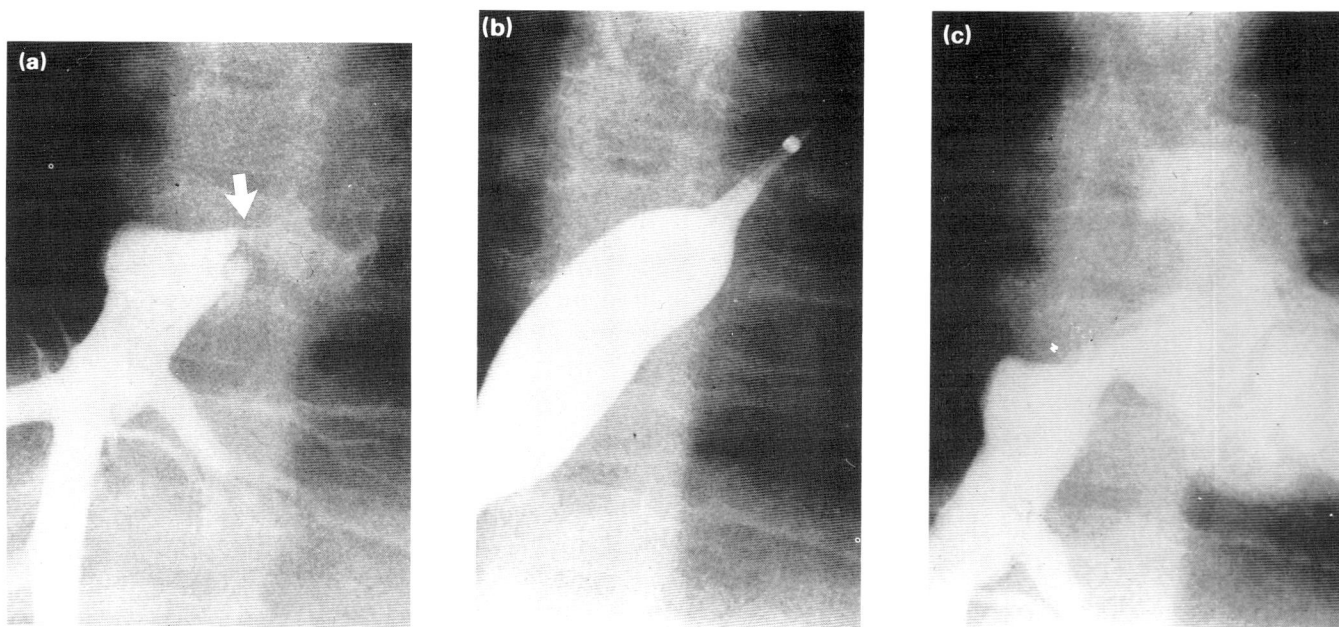

Fig. 5.8 Severe stenosis (arrow) of the lower limb of an atrial baffle inserted for the correction of complete transposition of the great arteries. Such stenoses respond well to balloon dilatation but require a balloon whose inflation diameter is several times that of the stenosis. In this example the inflated diameter of the balloon is ten times the diameter of the original stenosis. (a) Before, (b) during, and (c) after balloon angioplasty.

cut into small ($1-2\,\text{mm}^2$) pieces which are softened by being soaked in saline for 10 minutes before use. The pieces are placed in a 1 ml syringe, the plunger is replaced and the syringe filled with saline. The particles can then be flushed into the catheter. A slow, $2-5\,\text{ml}$ saline flush will then deliver the particles into the vessel. The result must be checked by injections of contrast medium since it is important to discontinue embolisation once vessel occlusion has been obtained; further embolisation after this point would result in the particles refluxing into other (unwanted) sites. An end-hole catheter can be used with a proximal balloon inflated to guard against reflux of particles to unwanted sites.

The technique is only suitable for embolisation of vessels terminating in a capilliary network — the particles would pass through an arteriovenous malformation comprising larger vessels. Gelfoam is resorbable so that occlusion is temporary unless thrombus forms and results in permanent occlusion.

Ivalon sponge may be cut into small fragments and flushed through the catheter. Somewhat larger vessels can be occluded and the occlusion is more permanent. Both gelfoam and Ivalon may be used as an adjunct to other embolisation techniques — spring coils or balloons.

Gianturco spring coils [37]

These consist of a spiral of fine wire incorporating dacron fibres (Fig. 2.14). When ejected from the containing cartridge and delivery catheter thrombus formation around the fibres results in vessel occlusion; coils of differing sizes are available (see Table 5.2)

The vessel to be occluded is selectively catheterised (position checked angiographically) and the delivery cartridge inserted into the hub of the catheter. The stiff end of a 0.025" or 0.038" guide wire serves to eject the coil into the lumen of the catheter. The guide wire is now reversed and the flexible end is used to push the spring coil through the catheter and to eject it into the vessel. The catheter must be matched to the size of the coil (slightly larger than the calibre of the coil; 6.5F for 0.038" calibre coils) and must not have side-holes as the coil might emerge (partially) through a side-hole. If the delivery catheter is too large the guide wire will jam beside the coil and delivery will be impossible.

Table 5.2 Manufacturers (Cook, Incorporated) specifications for Gianturco spring coils.

Calibre	Coil length (cm)	Coil diameter (mm)
0.025"	1.2—4.0	2.0—5.0
0.038"	1.0—15	3.0—10.0
0.052"	5.0—15.0	10.0—20.0

Hints

1 The extruded diameter of the coil must be about one-third larger than the diameter of the vessel to be occluded. A coil of the same diameter will assume a ring shape with potential for continuing central flow. A deformed coil provides most potential for occlusion. Too large a coil will tend to push the delivery catheter backwards and the coil may then embolise to an unwanted site.

2 The end of the delivery catheter should be free within the vessel; if it is impacted against the vessel wall it may be impossible to eject the coil.

3 The course of the delivery catheter should be as straight as possible. It may be impossible to deliver the coil through a catheter which follows a tortuous course. The catheter should be flushed before inserting a coil as thrombus within the catheter may prevent the coil passing freely through the delivery catheter. The patient should be heparinised for this reason.

4 On occasion the coil can only be partially ejected. There is then a danger that it might become detached as the catheter is removed; with resulting embolisation elsewhere than the desired site. A forceful 5 ml saline flush may serve to eject a jammed coil.

5 It may be necessary to place several coils in succession to achieve vessel occlusion.

6 Thrombus will take 15 minutes or so to form. Repeat angiography must therefore be delayed for this time before the result of embolisation can be assessed.

7 The delivery catheter seldom has the correct configuration for initial cannulation of the target vessel; the vessel may have to be engaged with other catheters or guide wires and these replaced, over an exchange guide wire, by the delivery catheter.

The system is cheap and easy to use but, as with all embolisation techniques, there is a danger that the coil might migrate through the pathological circulation if the vessels are large or if the delivery catheter becomes displaced. Medium-sized vessels can be occluded and the ideal vessel has significant length before narrowing or dividing. Examples of spring-coil embolisation are illustrated in Figs 5.9 to 5.11.

Detachable balloons

Silicone-filled, detachable, latex balloons employing a coaxial system have been developed by Debrun [38]. The balloons are tied to the end of the fine, central catheter using elastic thread. When in place and inflated the outer catheter is advanced and pushes the balloon off the end of the central catheter. The system has the advantage that balloons of many different sizes and configurations are available. In its original form it has the disadvantage that the balloons had to be prepared in advance by the physician; a tedious and difficult procedure. Preprepared, 'gold valve' (Kimal. Ingenor) balloons are now available but are not fully self-sealing so that they have to be filled with a two-part silicone gel with added opacifier; inflation is then irreversible if balloon placement is seen to be incorrect. However filling the balloon with dilute contrast medium may suffice since leaking is slow and thrombus formation may result in vessel occlusion before the balloon has collapsed.

The Bard–Parker (Becton–Dickinson) detachable mini-balloon embolisation system [33] has the advantages that (1) the balloon is available already prepared, and (2) the balloon is filled with dilute, radio-opaque, contrast medium which can be aspirated if the position is incorrect. When a satisfactory position has been achieved a deliberate action is needed to detach the self-sealing balloon. It is important to ensure that the tip of the catheter is free within the vessel. If the tip is impacted, the balloon will be bent back on itself as it emerges from the delivery catheter and inflation of the balloon will then be impossible.

Two sizes of balloon are available; a 1 mm balloon suitable for occluding vessels up to 4 mm in diameter and a 2 mm balloon for vessels up to 8 mm in diameter. The system requires a suitable introducer catheter of either 4.9F or 8.8F. The fine catheter which carries the balloon has to be flushed through the delivery catheter using a special delivery device (Fig. 2.13). The system is expensive and complicated to use.

Embolotherapy is a recent development (for the cardiologist, at least) and improved systems are under development which, hopefully, will make the procedure simpler than it is at present. None the less there will always be hazards associated with embolotherapy. Premature detachment or incorrect positioning of the device can lead to embolisation elsewhere in the systemic circulation. Even in pulmonary arteriovenous fistulae the communication may be so large that there is a real danger that the device will escape to the pulmonary veins and thence to the left heart [39]. An example of balloon embolisation is illustrated in Figs 5.9d and 5.9e.

TRANSCATHETER CLOSURE OF PATENT DUCTUS ARTERIOSUS (PDA)

Transcatheter closure of PDA using a wire and plug technique [40, 48, 54] has been practised for more than 15 years but has not gained wide acceptance. Briefly the technique involves passing a long (400 cm) guide wire (through a catheter) from the femoral artery through the PDA and into the main pulmonary artery. The guide wire is then snared with a transfemoral vein catheter and brought out through the right heart and femoral vein. An acorn-shaped plug is threaded over arterial end of the guide wire and followed by an end-hole catheter which is used to push the plug into position in the ductus. The plug has to be sized and shaped to fit the configuration of the ductus.

Recently an alternative technique has been developed which allows PDA closure by a transvenous approach. This technique is a development of the single (hooked) umbrella technique pioneered by Rashkind [41, 49]. Although, at present, use of the device is controlled by an FDA-approved experimental protocol there is no doubt that the successes already obtained [50–52] will lead to widespread clinical use in the near future. Since use of this device is not widely known a detailed description of the device and its use is given here (also see Acknowledgement on p. 78 at the end of this chapter).

The device (USCI Rashkind PDA occluder) consists of:
1 A double-disc prosthesis and lucite loader.
2 A catheter delivery system.

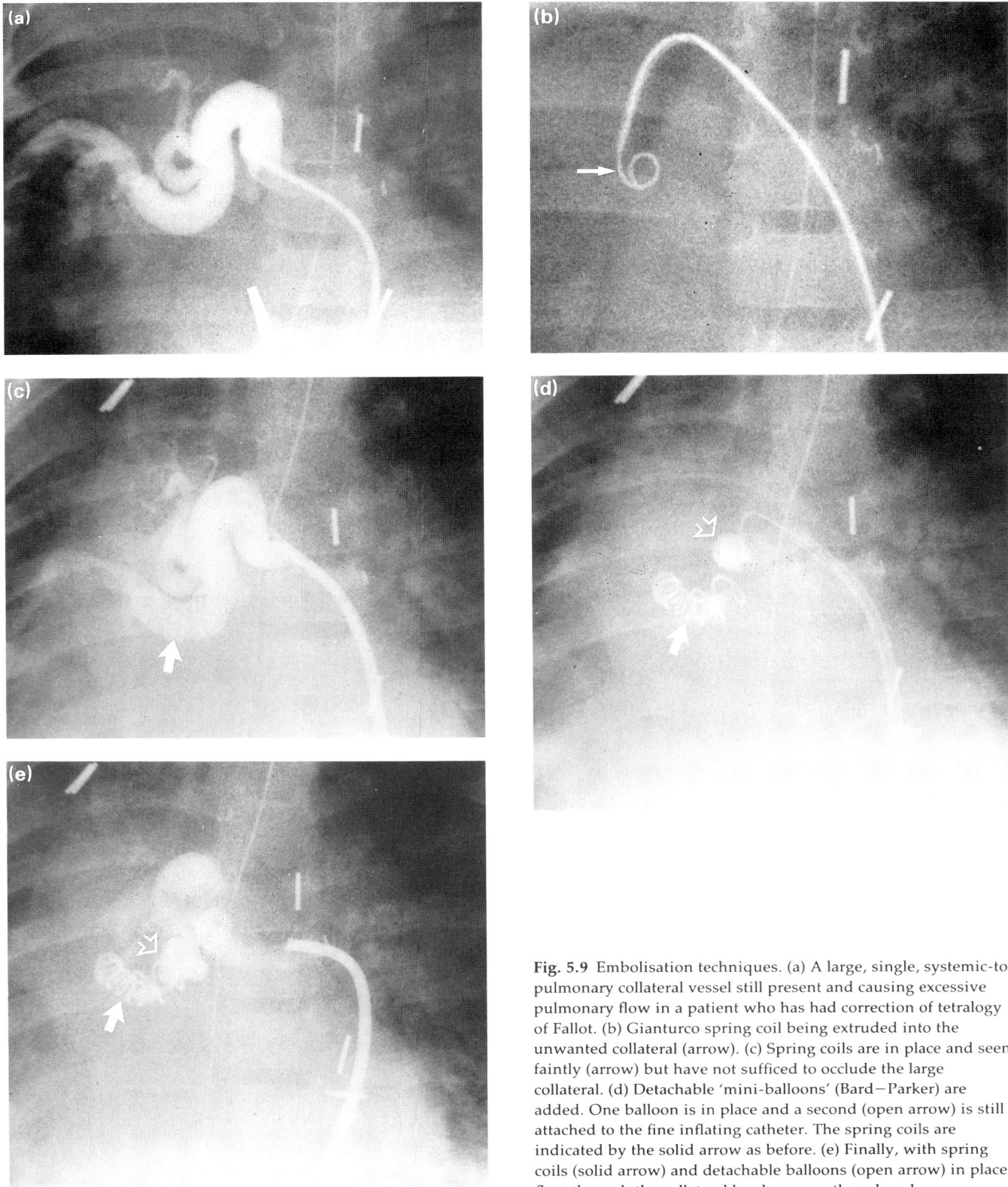

Fig. 5.9 Embolisation techniques. (a) A large, single, systemic-to-pulmonary collateral vessel still present and causing excessive pulmonary flow in a patient who has had correction of tetralogy of Fallot. (b) Gianturco spring coil being extruded into the unwanted collateral (arrow). (c) Spring coils are in place and seen faintly (arrow) but have not sufficed to occlude the large collateral. (d) Detachable 'mini-balloons' (Bard–Parker) are added. One balloon is in place and a second (open arrow) is still attached to the fine inflating catheter. The spring coils are indicated by the solid arrow as before. (e) Finally, with spring coils (solid arrow) and detachable balloons (open arrow) in place, flow through the collateral has been greatly reduced.

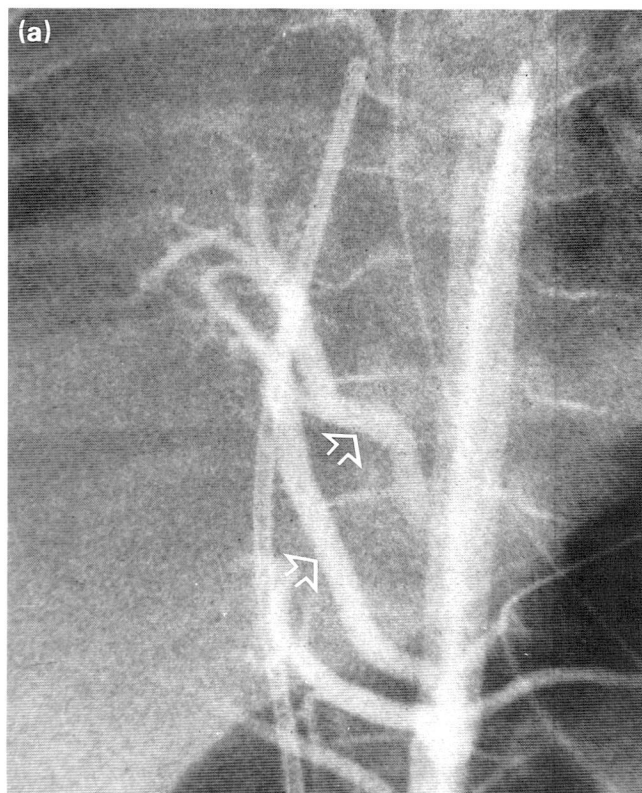

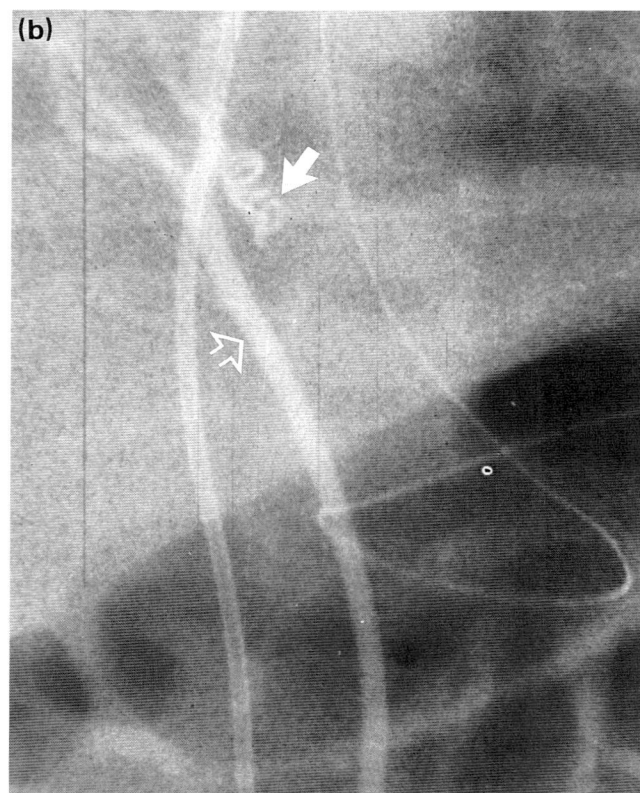

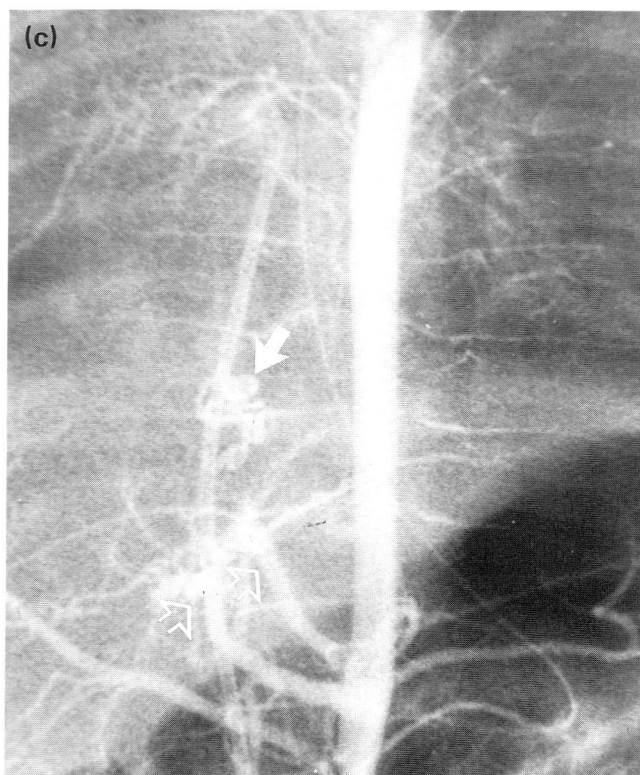

Fig. 5.10 Another example of spring coil embolisation. (a) Two anomalous systemic arteries (open arrows) supplying a sequestered segment in the right lower lobe. (b) Spring coils (solid arrow) have been placed in one of the anomalous vessels and the second vessel has been cannulated and the position checked by angiography (open arrow) prior to similar embolisation of this vessel. (c) Spring coils in place (solid arrow). An aortogram now shows that the two anomalous vessels (open arrows) are occluded distally.

The double-disc prosthesis

This consists of two polyurethane discs sewn to two opposing three- or four-arm spring assemblies. The individual arms are attached to the central spring mechanism and are 90° or 120° apart — resembling two opposed umbrellas. A small elliptical loop is built into the centre of the proximal disc to allow attachment to the delivery system. Each arm terminates in a fine eye and a prolene suture passes through the eyes of the distal disc. This suture passes through the centre of the lucite loader so that the discs can be drawn into the funnel-shaped opening of the loader — the distal disc with its arms folding forward, the proximal one with its arms folding

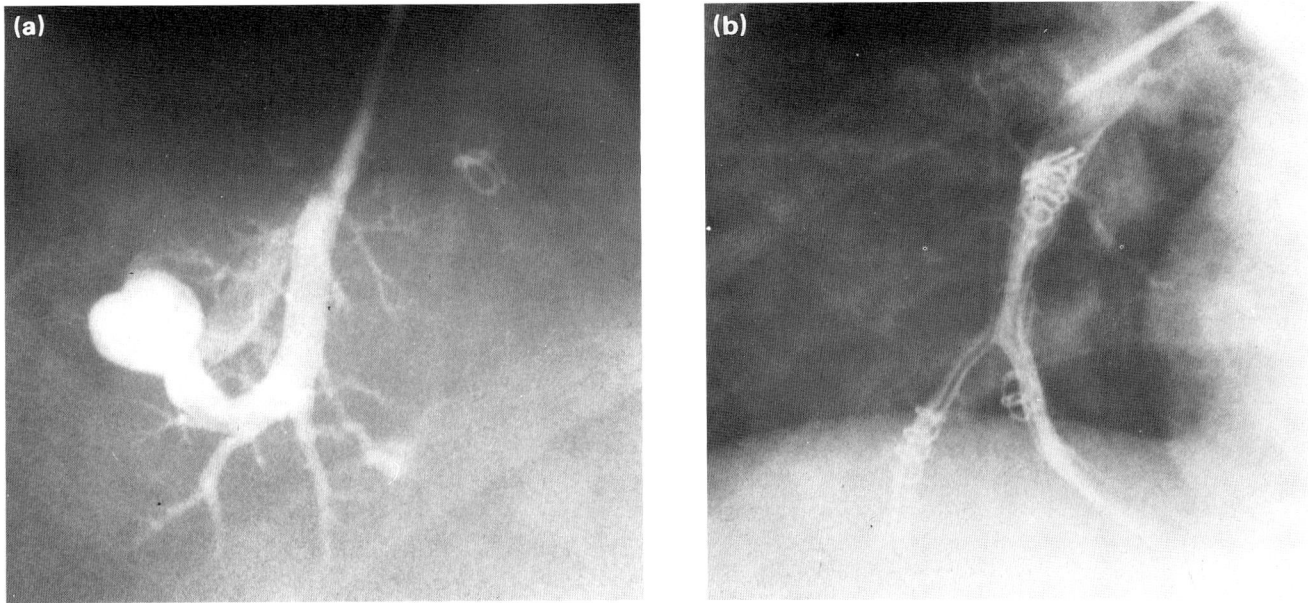

Fig. 5.11 Spring coil embolisation of a pulmonary arteriovenous fistula. (a) Angiogram of fistula; the artery and draining vein are seen. Coils are visible in another, nearby, arteriovenous fistula. (b) Coils in place; repeat angiogram shows almost complete vessel occlusion.

backwards. Two sizes of prosthesis are available — 12 mm and 17 mm in diameter respectively.

The delivery system (Fig. 5.12)

This consists of a coaxial assembly of:
1 A central fine wire terminating in a b-shaped knuckle (1). This fine central wire runs through:
2 A spring-coil delivery wire (2) at the distal end of which is welded a small tubular capture sleeve (3). The proximal end of the delivery wire is welded to a hollow steel rod (4) on which is mounted a 'pin-control clamp' and locking spring (5) which controls the position of the central wire and b-knuckle within the delivery wire and capture sleeve. Finally the delivery wire runs through:
3 An outer 8F, 85 cm long, delivery catheter at the distal end of which is a 1.7 cm long thin-walled stainless-steel delivery pod (6) (8F for the 12 mm device; 11F for the 17 mm device).

Assembly

The prosthesis is soaked in saline (or topical throm-bin — see below) for 5–10 minutes. The b-knuckle is engaged with the small loop attached to the centre of the prosthesis and the two held in opposition by one operator while a second operator pulls slowly on the pin-control clamp attached to the proximal end of the central wire thus drawing the loop and engaged b-knuckle into the capture sleeve. It is locked into position by a T-shaped spring locking device at the proximal end of the delivery system (6). The prosthesis is now drawn into the lucite loader by traction on the suture. When the prosthesis is fully collapsed within the narrow portion of the loader the delivery catheter is advanced over the coiled-spring guide wire so that the distal delivery pod is also within the loader. Traction on the spring guide (holding the catheter and delivery pod firmly within the loader) now draws the collapsed prosthesis into the delivery pod (where it can be locked into place by tightening an adjustable locking collar on the steel rod). The suture is now cut and withdrawn and the lucite loader discarded. The delivery system is now loaded.

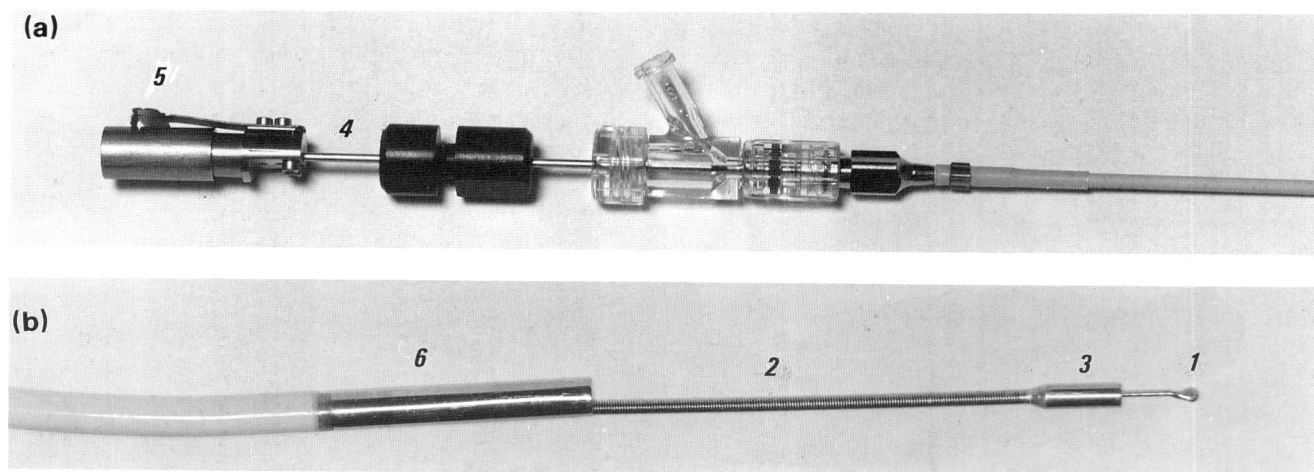

Fig. 5.12 (a and b) The USCI Rashkind PDA occluder. See text for explanation.

PDA CLOSURE USING THE RASHKIND PDA OCCLUDER SYSTEM

The delivery system is introduced and positioned via the femoral vein using a 48 cm long sheath and dilator [53]. An 8F sheath is used for the smaller (12 mm) prosthesis; an 11F sheath is needed for the larger (17 mm) prosthesis. An 0.038″ exchange guide wire is positioned across the PDA and well down the descending aorta (via a 7F, end-hole, balloon-tipped catheter) and the long sheath and dilator advanced over this guide until the end of the long sheath is through the PDA and in the descending aorta. The dilator is then removed leaving the sheath parallel to the axis of the duct with its tip in the aorta. An injection of contrast medium is made (either through the sheath or through a separate aortic pig-tail catheter) to determine whether the sheath has displaced the duct in a posterior direction. The delivery catheter is flushed through the side-port and the delivery pod inserted into the long sheath and advanced to the level of the tricuspid valve. At this point the locking collar can be loosened or re-positioned and the pin-control clamp and attached rod slowly advanced to push the prosthesis out of the delivery pod and into the sheath. The sheath acts as an extension of the delivery pod and the arms of the prosthesis will remain folded. This advance continues until the centre of the prosthesis is slightly posterior to the centre of the duct. This position is held while the sheath is slowly withdrawn until the distal arms are seen to open widely on the aortic side of the duct; the proximal arms must remain folded within the sheath, the tip of which is over the centre point of the prosthesis.

Gentle traction on the entire system should now cause the distal arms to flex inward as the device is pulled into the duct. The position of the prosthesis is held steady while further withdrawal of the sheath allows all proximal arms of the prosthesis to open fully at the pulmonary end of the duct.

At this stage the device is positioned but still held by the capture sleeve and is fully retrievable. The wire is now moved gently to-and-fro observing that the arms flex appropriately and that the device is not, therefore, free in the pulmonary artery or aorta. If the device is free the wire is retracted, pulling the prosthesis back into the sheath and delivery pod and allowing removal. If the position is satisfactory the pin-control clamp and wire are allowed to adopt a neutral position (to release any residual torque), the T-shaped locking spring is released and the pin-control clamp moved forward so as to eject the ring and b-knuckle from the capture sleeve thus releasing the prosthesis.

Hints

1 Ducts that are 4 mm or less in diameter at their narrowest point can be closed using the 12 mm prosthesis. Ducts that are 5–9 mm in diameter require the 17 mm device. It is unwise to attempt to close a duct which is more than 8 or 9 mm in diameter or which carries a very high flow. A small short duct with a funnel-shaped aortic ostium is most easily closed, although almost all PDAs may be closed with this technique.

2 The procedure requires the use of at least an 8F sheath and is thus limited to infants over 4–5 kg in weight. If the larger prosthesis is to be used, the femoral vein will have to accept an 11F sheath and this is unlikely in children under 8–10 kg.

3 Dislodgment of the prosthesis has resulted when irregularities on the b-knuckle have snagged the polyurethane foam disc. The device should be tested before use by drawing the knuckle across a coarse gauze — if the knuckle snags the device should be rejected.

Movement of the wire after release should not cause the prosthesis to move. If it does the knuckle has snagged the proximal disc. Advancing the sheath until it abuts the disc allows the prosthesis to be held in place while the knuckle is freed.

4 Dislodgment could also occur if the arterial catheter (used for angiography) snagged the aortic disc as it is withdrawn past the duct at the end of the procedure. A guide wire should be positioned in the arch or ascending aorta and all catheter withdrawal should be over this guide. A straight (e.g. Gensini or cut-off pigtail) may be used.

5 In order to cross a PDA the dilator/long sheath assembly should have a 90° terminal curve; the preset curve can be modified to 90° by moulding in boiling water. Similarly a 15° curve should be imparted to the delivery wire so that it lies smoothly within the natural curve of the duct. The T-spring locking device can be used to orientate the wire and the fat part of the b-knuckle should point towards the patient's back.

6 Early experience with the device included instances of partial closure. In order to reduce the incidence of residual shunts, Wessel [52] advises that the patient is not heparinised and the prosthesis is soaked in topical thrombin before use. 'Tamponading' the duct for a few minutes by advancing an inflated balloon against the proximal disc to reduce flow may also promote clot formation. To allow for clot formation, 15 minutes should elapse after the device has been released before aortography is performed to check on satisfactory closure.

7 Correct positioning of the prosthesis is crucial; as a rule the duct will be centred over the trachea on the lateral projection. Obviously preliminary aortography is mandatory in order that duct size, morphology and position can be determined before a decision is made about suitability for transcatheter closure. Note, however, that the presence of the long sheath dilator or the occluding device can alter the position of the duct — check by repeated test injections.

The development of an increasing variety of catheter-transportable devices opens up many possible uses. Partial pulmonary valvuloplasty may improve pulmonary flow in mixing situations (e.g. univentricular atrioventricular connection) with pulmonary stenosis without leading to pulmonary vascular disease and still obviating the need for a surgical shunt. A wide variety of congenital and iatrogenic cardiac lesions may be amenable to dilatation or occlusion and transcatheter closure of ASDs and ventricular septal defects (VSDs) is on the horizon. The subject has been reviewed by Fellows [42].

PERICARDIAL ASPIRATION

Although a number of alternative puncture sites have been described, the two most commonly used approaches are the xiphoid and the apical approach. Of these the xiphoid approach is more commonly used and regarded as the safer though inadvertent puncture of the thin-walled right atrium or ventricle is more hazardous than puncture of the thick-walled left ventricular apex. In practice the approach used is often dictated by the echocardiographic localisation of the major collection of pericardial fluid. It may be best to avoid the xiphoid approach in the presence of pulmonary (and right atrial and ventricular) hypertension.

The xiphoid approach

Premedication with atropine 0.6 mg (i.m. or i.v.) is advised and it is a sensible precaution to ensure that the patient's blood group is known and that cross-matched blood is available. The patient's shoulders should be supported by a pillow so that he is propped up at an angle of some 30°. The skin is cleaned and the area surrounding the chosen entry site is covered with sterile towels in the usual way. The skin is anaesthetised at the point of entry in the angle between the xiphoid process and the *left* costal margin. A small skin incision is made with the point of a no. 11 scalpel blade and the deep tissues anaesthetised using a 5 cm hypodermic needle. This and subsequent needle entry should be directed immediately beneath the left costal cartilage aiming at the left shoulder and at an angle of 30 to 40° to the frontal plane. A more vertically directed track might puncture the liver. The needle is now changed to an 8 to 10 cm long, thin-wall short bevel 18 gauge needle attached to a 10 ml syringe of 1% lidocaine. Following the same track, the tissues are slowly infiltrated with anaesthetic with intermittent suction to detect the moment of entry into the peri-cardial space. This moment may be felt as a sudden yielding sensation and will be accompanied by the aspiration of pericardial fluid. If the pericardial tap is for dignostic purposes only, fluid is aspirated into a sterile syringe and the procedure terminated. If pericardial drainage is required (e.g. for tamponade) a J-tip Teflon coated, 0.038″ guide wire is advanced through the needle until it lies free in the pericardial space. The needle is removed and a short, (25 cm long) Teflon, pigtail catheter (Fig. 3.4) advanced over the guide until it too lies well within the pericardial space. As a rule the Teflon catheter will be rigid enough to penetrate the tissues unaided, it's tip being straightened by the 0.038″ guide. Alternatively an 8F vessel dilator can be used to enlarge the track. The procedure is, of course, the standard percu-taneous, 'Seldinger' technique. The catheter can be fixed to the skin and, when aspiration is complete, connected to a sterile drainage bag for continuous drainage.

The apical approach

The position of the cardiac apex is determined by fluoroscopy in the AP projection using a metal in-strument to mark the position on the skin. The skin is anaesthetised about 2.5 cm lateral to the apex, a small incision made and the subcutaneous tissues anaesthetised exactly as for the xiphoid approach. The needle should traverse the intercostals *above* and not immediately below a rib as the intercostal arteries lie below the ribs and might be punctured. The needle is aimed at the back of the right shoulder — upwards, backwards and to the right. The course of the needle towards the apex can be checked by fluoroscopy. The rest of the procedure is exactly the same as for the xiphoid approach.

Hints

When clear straw-coloured fluid is aspirated there is little doubt that the pericardium has been entered. Problems arise when the fluid aspirated is heavily blood-stained or blood. Traditionally blood and blood-stained fluid are distinguished by (1) peri-cardial fluid does not clot — blood does, and (2) the haematocrit, pH and Po^2 of blood-stained pericardial aspirate are lower than that of the patient's mixed venous blood while the Pco^2 is higher.

But these results are not immediately available. Clues to the correct position of the needle/guide wire are:

1 A guide wire that is free within the pericardial sac will (usually) pass laterally to the left of the cardiac shadow; a right atrial or right ventricular position will be more medial. Always use fluoroscopy as an aid to the correct orientation and positioning of needles, guides and catheters.

2 The needle can be connected (via manometer tubing) to a pressure transducer and a right ven-tricular pressure trace is an indication to withdraw the needle and try again. Right atrial and pericardial pressures cannot, however, be distinguished with certainty.

3 The simplest check is to inject a little contrast medium through the needle. If the tip is in the pericardial space the contrast will be seen to pool inferiorly. If the needle is in a cardiac chamber the contrast will be seen to swirl and disappear.

The aspiration of pericardial fluid for tamponade should occupy 30 minutes or so; too rapid aspiration with a sudden increase in systemic venous return may lead to pulmonary oedema or acute right heart failure.

In the elective situation pericardial drainage can be combined with right heart catheterisation with monitoring of the haemodynamic benefit. The haemodynamic effects of cardiac tamponade are described in Chapter 16.

RETRIEVAL OF CATHETER FRAGMENTS

Catheter fracture during diagnostic catheterisation was a complication that could occur when a catheter was re-used and sterilised many times. It could also occur as the result of heat sterilisation of cardiac catheters. It is an almost unknown complication today as the result of the widespread use of disposable catheters and ethylene oxide sterilisation of re-usable catheters. Today, catheter fragments loose within the central circulation are most likely to be fragments of indwelling central venous catheters. The complication is most likely to occur with catheters that are introduced *through* a needle — the sharp bevel cuts through the catheter as it is being withdrawn. Guide wires may occasionally fracture and the fragment be lost within the circulation though safety wires should prevent this happening. All such fragments should be removed, non-surgically if possible, and a number of techniques have been developed for their transluminal recovery.

1 *Wire loop technique.* A fine (0.021'') exchange guide wire is doubled at a point 3 cm or so from its mid-point and the doubled wire passed, loop end first, through an 8F thin-wall catheter of the Cournand or Goodale–Lubin type. The catheter tip is placed near the catheter fragment and the loop extruded. If the free ends of the guide wire are now adjusted to the same length the kink that was formed when the guide wire was doubled will be with-drawn into the shaft of the catheter leaving a smooth, open loop protruding from the tip of the catheter. Attempts are then made to pass this loop over one end of the catheter fragment. If successful the catheter is advanced over the doubled wire thus trapping the fragment between the end of the catheter and the wire loop. The catheter is then withdrawn whilst keeping tension on both free ends of the guide wire. Final extraction of the fragment may require a limited cut-down at the entry site. This system has the advantage that the components are likely to be available, however unexpected the need for the procedure. A commercially available retrieval set of this type, the 'Curry intravascular retriever set' is available from Cook Incorporated (Cat. no. CRS−1) and is also available in a paediatric size (6.3F, Cat. no. CRS−2). Obviously it is only possible to remove a fragment by this technique if one end, at least, of the fragment is free and can be snared [43].

2 *Dotter intravascular retriever [44].* This device (Fig. 5.13) consists of a helical loop basket contained within an 8F catheter (Cook Incorporated Cat. no. DRS−1). Its action is very similar to the 'loop-snare' device described above; extrusion of the basket produces four wire loops and the chance of snaring the catheter

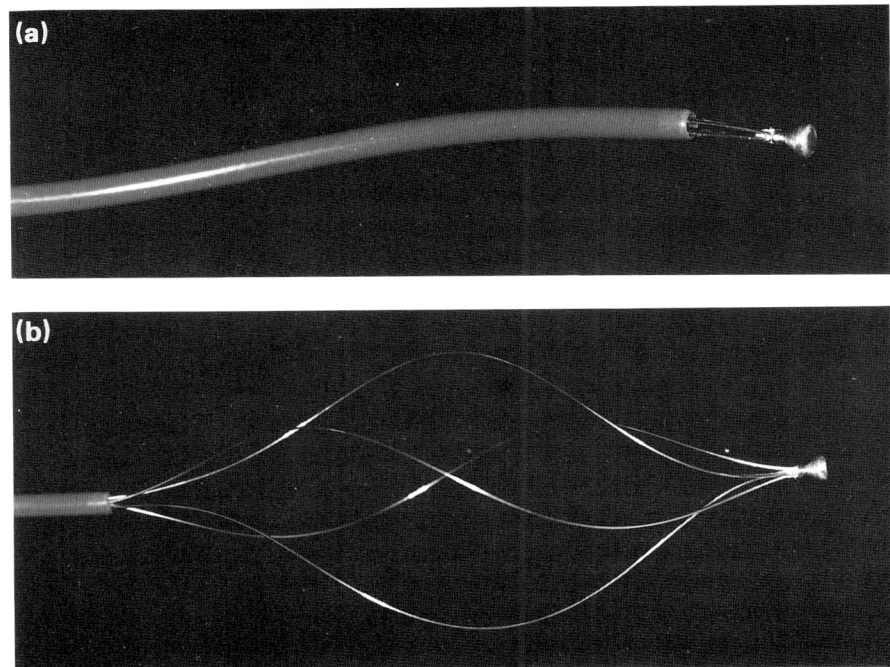

Fig. 5.13 Dotter intravascular retriever. (a) The helical basket is sheathed within the delivery catheter. (b) The basket has been advanced. When the catheter fragment has been snared, the basket is withdrawn to the original position (a), thus trapping the fragment and allowing retrieval.

fragment is thus improved. Again the technique will usually only succeed if an end of the fragment is free and can be snared.

3 Biopsy forceps can be used to grip a catheter fragment — providing it is not too thick — and may succeed when there is no free end of the fragment to be snared. Special gripping forceps are available (Cook Incorporated).

4 When the fragment is in a vessel, and not a cardiac chamber, a Fogarty or other balloon-tipped catheter can be manipulated past the fragment. If the balloon is then inflated it may be possible to draw the fragment back to a position from which it can be retrieved by a cut-down. Introducer sheaths can become detached from the hub and may still be accessible and removed by this technique.

The results of non-surgical catheter retrieval have been reviewed by Bloomfield [45].

ACKNOWLEDGEMENT

I am greatly indebted to Dr J. E. Lock, The Childrens Hospital, Boston, USA for reviewing the section on the use of the PDA occluder.

GENERAL READING

Lock JE, Keane JF, Fellows KE. *Diagnostic and interventional catheterization in congenital heart disease.* Boston, Martinus Nijhoff Publishing, 1987.
Abele JE. Balloon catheters and transluminal dilatation: technical considerations. *AJR* 1980;**135**:901.

REFERENCES

1 Rashkind WJ, Miller WW. Creation of an atrial septal defect without thoracotomy: palliative approach to complete transposition of the great arteries. *JAMA* 1966;**196**:991.
2 Park SC *et al.* A new atrial septostomy technique. *Cathet Cardiovasc Diagn* 1975;**1**:195.
3 Park SC *et al.* Clinical use of blade atrial septostomy. *Circulation* 1978;**58**:600.
4 Park SC *et al.* Blade atrial septostomy: collaborative study. *Circulation* 1982;**66**:258.
5 Kan JS, White RI, Mitchell SE, Gardener TJ. Percutaneous balloon valvuloplasty: a new method of treating con-

genital pulmonary valve stenosis. *New Engl J Med* 1982;**307**:540.
6 Pepine CJ, Gessner IH, Feldman RL. Percutaneous balloon valvuloplasty for pulmonic valve stenosis in the adult. *Am J Cardiol* 1982;**50**:1442.
7 Radke W *et al.* Percutaneous balloon valvotomy of congenital pulmonary stenosis using oversized balloons. *J Am Coll Cardiol* 1986;**8**:909.
8 Kan JS *et al.* Percutaneous transluminal balloon valvuloplasty for pulmonary valve stenosis. *Circulation* 1984;**69**:554.
9 Lababidi Z, Wu J-R, Walls JT. Percutaneous balloon aortic valvuloplasty; results in 23 patients. *Am J Cardiol* 1984;**53**:194.
10 Cribier A *et al.* Percutaneous transluminal valvuloplasty of acquired aortic stenosis in elderly patients: an alternative to valve replacement? *Lancet* 1986;**1**:63.
11 Cribier A *et al.* Percutaneous transluminal balloon valvuloplasty of adult aortic stenosis: report of 92 cases. *J Am Coll Cardiol* 1987;**9**:381.
12 McKay RG *et al.* Balloon dilatation of calcific aortic stenosis in elderly patients: postmortem, intraoperative, and percutaneous valvuloplasty studies. *Circulation* 1986;**74**:119.
13 Dorros G, Lewin RF, King JF, Janke LM. Percutaneous transluminal valvuloplasty in calcific aortic stenosis: the double balloon technique. *Cathet Cardiovasc Diagn* 1987;**13**:151.
14 Waller BF, Girod DA, Dillon JC. Transverse aortic wall tears in infants after balloon angioplasty for aortic stenosis: relation of aortic wall damage to diameter of inflated angioplasty balloon and aortic lumen in seven necropsy cases. *J Am Coll Cardiol* 1984;**4**:1235.
15 Helgason H *et al.* Balloon dilatation of the aortic valve: studies in normal lambs and in children with aortic stenosis. *J Am Coll Cardiol* 1987;**9**:816.
16 Safian RD *et al.* Postmortem and intraoperative balloon valvuloplasty of calcific aortic stenosis in elderly patients: mechanisms of successful dilation. *J Am Coll Cardiol* 1987;**9**:655.
17 Lock JE *et al.* Balloon dilatation angioplasty of aortic coarctation in infants and children. *Circulation* 1983;**68**:109.
18 Lababidi, Z, Daskalopoulos DA, Stoeckle H. Transluminal balloon coarctation angioplasty. Experience with 27 patients. *Am J Cardiol* 1984;**54**:1288.
19 Finley JP, Beaulieu RG, Nanton MA, Roy DL. Balloon catheter dilatation of coarctation of the aorta in young infants. *Br Heart J* 1983;**50**:411.
20 Evans VL, Nihill MR, Yousef SA. Balloon dilatation angioplasty for coarctation of the aorta in infants. *J Am Coll Cardiol* 1986;**7**:46A.
21 Saul JP, Keane JF, Fellows KE, Lock JE. Balloon dilation angioplasty of postoperative aortic coarctation. *J Am*

Coll Cardiol 1986;**7**:117A.

22 Kan JS *et al*. Treatment of restenosis of coarctation by percutaneous transluminal angioplasty. Circulation 1983;**68**:1087.

23 Lock JE *et al*. Percutaneous catheter commissurotomy in rheumatic mitral stenosis. *New Engl J Med* 1985; **313**:1515.

24 McKay RG *et al*. Percutaneous mitral valvuloplasty in an adult patient with calcific rheumatic stenosis. *J Am Coll Cardiol* 1986;**7**:1410.

25 McKay RG *et al*. Balloon dilatation of mitral stenosis in adult patients: postmortem and percutaneous mitral valvuloplasty studies. *J Am Coll Cardiol* 1987;**9**:723.

26 Al Zaibag M, Ribeiro P, Al Kasab S. Percutaneous balloon valvotomy in tricuspid stenosis. *Br Heart J* 1987;**57**:51.

27 Lock JE *et al*. Balloon dilatation angioplasty of hypoplastic and stenotic pulmonary arteries. *Circulation* 1983;**67**:962.

28 Ring JC *et al*. Management of congenital branch pulmonary artery stenosis with balloon dilation angioplasty. Report of 52 procedures. *J Thorac Cardiovasc Surg* 1985;**90**:457.

29 Lock JE *et al*. Dilation angioplasty of congenital or operative narrowings of venous channels. *Circulation* 1984;**709**:457.

30 Miller GAH. Balloon valvuloplasty and angioplasty in congenital heart disease. *Br Heart J* 1985;**54**:285.

31 Driscoll DJ, Hesslein PS, Mullins CE. Congenital stenosis of individual pulmonary veins: clinical spectrum and unsuccessful treatment by transvenous balloon dilation. *Am J Cardiol* 1982;**49**:1767.

32 Barth KH *et al*. Embolotherapy of pulmonary arteriovenous malformations. *Radiology* 1982;**142**:599.

33 White RI *et al*. Therapeutic embolisation with detachable balloons. *Cardiovasc Intervent Radiol* 1980;**3**:229.

34 Culham JAG, Izukawa T, Burns JE, Freedom RM. Embolisation of a Blalock-Taussig shunt in a child. *AJR* 1981;**137**:413.

35 Reidy JF, Baker E, Tynan M. Transcatheter occlusion of a Blalock-Taussig shunt with a detachable balloon in a child. *Br Heart J* 1983;**50**:101.

36 Grinnell VS *et al*. Transaortic occlusion of collateral arteries to the lung by detachable valved balloons in a patient with Tetralogy of Fallot. *Circulation* 1982;**65**: 1276.

37 Chuang VP, Wallace S, Gianturco C. A new improved coil for tapered tip catheter for arterial occlusion. *Radiology* 1980;**135**:507.

38 Debrun G *et al*. Detachable balloon and calibrated-leak

balloon techniques in the treatment of cerebral vascular lesions. *J Neurosurg* 1978;**49**:635.

39 White RI *et al*. Angioarchitecture of pulmonary arteriovenous malformations: an important consideration before embolotherapy. *AJR* 1983;**140**:681.

40 Porstmann W. Closure of patent ductus arteriosus by transfemoral approach. In: Kaufman HJ (ed.) *Progress in pediatric radiology* Basel, S. Karger, 1980;264—8.

41 Rashkind W. Transcatheter closure of atrial septal defects. In: Kaufman MJ (ed.) *Progress in pediatric radiology* Basel, S. Karger, 1980;269—71.

42 Fellows KE. Therapeutic catheter procedures in congenital heart disease: current status and future prospects. *Cardiovasc Intervent Radiol* 1984;**7**:170.

43 Curry JL. Retrieval of detached intravascular catheter or guide fragments — a proposed method. *AJR* 1969; **105**:894

44 Dotter CT, Rosch J, Bilbao MK. Transluminal extraction of catheter and guide fragments from the heart and great vessels: 29 collected cases. *AJR* 1971;**111**:467.

45 Bloomfield DA. The nonsurgical removal of intracardiac foreign bodies — an international survey. *Cathet Cardiovasc Diagn* 1978;**4**:1.

46 Commeau P *et al*. Percutaneous balloon dilatation of calcific aortic valve stenosis: anatomical and haemodynamic evaluation. *Br Heart J* 1988;**59**:227.

47 Cooper RS *et al*. Angioplasty for coarctation of the aorta: long term results. *Circulation* 1987;**75**:600.

48 Porstmann W *et al*. Catheter closure of patent ductus arteriosus: 62 cases treated without thoracotomy. *Radiol Clin North Am* 1971;**9**:203.

49 Rashkind WJ, Cuaso CC. Transcatheter closure of patent ductus: successful use in a 3.5 kg infant. *Pediatr Cardiol* 1979;**1**:63.

50 Rashkind WJ, Mullins CE, Hellenbrand WE, Tait MA. Nonsurgical closure of patent ductus arteriosus: clinical application of the Rashkind PDA Occluder System. *Circulation* 1987;**75**:583.

51 Lock JE *et al*. Transcatheter umbrella closure of congenital heart defects. *Circulation* 1987;**75**:593.

52 Wessel DL, Keane JF, Parness I, Lock JE. Outpatient closure of the patent ductus arteriosus. *Circulation* 1988;**77**:1068.

53 Bash SE, Mullins CE. Insertion of patent ductus occluder by trans-venous approach: a new technique. *Circulation* 1984;**70** (suppl II):II—285.

54 Kitamura S *et al*. Plug closure of patent ductus arteriosus by transfemoral catheter method. A composite study with surgery and a new technical modification. *Chest* 1976;**70**:631.

CHAPTER 6

The measurement of pressure and of oxygenation

THE MEASUREMENT OF PRESSURE

A fluid-filled catheter/manometer system is used for almost all routine diagnostic studies. In such a system the column of fluid (blood, saline) within the catheter transmits the pressure at the catheter-tip to the pressure transducer. The fluid is in contact with a stiff diaphragm within the transducer; changes in pressure cause the diaphragm to be displaced and this displacement generates an electrical signal which is amplified and then displayed or recorded on a suitable strip-chart recorder.

While adequate for most purposes such a fluid-filled system has some disadvantages. When pressure is applied to such a system the fluid within the system will oscillate due to the compliance of the catheter and connecting tubing and displacement of the diaphragm. The frequency of oscillation is the 'resonant (natural) frequency' of the system. Should the input (pressure) signal approach the resonant frequency of the system the output signal will be considerably amplified and the recorded signal will exceed the true pressure. In practice the oscillations of the fluid are damped as their energy is dissipated by friction within the system. In addition recording systems incorporate electronic damping circuits — usually with selectable degrees of damping. 'Optimal damping' for routine diagnostic purposes is obtained when the amplitude of the recorded signal matches the amplitude of the input signal up to frequencies of 20 Hz — the system is 'flat to 20 Hz'. Thereafter the ability of the system to accurately record higher frequencies is significantly impaired and an alternative recording system has to be employed. Thus for accurate measurement of the rate of change of pressure with time (dp/dt) a frequency response which is 'flat to 100 Hz' is needed and a catheter has to be used which does not rely on a column of fluid to transmit the pressure signal. Such catheters include those with a miniaturised pressure sensitive transducer mounted at the tip of the catheter — 'catheter-tip manometers'.

Recording systems which are used in catheterisation laboratories are designed for the purpose and the operator does not, as a rule, need to worry about the characteristics of the various components of the system. Those that are interested in more detail are referred to other texts such as *Principles of Clinical Measurement* [6]. However it is important that the operator recognises that the adequacy of the records obtained depends on the characteristics *of the whole system* — the catheter used, the presence of blood or air bubbles within the catheter or behind the membrane of a disposable transducer dome can all affect, profoundly, the performance of the system. Some of the errors that can creep in need special mention, therefore.

Zero errors. At the beginning of a study all the pressure transducers must be placed at the 'zero reference level' — usually mid-chest — and the transducer domes opened to atmospheric pressure. If the patient's position is changed during the study, for example if he is propped up on pillows, the position of the transducers must be re-adjusted and the system re-zeroed. At the same time the linearity of the system is checked using a column of fluid of adjustable height to provide hydraulic calibration; it is not sufficient to rely on the electrical calibration system provided by most commercial recording systems. 'Zero drift' can occur with time or as a result in temperature change and it is wise to check the zeroing and calibration of the system (hydraulically) whenever small gradients are being measured — at the tricuspid and mitral valves, for example.

'Catheter whip' and 'impact' artefact. Movement of the catheter within the heart and great vessels and intracardiac structures hitting the shaft of the catheter can both cause acceleration of the column of fluid within the catheter generating an artefactual signal that may be as much as 10 mmHg, in amplitude. These artefacts are difficult to avoid and are particularly liable to occur when the catheter is within the right ventricle or pulmonary artery or when its tip is within the left ventricle. Increasing the degree of electronic damping or damping the system by withdrawing blood into the catheter may help.

'End pressure artefact'. When blood flow ceases (e.g. during diastole) the kinetic energy of the flowing blood is converted into pressure and an artefactual pressure will be generated if an endhole catheter is being used with its tip pointing upstream; this is one reason for choosing catheters with side-holes (Goodale–Lubin or angiographic catheters).

'Over-' and 'under-damping'. Most importantly the operator must recognise over- and under-damping (Figs 6.1 to 6.3). These problems are inseparable from fluid-filled catheter-manometer systems. Even if everything has been done, in advance of the study, to ensure that the system is optimally damped ('flat to 20 Hz') the record obtained may be over- or under-damped. Different catheters are used, blood is present in the catheter and so on. The operator must recognise the exaggerated artefact of an under-damped tracing; even more importantly he must recognise an over-damped tracing. Over-damping causes smoothing and under-recording of atrial and arterial traces but is most easily recognised from the diastolic portion of ventricular tracings. Ventricular diastole becomes a smooth, downward, curve without a clearly identifiable early diastolic dip and end-diastolic point and a wave. Larger (no. 7 or 8F) catheters are less liable to cause both under- and over-damping than are the smaller sizes. Under-damping may be improved if contrast medium or blood is deliberately allowed to remain in the catheter. Most recording systems allow the amount of damping to be adjusted; this should be done until the record 'looks right'. Changing the position of the catheter within the chamber may improve the situation by removing whip, end-pressure and impact artefact. If all else fails subsequent analysis

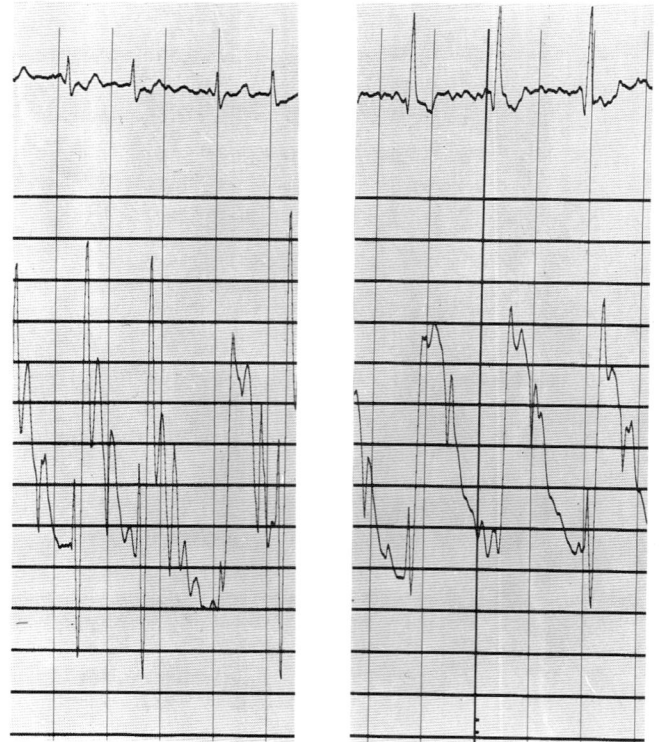

Fig. 6.1 Damping. Two records of pulmonary artery pressure; in the left-hand panel there are a series of high-frequency spikes characteristic of motion artefact in an under-damped recording. The record shown in the right-hand panel was obtained a few moments later after a blood sample had been withdrawn through the catheter. The quality of this second recording is much improved; simply drawing blood through a catheter can increase damping and improve an under-damped record.

of the pressure record should disregard the high-frequency, narrow, spikes that are characteristic of artefact.

Over-damping *must* be cured. Steps include careful inspection for air bubbles — not forgetting to check that there is fluid behind a disposable transducer-dome — and flushing the catheter or withdrawing blood to exclude bubbles or blood clot. Any suggestion of thrombus formation is an indication for heparinisation if this is not already part of the routine protocol. Manometer tubing (and the catheter) should be as short as possible. A fluid leak is another possibility — discard the defective equipment. If possible change the catheter to one of a larger internal diameter; no. 5F catheters often cause problems with over-damping, no. 4F almost always do. Finally check

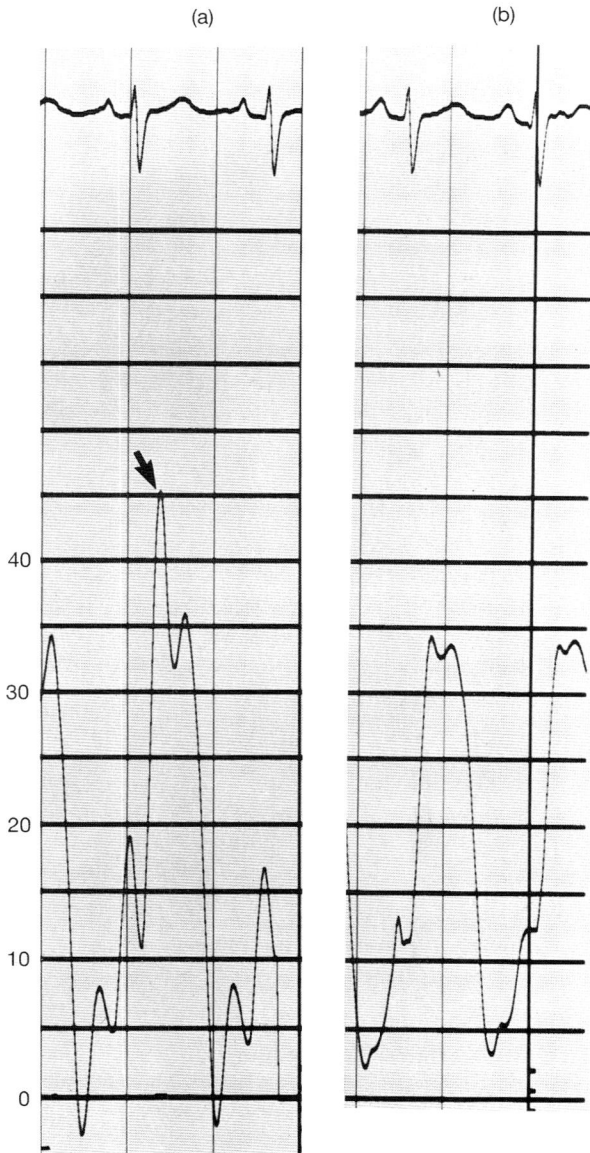

Fig. 6.2 Damping. Two recordings of right ventricular pressure; that shown in the left-hand panel is under-damped and a high-frequency spike (arrow) due to motion artefact makes right ventricular systolic pressure appear to be 45 mmHg. Damping was increased (electronically) and the recording repeated — right-hand panel. The true right ventricular systolic pressure is seen to be 34 mmHg, at the same time the sub-zero early diastolic pressure dip seen in the left-hand recording has been removed — it too was due to under-damping.

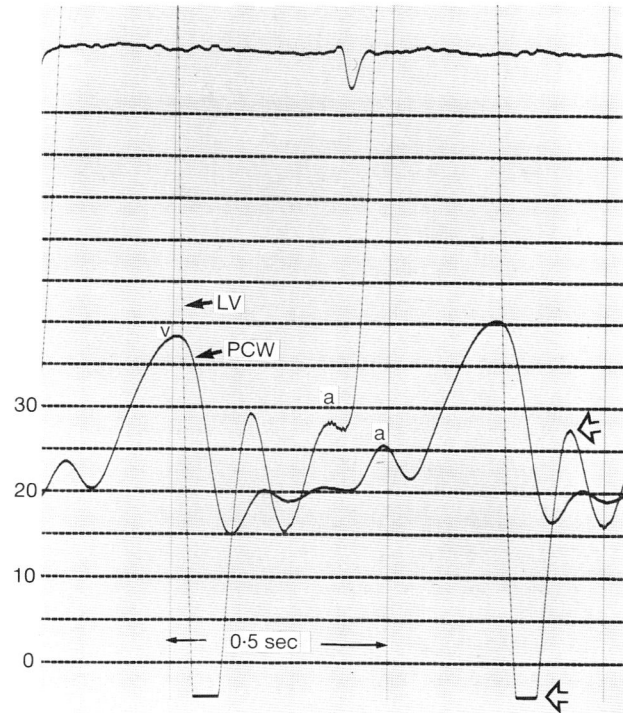

Fig. 6.3 Damping. Superimposed wedge (PCW) and left ventricular (LV) pressures recorded on the same scale. Wedge pressures are, almost inevitably, damped and this results in both diminished amplitude and delay (phase shift) of the pressure waves. Inspection of the a wave in the wedge pressure record shows it to be some 3 mmHg lower and delayed by 0.1 second and as compared with that recorded from the left ventricle. The left ventricular pressure recording is probably under-damped as evidenced by the sub-zero early diastolic dip followed by a rebound wave (open arrows).

that the recording technician has not, inadvertently, set the damping level too high.

Respiratory 'swing'. This is a problem if there is airways obstruction; for example in patients with obstructive airways disease (Fig. 6.4). A steady tracing can be obtained by asking the patient to stop breathing for a few moments. It is our practice to ignore, during pressure curve analysis, the short inspiratory pressure dips and to measure the record during the more prolonged, higher pressure, periods of expiration.

'Non-phasic' wedge pressure. Such a pressure is an unreliable indication of left atrial pressure. Attempts should be made to obtain a phasic record — perhaps by repositioning the catheter elsewhere in the pulmonary arterial tree.

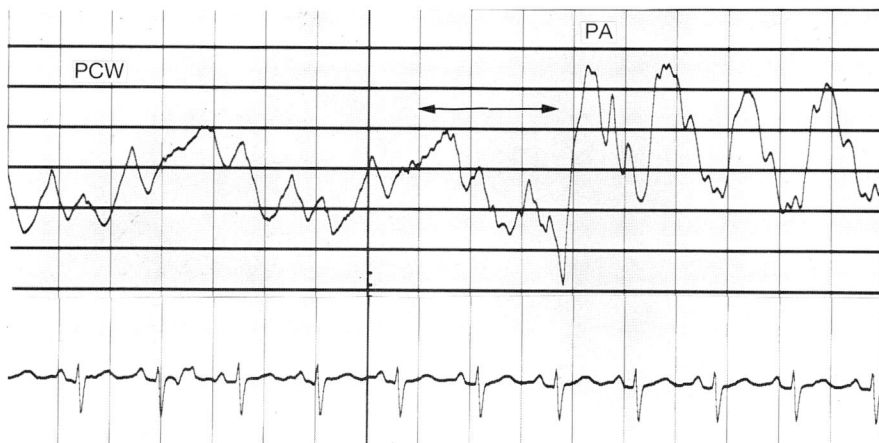

Fig. 6.4 Wedge pressure. At the left-hand end of this pressure recording there are two positive deflections (a and v waves) in each cardiac cycle characteristic of an atrial pressure. Artefact is superimposed between the arrows as the operator touches the catheter and pulls it from the wedged position until the tip is free within the pulmonary artery. At this point there is an *abrupt* change to an arterial waveform. These two features confirm that a valid record of the wedge pressure was being obtained. Note also the low frequency (every 5 seconds) variation in the wedge pressure due to changes in intrathoracic pressure ('respiratory swing'); respiratory swing is most marked in patients with obstructive airways disease.

THE DIAGNOSTIC USE OF PRESSURE RECORDS

During cardiac catheterisation the pressure trans-mitted from the tip of the catheter, together with the ECG, is continuously displayed on an oscilloscope. This display is in front of the operator and should be immediately beside the fluoroscopic display. The two displays enable the operator to see the position of the catheter within the heart or great vessels and, at the same time, to see the waveform and amplitude of the pressure at the catheter tip. The pressure trace provides help and diagnostic information in four ways:

1 *Waveform* (with amplitude). Since different wave-forms are obtained from within the atrium, ventricle and artery, the operator knows in which of the three possible sites the catheter tip is located — information that is not necessarily apparent from the fluoroscopic image (Fig. 6.5). Thus an atrial waveform indicates that the tip of the catheter is in the right or left atrium, the great veins or pulmonary veins or the coronary sinus. The amplitude may distinguish between right and left heart structures — certainly so if the two pressures are markedly different (Fig. 6.6).

A ventricular waveform (Figs 6.7 and 6.8) indicates that the catheter has entered right or left (or a single) ventricle and the amplitude may distinguish right from left — not always, however. An arterial trace (Fig. 6.9) indicates entry to the pulmonary or systemic

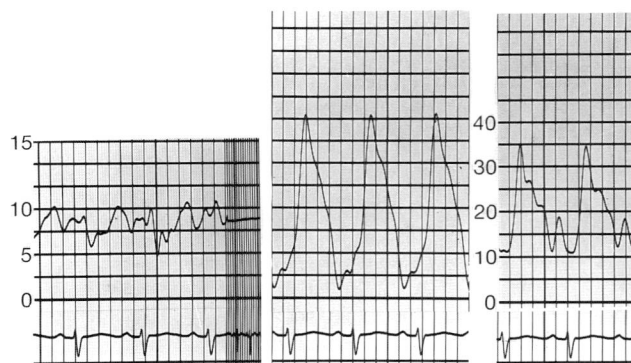

Fig. 6.5 Waveform as an indicator of catheter tip position. Right heart catheterisation recording, in sequence, an atrial pressure tracing showing a and v waves (left-hand panel), a ventricular pressure tracing from the right ventricle (middle panel) and an arterial pressure tracing from the pulmonary artery (right-hand panel).

circulation and, again, the amplitude may distinguish the two.

2 *Amplitude*. By itself the amplitude of the displayed pressure provides some diagnostic information. This may serve either to suggest a group of diagnostic possibilities or to exclude them. Thus a right ven-tricular systolic pressure of, say, 100 mmHg, may be due to right ventricular outflow obstruction, a ven-tricular septal defect (VSD) or many other possibilities but excludes a normal heart, uncomplicated atrial septal defect (ASD) and so on. Normal values for intracardiac pressures are given in Table 6.1.

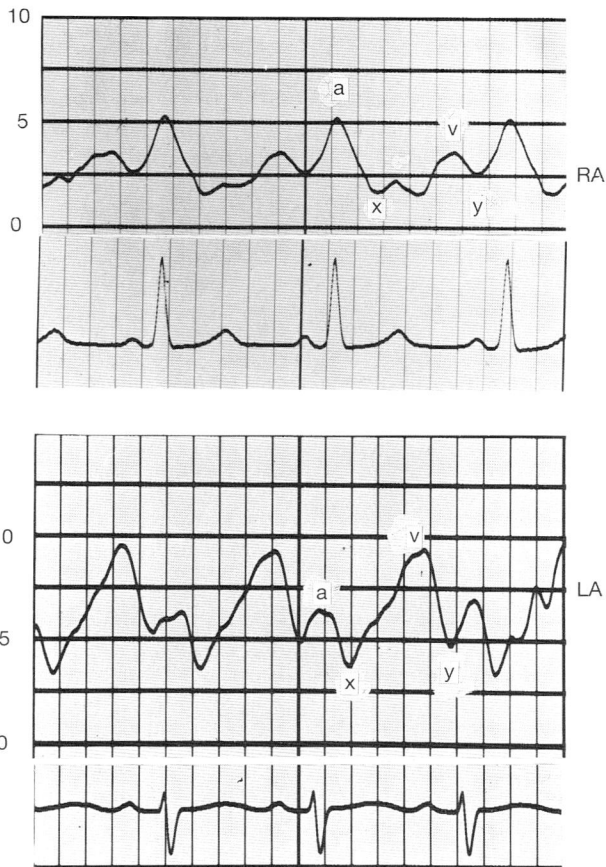

Fig. 6.6 Normal right (upper panel) and left (lower panel) atrial pressure records. Right atrial pressure is lower than the left atrial pressure and the a wave is dominant. The left atrial tracing exhibits a dominant v wave.

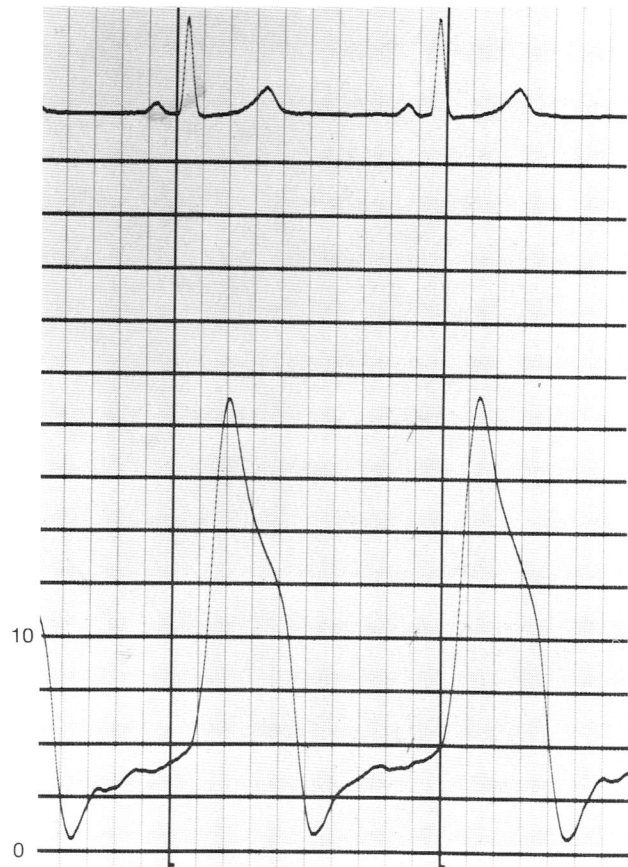

Fig. 6.7 Normal right ventricular pressure record. The systolic pressure is less than 30 mmHg and the waveform tends to be triangular. There is an early diastolic pressure which approaches zero and an end-diastolic pressure of less than 8 mmHg.

3 *Differential pressures.* The comparison between two pressures provides more information. Thus in the above example a pulmonary artery pressure of 15 mmHg while right ventricular pressure is 100 mmHg establishes right ventricular outflow obstruction (RVOTO) as the cause of the high right ventricular pressure. If pulmonary artery pressure is also 100 mmHg RVOTO is excluded but a VSD remains a possibility and more information will be needed to establish the diagnosis. It is the difference between two pressures, valve gradients for example, that enable us to quantify the severity of valve stenosis or to determine that an interatrial or interventricular communication must be small. Examples showing how comparison between two pressures is used to provide diagnostic information are shown in Figs 6.10 to 6.16.

4 *Abnormalities of waveform.* Perhaps surprisingly abnormalities of waveform are not very helpful in establishing the diagnosis. Certainly abnormalities of waveform may be recognised and may be associated with specific lesions; but there are many pitfalls and exceptions so that waveform analysis, by itself, is usually no more than a pointer towards a possible diagnosis.

The normal waveforms and the abnormal patterns that may be observed are described below.

WAVEFORMS

Right and left atrium

Normal right and left atrial pressure records display three positive deflections; 'a wave', 'c wave'

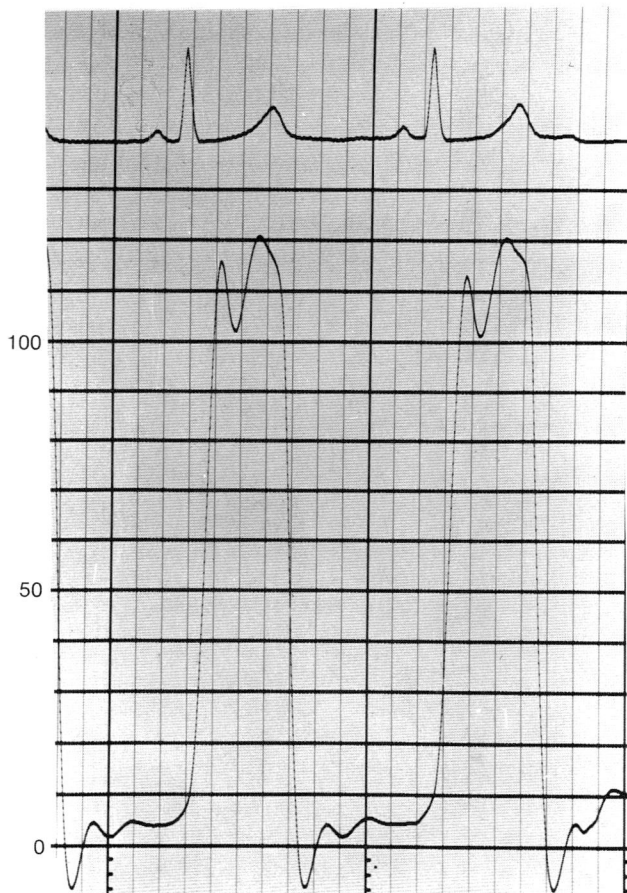

Fig. 6.8 Normal left ventricular pressure record. The waveform is more rectangular than is that obtained from the right ventricle. This record is slightly under-damped.

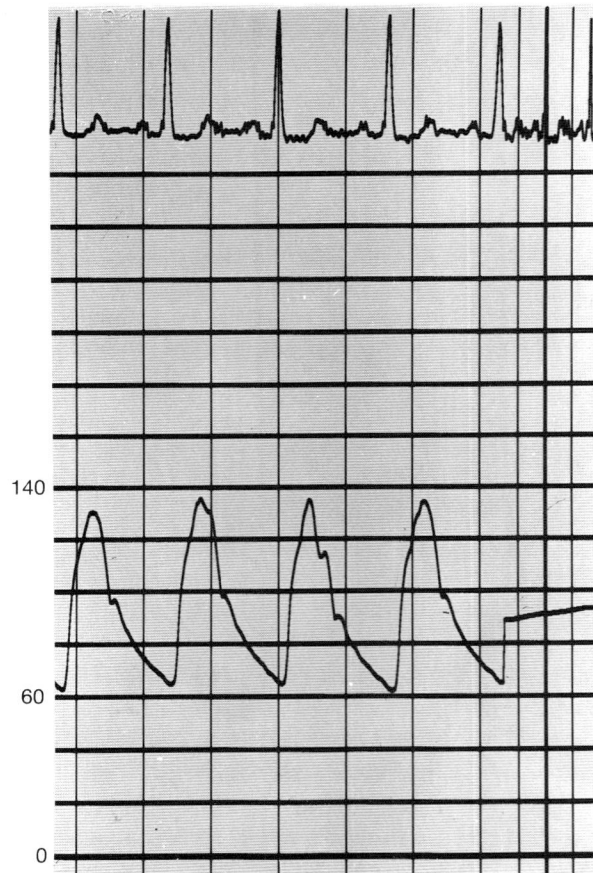

Fig. 6.9 Normal aortic pressure record. There is a rapid upstroke and the downstroke is interrupted by the dicrotic notch at the time of aortic valve closure. At the end of the phasic record electronic damping is increased to provide a record of *mean* aortic pressure.

and 'v wave', and three corresponding negative deflections; 'x descent', 'x'descent' and 'y descent' (Fig. 6.6). The a wave is due to atrial contraction (atrial systole); it begins at the apex of the P wave of the electrocardiogram and is followed by the x descent which is synchronous with atrial relaxation. Although atrial pressure is declining the atrium is filling (with the atrioventricular valve closed) from the capacitance vessels of the venous system. The x descent may be interrupted by a small positive deflection, the c wave which is synchronous with isovolumic ventricular contraction and, therefore, with the R wave of the electrocardiogram. The c wave is thought to be due to upward bulging of the tricuspid valve at this time. The c wave is followed

by the x descent; if there is no c wave the post-a-descent is labelled simply as the x descent. The x descent is interrupted by a positive deflection, the v wave which is due to continued atrial filling while the tricuspid valve is closed during ventricular systole. Finally, during early ventricular diastole, the ventricular pressure falls below the atrial pressure, the atrioventricular valve opens, blood leaves the atrium, rapidly, and the v wave is interrupted by the y descent. The y descent occurs soon after the T wave of the electrocardiogram. Normally the right atrial a wave is higher than the v wave; the reverse is true of left atrial pressure (Fig. 6.6). In the normal heart the right atrial a and v waves measure 2 to 8 mmHg and the mean right-atrial pressure is less

Table 6.1 Normal values for intracardiac pressures.

	mmHg	Range
Right atrium		
'a'	6	1—5
'v'	5	2—8
Mean	3	1—5
Right ventricle		
Systolic	25	15—30
End-diastolic	4	1—8
Pulmonary artery		
Systolic	25	15—30
Diastolic	9	5—12
Mean	15	9—16
Pulmonary arterial wedge (PCW)		
Mean	9	5—13
Left atrium		
'a'	10	4—16
'v'	13	6—21
Mean	8	2—12
Left ventricle		
Systolic	130	90—140
End-diastolic	9	5—12
Aorta		
Systolic	100—140	
Diastolic	60—90	
Mean	70—105	

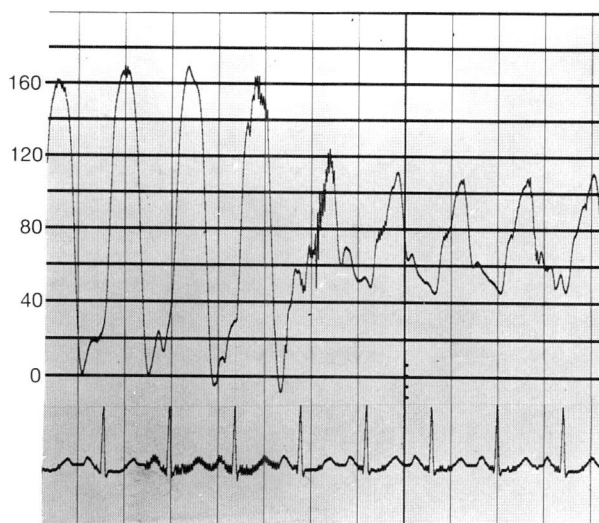

Fig. 6.10 Comparison between two pressure records: aortic valve stenosis. The catheter is withdrawn from the left ventricle to the aorta. There is a pressure drop of 50 mmHg as the waveform changes from a ventricular to an arterial tracing thus establishing that the site of obstruction is at valve level. Note the slow upstroke of the aortic pressure tracing, with an anacrotic notch and high frequency vibrations superimposed due to turbulence — often felt by the operator when he holds the catheter.

than 5 mmHg. In the left atrium the a and v waves may reach 16 mmHg and the mean pressure is 12 mmHg or less (Table 6.1).

Abnormal right and left atrial waveforms

1 *Arrhythmias.* Since the a wave represents atrial contraction it is absent in patients with atrial fibrillation. Complete heart block creates 'cannon waves' in the atrial pressure trace.

2 *Reduced ventricular compliance, atrial hypertrophy.* Prominent a waves suggest that there is powerful atrial contraction and the commonest cause is that the corresponding ventricle is hypertrophied and less compliant than usual (Fig. 6.17). In the right atrium this is most commonly seen when there is right ventricular outflow obstruction (e.g. pulmonary stenosis) and an intact ventricular septum. In the left atrium, aortic stenosis or hypertrophic cardiomyopathy are the commonest causes.

3 *Atrioventricular valve stenosis.* Mitral or tricuspid stenosis result in slow emptying of the corresponding atria; as a result the y-descent is prolonged (Fig. 6.15). The relationship between the height of the v wave and the duration of the y descent has been used to assess the relative degrees of mitral stenosis and incompetence [1] (see Chapter 15). More importantly a diastolic gradient develops between the atrium and ventricle. Normally there is rapid equalisation of atrial and ventricular pressure during early diastole. Normally the a wave is freely transmitted to the ventricle with no gradient between the atrial and ventricular a waves. This is not so when there is significant atrioventricular valve stenosis. The magnitude of the gradient is one variable in the calculation of valve area and the assessment of valve stenosis (see Chapter 15). Tricuspid stenosis is difficult to detect and may require a double-catheter (or twin-lumen catheter) technique; significant tricuspid stenosis is likely to be present when there is a mean diastolic gradient of 4—8 mmHg and a calculated valve area of less than 1.3 cm^2.

(a)   Aortic valve stenosis

(b)   Subvalvar stenosis

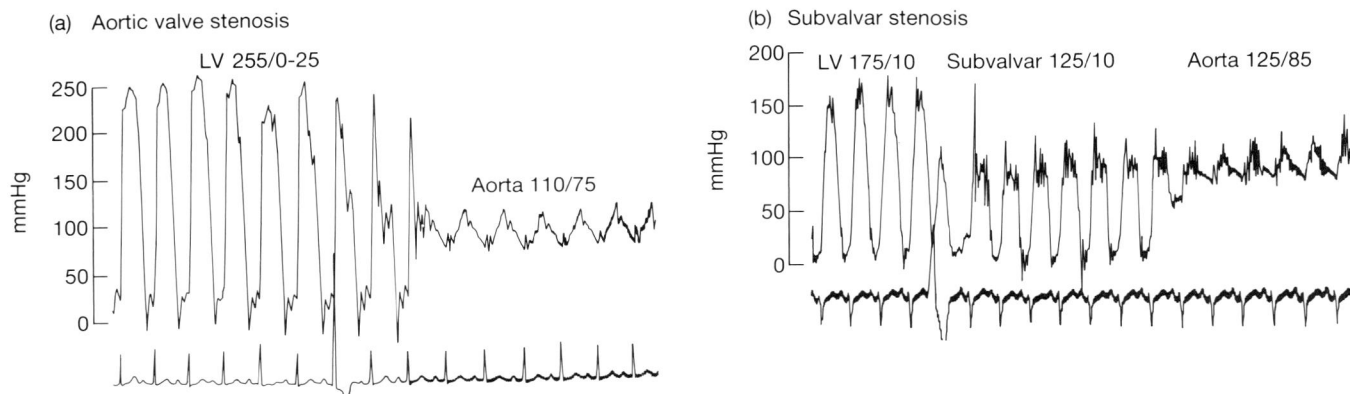

Fig. 6.11 Comparison between two pressures: records obtained during withdrawal of the catheter from the left ventricle to the aorta in (a) valvar and (b) subvalvar aortic stenosis. In subvalvar obstruction the pressure drop occurs at a time when the waveform is still that of a ventricle. No further fall in systolic pressure occurs as the catheter crosses the valve and the waveform changes to an arterial tracing.

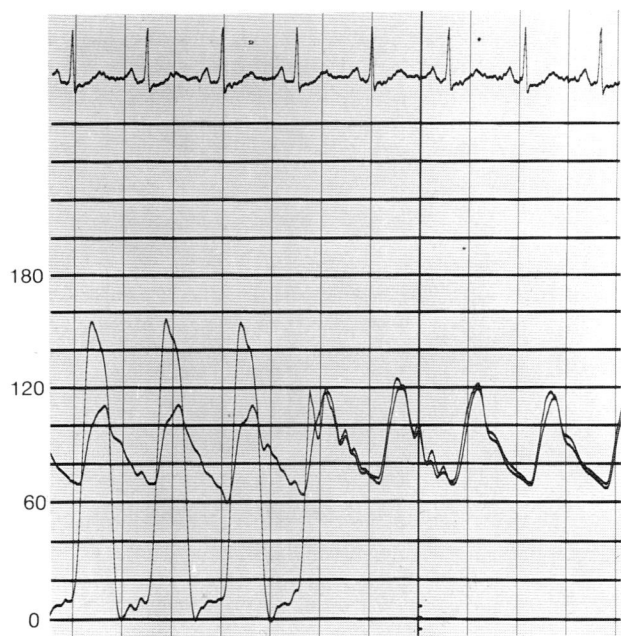

Fig. 6.12 Comparison between two pressures: aortic valve stenosis. At the left-hand end of the record simultaneous left ventricular and femoral artery pressures are being recorded, the left ventricular systolic pressure exceeds that in the femoral artery by some 45 mmHg. As the catheter is withdrawn from the ventricle the waveform changes to an arterial (aortic) waveform as the pressure drops thus establishing the diagnosis of aortic *valve* stenosis. Note that, with the catheter in the aorta, the arterial pressure rises and the true gradient is seen to be less than previously supposed — suggesting that the presence of a catheter across the valve had increased the degree of obstruction at the aortic valve.

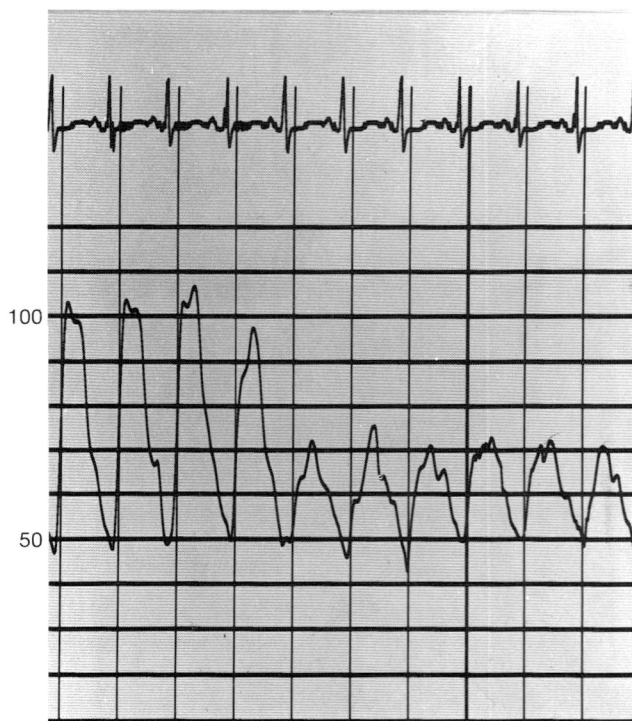

Fig. 6.13 Comparison between two pressures: coarctation of the aorta. The catheter is withdrawn from ascending to descending aorta and a pressure drop occurs as it crosses the coarctation.

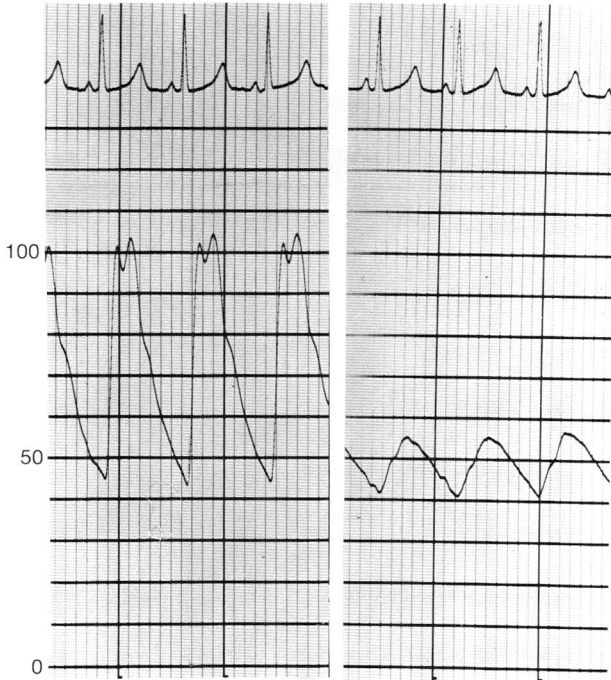

Fig. 6.14 Comparison between two pressures: coarctation. Left-hand panel: ascending aorta. Right-hand panel: descending aorta. Note the damped appearance of the descending aortic pressure with a slow upstroke and delayed (as well as lower) peak pressure as compared with the ascending aortic pressure.

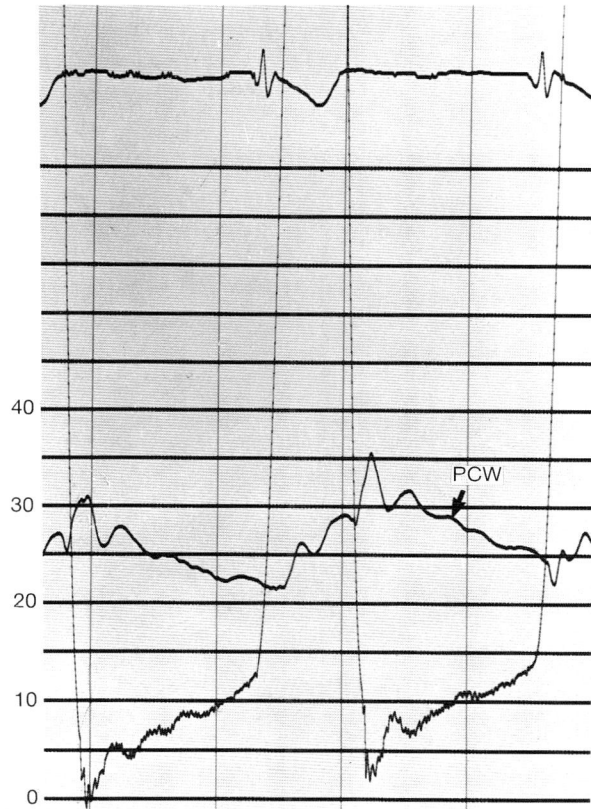

Fig. 6.15 Comparison between two pressures: severe mitral stenosis. The wedge (PCW) and left ventricular pressures are superimposed and recorded at the same sensitivity. There is a considerable gradient between the two pressures throughout diastole. Note the slow y descent in the wedge pressure tracing.

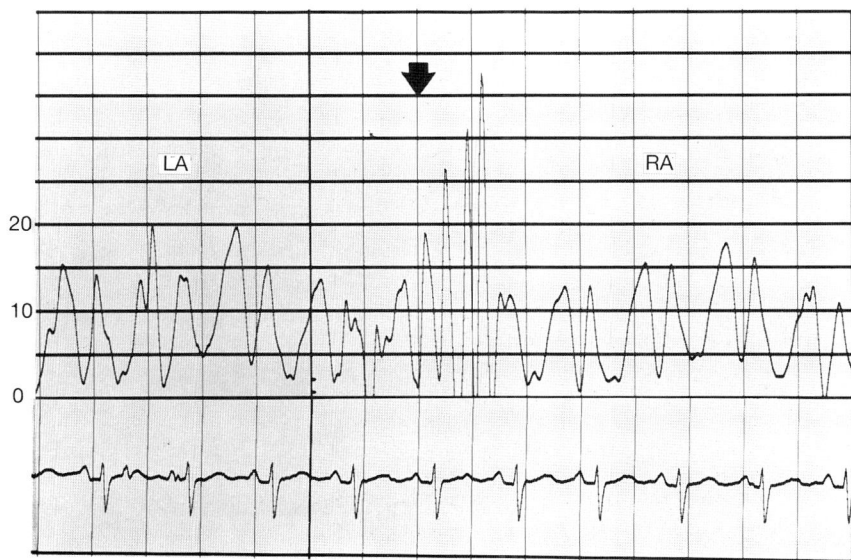

Fig. 6.16 Comparison between two pressures: atrial septal defect. The catheter has been withdrawn from the left (LA) to the right (RA) atrium. The two pressures are identical (left atrial pressure is normally higher) suggesting a free communication between the two atria. High frequency artefact is seen at the point (arrow) when the operator first touches the catheter to withdraw it from the left atrium.

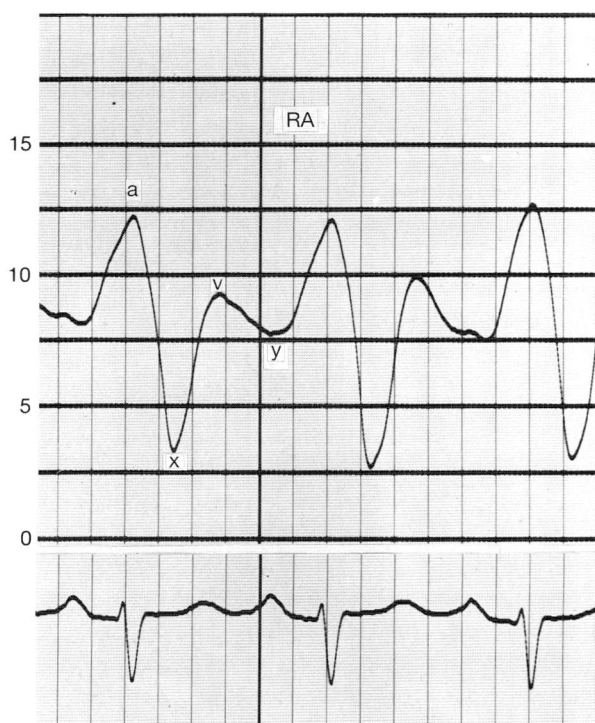

Fig. 6.17 Abnormalities of waveform. Right atrial pressure recording from a patient with severe (primary) pulmonary hypertension. There is a dominant, 12 mmHg, a wave characteristic of conditions with right ventricular hypertrophy and reduced ventricular compliance.

4 *Atrioventricular valve regurgitation.* This results in a systolic S wave in the atrial pressure trace. This wave begins earlier than the normal v wave and blends with it; indeed it is commonly referred to simply as the v wave. In severe tricuspid regurgitation the right atrial pressure trace may be almost indistinguishable from the right ventricular tracing. Severe mitral regurgitation also creates a large v wave — particularly if the left atrium is small or non-compliant as can occur in chordal or papillary muscle rupture. However there is a poor correlation between the height of the v wave and the severity of mitral regurgitation (see Chapter 15).

5 *Pericardial constriction and cardiomyopathy.* In these conditions the form of the atrial and ventricular diastolic pressure traces is of great diagnostic importance. The subject is discussed and pressure records are illustrated in Chapter 16.

6 *The indirect left atrial or 'wedge' pressure.* Left atrial pressure can be obtained if there is an ASD or patent foramen ovale (PFO) or may be obtained by retrograde catheterisation from the left ventricle. Often, however, the 'pulmonary capillary wedge pressure', or 'wedge pressure' is used as an approximation. In most patients, those with severe pulmonary vascular disease being the exception, the wedge pressure reflects the left atrial pressure with reasonable accuracy. A 'good' wedge pressure should be phasic; that is a and v waves with the corresponding x and y descents should be visible — if there is sinus rhythm. The pressure should differ from pulmonary artery pressure and, on withdrawing the catheter, there should be a sharp return to the pulmonary arterial waveform (Fig. 6.4). Usually there is some slight resistance initially until the catheter suddenly springs back to the left or right pulmonary artery. If blood sampling is attempted it is either impossible or fully saturated blood is obtained. Although mean left atrial pressure is accurately recorded the amplitude of the a and v waves is usually diminished. This is due to the damping effect of pressure being transmitted through pulmonary capillaries. As always damping results in *delay* as well as reduced amplitude. This delay is usually of the order of 0.1 second and should be allowed for when wedge/left ventricular gradients are being measured. It is often possible to see that the y descent does not coincide with the early diastolic left ventricular pressure — as it should — but is delayed by 0.1 second (Fig. 6.3).

Right and left ventricular pressures

A ventricular waveform consists of: (1) a rapid filling wave in early diastole during which some 60% of inflow occurs. This is succeeded by (2) a plateau or slowly rising pressure, during which 25% of inflow occurs, up to the point of inscription of (3) the a wave when atrial contraction contributes a final 15% of inflow. Pressure then rises steeply during isometric contraction (4) to be followed by a slowing of the rate of rise and then a decrease in pressure during (5) the ejection phase. Finally pressure falls sharply during (6) isometric relaxation to reach the lowest point of the pressure trace — the early diastolic pressure (Figs 6.7 and 6.8).

It is conventional to record early diastolic pressure, end-diastolic pressure (immediately following the a-wave) and peak systolic pressure. Depending on the frequency response of the system and the heart rate it may not be possible to distinguish a 'post-a' end-diastolic pressure; in this case the end-diastolic pressure is recorded as that immediately preceding the sharp upward rise of isometric contraction coincident with the R wave of the electrocardiogram.

Ventricular pressures are most easily distinguished from arterial pressures by the near-zero early diastolic pressure — obviously different from the pulmonary or aortic diastolic pressure. Normal right ventricular end-diastolic pressure is less than 8 mmHg and systolic pressure between 15 and 30 mmHg. Left ventricular end-diastolic pressure is less than 12 mmHg and systolic pressure between 100 and 140 mmHg (significantly less in neonates and infants).

ABNORMALITIES OF RIGHT AND LEFT VENTRICULAR PRESSURE

1 *Reduced ventricular compliance.* This causes abnormalities of ventricular diastolic pressure; the abnormalities that may be seen when this is due to pericardial or myocardial disease are discussed in Chapter 16. In addition to changes in the pattern of early filling there may be accentuation of the a wave if atrial contraction is powerful; most commonly seen in patients with aortic stenosis and severe left ventricular hypertrophy.

2 *Regurgitation at ventriculo-arterial valve.* As blood regurgitates into the ventricle the diastolic pressure rises steeply. In severe aortic regurgitation, left ventricular diastolic pressure may exceed the left atrial pressure resulting in premature closure of the mitral valve.

3 *Intracavity obstruction.* The characteristic abnormality produced by intracavity obstruction is a gradient which differs from that seen in valve stenosis in that the lower pressure distal to the obstruction still has a ventricular waveform (Fig. 6.11b). In the left ventricle the obstruction may be due to a fixed obstruction as in discrete, fibromuscular, subaortic stenosis. When the obstruction is dynamic, as in hypertrophic cardiomyopathy, a 'halt' on the upstroke of the ventricular pressure trace may be seen. The abnormalities of waveform associated with hypertrophic cardiomyopathy are described in Chapter 16. Intracavity obstruction of the right ventricle is common; tetralogy of Fallot being the obvious example. While it may be possible to demonstrate a low, ventricular-type, pressure beyond the infundibular stenosis (using an end-hole catheter) a severe stenosis at this site produces a low-pressure waveform of indistinct morphology.

4 *Congenital isolated hypoplasia of the right ventricle.* In this rare condition the right ventricular pressure trace is almost indistinguishable from the right atrial pressure tracing. Ventricular systole produces a narrow spike of low amplitude and the transmitted a-wave may be the dominant wave — seen in both right ventricle and pulmonary artery (Fig. 6.18).

Aortic and pulmonary arterial pressure

The normal arterial waveform begins to rise with the beginning of ejection at about the S wave of the electrocardiogram. The apex of the pressure pulse is more or less rounded and declines until interrupted by a small notch — the incisura or dicrotic notch — which signals closure of the ventriculo-arterial valve. Pressure then continues to decline more slowly, with run-off into the peripheral circulation until interrupted by the next systolic wave (Fig. 6.9).

The pressures that are reported are the highest (peak systolic) pressure, the lowest (diastolic) and the mean pressure. Mean arterial pressures are usually obtained electronically but can be calculated with reasonable accuracy from the phasic pressure trace. The mean pressure is given by the diastolic pressure plus one-third of the pulse pressure (i.e. one-third of the difference between the systolic and diastolic pressure). Normal values for systolic, diastolic and mean pulmonary artery and aortic pressures are given in Table 6.1.

It is normal for the peak peripheral arterial pressure, brachial or femoral artery for example, to exceed the peak central aortic pressure by up to 20 mmHg. This 'systolic peripheral amplification' is due to pressure waves being reflected from the peripheral vessels and branch points [2]. Although peak systolic pressure is amplified the diastolic pressure at the periphery is usually lower, the spike is narrower and the mean peripheral arterial pressure is the same as, or lower than, the mean central aortic pressure. This phenomenon is of importance; aortic valve gradients will be underestimated if left ventricular pressure is compared to peripheral arterial pressure. Aortic valve gradients must be measured between the left ventricle and the ascending aorta. Systolic amplification is most marked when left ventricular

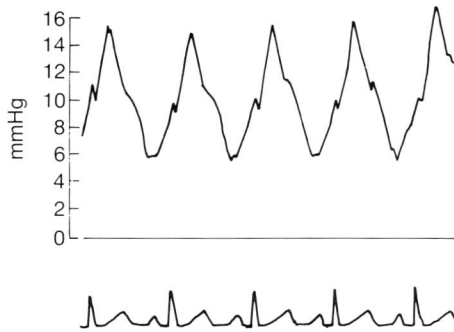

Fig. 6.18 Abnormalities of waveform. Right ventricular pressure in a patient with isolated congenital hypoplasia of the right ventricle. The transmitted a wave accounts for nearly 50% of the peak pressure and the right-ventricular contribution is a narrow spike. Systolic pressure is only 16 mmHg.

ejection is forceful and unimpaired and when peripheral resistance is high; aortic regurgitation and low output states with a constricted periphery are examples. Amplification is less when ejection is delayed; as in aortic stenosis. The combination of forceful early ejection with a halt as obstruction develops in hypertrophic obstructive cardiomyopathy gives the 'spike-and-dome' aortic pressure often seen in this condition (see Chapter 16).

In addition to amplification of the systolic pressure the onset of the upstroke of arterial pressure is progressively delayed towards the periphery.

ABNORMALITIES OF ARTERIAL WAVEFORM

1 *Aortic stenosis, pulmonary stenosis.* In aortic stenosis the rate of rise of aortic pressure is slowed and peak pressure delayed (Fig. 6.10). The rate of rise of aortic pressure depends on the heart rate but the upstroke of the aortic pressure pulse normally occupies less than 35% of ejection. In severe aortic stenosis the upstroke may occupy as much as 75% of the ejection time. Unfortunately the rate of rise of aortic pressure is an unreliable guide to the severity of aortic stenosis; in the elderly, in particular, the upstroke may be rapid despite severe aortic stenosis.

In aortic stenosis a notch appears on the upstroke — the anacrotic notch — and this is inscribed earlier as stenosis becomes more severe. High frequency vibrations may be seen on the upstroke of the pressure pulse (Fig. 6.10).

When aortic valve gradients are measured by

withdrawing the catheter from the left ventricle to the aorta it is sometimes noticed that the first one or two aortic pressure pulses are of lower amplitude than subsequent ones (Fig. 6.12). This may be because they have been preceded by a series of ectopic beats from which the output is now recovering; ectopics must not be used in gradient calculations. However this phenomenon may be present after an ectopic-free pull-back. It may be due to a venturi effect just above the valve — abolished with further pull-back — or it may be due to the catheter itself having further reduced the valve area while it was across the valve [3]. Whatever the cause aortic valve gradients must be reported by comparing left-ventricular pressure with the later higher aortic pressure pulses.

Pulmonary valve stenosis distorts the pulmonary arterial trace and makes interpretation difficult; in both aortic and pulmonary stenosis it is the *gradient* across the valve which is important in assessing severity.

2 *Aortic regurgitation.* This lesion produces a wide pulse pressure with a low aortic diastolic pressure. In severe aortic regurgitation there may be equalisation of aortic diastolic and left ventricular diastolic pressures ('diastasis') in late or even mid-diastole. Premature mitral valve closure has been mentioned above.

3 *Pulmonary regurgitation.* This is a rare lesion unless surgically induced following outflow tract reconstruction. Pulmonary arterial pressure may be difficult to distinguish from right ventricular pressure. In the syndrome of congenitally absent pulmonary valve there is usually outflow tract obstruction (stenosis) as well as pulmonary regurgitation.

4 *Peripheral pulmonary artery stenosis and pulmonary artery banding.* In these conditions pulmonary artery pressure proximal to the constriction can appear very like right ventricular pressure since diastolic pressure is very low. This finding can be a source of confusion — the catheter appears to be in the pulmonary artery, as judged by fluoroscopy, and yet the pressure still appears to be that found in the right ventricle.

5 *The effect of peripheral resistance.* A low peripheral resistance results in a wide pulse pressure. The 'run-off' due to aortic regurgitation is an example already discussed but patent ductus arteriosus (PDA), coronary-cameral fistula and other large systemic-to-pulmonary shunts are further examples.

The normal pulmonary circulation is a low resistance circulation; in large VSDs pulmonary arterial and systemic arterial *systolic* pressures are identical but, if pulmonary resistance is low, pulmonary artery *diastolic* pressure (and therefore mean pressure) is lower. As pulmonary vascular resistance rises the diastolic pressure rises until aortic and pulmonary arterial pressures are identical in both systole and diastole — a sure sign of inoperability due to severe pulmonary vascular disease.

6 *Low output states — shock.* When there is a low cardiac output, small stroke volume and intense peripheral vasoconstriction the peripheral pulse has a sharp upstroke, is of low volume (small area under the curve) and there is likely to be a tachycardia.

7 *Coarctation and supravalve aortic stenosis.* A significant coarctation results in a lower peak systolic pressure distally (gradient) with a damped pressure trace and a delayed peak pressure. Proximal to the coarctation the pulse pressure may be wide (and there may be hypertension) (Figs 6.13 and 6.14). Similar findings accompany supravalve aortic stenosis but the pressure gradient will be detected in the ascending aorta.

8 *Mitral regurgitation.* In severe mitral regurgitation, particularly when of recent onset (e.g. chordal rupture), the left atrial v wave may be so large that it is superimposed on the pulmonary arterial tracing as a second, narrow, spike. This v wave may be higher than the pulmonary artery systolic pressure but the area under the curve in the wedge pressure tracing (and therefore the mean pressure) is less.

OXYGENATION

Blood that is completely free of oxygen is dark maroon in colour and has an oxygen tension, saturation and content of zero. On exposure to air, the tension in the plasma rises and the haemoglobin changes colour as its oxygen content increases, (Fig. 6.19). The relation between tension and saturation (the oxygen dissociation curve of haemoglobin) is determined by the type of haemoglobin present. Colour is a direct index of the percent saturation of haemoglobin with oxygen but, like saturation, is mainly informative in the venous range, (P_{O_2} <60 mmHg). Above that value, wide swings in oxygen tension have little effect on saturation. Oxygen content is the product

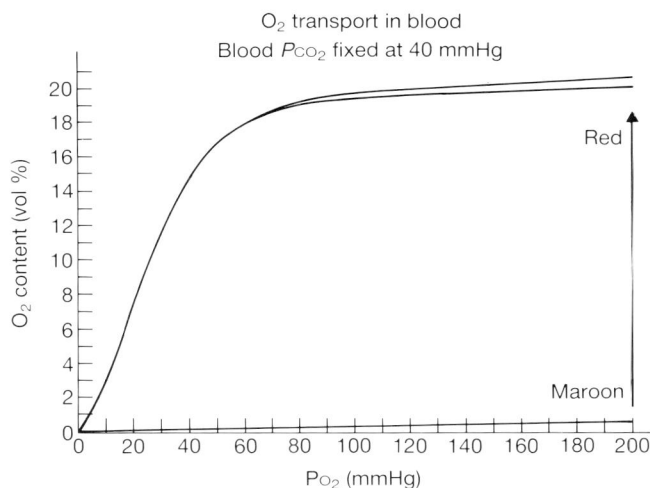

Fig. 6.19 The amount of oxygen carried in blood with a haemoglobin content of 15 gm % at a fixed P_{CO_2} of 40 mmHg. The lowermost curve shows the oxygen in simple solution, which rises linearly with P_{O_2}. The middle curve shows the amount combined with haemoglobin. The uppermost curve shows the sum of the two. The arrow to the right of the graph is a reminder that the colour change in blood is most informative over the steep part of the oxygen-dissociation curve.

of percent saturation and the total amount of haemoglobin present. Saturation, content and tension are three separate indices of blood oxygenation, with different uses in cardiology. Blood colorimeters are used to map the distribution of blood streams of differing saturations, oxygen content analysers are employed for accurate determinations of blood flows, and oxygen tension sensors are used to measure right-to-left shunts precisely.

Any such measurement is only as good as the sample on which it is based. Blood should be drawn slowly and evenly, over a period of about one minute, into tightly-fitting syringes. The syringes should be made of clear plastic or ungreased glass. Ideally, samples from arterial and venous sites should be taken simultaneously. These precautions minimise errors due to fluctuations in blood gas content with the respiratory cycle, and avoid absorption of dissolved gas by grease. Immediately after the samples are drawn, the syringes should be up-ended and gently tapped until all bubbles are expelled. Where possible the samples should be analysed directly. If this is impractical, they should be stored in capped syringes on crushed ice until an analyser is available. If the delay exceeds one hour, the result of the analysis will not be reliable.

THE MEASUREMENT OF OXYGEN SATURATION

Devices that measure oxygen saturation are called oximeters. They sense the absorbtion of light by the sample, at several wavelengths which characterise various states of haemoglobin, (deoxy-Hb, oxy-Hb, met-Hb, carboxy-Hb). Usually they haemolyse the sample first to reduce scattering errors. This takes 30 seconds or so, and the analysis takes a few seconds more. Measurements can be done on samples of 1 ml or less and can be repeated at intervals of a minute or so. In the catheter laboratory, saturation studies are used to detect, localise and quantitate intracardiac shunts, and to obtain approximate estimates of cardiac output by the Fick method.

Intracardiac shunts

LEFT-TO-RIGHT SHUNTS

When searching for a left-to-right shunt the operator takes a series of samples (oximetry run) from a number of sites within the heart and great vessels. These sites are:
1 Main pulmonary artery (and left and right pulmonary artery if a PDA is suspected).
2 High right ventricle (outflow).
3 Low right ventricle (inflow).
4 Low right atrium.
5 Mid right atrium.
6 High right atrium.
7 Low superior vena cava (SVC).
8 High SVC.
9 High inferior vena cava (IVC).
10 Low IVC (at L4 or L5 level).
Naturally there are many other sites from which samples may need to be taken and the above series need not be adhered to religiously; sampling sites are dictated by the abnormality being studied.

Left heart samples may be taken from the pulmonary veins, the left atrium, the left ventricle and the ascending and descending aorta or a peripheral artery. The oxygen saturation of samples taken from the pulmonary vein are usually one or two percentage points higher than those taken from the aorta.

The effect of a left-to-right shunt is to cause an increase in saturation at, or just beyond, the site of the intracardiac communication. The increase is commonly referred to as a 'step-up'. But the oxygen saturation of blood within the right heart is not uniform so that we have to define a significant step-up as an increase in saturation that exceeds the normal variability that is observed between samples taken from different sites in the right heart and within a right heart chamber. This variability is greatest between the cavae and right atrium and, as a result, within the right atrium. Saturation within the superior cava is close to, but usually slightly less than, the true 'mixed' venous saturation. Inferior caval blood contains two streams; blood of low saturation entering from hepatic veins and blood of considerably higher saturation from renal veins. Lastly coronary sinus blood, entering the low right atrium, is of very low saturation. As these streams of different saturation cross the tricuspid valve there is some mixing so that right ventricular blood tends to be of more uniform saturation than right atrial blood. Further mixing takes place at the pulmonary valve so that, in the absence of an intracardiac shunt, the pulmonary artery sample provides the best estimate of true mixed venous saturation.

It has been estimated that a difference in saturation of at least 7% between the superior cava and right atrium is needed before we can assume left-to-right shunting at atrial level. A difference of 5% is needed between the right atrium and ventricle and between right ventricle and pulmonary artery before we can assume shunting at ventricular or pulmonary arterial level [4, 5]. But the situation in practice is rather different; we do not depend on oximetry alone to detect shunts — they are likely to be confirmed, or disproved, by angiography. Because the step-up is less than the above does not mean that there is no shunt — only that it is not detectable with certainty by oximetry. And we can use intelligence and experience rather than a blind faith in numbers. For example the saturation in the mid-lateral right atrium is usually no higher than the right ventricular saturation (it is the best 'average atrial sample'); the high-right atrial sample is usually a few percentage points lower. If we find a higher saturation in mid right atrium than anywhere else in the atrium or cavae the probability of an ASD being present is high. If the high right atrial position yields blood which is more highly saturated than any other atrial sample a 'sinus venosus defect' or anomalous pulmonary venous drainage are high on the list of probabilities — to be confirmed angiographically. If an atrial sample is of higher saturation than even that from the low-inferior cava (renal veins) we can be certain that there is an atrial level shunt. Conversely it would be unwise to assume an atrial shunt on the basis of an atrial sample of lower saturation than low IVC — though one may be present.

From the discussion above it is apparent that there are pitfalls in the interpretation of saturation data. The streaming of blood of different saturations is just one. Others are: (1) samples taken from a peripheral arm vein are often of very high saturation. This may be because the arm is resting during catheterisation — whatever the reason it is a normal phenomenon and should not stimulate a search for a non-existent AV malformation. (2) Because of 'streaming' the step-up due to a VSD may not be detected until pulmonary artery level; that due to an ASD may not be detected until ventricular level. (3) If a PDA is present the saturation in the left pulmonary artery will be significantly higher than in the main or right pulmonary artery; samples must be taken from both pulmonary arteries and averaged in order to calculate shunt size. (4) Because of the shape of the oxygen dissociation curve measurements of *saturation* are a more sensitive measure of oxygen content than are measurements of oxygen *tension* (Po_2) in the 'venous range', that is below 60–70% saturation. In the 'arterial range' Po_2 measurements are more sensitive; large increases in Po_2 are associated with smaller changes in saturation. This is of great importance when high levels of inspired oxygen are given to investigate the effect on pulmonary vascular resistance. Under these circumstances oxygen *content* must be measured directly or derived from measurements of oxygen *tension*. This subject is discussed further, at the end of this chapter. (5) The normal value for pulmonary arterial saturation is about 75%. It is not safe to assume that there can be no left-to-right shunt because a saturation of this order is obtained; the cardiac output may be low and mixed venous saturation may be very much lower (see example below). (6) Finally it must be noted that, while left-to-right shunts are most readily detected from saturation data, measuring the actual volume of the shunt flow requires measurement of the *oxygen content* of pulmonary arterial and pulmonary venous blood. Oxygen content is determined by the oxygen capacity (haemoglobin level) as well as the percent saturation. Moreover shunt ratios (QP/QS) are influenced by the systemic flow so that a given

step-up between say 60 and 70% implies a lower QP/QS ratio than does the same step-up between say 80 and 90% [4]. The way that pulmonary and systemic flow and shunt size is calculated from measurements of oxygen saturation is described in Chapter 11.

RIGHT-TO-LEFT SHUNTS

Systemic arterial saturation is normally 95% or higher. A lower value indicates either true, intracardiac, right-to-left shunting or that there is pulmonary venous desaturation. Pulmonary venous desaturation also implies right-to-left shunting but of a different type — intrapulmonary shunting of blood away from air-containing alveoli. The causes for such intrapulmonary shunting that concern the cardiologist are;
1 Hypoventilation — especially in oversedated infants and children or those under anaesthesia.
2 'Lung disease' with defective gas transfer.
3 Pulmonary oedema, e.g. in patients with severe left heart lesions such as mitral stenosis.
4 Massive pulmonary embolism.
5 Pulmonary arteriovenous fistula.

Sedation as a cause of hypoventilation can lead to important problems in studying infants and children; it is for this reason (among others) that we prefer to employ general anaesthesia in the majority of paediatric studies. If used, general anaesthesia must be accompanied by intubation and good hand or mechanical ventilation with 33% O_2. An arterial sample taken for blood gas estimation early in the study will serve to check that ventilation is adequate — and corrected if necessary.

Hypoventilation in adults may be due to sedation — we do not routinely sedate adults — or to the supine position. Patients with severe left heart lesions are best studied while propped up as much as is possible. Hypoxaemia due to any of the causes above (except pulmonary AV fistula) will be reduced or abolished by giving oxygen by face mask; if hypoxaemia persists right-to-left intracardiac shunting must be suspected.

Pulmonary vein saturation is usually a few percentage points higher than left ventricular and systemic arterial saturation. Since it is not always possible to catheterise the pulmonary veins it is conventional to assume a pulmonary venous saturation of 97%. Pulmonary vein saturation cannot be *lower* than systemic arterial saturation (i.e. if systemic artery saturation = 100% then assume pulmonary vein saturation = 100%). If there is reason to suspect pulmonary venous desaturation (e.g. pulmonary oedema, uncorrected hypoventilation) and no reason to suspect intracardiac shunting then assume pulmonary venous saturation to be one or two percentage points higher than systemic arterial saturation.

Left ventricular blood is of lower saturation than pulmonary vein blood because of the drainage of some coronary venous blood directly into the left ventricle via Thebesian veins.

The way in which the magnitude of right-to-left shunts and bidirectional shunts is calculated from saturation data is described in Chapter 11.

The example of catheterisation data obtained in a case of congenital heart disease may serve to illustrate the diagnostic use of pressure and saturation measurements (Table 6.2).

In Table 6.2 the information is listed in the order in which it was obtained. The first four items of information (Step 1) tell us:

1 That there is pulmonary hypertension but do not tell us why — it might be due to high resistance in the pulmonary circulation, to a high flow in the pulmonary circulation or to a combination of high flow and resistance (but see later).

2 There are likely to be two ventricles and an intact ventricular septum since pulmonary arterial and aortic pressures differ significantly.

3 There is normal 'streaming' — that is pulmonary arterial saturation is less than aortic so there is preferential flow of systemic venous blood to pulmonary artery and pulmonary venous blood to aorta — thus excluding a diagnosis of 'complete transposition' since the reverse is true in this condition.

4 There is right-to-left shunting (or possibly hypoventilation and pulmonary venous desaturation).

5 Since pulmonary arterial saturation is normal, pulmonary flow is not increased and the pulmonary hypertension is due to increased (total) resistance. All this information can be deduced from pressure and saturation measurements in just two sites.

At Step 2 we find the mean wedge pressure to be increased so that a high pulmonary venous pressure is at least part of the cause of the pulmonary hypertension. At Step 3 an oximetry run tells us that, despite the normal pulmonary flow implied by a normal pulmonary arterial saturation (Step 1), there *is* a left-to-right shunt — at atrial level. The low

Table 6.2 Patient breathing room air.

Step	Site	Pressure (mmHg) Syst	Mean	Saturation (%)
1	Pulmonary artery	100		75
	Ascending aorta	75		85
2	Wedge		20	
3	Pulmonary artery			75
	Right ventricle			75
	Right atrium			75
	Superior vena cava			30
4	Left atrium		5	85
5	Inferior vena cava			95

(30%) superior caval saturation suggests that the cardiac output is low.

Then at Step 4 we find that, despite the high wedge pressure, left-atrial pressure is low so that there must be obstruction of pulmonary veins between the two sites. There is desaturated blood in the left atrium so that there is a right-to-left shunt at atrial level as well as a left-to-right shunt (again provided there is not hypoventilation and pulmonary venous desaturation). At this stage we can synthesise all this information and produce a probable diagnosis of infradiaphragmatic *total anomalous pulmonary venous drainage* (TAPVD). Arterial desaturation with bidirectional atrial shunting is compatible with TAPVD. So is an intact ventricular septum and pulmonary hypertension (in the neonate). Most cases of TAPVD (supracardiac and cardiac level drainage) have a pulmonary arterial saturation that is the same as, or higher than, aortic saturation. In infradiaphragmatic TAPVD the highly saturated IVC blood streams across the atrial septum to reach the left heart while SVC blood of low saturation streams across the tricuspid valve to reach the right ventricle and pulmonary artery. Finally obstruction to pulmonary venous return (within the portal circulation) is to be expected in infracardiac TAPVD.

Having deduced the anatomy we check by sampling IVC blood (Step 5) and find that, as expected, the saturation is very high. Having made the diagnosis, on haemodynamic grounds, we are in a position to perform angiography with the appropriate site of injection (pulmonary artery) and are careful to include the upper abdomen in the field and to continue filming for much longer than usual as pulmonary venous return slowly opacifies the portal circulation and then the IVC.

The measurement of cardiac output (Fick)

The way in which saturation data is used to calculate cardiac output by the Fick method is described in Chapter 11. Estimation of 'mixed venous' saturation in the presence of a left-to-right shunt poses problems. These, and the various formulae which have been used to estimate mixed venous saturation, are also described in Chapter 11.

THE MEASUREMENT OF OXYGEN TENSION

Conventional 'blood-gas analysers' measure the P_{O_2}, P_{CO_2} and pH of a small sample of blood, using electrodes. The oxygen tension is measured with a polarographic electrode, i.e. one which applies a specific voltage (0.6 v) to the sample and measures the current produced by the ionisation of oxygen. The current is proportional to the oxygen content of the plasma, which is linearly proportional to the oxygen tension. Because the current damages other constituents of plasma, particularly proteins, which would accumulate on the electrode and alter its sensitivity, the sensor is separated from the sample by a thin gas-permeable membrane which is disposable. Most devices are accurate to $\pm 2\,mmHg$, have a 90% response time of some 30 seconds, require about 1 ml of sample, and measure its P_{CO_2} and pH with other electrodes, at the same time.

Measurements of oxygen tension are most useful in the assessment of the gas-exchanging property of the lung, and the estimation of right-to-left shunts. Gas exchange in any alveolus is governed by two 'conservation of matter' equations. The first of these, known as the alveolar ventilation equation, simply says that the P_{CO_2} in an alveolus is proportional to the CO_2 excreted through it (V_{CO_2}), and inversely proportional to the flow of CO_2-free gas that is sweeping it away (V_A), i.e:

$$P_a_{CO_2} = kV_{CO_2}/V_A,$$

where k is simply the constant of proportionality (see Chapter 11 for further details).

The second relation, known as the alveolar air equation, says that the P_{O_2} in the alveolus equals the P_{O_2} in moist inspirate ($P_i_{O_2}{}^*$), minus the $P_a_{CO_2}$ divided by the ratio of CO_2 output to oxygen uptake (R). The asterisk in the symbol $P_i_{O_2}{}^*$ indicates that the moisture in breath has been taken into account. In effect, the division converts $P_a_{CO_2}$ into the fall in P_{O_2} due to oxygen uptake. There are two forms of the equation. The simplest, which is quite satisfactory for most purposes, is:

$$P_a_{O_2} = P_i_{O_2}{}^* - P_a_{CO_2}/R.$$

The more accurate form, which takes account of small effects due to the presence of nitrogen as an inert diluent, is used for research purposes:

$$P_a_{O_2} = P_i_{O_2}{}^* - P_a_{CO_2} (F_i_{O_2} + (1-F_i_{O_2})/R),$$

where $F_i_{O_2}$ is the fractional concentration of oxygen in the inspirate (0.2093 when the inspirate is air; 1.00 when it is 100% oxygen).

The alveolar air equation is important in cardiology, because it allows the investigator to calculate the oxygen tension in pulmonary venous blood, even when the pulmonary veins are not accessible and direct sampling is therefore impossible. For example, an unsedated adult patient undergoing catheterisation while breathing air, has a systemic arterial P_{CO_2} of 32 mmHg an arterial P_{O_2} of 73 mmHg, and an arterial pH of 7.42. What should the P_{O_2} of pulmonary venous blood be? Firstly, we note the arterial P_{CO_2} is low, but the pH is normal. Therefore it is unlikely that ventilation is being driven by significant hypoxia and more probable the patient is hyperventilating from anxiety. This would normally raise $P_a_{O_2}$, so the value of 73 mmHg is definitely low. The barometric pressure is normal, say 760 mmHg. As air enters the patient's mouth and nose it is warmed and wetted, so that it is saturated with water vapour at 37°C by the time it is halfway down the bronchial tree. So the partial pressure of dry air in the wet mix will be (760−47=) 713 mmHg. We know 21% of this is oxygen, and can quickly calculate the moist inspired P_{O_2} ($P_i_{O_2}{}^*$) as 10%+ 10%+1%, i.e. 71+71+7 = 149 mmHg. Assuming a respiratory exchange ratio of 1.0, as we think the patient is hyperventilating acutely, we calculate the alveolar P_{O_2} as:

$$P_a_{O_2} = 149 - 32/1.0 = 117\,mmHg.$$

Normally there is an alveolar−pulmonary venous P_{O_2}

gradient of 10 to 15 mmHg, due to slight mismatching of blood to air flow through the lung as a whole, so we would expect this patient's pulmonary venous P_{O_2} to lie between 102 and 107 mmHg. Therefore there is a shortfall in systemic arterial blood of some 50 mmHg. Could this be due to a right-to-left shunt? To discover this, we take advantage of the flatness of the oxygen-dissociation curve at high P_{O_2}. In this range, small changes in content, introduced by the shunt, produce large swings in P_aO_2. The patient is given 100% oxygen to breath, for 10 minutes or so, and a repeat arterial sample is taken. The P_aCO_2 is still 32 mmHg, and the pH has not changed, but the P_aO_2 has risen to 371 mmHg. What does this mean? The pulmonary venous P_{O_2} is calculated as before:

$$P_aO_2 = 713 - 32/1.0 = 681\,mmHg.$$

Allowing a 10 mmHg gradient as before, we would expect the pulmonary venous P_{O_2} to be 671 mmHg, but it is 300 mmHg lower. This suggests a 15% right-to-left shunt, since for a normal cardiac output and metabolic rate at rest, each 1% of shunt drops the systemic arterial P_{O_2} by 20 mmHg. To check this, it is better to obtain simultaneous blood samples from the pulmonary and systemic arteries, determine their contents directly (see below), then estimate the content of idealised pulmonary venous blood and calculate the true shunt fraction as described in Chapter 11.

THE MEASUREMENT OF OXYGEN CONTENT

If precise measurements of cardiac output or shunt fractions are required, it is better to measure the oxygen content of the blood samples than estimate them. It can be obtained in three ways: from blood gas tensions and haemoglobin; from oxymetry and haemoglobin content; or by direct determination using a content analyser. There are good and bad points about each approach.

Blood gas analysers are reasonably rapid instruments that are fairly simple to use. The same is true of haemoglobinometers, which measure haemoglobin content. If the P_{O_2}, P_{CO_2} and pH of a blood sample are known, the shape of its haemoglobin–oxygen dissociation curve, which is sensitive to pH and P_{CO_2}, can be *estimated*. This estimation assumes that the haemoglobin is normal, and will be in error if the red cell 2−3 DPG content is abnormal, the haemoglobin is of an odd type, or if it includes unusual amounts of methaemoglobin or carboxyhaemoglobin. The oxygen saturation can then be derived from the estimated curve and the measured P_{O_2}. The content itself is then estimated, as the product of saturation and estimated or measured haemoglobin content, assuming each gram of haemoglobin, when fully saturated, carries 1.34 ml O_2 (STPD). Modern blood gas analysers, complete these calculations automatically, making the same assumptions, and so are as vulnerable to errors of assumption.

Oximeters measure haemoglobin saturation directly, by spectrophotometry, and usually also calculate the methaemoglobin, carboxyghaemoglobin and total haemoglobin content. They are not sensitive to the amount of oxygen in physical solution in plasma and red cell water. At oxygen tensions above 100 mmHg, the amount of oxygen in solution is significant, particularly in the calculation of right-to-left shunts. It increases by 0.3 ml/100 mmHg and so may add a good 2 ml O_2/100 ml blood to the total arterial content, when breathing pure oxygen. As the normal arteriovenous extraction is 5 ml/100 ml, ignoring the extra 2 ml introduces a substantial error. Details of the appropriate calculations are given in Chapter 11.

Oxygen content meters displace the gas from solution and measure it volumetrically, or consume it hydrolytically and measure the current required. Both procedures require skilled technicians who have kept in practice. In such hands, they provide absolute measures of oxygen content, vulnerable only to errors of calibration and sampling.

REFERENCES

1 Owen SG, Wood P. A new method of determining the degree or absence of mitral obstruction: an analysis of the diastolic part of indirect left atrial pressure tracings. *Br Heart J* 1955;**17**:41.
2 Murgo JP, Westerhof N, Giolma JP, Altobelli SA. Aortic input impedance in normal man: relationship to pressure waveforms. *Circulation* 1980;**62**:105.
3 Carabello BA, Barry WH, Grossman W. Changes in arterial pressure during left heart pullback in patients with aortic stenosis: a sign of severe aortic stenosis. *Am J Cardiol* 1979;**44**:424.

4 Antman EM, Marsh JD, Green LH, Grossman W. Blood oxygen measurements in the assessment of intracardiac left to right shunts: a critical appraisal of methodology. *Am J Cardiol* 1980;**46**:265.

5 Freed MD, Miettinen OS, Nadas AS. Oximetric detection of intracardiac left-to-right shunts. *Br Heart J* 1979;**42**: 690.

6 Sykes MK, Vickers MD, Hull CJ. *Principles of Clinical Measurement*. Oxford, Blackwell Scientific Publications, 1981.

Angiography

PART I: X-RAY EQUIPMENT AND RADIATION PROTECTION

It is the purpose of this section to describe the basic principles of the X-ray equipment used for angiography. It is not intended to be an exhaustive description of the physics or design of modern angiographic equipment, but rather a guide to the user.

Cine fluoroscopic apparatus

THE X-RAY TUBE

Electrons from the cathode of an X-ray tube (Fig. 7.1) strike the tungsten anode to produce X-rays. The number of photons of X-rays (quanta) produced by a tube depends on the current flowing through the tube (mA). This is regulated by the heating of the source of the electrons, the cathode. The filament of the cathode is heated by an electric current which can be controlled — the filament current. By turning the control marked 'mA' on the control panel, the filament current is altered, thus varying the number of electrons produced by the cathode to bombard the anode. The passage of electrons through the tube produces a current — the tube current.

The energy of the X-rays, that is their penetrating power, is altered by varying the speed at which electrons strike the anode. This speed depends on the potential across the X-ray tube — the kilovoltage (kV). This potential is produced from the alternating current provided by the electrical mains which is converted into a direct current by transformers in the generator (Fig. 7.2). The generator also smooths the current so that the potential remains as constant as possible (a simple conversion of alternating to direct current produces pulses). Nevertheless the kilovoltage is never completely constant, especially

when switching circuitry is used to pulse the tube, and the kilovoltage referred to is the peak kilovoltage (kVp) achieved in each cycle.

The anode and cathode are situated in a tube (the insert), usually of glass, in which there is a vacuum (Fig. 7.1). The tube encloses a mechanism to allow rotation of the anode and, if used, a grid. The tube is surrounded by oil for electrical insulation and for cooling and is contained within a metal housing. A thermal cut-out is incorporated within the housing to protect the tube and casing from over-heating.

The production of X-rays at the anode generates a considerable amount of heat. It is this heat generation which limits the use of the tube. To help spread the local heat the anode is rotated rapidly (up to 10 000 rpm) so that only a small part of the anode is being used at any one moment. In heavy duty tubes, such as those used for angiography, the

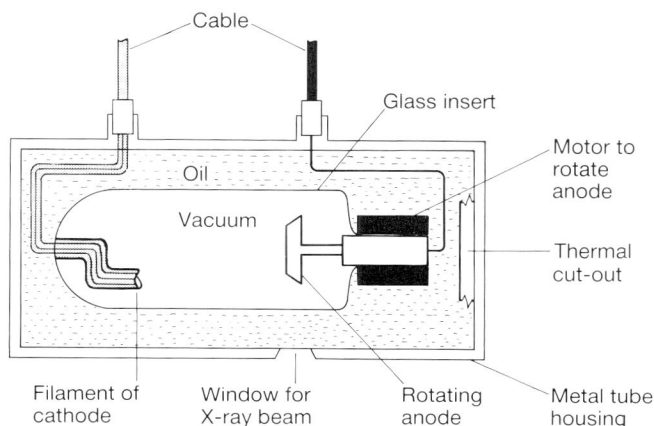

Fig. 7.1 Diagram of a rotating anode X-ray tube.

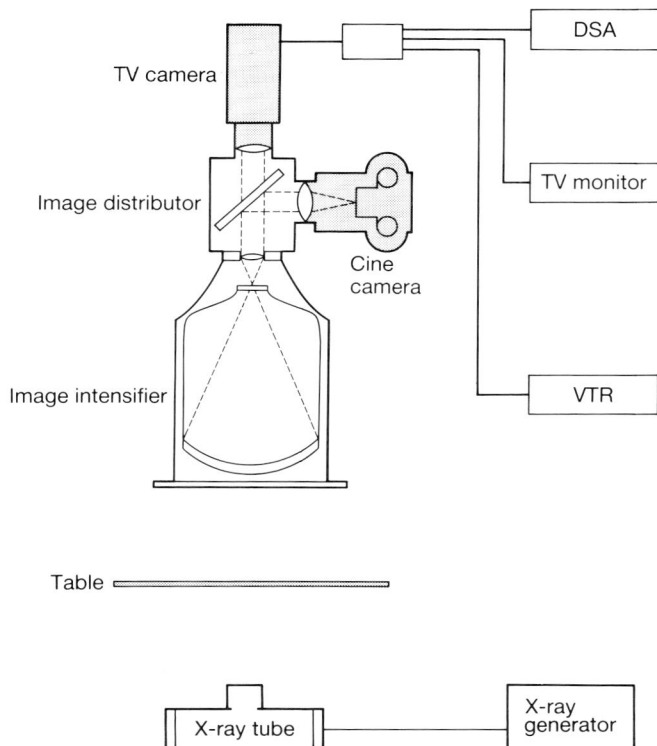

Fig. 7.2 Diagram of equipment of angiography.

diameter of the anode is made as large as possible. Even so, if it were visible, the anode would be seen to become red hot during an average working day. The X-rays are produced at the focal spot (usually 0.6 or 1.0 mm). The smaller the focal spot, the sharper the image, but the heat is produced over a smaller area. The tube 'rating' is calculated by the manufacturers and is provided as a chart of the exposure levels at different tube currents (mA) and energies (kV), and for different focal spot sizes, which may be used without damaging the anode. Rapid serial exposures, such as are used in cine angiography, produce considerable heat which must be given time to dissipate to avoid melting the anode. Heat damage to the anode causes pitting of the surface with subsequent erratic production of X-rays. The exposure limits in modern apparatus are incorporated into the generator and switching mechanism and automatic cut-outs come into action to safeguard the tube.

The angle of the anode determines the size of the *actual* focal spot so that, for a given *effective* focal spot, the actual focal spot may be increased by using a shallower target angle. (Fig. 7.3). For a given amount of heat energy the temperature rise at the target is determined by its area, thus a larger focal spot with a wider beam of electrons increases the potential loading of the tube by this simple method without loss of definition of the image. However the shallower the angle on the anode the narrower the beam of X-rays produced for a given electron beam width. A 6 to 7° angle will cover a 23 cm (9 in) intensifier but a 12° angle is needed to cover a 36 cm (14 in) radiographic field. The loading capacity of the tube is greatly increased with a 6° target angle compared with a 12° angle.

Cine angiography uses 'pulsed' X-rays — note that X-rays are not produced while the camera shutter is closed — as a result the patient is not needlessly exposed to 'unused' X-rays. Most manufacturers achieve this by electronic control within the generator but some use a 'grid' control inserted between the cathode and the anode within the tube. The grid is given an intermittent negative charge (bias) to stop the flow of electrons to the anode, the tube being used as an on/off switch to provide the pulses of X-rays. However this method of secondary switching may restrict the output of the tube and the voltage required to stop the electrons may be higher than the voltage required to produce X-rays.

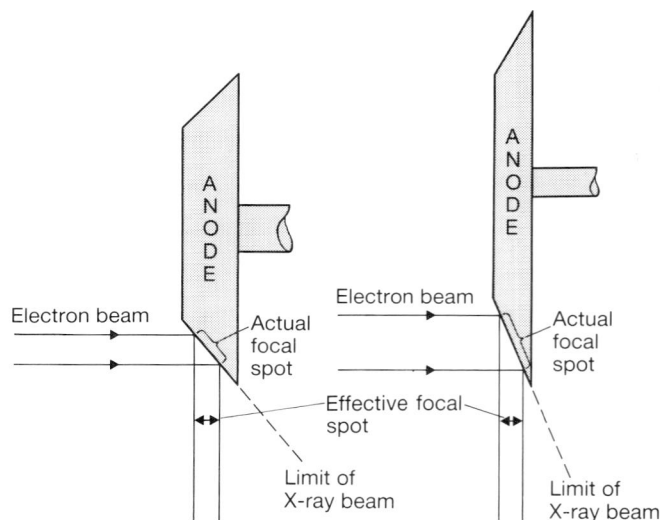

Fig. 7.3 Diagram showing how a shallow target angle on the anode of an X-ray tube may increase the actual focal spot size without affecting the effective focal spot. Note that the shallow angle on the anode reduces the limit of the X-ray beam, thus reducing its width. Near this limit, the intensity of the beam falls off.

IMAGE INTENSIFIER

As cine film is sensitive to light and less so to X-rays, the radiographic image must be transformed into a light image by an image intensifier. The X-ray beam falls on the input phosphor (usually caesium iodide) of the intensifier where it is converted into a light image (Fig. 7.4). This light image is then transformed into an electron image by the photo cathode which is in intimate contact with the input phosphor. The electrons produced are accelerated through the intensifier by a difference in potential across it, usually about 25 kV. The beam of electrons is focussed on the output phosphor where it is converted back into a light image. This light image is much brighter than the input image because of gain by the acceleration of the electrons and by minification. A 23 cm (9 in) input is intensified 81 times when minified to a 2.5 cm (1 in) output phosphor. The gain through electron acceleration is usually about 50 times but a total brightness gain of over 4000 may be achieved. Unfortunately, in spite of many devices for correction, the image intensifier distorts the image slightly, particularly around the periphery, due to some flaring of the electron beam. Thus the image of a mesh will be seen to be larger, slightly blurred and distorted at the edge (pin cushion effect). In addition, there is some loss of brightness and of resolution at the periphery (vignetting). The geometric distortion can be corrected to some extent by the collector lens of the outlet of the intensifier.

From the collector lens system the image falls on the image distributor which splits the light beam to the television and to the cine (or 100 mm) camera.

Image intensifiers vary in size. They are measured according to the diameter of the input phosphor and range from 12 cm to over 35 cm. The smaller the intensifier the greater the magnification of the image. The area of the patient covered by the intensifier is always slightly less than the area of the input because the X-ray beam is divergent, and a certain degree of magnification occurs depending on the distance of the object X-rayed (the patient) from the input phosphor (Fig. 7.5). This magnification is usually about 1.3 : 1 in angiography so that the maximum area of the heart that can be covered is 20–30% less than the area of the input phosphor. Further the magnified image of a smaller intensifier loses the advantage of increased brightness by minification. Thus to obtain the same degree of light

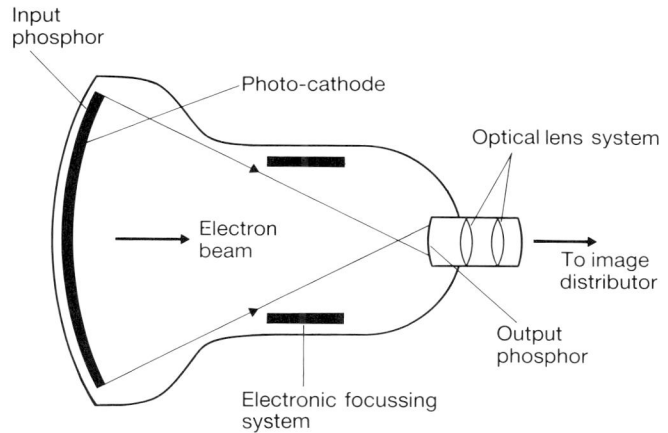

Fig. 7.4 Diagram showing cross-section of an image intensifier.

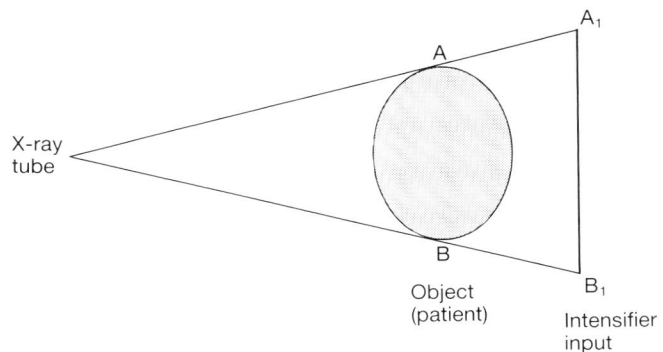

Fig. 7.5 The object A–B in the patient is magnified to A_1–B_1 at the input phosphor of the intensifier (or radiographic film). The magnification is less if the X-ray tube is further away, or A–B is closer to A_1–B_1.

output, assuming electronic gain is the same, the amount of radiation will have to be increased with the smaller intensifier. This amounts to a three-fold increase in dose of radiation when a 12 cm intensifier is used instead of a 17 cm intensifier. There is no doubt, though, that the resolution of the smaller intensifier is better than of the larger; detail of the magnified objects on the resulting cine film is clearer. The noise to signal ratio is reduced and there is less distortion of the image from the pin-cushion effect and vignetting. With a smaller field a shallower target angle and a higher tube rating may be used (see Table 7.1).

Most modern image intensifiers have multiple (dual or triple) modes providing a choice of field size. Field sizes are controlled electronically and can be altered easily by a switch on the control panel.

Table 7.1 Comparison of the large and small fields on an image intensifier.

	Large field	Small field	
Magnification	↓	↑	
Resolution	↓	↑	
Noise-to-signal ratio	↑	↓	Advantages of small field
Distortion of image	↑	↓	
Tube rating	↓	↑	
Brightness	↑	↓	
Radiation dose (to maintain brightness)	↓	↑	Disadvantages of small field

Nevertheless it must be remembered that the smaller the field size used, the greater is the radiation to the patient. When the field size is changed collimation (coning) of the X-ray beam must be changed so that unnecessary radiation of the patient not covered by the field of vision does not occur and scattered radiation is reduced. This is automatic on modern apparatus, allowing for both change in field size and change in the distance of the intensifier from the patient. However on older machines the operator will be required to adjust the coning when the field size or the position of the intensifier is changed.

The size of intensifier to be chosen will depend on the type of work undertaken. A 12 cm intensifier gives excellent magnification of coronary arteries but may not cover a ventriculogram in an adult if the left ventricle is enlarged. Coronary arteriography with this size of intensifier may require 'panning' with attendant problems of movement and of brightness control. Neonates require as much magnification as possible in order to see detail and a small intensifier is ideal. For larger children and adults a larger field is needed to include the pulmonary arteries, the arch of the aorta and lungs. If the apparatus is also used for peripheral angiography and digital subtraction angiography of the pulmonary or systemic arteries a 35 cm intensifier may be needed. This large intensifier is more cumbersome and more difficult to manoeuvre into all the projections required for investigation of the heart than are the smaller intensifiers. It may be difficult to get the intensifier close to the patient in angled views. For a cardiac laboratory studying both adults and children a compromise of a 27, 17 and 14 cm multiple mode intensifier is ideal though a dual field, 27 and 17 cm intensifier will suffice for most patients.

An X-ray beam is made up of quanta ('packets' of X-rays) which are not uniformly distributed. Thus if the intensification of the image is increased too much and the radiation beam consequently reduced these quanta become visible and the image is degraded by 'quantum mottle' (or noise). The number of photons striking the input phosphor of the image intensifier should be sufficient to eliminate the statistical fluctuation of quanta. A uniform, noise-free, image will then be achieved.

IMAGE DISTRIBUTOR

The image from the collector lens of the output of the image intensifier passes through a mirror system for distribution to the television camera, the cine camera and, possibly, a roll film or 100 cm cut film camera. The distributor splits the light beam so that the appropriate brightness falls on the different cameras. When fluoroscopy alone is being used the light beam from the image intensifier is directed to the television camera but when the cine or 100 mm camera is in operation the mirror system of the image distributor is switched so that the light beam is split and about 90% is reflected into the camera lens and 10% into the television camera. In order that the television image is kept at the same brightness during cine radiography as during fluoroscopy the radiation has to be increased by a factor of ten. The image being filmed can then be viewed simultaneously on the visual display unit and recorded on a video-tape recorder.

TELEVISION CAMERAS

Television cameras are of two types. In the plumbicon camera the photo conductor on the face of the tube is lead monoxide; in the videcon camera it is antimony trisulphide. The videcon camera has a time-lag with persistence of the image. The plumbicon has much less time-lag so that image blurring due to persistence of the previous image is much less — though at the expense of a slightly noisier signal. It is the plumbicon camera which is most commonly used for angiography.

The television camera produces an image which is displayed on a monitor screen. For most purposes a system using 525 lines is adequate but high resolution (1023 to 1049) line systems are needed for interventional procedures such as coronary angioplasty.

ROLL AND CUT FILM CAMERAS

A 70 or 105 mm roll film camera may be attached to the side-arm of the image distributor. Images can be obtained at up to 12 per second with a roll film camera and up to six per second with a cut film camera. This type of image recording is favoured by some cardiologists and is of particular value when large field sizes and large intensifiers are used.

CINE CAMERA

The brightness of the image intensifier has to be increased during cine filming as the film is exposed to light for short periods only — the shutter is closed for 50—60% of the cycle to allow transport of the film. Cine cameras using 35 or 16 mm film are available. Image detail is better with the larger film but camera speeds of 12—150 frames per second are less than those which can be achieved (25—200 f.p.s.) with a 16 mm camera; 35 mm film is much more commonly used than 16 mm film.

The X-ray beam is pulsed so that when the camera shutter is closed the X-ray beam is interrupted and radiation to the patient is minimised. The pulse rate is related to the frequency of the alternating current supply. Thus, in the UK, rates of cine filming in common use are 12.5, 25 and 50 f.p.s. When the slower speeds are used wider pulses (up to 8 ms) with fewer X-ray quanta can be used with the same exposure of the film. In cine angiography 50 frames per second is ideal for viewing and is necessary for rapidly moving infant hearts. However, in order to reduce radiation dose, 25 f.p.s. can be used for such investigations as coronary arteriography though, in viewing, cine flicker is much more noticeable. Pulse widths are up to 4 ms for 50 f.p.s. and up to 8 ms for 25 f.p.s. Higher speeds of 100—200 f.p.s. are unnecessary for routine diagnostic purpose but may be of value in research.

The brightness of the image is controlled either by a light sensitive cell within the image distributor or by measurement of the current across the image intensifier. The tube current (mA) or, more usually, the potential (kV) are automatically adjusted to provide a uniform amount of brightness during fluoroscopy. If the amount of light reaching the camera alters, during cine filming, the pulse width can be automatically varied by a similar feed-back mechanism. During fluoroscopy this 'automatic brightness control' allows an image to be obtained when the field of view changes from an area in which there is considerable absorption of X-rays (over the spine, for example) to an area of relatively less X-ray absorption (over the lungs, for example) without 'flaring' of the television image. Similarly, during a cine run, injected contrast medium may cause a considerable drop in the number of photons reaching the image intensifier; adjustment of either the kV or the pulse width (or both) may be necessary to prevent under-exposure of the cine film. On modern angiographic apparatus the required exposure is estimated automatically by two or three small exposures in the 'run up' after the cine camera has started moving and just before the exposures begin. In older apparatus it is necessary to simulate the exposure, manually, for a few seconds before cine filming to obtain the correct factors. Automatic brightness control is almost instantaneous though a noticeable lag period was invariably present in older apparatus. It is essential that the operator understands this automatic control; the apparatus will adjust to the *overall* brightness of the image and it may be that the region of interest lies in one of the more dense areas. For example if, during coronary arteriography, a large part of the lung is included in the field the contrast medium within the denser image of the heart may not be visible since the light sensor will be activated by the bright lung fields and adjust the brightness accordingly. It would, in this instance, be important to exclude as much as possible of the lungs from the field before the cine run. It is for this reason that 'panning' may not be successful as the field moves to include the bright lung field. It can be seen therefore that collimation (coning) of the X-ray beam is of great value in obtaining the best image of the field of interest. Some angiography machines are fitted with a semi-transparent, 'cardiac shaped', radiation filter which can be adjusted to coincide with the heart border. Collimation is also of importance in reducing the area of the patient being irradiated and in improving the image by reducing the amount of scattered radiation.

BIPLANE CINE ANGIOGRAPHY

For biplane cine angiography two X-ray tubes, two image intensifiers and two cine cameras are needed. These are mounted on suspensions on either side

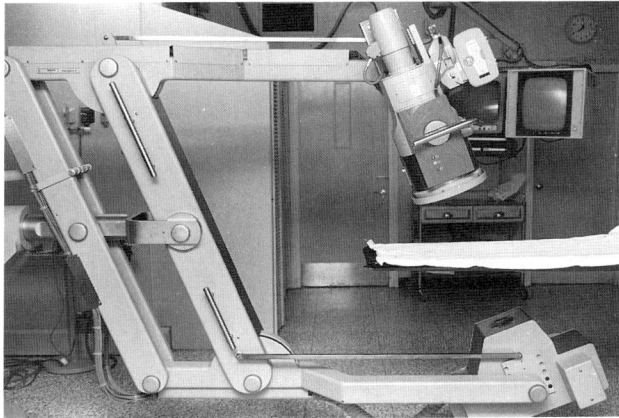

Fig. 7.6 Parallelogram type of suspension for the X-ray tube (under couch) and image intensifier/cine camera assembly (over couch) allowing angulation in two planes (Phillips 'Polydiagnost C').

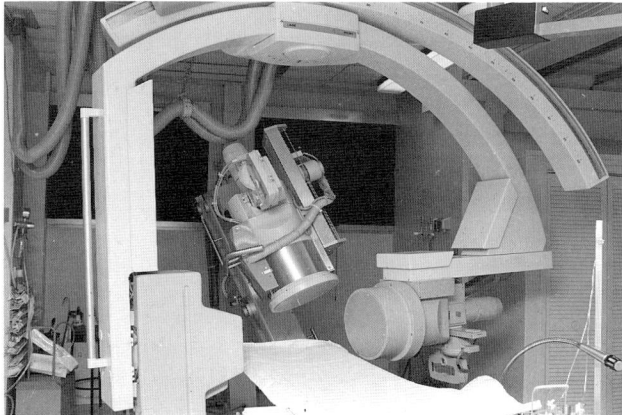

Fig. 7.7 Biplane suspension incorporating the 'Polydiagnost C' and a second tube/intensifier suspension (Phillips 'L-arc').

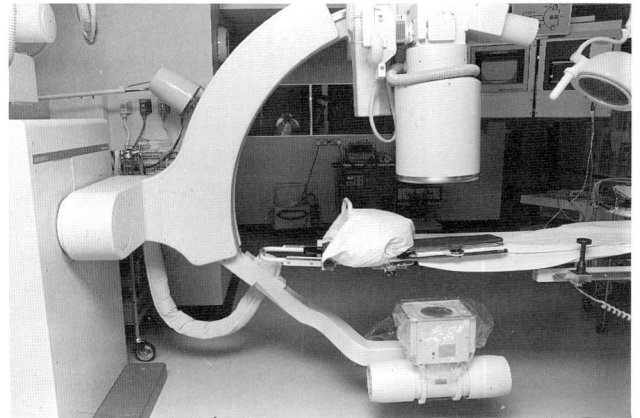

Fig. 7.8 Single plane, C-arm suspension for the X-ray tube and image intensifier (Siemens 'Coroscop C').

and above and below the catheter table in such a way as to interfere with the procedure as little as possible (Figs 7.6, 7.7 and 7.8). Nevertheless, because of the weight and necessary size of X-ray tubes and intensifiers, they occupy valuable space around the patient. In modern systems the two planes rotate about a common central point, the isocentre, though at the extremes of angulation this may be difficult to achieve. This facility makes setting up for cine angiography much easier and quicker than was the case when the two planes did not share an iso-centre and each had to be set up independently.

During the cine run the generator provides the pulses of X-rays for each plane alternately and the

cameras have to have their shutter movements interphased so that one shutter is closed when the X-rays are being produced by the tube of the other plane. This is necessary to prevent scattered radiation from one plane fogging the cine film of the other plane. Adjustment of this alternate pulsing and shutter closure is critical and the success of biplane cine filming depends upon it.

CINE FRAMING

The cine camera exposes a rectangle measuring 18 × 34 mm on 35 mm film. As the output phosphor of the image intensifier is circular there is a mismatch of framing. If the whole circle is within the cine frame, 'under-framing', there is a considerable waste of unexposed cine film. Similarly, if the cine frame is entirely within the circle, 'over-framing', about 40% of available image is not photographed. In most angiographic systems a compromise, 'maximal horizontal framing', is used. There is a certain degree of over-framing and the operator must remember that not all that he sees on the television monitor will be photographed on the cine film: some of the picture at the top and bottom of the circle will be cut off (Fig. 7.9).

CINE FILM PROCESSING

Automatic processors for cine film are now used universally. Cine film passes through a developer tank, is fixed, washed and then dried. The developer and fixer are automatically replenished from feeder

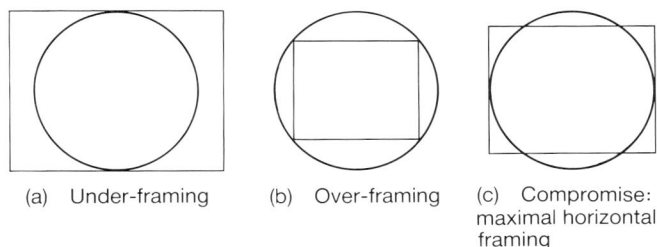

(a) Under-framing   (b) Over-framing   (c) Compromise: maximal horizontal framing

Fig. 7.9 Cine framing.

tanks. Variables involved in this process include the speed at which the film passes through the tanks, the temperature of the developer, the type of developer, etc.

The type of film used and the processing chemicals should be selected to achieve what is desired. The faster the film used the shorter the exposure needed, but the result will be a more grainy picture. If the film is very fast some of the graininess may be due to quantum mottle.

Slow film may give better definition but will require either a longer exposure, which may not be possible at the cine speed selected, or more X-ray quanta to provide a brighter image. The light reaching the film may also be adjusted, to some extent, by alteration of the diaphragm (F number) on the cine camera.

In the UK types of film in common use for cine angiography are Scopix RPIC (Agfa−Gevaert) and CFE (Kodak). The film manufacturers will recommend the correct chemicals for processing their film. There are, however, daily variations in the temperature and state of the chemicals and it is important to introduce quality control of film processing. A strip of pre-exposed film, with steps of grey levels, is obtainable from film manufacturers. A strip should be put through the processor, each day, and density measurements made with a densitometer to construct a density/exposure ('characteristic') curve (Fig. 7.10). To construct a characteristic curve the densitometer readings are plotted on the vertical axis against the log of the relative exposure on the horizontal axis. In the case of the film-strip the manufacturers will provide numbers for the log of the relative exposure to correspond to each grey level on the strip. Alternatively, a film-strip can be constructed by exposing a step wedge. A step wedge is made of aluminium and the thickness of each step

is known; thus the relative exposure of each step can be calculated from the thickness.

The lowest density of the film when no exposure has occurred is the basic fog level. At the upper limits of density further exposure has little effect and the curve flattens off. The useful range of density is therefore on the straightest portion of the curve. The gradient of the straight line portion of the characteristic curve is known as 'gamma'. However, as it is often difficult to define a straight line portion of the curve, gamma is difficult to measure and an 'average gradient' is now more commonly used. The most useful part of the characteristic curve lies between a density of 0.25 plus base fog and 2.0 plus base fog (Fig. 7.11). The average gradient will give an indication of the magnitude of radiographic contrast one can expect in the image. For cine angiographic film the average gradient is ideally 1.6 but a small variation may be permitted for individual preference. The gradient should not vary by more than 0.075. The steeper the curve (higher gamma or average gradient), the more contrast is obtained from smaller variations in exposure. The flatter the curve (lower gamma or average gradient), the less contrast is obtained. Factors affecting density and gamma are listed in Table 7.2.

Developer exhaustion is caused by insufficient replenishment and oxidation by air. The processor must be cleaned regularly as deposits of chemical form in the tank and then are deposited on the film. When the processor is cleaned once a week, fresh developer should be made up as even unused developer in the replenishing tank will have become

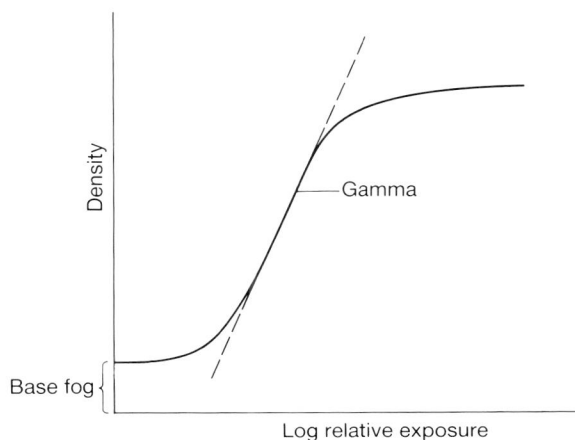

Fig. 7.10 Characteristic curve for a film and development combination showing gamma.

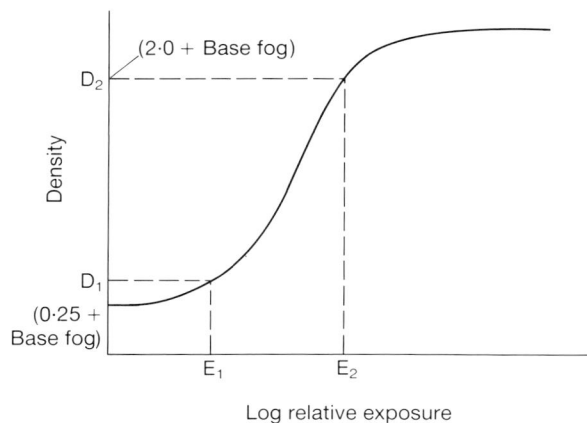

Fig. 7.11 Characteristic curve showing how average gradient is obtained:

$$\text{Average gradient} = \frac{D2 - D1}{E2 - E1}$$

Table 7.2 Showing effect of changes in developer.

	Film		
	Base fog	Density	Gamma or average gradient
Developer temperature raised	↑	↑	↓
Developer exhaustion	no change	↓	↓
Transit time increases (longer development time)	↑	↑	↓
Developer concentration increases	↑	↑	↓

Table 7.3 Summary of factors influencing the final cine film.

	Fixed by type of apparatus, etc.	Varied by service engineers	Varied by operator
Tube current (mA)		±*	±*
Tube kilovoltage (kV)		±*	±*
Dose rate		+	
Image intensification	+		
Field size			+
Pulse width			+
Cine speed (f.p.s.)			+
Film speed	+		
Camera diaphragm (F stop)		+	
Developer temperature			+
Processing speed			+
Developer	+		

* Dependent on make of apparatus.

oxidised and, therefore, exhausted. A summary of the factors influencing the final film quality is given in Table 7.3.

FILM CHANGERS

For most purposes cine angiography provides the best method for imaging the heart but there are limitations on the field size and on the resolution of fine structures. The pulmonary vessels, particularly the peripheral vessels, are better seen on conventional radiographic film so that a rapid film changer may be needed for good quality pulmonary angiography. Two commonly used rapid film changers are the AOT (Elema) and the Puck (Fig. 7.12) but others are available. Both the AOT and Puck are capable of using $35 \times 35\,$cm cut radiographic film — adequate to cover both lung fields in all but the largest patients. Angiography of other parts of the body, the abdomen for example, is possible with these changers. Up to six exposures per second and a maximum of 30 exposures can be achieved with the AOT changer. The Puck changer, which is smaller, allows only 20 exposures at a maximum exposure rate of four per second. Each of these changers incorporates a pair of intensifying screens. The films are transported from the magazine to lie between the intensifying screens which come together to clamp the film during the exposure. Close proximity of the intensifying screen and the film is

necessary to give good definition. After the exposure is made the screens separate and the film is transported into a receiver before the next film arrives between the screens. This mechanical transport depends upon the rigidity of the films; any buckling or slight maladjustment leads to jamming of the apparatus, a fault to which all film changers are prone, especially at the faster exposure rates.

VIDEO TAPE RECORDING

The television signal can be recorded on video tape or disc. Unlike cine film, video systems have immediate playback capability; the operator can review

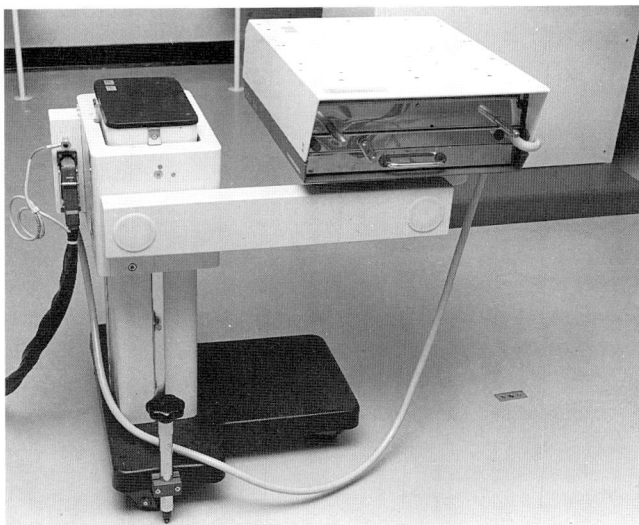

Fig. 7.12 'Puck U4' large format cut-film changer (Siemens—Elema).

immediately the angiogram just performed. As the video signal is taken from the television monitor a record can be made during fluoroscopy and there is no need for the additional radiation exposure needed for cine filming. Why then is video recording not used for documenting the images? Why use cine film? The first reason is that although rapid video playback provides an image as clear as that provided by cine filming this is not the case when a single frame (stop motion) is observed — detail is then not nearly as good as that of cine film. Video playback is not as easily manipulated backwards and forwards as is the viewing of cine film on a suitable analyser. Cine film is more robust than magnetic tape and is likely to retain a better image after several years storage. Images are, at present, stored in analogue form since the capacity of analogue storage is greater than that of digital storage. It is likely, however, that this limitation will soon be overcome; as video and optical disc recording systems improve these disadvantages are likely to disappear and the future of angiography will be with a filmless catheterisation laboratory.

CINE VIEWING

Cine film should always be viewed under the best conditions. A darkened room and a suitable projec-

tion screen are essential. Film analysers of the 'Tagarno' type allow immediate stopping of the cine and variable speed viewing both backwards and forwards. Frame counting is provided and attachments allow a camera to be fitted to make still photographs of a single frame or to permit computer assisted analysis of the image. Other film analysers include the 'Vanguard' and the 'Cipro'.

Regular servicing is essential and should include cleaning of the lenses and centring the projection bulb. Deterioration in quality of the final image may be due to defects in the viewer and not to fall off in film quality.

QUALITY CONTROL AND SERVICING

Regular servicing of the whole system is essential. This is usually performed by a service engineer from the company providing the equipment. Amongst the items the engineer should check are: the radiation output of the tube, focal spot size, alignment and collimation of the beam, automatic brightness control, resolution of the image intensifier and television chain, brightness gain of the intensifier (conversion factor), focussing of the television and cine cameras, aperture of the cine camera, mechanical stability of the suspension and the table, integrity of cables and wires (particularly the high tension cables to the tube), safety interlocks and the cameras and camera motors. Any minor faults that occur, even if intermittent, should be noted by the radiographer in a 'faults' book so that the engineer can correct them on his next visit. More serious faults which may damage the apparatus or be hazardous to the patient or staff should be dealt with as soon as possible and it may be necessary to confirm with the manufacturers that it is safe to continue to use the equipment before the fault can be repaired.

DIGITAL ANGIOGRAPHY

Simple subtraction angiography can be performed photographically on conventional radiographic film. A positive 'mask' of the image taken before the injection of contrast medium is superimposed on the film taken after the injection. In the resulting image background shadows of the spine, ribs and so on are obscured and the vessels containing contrast medium are highlighted. This subtraction is more easily, rapidly and accurately performed by digitising the electronic signal from the image intensifier—television chain. Such a system allows computer manipulation of the images for greater detail than can otherwise be obtained. In particular, digital subtraction angiography (DSA) provides clearer images of vessels as overlying structures are 'subtracted'. Systems are now available for this process to operate in a continous (cine) mode up to 50 frames per second with viewing in real time on a monitor. For the best images there must be as little movement as possible of the subtracted structures between the mask and the full image. In cardiac work this can be achieved by 'gating'; that is by timing the images in relation to the electrocardiogram so that exposures are made at the same time in each cardiac cycle. When gating is used the image acquisition time is long and the method is unsatisfactory for this reason. Subtraction is better achieved if the mask is taken from an average of images prior to the injection of contrast medium.

Digital imaging offers several advantages as well as subtraction. It is possible to manipulate the image after acquisition by edge enhancement and by variation of the grey levels and the range of grey levels. Computer evaluation of cardiac images allows calculation of ejection fraction, assessment of regional wall motion and estimation of the severity of coronary arterial stenoses. Such 'quantitative angiography' is discussed in the next chapter.

Radiation protection

By 1902, 7 years after Roentgen discovered X-rays, the harmful effects of radiation were recognised when a worker in a factory making X-ray tubes had developed cancer on the hand. Detailed studies of the effects of radiation were made in the 1920s and in 1928 internationally accepted standards for measuring radiation exposure and recommendations for protection were made. In 1957 a code of practice for protection of persons against ionising radiation arising from medical and dental use was published by the Ministry of Health in the UK and, until 1984, this formed a practical guide to radiation protection in all hospitals in the United Kingdom. Because of directives from Euratom — the EEC commission on radiation — *The Ionising Radiation Regulations* 1985

[1, 2] were passed under *The Safety at Work Act* 1974. These concern protection of radiation workers in both industry and medicine. More recently *The Ionising Radiation (Protection of Persons Undergoing Medical Examination or Treatment) Regulations* 1988 have been introduced requiring all persons using ionising radiation in medicine and dentistry to have training in radiation protection. The regulations are particularly concerned with protection of the patient. Hospital authorities are to make certain that anyone exposing a patient to ionising radiation has had such training before being allowed to use X-ray equipment. There are further rules for persons injecting radioisotopes.

BIOLOGICAL EFFECTS OF RADIATION

Ionising radiation damages body cells to a varying degree [3]. Radiation alters the chemical structure of DNA and may damage one or both strands of the double helix of DNA. Cellular enzymes may, or may not, succeed in repairing this damage. Thus the cell may not be able to produce viable daughter cells on division so that cell death occurs. Alternatively the damaged cell may be able to produce daughter cells to which the DNA error is transmitted. Descendant cells may then malfunction in the same way as the damaged cell. Effects resulting in cell death are related to the dose of radiation and are termed 'non-stochastic'. The hereditary and carcinogenic effects of radiation in which the dose determines a probability rather than a certainty of the effect occurring are termed 'stochastic'. Thus radiation may:
1 kill cells (non-stochastic effect), or
2 cause multiplication of damaged germ cells resulting in offspring with inherited abnormalities (stochastic effect), or
3 cause multiplication of damaged cells which are inadequately controlled by normal body processes so that cancer results (stochastic effect).

Non-stochastic effects

Tissue damage caused by radiation depends on several factors including the dose of radiation, the time over which injury occurred and the sensitivity of the particular cell. Cells which are particularly sensitive are those in the developing embryo, in the testis and ovary and in the lens of the eye in which cataract may be induced with relatively small doses of radiation. For other tissues the threshold for any clinically detectable non-stochastic effect is substantially higher. Skin burns may occur and it has been known for cardiac patients to suffer a first degree burn (erythema) following long periods of fluoroscopy for pacemaker insertion.

Stochastic effects: genetic

Though there is good evidence in animals of the genetic effects of radiation no reliable data are available, in the human, on which an estimate of risk can be made. Estimates have been made following the atomic bombing of Hiroshima and Nagasaki but, as the doses received are only estimates, the results cannot be regarded as wholly reliable and extrapolation from animal experiments seems, perhaps, a better method.

Stochastic effects: the induction of cancer

There is no doubt that irradiation can cause malignant change in the human. There is a higher incidence of cancers and other tumours in patients who have received radiotherapy than in the control population; occupational cancers have occurred in uranium miners, radium workers and the medical profession in the early days of X-ray use. The induction of malignant disease by the diagnostic use of X-rays has been reported. Women who underwent collapse therapy for pulmonary tuberculosis and had repeated fluoroscopic procedures showed a higher incidence of breast cancer in the subsequent 15 to 45 years than did the control group [4]. A higher incidence of leukaemia has been reported in children who were irradiated *in utero* [5, 6]. There is also evidence from Hiroshima and Nagasaki that doses of radiation which cause no immediate symptoms have caused an increased incidence of cancer in subsequent years.

PROTECTION OF THE PATIENT

A Measures under the control of the medical and radiographic personnel

1 The irradiation of patients must be no more than is necessary to produce a satisfactory result. Ionising radiation should not be used if the information needed can be obtained equally well by other means.

2 Care must be taken to minimise radiation to sensitive tissues such as the gonads and bone marrow. Gonad shields should be used if possible.
3 The X-ray beam should be collimated so that only the area of interest is included in the field of irradiation. This is especially important in children. The field should always be slightly smaller than the film size in radiography or serial filming (for cine see 'cine filming' above).
4 The dose received during fluoroscopy and cine angiography is high. Fluoroscopy should not be used if the same information can be obtained by radiography. Image intensification must always be used.
5 The duration of fluoroscopy and of cine runs should be as short as possible. During catheterisation the operator must only employ fluoroscopy when he is actively moving the catheter and watching the screen. It is important to record the time of fluoroscopy and the mA used during each procedure. It is advisable to set a limit of mA × time for the laboratory beyond which fluoroscopy is only continued in exceptional circumstances and with the permission of the laboratory director. 30 mA minutes is a good upper limit and most procedures should be completed with far less fluoroscopy time.

B Measures for protection incorporated in the apparatus

1 The apparatus must be designed so that the patient cannot be irradiated inadvertently.
2 The image intensifier and television system should be of such quality, both in design and maintenance, as to give the best possible image with the least possible radiation (i.e. the lowest mA).
3 The cine film used should be the fastest consistent with satisfactory results.
4 Automatic collimation to the field size is preferred when the intensifier has multiple fields.

PROTECTION OF STAFF

Most of the measures which reduce radiation to the patient also reduce the dose to the staff.

A Primary irradiation

'No person, other than a person undergoing examination, should be exposed to the useful beam of the
X-ray equipment' [2]. Thus under no circumstances
should the operator's hands be visible on the television screen during catheterisation. Careful collimation of the beam to the field size is important;
when a small field of the image intensifier is being used the beam, if not collimated, will be ir-
radiating the area around that which is visible and
the fingers of the operator or anaesthetist may be
being irradiated without it being evident on the
television screen.

B Secondary irradiation (scattered radiation)

When X-rays pass through a person or an object not
only are ions produced but also new X-rays with a
longer wavelength. These X-rays scatter in all directions from the field of radiation (Fig. 7.13) and it is
this secondary radiation which accounts for the exposure of staff in a catheterisation laboratory. A
system of work and local rules for the protection of
staff must be written and all persons working in the
laboratory must be familiar with these rules for their
own protection (a requirement of *The Ionising Radiation Regulations* 1985). This system of work should
include the following:
1 Only those persons whose presence is essential
should remain in the procedure room while radiological examinations are being carried out. Thus
recording equipment, and the technicians operating
it, should be housed in a separate, shielded, monitoring room.
2 The operator and others should stand as far as is
practical from the useful beam. Radiation intensity
decreases as the square of the distance from the
source: i.e. at 6 feet (1.8 m) from a source of radiation
the dose received is not half that at 3 feet (0.9 m) but
one-quarter and, at 12 feet (3.6 m) is one-sixteenth.
3 Protective clothing must be worn by all persons
in the catheterisation laboratory while a procedure
involving ionising radiation is being performed.
Protective clothing consists of approved lead aprons
with a lead equivalent of at least 0.35 mm for all
persons and a thyroid collar and lead glass spectacles
for the operator and assistant. Lead gloves are obviously impractical whilst catheterising but it must be
remembered that the extremities are more exposed

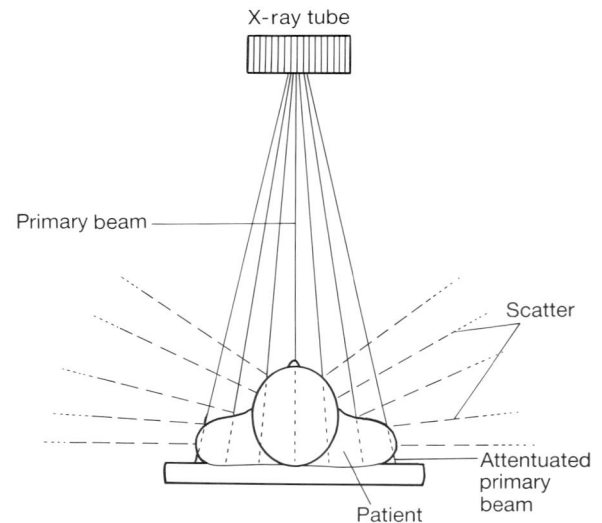

Fig. 7.13 Diagram showing the radiation scattered in all
directions when the primary beam, or the beam after it has
passed through the patient (attenuated beam), reaches the patient
or the table.

and should be kept away from the irradiated field as
much as possible.
4 The design and construction of X-ray apparatus in
catheterisation laboratories must incorporate protective devices and barriers such as warning lights,
safety and interlocking switches, beam collimation,
lining of walls, floors and ceilings if they are not of
adequate thickness and lead glass windows to protect not only those present in the room but also
persons working in adjacent rooms and corridors.

RADIATION MONITORING

The dose of radiation received by personnel may be
measured by estimating the degree of blackening of
photographic film, by estimation of colour change in
thermoluminescent powder such as lithium fluoride
(TLD) or by pen-type ionising chambers. It is advisable that all personnel in the catheterisation laboratory are monitored, the photographic or TLD badge
being processed at monthly intervals. The dose received should be recorded and a record kept for
each person during their lifetime. This record is
passed on to any new employer. The dose limit at
present in force in the UK for the effective dose
equivalent for the whole body for employees aged
18 years or over is 50 millisieverts (mSv) in any one
year. Nearly all personnel working in catheterisation

laboratories receive only a small fraction of this maximum permissable dose. The highest doses are received by those working closest to the patient, that is the persons manipulating the catheters; for them doses can approach the maximum permissable level — particularly for certain organs such as the lens of the eye, the thyroid and the hands for which there are other specified limits (hands 500 mSv per year, lens 150 mSv per year). Periodical assessment of doses should be made by placing monitoring badges around the room and on different parts of the operators body — hands, forehead and feet. A survey can then be made of the scattered radiation so that protective screens can be designed to fit around the X-ray apparatus if necessary. A balance has to be reached between causing the least obstruction to the procedures being performed and the safety of the staff.

RADIATION PROTECTION ADVISOR

Under *The Ionising Radiation Regulations* 1985 every employer (i.e. hospital or institution) using X-rays or other ionising radiation must appoint a radiation protection advisor whose duties will include giving advice on:

1 Restriction of exposure and maintenance of engineering controls for such restrictions.
2 Identification of areas in which there is a high dose rate (controlled area = dose rate more than 7.5 μSv per hour).
3 Control of access to these areas.
4 Dosimetry and monitoring.
5 Drawing up written systems of work and local rules.
6 Selection of radiation protection supervisors.
7 Investigation of high exposures and over exposures.
8 Training.
9 Deciding whether it is possible to restrict the exposures of female employees to ionising radiation.
10 Prior examination of any plans for new plant or new premises or modification to existing plant or premises from a radiation aspect.
11 Other aspects of radiation protection.

GENERAL READING

Forster E. *Equipment for diagnostic radiography.* Lancaster, MTP Press, 1985.
Jenkins D. *Radiographic photography and imaging processes.* Lancaster MTP Press, 1980.
Pochin E. *Nuclear radiation: risks and benefits.* Oxford Clarendon Press, 1983.

REFERENCES

1 Statutory Instruments (1985) No 1333: *The Ionising Radiation Regulations* 1985, HMSO London.
2 Approved Code of Practice: (1985): *The Protection of Persons Against Ionising Radiation Arising From Any Work Activity: The Ionising Radiation Regulations* 1985 HMSO London.
3 Russell JGB. How dangerous are diagnostic X-rays? *Clin Radiol* 1984;**35**:347.
4 Myrden JA, Hiltz JE. Breast cancer following multiple fluoroscopies during artificial pneumothorax treatment of pulmonary tuberculosis. *Canad Med Ass J* 1969;**100**: 1032.
5 Stewart A, Kneale GW. Radiation dose effects in relation to obstetric X-rays and childhood cancers. *Lancet* 1970; **1**:1185.
6 Diamond EL, Schmerler H, Lilienfeld AM. The relationship of intra-uterine radiation to subsequent mortality and development of leukemia in children. *Am J Epidemiology* 1973;**97**:282.

Angiography

PART II: TECHNIQUES

The term 'selective angiography' refers to X-radiography during the injection of radio-opaque contrast media into blood vessels; the term angiocardiography may be used to include injection into both vessels and cardiac chambers. More specific terms such as ventriculography, aortography, coronary arteriography and the like have meanings which are self-explanatory. Coronary arteriography, aortography and pulmonary arteriography are discussed elsewhere; this section is concerned with general principles and with ventriculography; the term 'angiography', though not strictly accurate, is widely used and will be used here.

Radio-opaque contrast media

Contrast media used in cardiac angiography are either the conventional ionic media or the newer, 'non-ionic' or 'low osmolar' media introduced in the early 1980s.

CONVENTIONAL IONIC MEDIA

These are water soluble salts of tri-iodinated substituted benzoic acids. The acids (anions) in commonly used media are diatrizoic acid, iothalamic acid or metrizoic acid. These acids are combined with a cation which is usually sodium or methylglucamine (meglumine). Calcium and magnesium ions may be substituted for some of the sodium ions. Various formulations have been developed in the continuing search for the ideal contrast medium. The ideal medium would be non-toxic and have high radio-opacity. In practice the radio-opacity that can be obtained depends not only on the iodine content but also on the viscosity of the medium; the more viscous the medium is the more difficult it is to inject an adequate volume through the long, thin, catheter. Sodium salts are less viscous than meglumine salts; unfortunately formulations with a high sodium content are more toxic. Conversely formulations with a low (<140 mmol/l) sodium content are more liable to precipitate ventricular fibrillation during coronary arteriography — as was found when the formulation of Renograffin was altered (temporarily) to one containing almost no sodium ions [1]. Contrast media for coronary arteriography should have a sodium content between 140 and 190 mmol/l.

Apart from toxicity (due to the cations) the other great drawback to conventional ionic media is their high osmolality in solution. The osmolality of conventional media varies between 1400 and 2400 mOsm/kg; the osmolality of blood is about 300 mOsm/kg. This high osmolality is responsible for many of the undesirable effects of contrast media. Clinically important effects include:

1 Shift of fluid from the red cells into the plasma with resulting erythrocyte deformation [2]. This can result in acute haemolysis in patients with sickle cell disease [3]. Deformed red cells pass less easily through the capillaries and the resulting (temporary) increase in effective pulmonary vascular resistance may contribute to the well known risk associated with angiography in patients with severe pulmonary vascular disease [4] — patients with primary pulmonary hypertension, for example.

2 Shift of extravascular fluid into the circulation resulting in hypervolaemia [4]. This hypervolaemia can lead to worsening heart failure and pulmonary oedema in patients with an already critically reduced reserve. The effect is particularly important in neonates and infants in whom a severe volume load

is already present and in whom relatively large amounts of contrast medium are needed for adequate demonstration of the anatomy; it is for this reason that angiography carries a high risk in neonates with persistent truncus arteriosus.

3 Peripheral vasodilatation. This effect of the hyperosmolar media is responsible for the sensation of heat ('hot flush') experienced by all patients immediately following angiography. Some patients find this distressing but the importance of the vasodilatation is its potentially lethal effect in patients with a low, fixed cardiac output. Since output cannot be increased to compensate for the vasodilatation there is a period of hypotension during which coronary perfusion is impaired. Patients at risk include those with massive pulmonary embolism, those with critical aortic stenosis and those with severely impaired left ventricular function.

4 Depressed myocardial function [5]. All contrast media cause some depression of myocardial function — particularly the conventional ionic media. The effect is temporary but can be significant; patients with severely impaired myocardial function are at risk during angiography and 'non-ionic' media (see below) should be used in such patients.

5 Rhythm disturbances. Conduction disturbances — bradycardia, AV block and asystole — are not uncommon during coronary arteriography. These effects are temporary and almost invariably self-limiting. Ventricular tachycardia or fibrillation occurs occasionally and demands immediate treatment by DC countershock.

6 Nephrotoxicity [6]. The risk of nephrotoxicity is negligible in patients with normal renal function but may be significant in those with impaired renal function [7]. High risk patients include those with diabetes, with myelomatosis and patients with a plasma creatinine above 2.5 mg/100 ml [8]. The risks of angiographically induced nephrotoxicity may have been overstated in the past [9] but angiography is contraindicated in patients with renal failure.

7 Anaphylactoid reactions. These reactions to contrast media are, fortunately, exceedingly rare; fatal reactions have been estimated to occur in less than 1 in 10 000 examinations [10]. When anaphylactoid reactions do occur the clinical picture is of shock (severe hypotension) with bronchospasm, laryngeal and pulmonary oedema and seizures. The reaction almost always occurs within a minute or two of the injection of contrast medium but may be delayed by

up to 30 minutes. Resuscitation will involve endotracheal intubation and ventilation, i.v. adrenaline (epinephrine) 2.5—5 ml of 1 : 10 000 solution, fluid expansion with i.v. fluids (dextran) — and elevation of the legs.

Patients with a history of allergy or asthma have a risk of developing a reaction to contrast media which is twice that of the general population; those with a history of a previous reaction to contrast media are at three-fold risk [10]. However, many patients give a history of a previous 'reaction' (often following intravenous pyelography) and yet experience no problems during subsequent angiography. Testing by a small preliminary injection is of no predictive value and serious anaphylactoid reactions have followed such test injections. It appears that the incidence of reactions is greater with intravenous than with intra-arterial or central injections.

It has been suggested that the incidence of anaphylactoid reactions in 'at risk' patients can be reduced by prior premedication [11] and elaborate regimes have been proposed (e.g. prednisolone 50 mg orally 12 hours and 4 hours before the study together with hydrocortisone sodium succinate 100 mg i.v. immediately before the study). The evidence that premedication with steroids can reduce the incidence of reactions is uncertain and there is, as yet, no definite evidence that non-ionic media are less likely to cause an anaphylactoid reaction; indeed evidence will be hard to obtain in view of the rarity of such reactions. Despite this, my practice in 'at risk' patients, is to give hydrocortisone sodium succinate 100 mg i.v. immediately before the study and to use a non-ionic medium.

8 Urticarial reactions. These reactions are presumably histamine-mediated and milder forms of the above anaphylactoid reactions. They are not uncommon and usually take the form of mild itching together with wheals on the face and chest. It is our practice to give an antihistamine (chlorpheniramine maleate, Piriton, 10 mg i.m.) when these reactions are observed.

9 Nausea, headache. These effects of contrast media are common. Though short lasting they are distressing; voluntary hyperventilation provides the most effective relief of nausea. The headache (but not the nausea) is dose-related and more likely to follow ventriculography than other angiographic investigations. It is not possible to predict which patients will experience these side effects. It is

largely because nausea is common that patients are studied while fasting.

10 Endothelial damage. Though reversible, endothelial damage may be responsible for cerebral oedema and neurological dysfunction. The complication is most likely to occur when an excessive amount of contrast medium has entered, selectively, the cerebral circulation. Repeated attempts to opacify an internal mammary graft, with contrast medium escaping into the vertebral artery, have resulted in cortical blindness [12, 13]. Though terrifying for patient and physician alike the condition resolves within 24 hours.

Venous thrombosis can result from peripheral vein injections; cardiologists, who are unused to venography, should be reminded to aspirate any contrast medium that may have been injected into a peripheral vein or to flush the vein with saline after the injection of contrast medium. Cerebral venous thrombosis is a rare but lethal complication of angiography which can occur in very cyanosed, polycythaemic, patients with congenital heart disease. Such patients should be well hydrated before the study and fluids given in quantity on return to the ward.

11 Pain. Central injections are not painful but injections into peripheral arteries can cause exquisite pain — the cardiologist must remember this if he wishes to retain the confidence of his patients.

NON-IONIC, LOW OSMOLAR, CONTRAST MEDIA

That most, if not all, of the side-effects of contrast, media listed above are the result of the high osmolality of conventional media has stimulated the development of media with a lower osmolality (600–850 mOsm/kg). These newer media include metrizamide (Amipaque), iopamidol (Isovue, Niopam), iohexol (Omnipaque), iopromide (Ultravist) and a low osmolar, ionic, medium — sodium and meglumine ioxglate (Hexabrix). Of these agents metrizamide is prohibitively expensive and, in the UK all are four to five times as expensive as conventional agents — 20 times as expensive in the USA [14]. It has been estimated that if all conventional media were replaced by low osmolar media the additional cost in the UK would be £10 000 000 per year [15]. A further disadvantage of the newer media is that they tend to be more viscous than the equivalent conventional media; thus, though the iodine content per unit volume is the same as for conventional media, the amount of iodine (and, therefore, radio-opacity) that can be delivered through the catheter in unit time may be less. Since the newer media tend to be used in neonates and infants, in whom fine catheters are needed, this increased viscosity can be a considerable drawback. Viscosity is less if the contrast medium is warmed to body temperature; this should be done with all media but is of particular importance if the newer media are used.

Apart from increased cost and viscosity the low osmolar media have considerable advantages. There is no doubt that they cause fewer side-effects than conventional media [16, 17]; the hot flush and nausea are minimal, haemodynamic effects are less and there is less myocardial depression. Pain on injection into peripheral vessels is virtually absent and thrombosis of peripheral veins less frequent. It is probable, but unproven, that they are less liable to cause anaphylactoid reactions. At present these low osmolar agents should be reserved for use in the following categories of patient:

1 Sick neonates and infants — especially those with heart failure due to a severe volume load (e.g. persistent truncús arteriosus).

2 Patients with sickle-cell disease.

3 Patients with impaired renal function; diabetic nephropathy, myelomatosis.

4 Patients with critical aortic stenosis; for pulmonary arteriography in patients with acute massive pulmonary embolism or primary pulmonary hypertension.

5 Patients with severely impaired left ventricular function.

6 Patients with a history of allergy or who have had a previous reaction to contrast medium.

7 And, possibly, for coronary arteriography in patients with unstable angina or a history of arrhythmias.

PREVENTION OF COMPLICATIONS DUE TO CONTRAST MEDIA

The incidence of complications due to contrast media will be reduced if the following rules are followed:

1 The total amount of contrast medium given during one study should not exceed 4 ml/kg body weight (5 ml/kg if low osmolar medium is used).

2 A low osmolar (non-ionic) medium should be used in high risk patients — as defined above. If possible avoid angiography altogether in high risk patients — especially those with primary pulmonary hypertension. Angiography is contraindicated in renal failure.

3 Be careful not to inject large quantities of contrast medium close to the origins of the head and neck vessels.

4 Consider using steroid premedication in patients with a history of allergy or previous reactions to contrast media.

5 Ensure good hydration in very polycythaemic patients — before and after the study. Consider prior haemodilution.

6 Avoid injecting into peripheral arteries; aspirate contrast medium from peripheral veins and flush with saline.

Table 7.4 Commonly used contrast media.

Composition	Proprietary names (manufacturer)
Sodium and meglumine diatrizoate	Renografin 76 (US, Squibb) Urografin 370 (UK, Schering)* Hypaque (Winthrop)
Sodium and meglumine iothalamate	Conray (US, Mallinckrodt; UK, May and Baker)
Sodium, calcium, magnesium and meglumine metrizoates	Isopaque 440 (Nycomed)* Triosil (Glaxo)
Sodium and meglumine ioxaglate	Hexabrix (UK, May and Baker)
Iopamidol	Niopam (UK, Merck) Isovue 370 (US, Squibb)
Iohexol	Omnipaque (UK, Nycomed; US, Winthrop—Breen)*
Iopromide	Ultravist (Schering)

*These media are currently employed at the Brompton Hospital.

Name	Viscosity		Osmolality
	20°C	37°C	
Urografin 370	18.5	8.9	1700
Isopaque 440	13.3	6.6	
Omnipaque 350	23.3	10.6	780

The numbers 370, 440 and 350 after the proprietary names in Table 7.4 refer to the iodine concentration (mg/ml). Urografin 370 (Renografin 76 in the US) is the most widely used medium for coronary arteriography in view of its proven low arrhythmogenicity; the relatively high viscosity is of little importance in coronary arteriography where no more than 3 to 8 ml need to be injected over 1 second. Urografin is also often used for ventriculography in adults.

Isopaque 440 is our preferred medium for ventriculography and general angiography — especially in infants and children. Its high iodine content and relatively low viscosity provide excellent radio-opacity.

Omnipaque 350 is used in high risk patients. The high (23.3) viscosity at 20°C falling to 10.6 at 37°C emphasises the importance of prewarming this contrast medium.

The complications which can occur following angiography are not all due to the effects of contrast medium, they also include simple mechanical effects of a high pressure emergent jet which can damage the myocardium or vessel wall. This usually occurs when the catheter tip is close to the myocardium and is not free to move or is wedged beneath trabeculae. The resulting 'intramyocardial injection' (Fig. 7.14) is usually small but can be extensive and even rupture

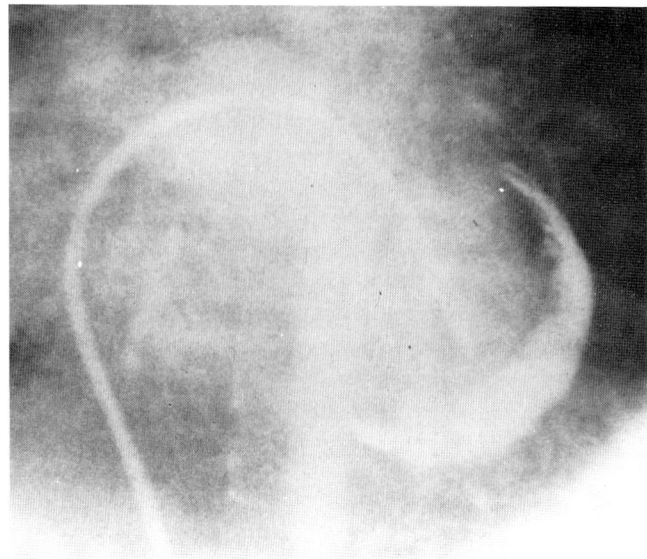

Fig. 7.14 Intramyocardial injection of contrast medium which has extended into the pericardial space.

through to the pericardial space. In a vessel it may cause a local dissection. The patient complains of chest pain and ECG changes (S-T elevation) may be alarming but in most instances resolution, as judged by the fluoroscopic appearances, occurs within minutes without sequelae. The incidence of this complication will be reduced by following certain rules for safe angiography:

1 Angiographic injections should always be preceded by a small hand injection ('scout injection') of contrast medium to determine that the catheter tip is free and not wedged between trabeculae.

2 Single end-hole catheters should not be used; there should always be additional multiple side-holes. The practice of using a single 'Sones' type of cathether for both coronary arteriography and ventriculography is liable to result in intramyocardial injections.

3 The force of the emergent jet can be reduced by choosing the largest bore of catheter that is convenient, by selecting the lowest injection pressure compatible with the desired delivery rate and by choosing a catheter with multiple side-holes.

The emergent jet has a second mechanical effect which is to cause the catheter to straighten or, if there is an unopposed end-hole, to recoil. This catheter movement may result in its displacement from the chosen site — even to another chamber — but is not likely to cause a complication other than a salvo of ectopic beats.

There is always a possibility of air embolism whenever an injection is made through a catheter; this potential complication of angiography is avoided by attention to technique when filling the angiographic injector pump — see below.

Angiographic injectors

The injection of a large volume of contrast medium through an angiographic catheter requires a power-driven syringe. Two types of injectors are currently available; pressure-controlled injectors and flow-controlled injectors (Fig. 7.15) such as the 'Viamonte–Hobbs' [18]. Pressure-controlled injectors allow the operator to preselect the volume of contrast medium to be injected and the pressure developed within the syringe. The rate at which the contrast medium is injected cannot be selected and is determined by the viscosity of the medium and the length and internal diameter of the catheter. Although it is

possible to construct tables relating flow rate to pressure for each size and type of catheter (and hence to choose the appropriate pressure for the desired rate of flow) pressure-controlled injectors are obsolete and have been replaced by flow-controlled injectors. These allow the operator to select the total volume to be injected and the rate of injection (ml/sec). A microprocessor determines the pressure needed to achieve the desired rate of flow. The maximum allowable pressure can be preset — usually at 1000 p.s.i. though as a rough guide 100 multiplied by the French gauge of the catheter will provide an adequate flow rate while avoiding the possibility of rupturing the smaller and thinner catheters. (e.g. 500 p.s.i. (3450 kPa) for a no. 5F catheter). The injectors incorporate a warming device designed to keep the contrast medium at body temperature — and thus to reduce its viscosity. While adequate to maintain the temperature of the injectate the warming jacket is not designed to warm cold contrast in a short time. Thus it is good practice to hold a day's supply of contrast medium in a cabinet which is thermostatically maintained at 37°C. The syringe of the injector is transparent and is filled with contrast medium while in a vertical position. The movement of the plunger is then reversed to expel all air before the injector is returned to a slightly 'nose-down' position for connection to the catheter. Once the hub of the catheter is firmly attached to the Luer-lock of the injector the plunger is again withdrawn *slowly* until a little blood is aspirated into the syringe. This procedure is important as it avoids the possibility of air embolism. Any air trapped in the catheter will be aspirated and seen in the syringe. If a significant air bubble is present the procedure should be repeated. However a small amount of air is permissable *provided* that (1) the syringe is kept in a nose-down position (so that the air is against the plunger and remote from the catheter), (2) the volume of contrast medium held in the syringe significantly exceeds the volume to be injected. Injector pumps incorporate a safety stop which should be set at 2 ml more than the selected injection volume. (The 2 ml margin allows for the catheter volume and the safety stop allows for inadvertent mis-setting of the volume to be injected.) The volume of the catheter can be significant in relation to the volume to be injected in paediatric work when the total volume to be injected may be no more than 3 or 4 ml. In such cases it is wise to prefill the catheter with contrast

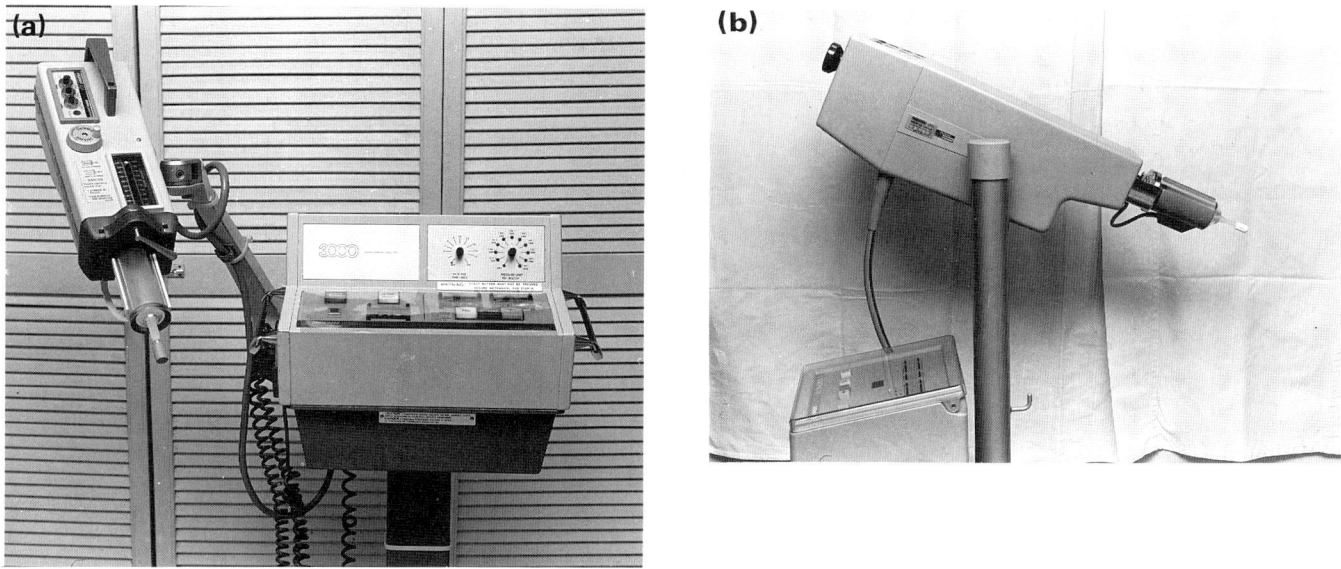

Fig. 7.15 Two flow-controlled angiographic injectors: (a) 'Angiomat 3000 Viamonte—Hobbs' injector, (b) 'Simtrac DH' injector (Siemens).

medium by gently advancing the plunger so as to expel 1 or 2 ml before 'arming' the injector for the powered injection. In some laboratories a length of transparent, high pressure, 'angiographic tubing' is used to connect the catheter to the injector. We prefer to connect the catheter directly so as to minimise the number of connections that might become detached.

Angiographic catheters

These are described in Chapter 2: 'The tools of catheterisation'.

Angiographic projections

Conventional nomenclature, as used by radiologists, defines the projection in terms of the direction of the X-ray beam from tube to intensifier (or film). Thus with the tube behind the patient and the film in front a postero-anterior (PA) film is obtained. In cardiac radiology a different nomenclature is generally adopted. This defines the projection in terms of the position of the image intensifier. The view is described in terms of what the operator would see if his head was in the same position as the intensifier. Thus if the intensifier is tilted 30° towards the patient's head we obtain a '30° cranial view'. Tilted towards the patient's feet we obtain a 'caudal view'.

In the transverse plane angulation is measured from the midline; with the intensifier tilted 30° to the patients left we obtain a '30° left (anterior) oblique view' (LAO), 30° to his right and we have a '30° right (anterior) oblique' (RAO). With modern equipment we can angulate the intensifier and tube in both the sagittal and transverse planes at the same time. The combined views produce right and left oblique cranial and right and left oblique caudal projections. In paediatric cardiology especially, two of these combined views have become known as the four chamber and 'long axis' projections. These views require some explanation. Ventricular septal defects (VSD) may be in the inlet septum when they lie relatively posteriorly, or in the membranous septum when they lie relatively anteriorly. Subarterial defects in the outlet septum are the most anteriorly positioned of all. Since the right ventricle is 'wrapped around' the left ventricle the ventricular septum is not a straight structure but extends in an arc of 100°. Reference to the diagram (Fig. 7.16) shows that to profile defects in the membranous septum the X-ray beam must be at approximately 75° LAO; this orientation will place the defect at right angles to the beam. Posterior (inlet septal) defects will be profiled if the beam is at approximately 25° LAO while anterior (subarterial) defects in the outlet septum require a 90° LAO (left lateral) projection to be correctly profiled. Not only is the ventricular septum curved but it, and the left ventricle are also directed anteriorly, inferiorly and to the left. As a result the ventricular septum will be foreshortened unless cranial angulation is added to the X-ray projection. While the long axis of the left ventricle is orientated anteriorly, inferiorly and to the left it is orientated more anteriorly than leftward; thus views which approach the frontal projection require steeper cranial angulation than do views which approach the lateral projection. Putting all this together we see that to profile posterior inlet defects we need to add steep (45°) cranial angulation to the relatively shallow (25°) LAO projection. This view also profiles the interatrial septum and separates all four cardiac chambers; it is commonly known as the 'four chamber view'. To profile anterior (perimembranous) defects we need to add less (25°) cranial angulation since the steep (75°) LAO projection is approaching the lateral view. This is the 'long axis' view. Subarterial defects will be profiled in a right or left lateral projection [19–22].

While the above views serve to profile VSDs they are not the views that are used for ventriculography in adult patients with acquired heart disease. If single plane left ventriculography is employed a 30° RAO projection is commonly chosen though consideration of the above would suggest that adding some caudal angulation would reduce the foreshortening that must result from the leftward orientation of the ventricle. This view profiles the mitral valve and will demonstrate aneurysms of the anterior wall of the ventricle. Anterior apical and inferior segmental wall motion can be assessed but the posterior segment is obscured. Ideally therefore, left ventriculography should be performed with biplane filming using both right and left oblique views. The left oblique view allows assessment of posterior segmental wall motion, the aortic valve is well seen and some of the septum is profiled. Although biplane ventriculography with a 30° RAO and 60° LAO projection provides good otthogonal visualisation of the left ventricle there is still some foreshortening. This will be minimised if 15° caudal angulation is added to the RAO and 15° cranial angulation added to the LAO. In the adult biplane filming has one disadvantage — film quality may be somewhat impaired by scatter of X-rays from the contralateral tube. It is also slightly more time consuming and of course requires expensive biplane

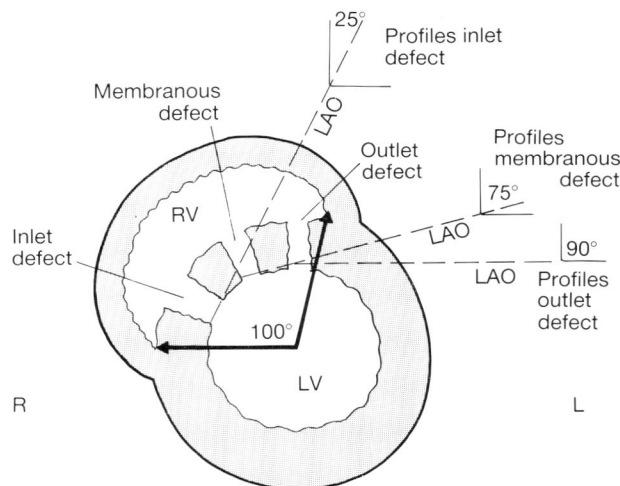

Fig. 7.16 The different positions of defects in the curved ventricular septum determines the degree of angulation of the X-ray beam needed to profile each type of defect.

equipment. Radiation to laboratory personnel is also increased.

Ventriculography

Left ventriculography is probably the most frequently performed angiogram. The correct catheter for ventriculography is one with multiple sideholes; the choice of catheter is discussed in Chapter 2 but there is no doubt that, in adult work at least, the pigtail ventriculography catheter is the catheter of choice. Alternatives include the NIH and Eppendorf and these catheters are ideal for right ventriculography. In paediatric work, a balloon-tipped angiographic catheter (Swan–Ganz or Berman) may be used though pigtail catheters are available in small sizes suitable for infants and children — as is the NIH. For adult work a no. 8F catheter is needed but a no. 7F may have to be accepted if the brachial approach is used and the artery too small to accept a larger catheter. Thin-wall catheters will allow a higher flow rate but lack the wire mesh that facilitates catheter manipulation.

The ideal position for the catheter tip is in the mid-cavity. This position may be impossible to hold as it may result in repeated ventricular ectopic beats; if so the catheter must be positioned in the inflow tract of the left ventricle just in front of the posterior leaflet of the mitral valve. This position in the inflow tract is usually 'quiet' — that is to say ectopic beats are few or absent; it has the disadvantage that mitral valve function may be disturbed with resulting spurious mitral regurgitation. A second disadvantage is that the ventricular apex may be inadequately opacified. An apical position is undesirable; ectopic beats are likely to be troublesome and, in patients with prior myocardial infarction, there is a danger of dislodging mural thrombus. For right ventriculography the ideal catheter position is in the trabecular (apical) portion of the ventricle or, if ectopic beats are a problem, the outflow portion may have to be selected.

Ventriculography, indeed all angiography, must be preceded by a small ('scout') injection of contrast medium. Three to 5 ml injected by hand are all that are needed. The purpose of scout injections is to ensure that the catheter is correctly positioned and that the tip of the catheter is not trapped among trabeculae — a position that might lead to an intramyocardial injection (Fig. 7.14).

INJECTION VOLUME AND RATE OF INJECTION

As a rough guide to the volume of contrast medium and the rate of injection the aim should be to inject somewhat less than the ventricular stroke volume in one cardiac cycle. In neonatal and infant studies this may be not more than 4 to 5 ml or roughly 1 ml/kg. In adult studies 30 ml injected at 15 ml/sec is appropriate. The volume must be increased when the ventricle is volume loaded because of mitral or aortic regurgitation or left-to-right shunting. When the ventricle is of small volume, as in pulmonary atresia with intact ventricular septum, the volume injected must be small — less than 1 ml/kg. When the ventricle is enlarged because of impaired myocardial function the volume injected does not need to be increased since the stroke volume is small and the whole cavity will opacify over several cardiac cycles.

PRECAUTIONS

1 Ventriculography carries an increased risk when myocardial function is severely impaired. If this is known to be the case from prior clinical or echocardiographic studies but ventriculography is mandatory it is wise to use a non-ionic low osmolar medium (see above). Preparation should include energetic diuretic therapy. A mean wedge pressure

in the region of 40 mmHg, should warn the operator that acute pulmonary oedema may well ensue as ventricular function is further depressed and an osmotic hypervolaemia results from the action of contrast medium. A raised left ventricular end-diastolic pressure of the same order is another, less reliable, warning. If the high risk patient develops an irritating cough during the study this is an almost infallible warning that acute pulmonary oedema is imminent; the study must be brought to a rapid conclusion so that the patient can be allowed to sit up. It may be necessary to give frusemide (Lasix) 5−10 mg i.v.

2 Always obtain a video record during the ventriculogram. View the VTR record to ensure that an adequate study has been obtained before withdrawing the catheter from the ventricle — unless it is stimulating multiple ectopic beats.

3 Mechanically induced ventricular ectopics are common during ventriculography. Very rarely ventricular tachycardia or fibrillation will ensue; the catheter must be withdrawn immediately to the aorta and sinus rhythm restored by immediate DC countershock. A bolus dose of i.v. lignocaine (lidocaine, xylocaine) 1 mg/kg may also be given.

4 While the operator must always be prepared to quickly withdraw the catheter if something untoward occurs it is unlikely that he can react quickly enough to abort the intraventricular injection. For this reason it is not our practice to keep hold of the catheter during the injection — a practice that some recommend. Instead the operator should remember that the radiation to which he is exposed decreases as *the square* of the distance from the X-ray source — and stand well back! Unfortunately this is not possible during coronary arteriography when the operator has to hold the catheter to maintain its position in the coronary ostium.

REFERENCES

1 Snyder CF, Formanek A, Frech RS, Amplatz, K. The role of sodium in promoting ventricular arrhythmia during selective coronary arteriography. *Am J Roentgenol* 1971;**113**:567.

2 Dawson P, Harrison MJG, Weisblatt E. Effect of contrast media on red cell filtrability and morphology. *Br J Radiol* 1983;**56**:707.

3 Rao AK, Thompson R, Durlacher L, James F. Angiographic contrast agent-induced acute hemolysis in a patient with hemoglobin SC disease. *Arch Intern Med* 1985;**145**:759.

4 Hayward R, Dawson P. Contrast agents in angiocardiography. *Br Heart J* 1984;**52**:361.

5 Kloster FE, Friesen WG, Green GS, Judkins MP. Effects of coronary arteriography on myocardial blood flow. *Circulation* 1972;**46**:438.

6 Grainger RG. Renal toxicity of radiologic contrast media. *Br Med Bull* 1972;**28**:191.

7 Swartz RD, Rubin JE, Leeming BW, Silva P. Renal failure following major angiography. *Am J Med* 1978;**65**:31.

8 D'Elia JA *et al.* Nephrotoxicity from angiographic contrast media. A prospective study. *Am J Med* 1982;**72**:719.

9 Cramer BC *et al.* Renal function following infusion of radiologic contrast material: a prospective controlled study. *Arch Intern Med* 1985;**145**:87.

10 Shehadi WH. Adverse reactions to intravascularly administered contrast media. *Am J Roentgenol* 1975;**124**:145.

11 Myers GE, Bloom FL. Cimetidine (tagamet) combined with steroids and H1 antihistamines for the prevention of serious radiographic contrast material reactions. *Cathet Cardiovasc Diagn* 1981;**7**:65.

12 Vik-Mo H, Todnem K, Folling M, Rosland GA. Transient visual disturbance during cardiac catheterization with angiography. *Cathet Cardiovasc Diagn* 1986;**12**:1.

13 Horowitz NH, Werner L. Temporary cortical blindness following angiography. *J Neurosurg* 1974;**40**:583.

14 Wolf GL. Safer, more expensive, iodinated contrast agents. How do we decide? *Radiology* 1986;**159**:557.

15 Grainger RG. Annotation: radiological contrast media. *Clin Radiol* 1987;**38**:3.

16 Gertz EW *et al.* Clinical superiority of a new non-ionic contrast agent (Iopamidol) for cardiac angiography. *J Am Coll Cardiol* 1985;**5**:250.

17 Bettmann MA *et al.* Contrast agents for cardiac angiography: effects of a non-ionic agent, vs. a standard ionic agent. *Radiology* 1984;**153**:583.

18 Viamonte M, Hobbs J. Automatic electric injector: development to prevent electromechanical hazards of selective angiocardiography. *Invest Radiol* 1967;**2**:262.

19 Bargeron LH *et al.* Axial cineangiography in congenital heart disease. Section 1. Concept, technical and anatomic considerations. *Circulation* 1977;**56**:1075.

20 Elliott LP *et al.* Axial cineangiography in congenital heart disease. Section 2. Specific lessions. *Circulation* 1977;**56**:1084.

21 Fellows KE, Keane JF, Freed MD. Angled views in cineangiocardiography of congenital heart disease. *Circulation* 1977;**56**:485.

22 Santamaria H *et al.* Angiographic differentiation of types of ventricular septal defects. *AJR* 1983;**141**:273.

Quantitative angiocardiography and the assessment of ventricular function

INTRODUCTION

The assessment of ventricular function has been essential in the investigation and description of the function of the normal heart, and it is central both to the characterisation of specific cardiac disease states and to the evaluation of the cardiac actions of pharmacological agents. However, it is used primarily in day to day clinical cardiological practice in the complete assessment of an individual patient and in the determination of therapeutic options and prognoses. This chapter confines itself to invasive and angiographic techniques, and while some methods of assessment may be more appropriate for one or other of the above purposes, it is the aim of this chapter to discuss the most commonly used methods, their theory and practice, and indicate their relative usefulness in clinical cardiology.

An ideal measure of left ventricular function would have the following characteristics: it would be easy to perform and have high sensitivity, specificity and reproducibility. It would provide assessment of regional performance, be independent of preload and afterload, be quantitative and qualitative, and be of prognostic value. Furthermore it would accurately predict the performance under stress without having actually to stress the patient. Unfortunately no such ideal has yet been achieved, but the value of existing techniques may be viewed with such an ideal in mind.

Presently the methods of analysis of ventricular function fall conveniently into two broad approaches; first, the derivation of indices that attempt to define global ventricular function in terms of a single unique number, and second, the analysis of

ventricular wall motion. The former mainly comprises angiographically derived volume data or intraventricular pressure data and their relationship, individually with time or with each other. Thus this approach can be further divided into the derivation of indices that describe ventricular performance as a pump (ejection phase indices), for example cardiac output, stroke work, ejection fraction, and those that describe it in terms of myocardial contractility (isovolumic indices). This latter group attempts to extrapolate to the intact man indices used to describe force—length—time relationships in isolated cardiac muscles preparations. Examples are max dP/dt and V_{MAX}. While each method yields useful results, it has become clear that no single index of ventricular function is comprehensive, each has practical and theoretical limitations and for the most sensitive assessment a combination of different methods is required [1, 2].

The failure of any single measurement adequately to describe ventricular function prompts further research into the second approach; the qualitative and quantitative analysis of ventricular wall motion from angiographic images. This concerns analysis of regional ventricular motion and its relationship spatially and temporally with other ventricular areas or with fixed reference points. Analysis of wall motion in three dimensions has also attracted a lot of interest. Rapidly advancing computer technology, in particular digital imaging, image processing and colour graphics, has provided the tools for complex image analysis and for the presentation of the large volumes of resulting data.

Both broad approaches may be further divided by their application to systolic and diastolic ventricular function of both left and right ventricles.

SYSTOLIC FUNCTION

Simple measures of ventricular performance

STROKE WORK, VENTRICULAR FUNCTION
CURVES AND END DIASTOLIC PRESSURE

Stroke work is the amount of work measured in gram metres (g m) or kilogram metres (kg m) that is performed by the ventricle in each beat. It can be divided into the useful work i.e. that used in expelling and propelling blood from the ventricle, and non-useful work, that expended in heat and overcoming friction and viscosity. Useful work is easier to measure than non-useful work (see also the section on pressure volume loops). Ventricular function curves are plots of stroke work or stroke volume against ventricular filling pressure.

Ventricular function curves depend upon two fundamental principles of muscle physiology. First, that the degree to which contractile elements stretch at end diastole (*preload*) is directly related to the filling pressure; and second, that the amount of work generated is linearly related to the degree of muscle stretch [3]. The combination of the two results in a relationship between filling pressure and stroke work which takes into account changes in either of the fundamentals that may occur in ventricular failure. The slope of this curve represents the state of myocardial performance. Changes in the inotropic state will move the function curve upwards and to the left or down and to the right (Fig. 8.1). At least

two sets of data points are required in order to construct such a slope, but interventions designed to provide the extra points such as acute volume loading or acute pressure loading result in concomitant changes in the inotropic state, ventricular compliance and afterload, thus invalidating the derived slope. However, Bradley [4] measured ventricular stroke work at various preloads, (in this case effected by repeatedly removing aliquots of blood) in a selection of patients with different circulatory derangements and described a fan-shaped arrangement of function curves (Fig. 8.2) with an approximately common origin. Thus he was able to construct general stroke work equations for left and right ventricles:

$$W_L = \frac{(b - 13)P_L + 10b - 130}{a + 10} + 13 \qquad (1)$$

General stroke work equation for the left ventricle where W_L is the left ventricular stroke work in gram metres, P_L is the left ventricular filling pressure in mmHg measured from the sternal angle and a and b are the x and y coordinates of any single point on the equation.

$$W_R = \frac{bP_R + 10b}{a + 10} \qquad (2)$$

General stroke work equation for the right ventricle where W_R is the right ventricular stroke work in gram metres, P_R is the filling pressure in mmHg measured from the sternal angle and a and b are the x and y coordinates of any single point on the equation.

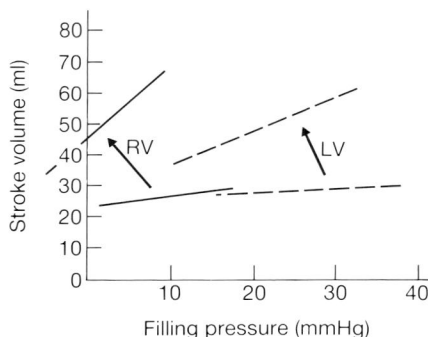

Fig. 8.1 Left and right ventricular function curves shifted upwards and to the left after infusion of isoprenaline in a patient with an acute anterior myocardial infarction. This represents an increase in myocardial contractility. With kind permission of RD Bradley.

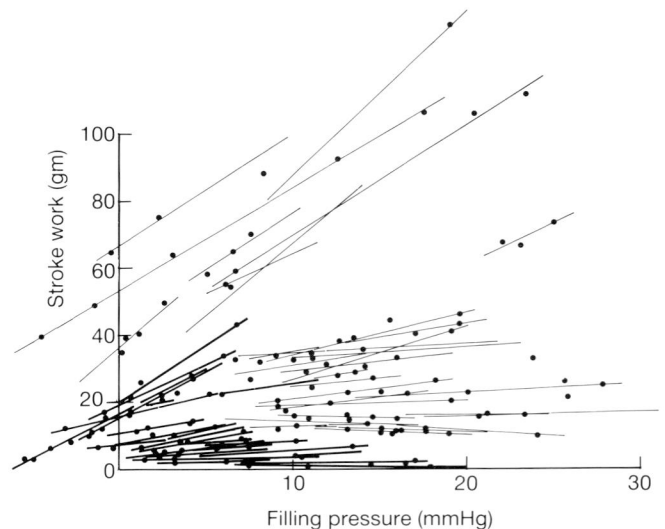

Fig. 8.2 Stroke work equations of the left and right hearts of a number of patients ranging from normal to extremes of dysfunction [4]. With kind permission of RD Bradley and Edward Arnold.

Thus if only a single value for stroke work is known at a given preload, the slope and the intercept of the equation can be simply derived.

The measurements are easy to make, using either dye dilution or thermal dilution techniques for measurement of stroke volume (Chapter 10), a right atrial pressure catheter, systemic arterial pressure catheter, and an indirect measurement of left atrial pressure using either pulmonary artery diastolic [119] or pulmonary artery wedge pressures. The values for stroke work (from equations 3a and 3b) and filling pressure can then be substituted in equations 1 or 2 (note that the right atrial pressure is measured from the sternal angle):

$$W_L = (MAP - AP_L) \times SV \times 1.36.10^{-2} \quad (3a)$$

$$W_R = (MAP - AP_R) \times SV \times 1.36.10^{-2} \quad (3b)$$

Equation for the calculation of stroke work where MAP is the mean systemic arterial pressure, AP_L and AP_R are the left and right mean atrial pressures, SV is the stroke volume and $1.36.10^{-2}$ is a constant for converting from mmHg ml to gram metres.

Of course these equations are physiological generalisations and therefore approximations. Nevertheless such a measure of ventricular function has its use in clinical practice, especially in the critically ill patient where it can be used as a means of monitoring progress and for its prognostic value; those patients with left ventricular stroke work intercepts of less than 13 g m/beat die due to inadequate blood flow.

Conclusion

Stroke work and the construction of ventricular function curves provide a very general assessment of ventricular function and it should be noted that this method only measures useful work generated. It neither takes account of changes in afterload, although these may be insignificant in the face of severe ventricular dysfunction, nor distinguishes between valvular and myocardial disease.

End-diastolic pressure (EDP)

Definition and measurement

EDP should be recorded after the a wave of atrial contraction at the z point. This is the short period following atrial contraction when atrial and ventricular pressures are the same in normals and which occurs an average of 0.052 seconds after the onset of the QRS complex of the electrocardiogram (ECG) [7]. This is commonly taken as the ventricular pressure at the time of the peak of the R wave. Deviations from this technique can lead to inter-observer errors and detract from any value of EDP measurement.

It has been known since 1920 [5] that the failing ventricle dilates and that the EDP of the dilating ventricle rises. Until suitable methods for measuring ventricular volume *in vivo* were available the EDP was the best indirect method of assessing this dilatation. It continues to be used as an easily obtained guide to ventricular performance. However it is not very reliable, indeed Rackley [6] found no relation between left ventricular EDP and end-diastolic volume (EDV) in a variety of cardiac disease states.

The diastolic pressure—volume equation extrapolated from the pressure—length relationship, is similar to the ventricular function curve, being moved left or right by changes in ventricular compliance rather than contractility. As can be seen in Fig.8.3, at any given level of myocardial compliance there may be large changes in EDV with small changes in EDP. EDP is therefore not a very sensitive measure of EDV when EDP is in the normal range or slightly elevated. Just as a single measure of filling pressure does not give the ventricular stroke work because of possible changes in the inotropic state, a single measure of EDP does not accurately reflect volume or tension because of possible changes in ventricular

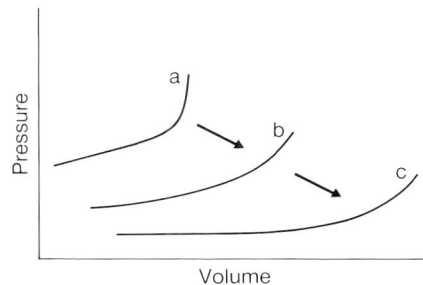

Fig. 8.3 Diastolic pressure/volume relations demonstrating increasing compliance from a to b to c. In a compliant ventricle volume can increase considerably with little change in end-diastolic pressure.

compliance. Thus in patients with primary or secondary left ventricular hypertrophy and a normal EDV, the EDP may be raised, sometimes to levels of twice the upper limit of normal [8]. Likewise a volume overloaded normal ventricle may have an elevated EDV but a normal EDP. EDP measurements are further confounded by the fact that they are measured relative to atmospheric pressure and not pericardial pressure, and pericardial disease itself may cause alterations in EDP.

Conclusion

Despite its poor performance as an index of ventricular function, including that of the right ventricle [9], EDP has been shown to be a reasonably sensitive but highly non-specific determinant of severe cardiac disease [1, 10]. The sensitivity of EDP alone to identify less severe cardiac disease can be increased by measuring it during isometric exercise when EDP in normal subjects does not change significantly [11]. Pre- and postventriculography measurements also enhance the sensitivity of EDP; increases in post-ventriculography measurements indicate myocardial disease.

Measures of volume or dimension

End-systolic volume (ESV)
End-diastolic volume (EDV)
Ejection fraction (EF)
Mean normalised systolic ejection rate (MNSER)
Velocity of circumferential fibre shortening (V_{CF})

The techniques for the measurement of left ventricular volume and their limitations are dealt with in detail in a following section. Here a short explanation of the basic principles will suffice to appreciate the value of the described indices.

Measurements of ventricular volume are based on the assumption that the ventricle approximates to a simple geometric figure, an ellipsoid in the case of the left ventricle and a triangular-based pyramid [12] in the case of the right ventricle. Using either monoplane or biplane angiography, volumes can be calculated by the application of an appropriate formula to specific dimensions of the projected image of the ventricle, which appears as an ellipse (left ventricle) or a triangle (right ventricle). For

shapes that do not conform to standard geometric models other methods of planimetry have been devised [13]. Calibration of the images is performed by knowledge of the camera geometry or filming of a reference figure. Errors can be introduced by optical distortions, calibration techniques, geometric assumptions and in the final analysis of the images.

End-systolic and end-diastolic volumes

For definition and measurement see also section on volume measurement. End-systolic volume (ESV) is commonly taken as the volume at minimum ventricular dimension rather than when the semi-lunar valve is seen to close on angiography, or at the time of the incisura on the intraventricular and aortic pressure recordings. EDV may be taken as the largest ventricular dimension, but it is quite easy and more accurate to time it with the R-wave of the ECG. This excludes errors introduced by incoordinate motion which make estimation of minimum and maximum dimensions difficult unless all frames of a cardiac cycle are objectively analysed.

Volume overloaded ventricles such as those found in patients with valvular insufficiency or congenital heart disease have large stroke volumes and increased ESV and EDV but they may have normal myocardial contractility. Similarly severely diseased ventricles may have normal ESV or EDV with grossly abnormal myocardial function [14−17]. Despite this, values of EDV and ESV for specific cardiac lesions have been published [17−19] Normal values for EDV vary from $70\pm20\,\mathrm{ml/m^2}$ to $82\pm11\,\mathrm{ml/m^2}$.

EDV is marginally raised in mitral valve stenosis and aortic valve stenosis and markedly increased in mitral regurgitation, aortic regurgitation and primary myocardial disease. The degree of increase of EDV in mitral regurgitation and aortic regurgitation is directly proportional to the regurgitant volume [19]. ESV alone has been used as a prognostic indicator in surgery for chronic left ventricular volume overload in valvular regurgitation. It predicts both postoperative left ventricular function and perioperative mortality [20]. It has recently been shown to be the major determinant of survival after recovery from myocardial infarction, being superior to both ejection fraction and EDV [21]. Either volume may be normalised for body surface area to create the indices ESV index (ESVI) and EDV index (EDVI) which provide more useful comparative measures.

Conclusion

The ESVI does provide an indicator of severe myocardial dysfunction and it is easy and quick to measure. However neither ESV nor EDV, alone and out of context, is a very sensitive index of ventricular function but the relationship between them, the *ejection fraction*, is.

Ejection fraction (EF)

Definition and measurement

The ejection fraction (EF) is the proportion of the EDV that is ejected in systole:

$$EF = \frac{EDV - ESV}{EDV} \qquad (4)$$

Equation for the calculation of ejection fraction.

Values for the normal EF vary according to whether monoplane or biplane angiography has been used. In adults an average value for left ventricular ejection fraction in studies using biplane methods is 0.66 with a range of 0.58 to 0.72; and in children less than two years 0.42 ± 0.10 [22]. With monoplane studies the average is slightly increased to 0.68 with a range of 0.60 to 0.76. An ejection fraction of <0.4 indicates significant myocardial depression and an ejection fraction of <0.25 suggests very severe myocardial dysfunction and a poor prognosis.

As a ventricle dilates under the influence of a higher filling pressure and is able to accommodate a greater volume, so the tension in the ventricular wall rises. The application of this relationship (Laplace's law, equation 8a) to cardiac structure and function was first made by Woods [23] in 1892 and has been explored extensively since then in the analysis of ventricular wall stress (see below). Consequently a dilated ventricle, for a given degree of fibre shortening, produces a larger stroke volume than a normal sized ventricle but at considerably increased energy expenditure as indicated by increased myocardial oxygen consumption [24] and increased stroke work [16]. The prolonged increase in tension also has a detrimental effect on the velocity of contraction of the contractile elements [25]. Thus the volume overloaded ventricle initially produces a larger stroke volume and a normal or slightly increased ejection fraction; but progressively in-

creasing tension and consequent decrease of fibre shortening rate finally result in a smaller stroke volume and decreased ejection fraction [26]. A reduced ejection fraction can therefore be seen as a good marker of additional myocardial disease in the volume overloaded ventricle.

Ejection fraction does not distinguish between forward and backward flow in valvular heart disease. However if the forward stroke volume, measured by indicator dilution technique (Chapter 10), is taken into account, and if the heart rate is the same for both measurements, the regurgitant and forward fractions can be calculated according to equation 5:

$$RF = \frac{SV_{angiographic} - SV_{indicator}}{SV_{angiographic}} \qquad (5)$$

Conclusion

Notwithstanding the errors that may occur in angiographic determinations of volume (see below), the ejection fraction is a widely used, easy to perform, relatively sensitive indicator of left ventricular disease [2] and the experienced interpreter can make a very good estimate of ejection fraction from the subjective analysis of the ventriculogram. Ejection fraction is also accepted as a useful and readily measurable index in other modes of investigation, for example nuclear cardiology and echocardiography.

RIGHT VENTRICULAR EJECTION FRACTION

Ejection fraction of the right ventricle in normals has been studied by a number of authors using different techniques of volume estimation from angiograms, both monoplane and biplane [27–30]. It has been shown that it is significantly lower than that of the left ventricle [31] although the stroke volume [32] and stroke index [31] are the same.

Ejection rate

Definition and measurement

The rate at which blood is ejected from the ventricle during systole. This is the same as the rate of change of ventricular volume (dv/dt) during systole and can be measured either instantaneously or as a mean value. The left ventricular systolic ejection rate is equal, provided there is no valve incompetence, to systolic aortic blood flow.

Instantaneous ejection rate or dV/dt is obviously more difficult to measure since it requires many measurements of ventricular volume per cardiac cycle. Peak dV/dt is not a reliable measure of cardiac function but when normalised to EDV it shows a good correlation with peak normalised velocity of circumferential shortening rate (peak V_{CF}) [33]. An easier measure to make is mean normalised systolic ejection rate (MNSER):

$$MNSER = \frac{EF}{ET}$$

Equation for the calculation of mean normalised ejection rate where EF is ejection fraction and ET is ejection time.

Conclusion

The normal range for MNSER was first published by Peterson *et al.* [2] in 1974 who showed it to correlate well with EF and mean V_{CF} ($r = 0.87$ and 0.79 respectively).

Velocity of circumferential fibre shortening

Definition

This is commonly taken to be a measure of myo-cardial contractility but can be seen as another indirect means of expressing a rate of change of ventricular systolic volume. It is measured according to the following formula:

$$mean\ V_{CF} = \frac{EDD - ESD}{EDD \times ET} \quad (6)$$

Equation for velocity of circumferential fibre shortening where EDD and ESD are the maximun transverse diameters in the right anterior oblique (RAO) projection of the left ventricle at end-diastole and end-systole respectively.

An alternative method involves calculating the mid-wall circumference at the level of the maximum diameter from the area of the ventricle derived from area—length analysis (see page 142) in the RAO projection according to the following equation:

$$C = \frac{4A}{L + \pi h} \quad (7)$$

Equation for the calculation of mid-wall circumference where C is the circumference at the level of mid-ventricular wall, L is the maximum chord length, A is the projected area and h is the wall thickness.

Clearly V_{CF} measures velocity of fibre shortening only for a specific point of the ventricular wall and takes no account of regional variations. Therefore, as an index of contractility, extrapolation to the whole ventricle is suspect. Furthermore any increase in afterload that delays systolic emptying, for example hypertrophic obstructive cardiomyopathy or aortic valve stenosis, will cause a fall in V_{CF} despite normal myocardial contractility and a normal EF.

Conclusion

Velocity of circumferential fibre shortening is critically afterload-dependent.

Measures of pressure and volume combined

Pressure—volume ratio
Elastance (E)
Wall stress (σ)

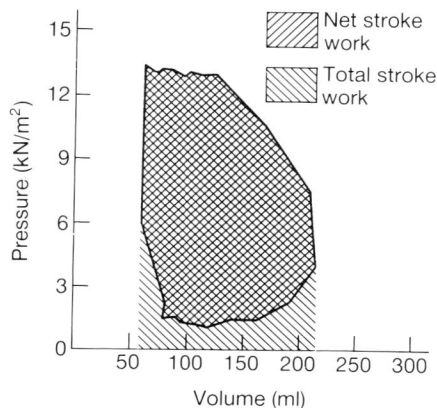

Fig. 8.4 A pressure/volume loop for the normal left ventricle. With kind permission of Dr MM Webb-Peploe.

Indices of the end-systolic pressure—volume relation are measures of myocardial contractility, and while wall stress is a measure of mechanical loading, its relationship with fibre length is also a good reflection of myocardial contractility. A major problem with isovolumic indices of contractility, e.g. maximum dP/dt (see below) is eliminating their dependence upon preload. An advantage of the pressure–volume indices is that they have been shown to be independent of preload [34–35].

Pressure–volume relationship

Definition and measurement

The ratio of instantaneous ventricular pressure and instantaneous ventricular volume. A pressure–volume loop (Fig. 8.4) may be constructed by recording simultaneous pressure and volume measurements throughout a cardiac cycle. A high frequency response (25–200 Hz) catheter tip micro-manometer, for example a Millar, Gaeltec or Camino catheter, is used for pressure measurement and either monoplane or biplane ventriculography for volume measurement, although radionuclide methods may also be used for volume estimation [36].

The resulting loop can be used as an accurate measure of stroke work, the net stroke work being represented by the area enclosed by the loop, and the area below the loop representing the diastolic work of ventricular distension. The area is measured in millilitre mmHg but can be converted to kilogram metres by multiplying by 1.36 (converting mmHg to centimetres of water) and dividing by 100 000.

While the loop may have characteristic shapes in different disease states (Fig. 8.5) [37], and its diastolic portion be used in measuring ventricular

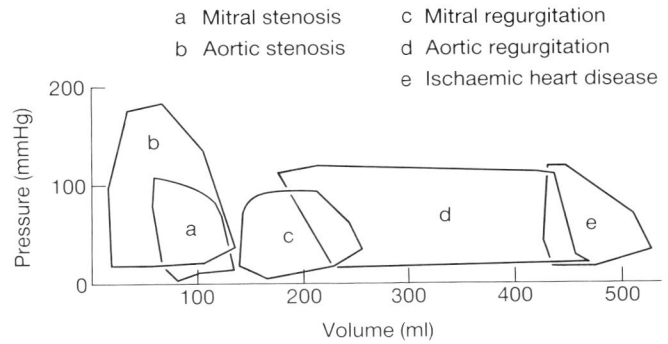

Fig. 8.5 Pressure/volume loops of five patients with various loads on their left ventricles [37].

compliance (see section on diastolic function), it does not in itself represent a measure of contractility. However if pressure–volume loops are constructed at different levels of ventricular loading, using infusions of vasodilators or vasoconstrictors, it has been shown that there is a linear relationship between isochronal instantaneous pressure–volume plot points, which becomes maximal at end systole (Figs 8.6a and 8.6b). Suga and Sagawa termed the slope of this end-systolic relationship the maximal elastance (E_{MAX}) and demonstrated, in a canine model, that given a constant heart rate and constant contractile state, it is not influenced by changes in preload or afterload [38].

Elastance

Definition

Elastance (E) is measured in mmHg per ml and is the relationship:

Fig. 8.6 (a) Pressure/volume loops created under various loading conditions. Control, and with infusions of methoxamine and nitroprusside. (b) The time-varying elastance. The isochronal points in each of the loops have been connected, the slope of the resulting line representing elastance. Note that this is maximal at end systole (E_{MAX}) [38]. With kind permission of Dr MR Starling.

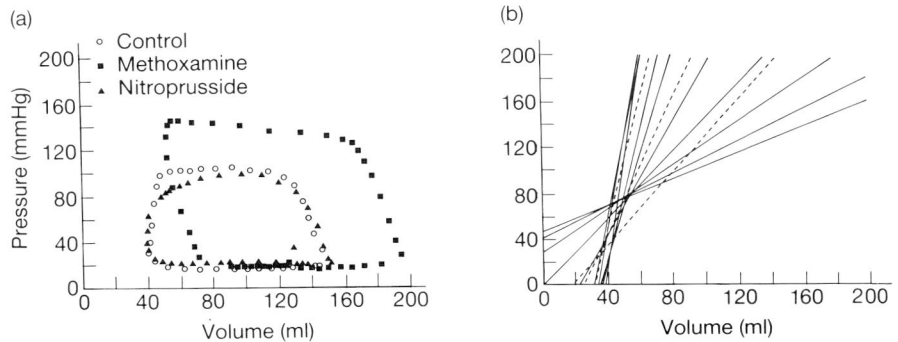

$$\frac{\text{(Instantaneous ventricular pressure)}}{\left(\begin{array}{c}\text{Instantaneous} \\ \text{ventricular volume}\end{array}\right) - \left(\begin{array}{c}\text{Volume at} \\ \text{zero pressure}\end{array}\right)}$$

The maximal time varying elastance is E_{MAX} (Figs 8.6a and 8.6b) and represents a load-independent measure of ventricular contractility. Unfortunately the zero pressure intercept, (volume at zero pressure) V_0 varies from ventricle to ventricle so that the state of myocardial contractility in any given patient cannot reliably be determined from a single end-systolic pressure–volume measurement. At least three recording under different loading conditions must be made and the isochronal end-systolic co-ordinates joined. The volume at zero pressure, V_0, can then be extrapolated and the slope taken as E_{MAX}. There have been attempts to normalise E_{MAX} so that a single end-systolic pressure–volume recordings might be representative. It has recently been reported that left ventricular E_{MAX} in man may be normalised to left ventricular mass [39].

The definition of end-systole itself is a moot point. It may be defined as zero aortic flow as determined by the aortic pressure dichrotic notch or by the incisura of the intraventricular pressure trace, but it may also be defined as the maximum pressure–volume ratio, minimum dP/dt, or as minimum dimension or volume on the ventriculogram. These definitions of end-systole have been shown to underestimate E_{MAX} [39]. It may be more satisfactory to consider end-ejection, as recognised by semi-lunar valve closure, rather than end-systole, as determined by any haemodynamic measurement. This would be particularly applicable to the right ventricle as it has been noted that ejection may continue after the time of the maximum pressure–volume ratio [40].

Conclusion

Accurate measurement of time varying elastance in man is complex, involving fixed rate pacing and changes of loading conditions. While it may be the closest to an ideal load-independent measurement of ventricular contractility it is clearly not practical for everyday use. Other indices of end-systolic pressure–volume relations [41] using peak ventricular pressure suffer the same drawbacks.

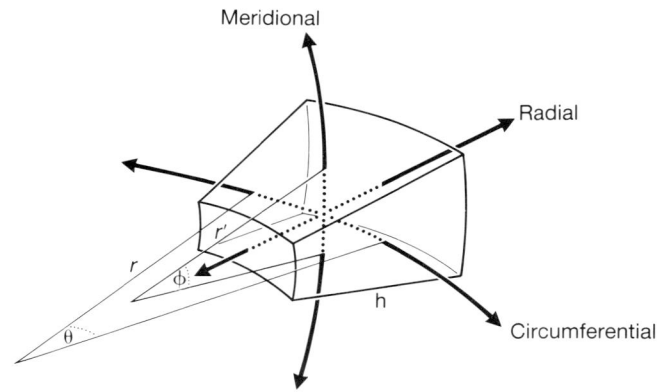

Fig. 8.7 Wall stress in a thick-walled ellipsoidal model. Stress is resolved into its three components, circumferential, meridional and radial. Where h is wall thickness, r and r' are the circumferential and meridional radii respectively and θ and φ are the circumferential and meridional arcs respectively.

Wall stress

Definition

Stress is defined as force per unit cross-sectional area and is measured in dynes (or μN) per cm^2. Stress can be resolved into three orthogonal components; circumferential — around the short axis; meridional — around the long axis; and transverse — in the direction of the radius through the thickness of the wall (Fig. 8.7). The calculation of wall stress requires the simultaneous measurement of intraventricular pressure and volume just as for the above pressure–volume relations. However, only end-systolic or end-diastolic estimates of stress are used. Thus such high frequency response manometers that are needed for the calculation of elastance are not necessarily required for measuring wall stress.

Ventricular wall stress would be the best measure of the force the ventricle produces during systole (afterload) and the level of passive loading in diastole (preload). However no suitable means as yet exists for the direct measurement of global or local wall stress in man, and in order to determine estimates of wall stress a large number of assumptions about the geometric and physical properties of the ventricle have to be made.

The direct application of Laplace's law (equation 8a), which states that the tension (stress) in the wall of a sphere is directly related to the product of the radius of the sphere and the pressure within it, assumes the ventricle to be of notional wall thickness, while further derivations (equation 8b) [42] require a wall thickness to be less than a tenth of the radius. This is not the case even at end-diastole in a dilated ventricle and certainly not during systole. However, the use of derived equations for a thick-walled ventricle (equations 8c and 8d) appears to confer no significant advantages in the calculation of wall stress [43, 44].

The ventricle may be assumed to be represented by a sphere, a prolate ellipsoid [45] or a general ellipsoid [43]. An ellipsoid is a good approximation especially at end-diastole. In dogs, calculated wall stress using an ellipsoid rather than a spherical model correlated well with direct measures using an implanted force gauge [46]. However, the diseased ventricle can become distorted in such a way that it is not well represented by any single geometric primitive. Other assumptions include:

1 That there is a linear stress — strain relationship (elastic modulus) of the ventricular wall — whereas it is most likely to be an exponential one.
2 That the ventricular wall is isotropic — in other words that the elastic modulus is the same in all directions.
3 That the ventricle is homogeneous — the elastic properties are constant throughout the myocardium.
4 That ventricular wall deformation is symmetrical about defined axes so that shear forces and bending moments can be ignored.

Yet the ventricle is an irregularly shaped, thick-walled, inhomogeneous membrane with shear forces that vary throughout the ventricle — as well as with time as the orientation of muscle fibres changes during the cardiac cycle.

Although there have been attempts to take into account the thick-walled, anisotropic and inhomogeneous nature of the ventricular wall [43, 47] the true distribution of the inhomogeneity remains elusive:

$$P = \frac{WT_1}{r_1} + \frac{WT_2}{r_2} \quad (8a)$$

Laplace's law where r_1 and r_2 are the principal radii of curvature, WT_1 and WT_2 are the principal wall tensions and P is the pressure.

$$\sigma = \frac{Pb(2a^2 - b^2)}{h(2a^2 + bh)} \quad (8b)$$

Equation for the calculation of wall stress: Falsetti's method. Falsetti's derivation from Laplace's law of circumferential stress in a thin-walled ventricle where σ is circumferential wall stress, P is cavity pressure, a and b are the major and minor semi-axes respectively and h is the wall thickness.

$$\sigma_\phi = \left(\frac{Pb}{2h}\right)\left(\frac{1-h}{2b}\right)^2 \quad (8c)$$

$$\sigma_\theta = \left(\frac{Pb}{h}\right)\left(1 - \frac{b^2}{2a^2} - \frac{h}{2b} + \frac{h^2}{8a^2}\right) \quad (8d)$$

Equation for the calculation of wall stress: thick walled method. Mirsky's simplified equations for a thick-walled ellipsoid, where σ_θ and σ_ϕ are the circumferential and meridional stresses respectively, P is the cavity pressure, h is the wall thickness and a and b are the mid-wall semi-major and semi-minor axes respectively [48].

Regardless of which formula is used, end-systolic circumferential wall stress adheres consistently to the following trends in different cardiac disease states: it rises in dilated cardiomyopathy, aortic regurgitation, mitral stenosis and marginally in mitral regurgitation, but falls in aortic stenosis [49]. This might be expected since as can be seen in the above equations, there is an inverse relationship between wall thickness and wall stress. Ventricular hypertrophy would therefore appear to be a suitable compensatory mechanism to maintain normal wall stress despite increases in afterload or radius. This may in part explain the variation in wall thickness in different areas of the ventricle. Those areas with a large radius of curvature and therefore a higher wall stress, for example the equatorial free wall, have a greater wall thickness than areas with a small radius of curvature and consequently lower stress, for example the apex.

Finite element analysis

The finite element method of analysis avoids the necessity for complex mathematical models to allow for anisotropy, inhomogeneity and variations in wall thickness and radius of curvature.

It involves the division of the ventricle into longitudinal and transverse sections based on single plane [50] or biplane [51] ventriculograms. This is done by marking the endocardial and epicardial long axis silhouettes with evenly spaced points and interpolating a circumference at each point either by using additional long axis views (biplane) or by rotating about the long axis one hemi-silhouette. This results in a finite number of polyhedral wall sections (elements) of known thickness, and radius of curvature (Fig. 8.8). This technique has provided insight into local ventricular wall stress unobtainable by the geometric methods described above. For

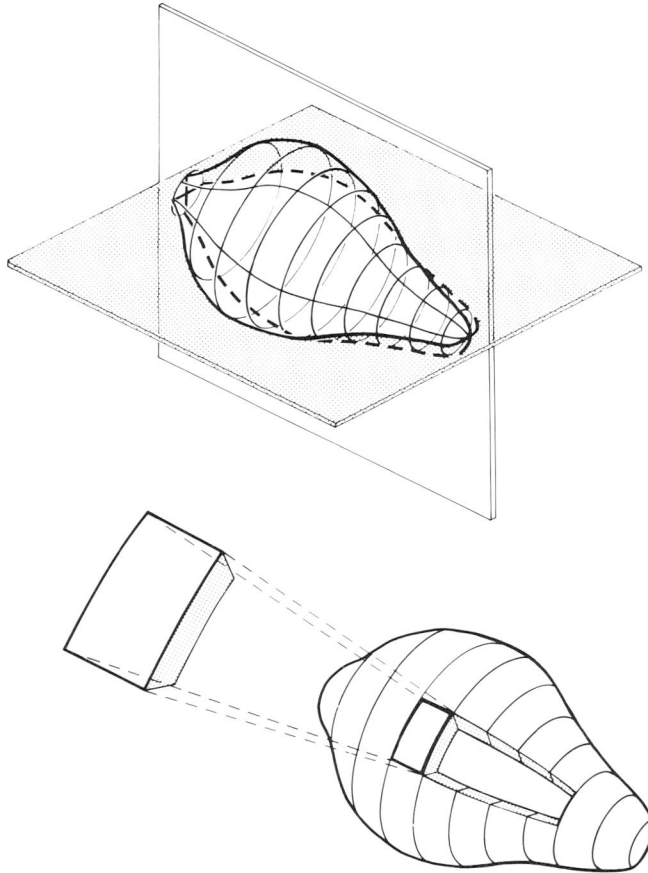

Fig. 8.8 Finite element analysis of biplane ventriculograms to establish local wall stress. Each 'element' is a polyhedral segment of the wall, of known circumferential and meridional radii of curvature, and known wall thickness.

example Gould [50] found that the linear stress distribution across the wall from endo- to epicardium was reversed when the curvature of the wall was reversed. However even with powerful computer resources available such techniques are very time consuming and at present only suitable for research purposes.

Conclusion

Reliable measures of local wall stress are too complex and too difficult to measure at present. Therefore, for routine clinical use, calculations of mean, global, circumferential wall stress using internal diameters and simplified equations must suffice (equations 8b, 8c and 8d).

Wall stress—length relation

The combination of the decreasing ventricular radius and increasing wall thickness that occurs during systole means that peak wall stress occurs earlier in systole than peak intraventricular pressure. Thus any cause of diminished velocity of fibre shortening will result in an increase in wall stress. This inverse relationship between end-systolic wall stress and velocity of fibre shortening provides a means of assessing myocardial contractility that is probably preload-independent [35].

Isovolumic indices of contractility

Max dP/dt
$(dP/dt)/P$
V_{MAX}
V_{PM}

Definitions

These indices are all measures of the rate of change of intraventricular pressure during the isovolumic contraction phase of systole. They are extrapolated from studies of isolated muscle preparations and are designed to measure contractility by identifying the position of the ventricle in question on the force-velocity length curve.

The creation of these indices requires a large number of assumptions to be made about myocardial function. It is assumed that there is no myocardial fibre shortening during the isovolumic contraction phase. The 'two-element' model for cardiac muscle is also assumed. In this model the myocardium is considered to consist of a contractile element and an elastic element in series together. It is suggested that any shortening of the contractile element is compensated by the stretching of the series elastic element with a resulting increase in wall tension and a rise in the intracavity pressure. As can be seen from the above section on wall stress, if a cavity is assumed to be of notional wall thickness and the fibre length (cavity dimension) does not change then the pressure developed represents developed wall stress. Thus dP/dt can be seen to represent the rate of change of wall stress. This theoretical justification for the derivation of these indices from pressure measurements only is cor-

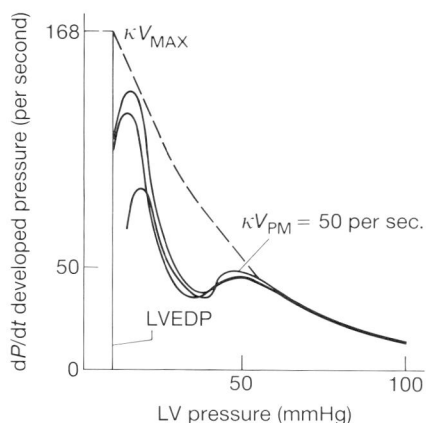

Fig. 8.9 Plot of dP/dt (developed pressure) against left ventricular pressure. The decline of $dP/dt/DP$ has been extrapolated back with an exponential function to find κV_{MAX}. The alternative index κV_{PM}, the peak value of $dP/dt/DP$, is shown.

roborated by clinical validation. Mirsky *et al.* [52] in 1971 found a correlation coefficient of 0.92 between V_{MAX} calculated by pressure alone and V_{MAX} calculated from wall stress measurements.

When dP/dt is normalised to ventricular pressure it represents the velocity of contractile element shortening (equation 9):

$$V_{CE} = \frac{(dP/dt)}{\kappa P} \qquad (9)$$

Velocity of contractile element shortening (V_{CE}) *where* (dP/dt) *is the gradient of the pressure rise,* κ *is a stiffness constant and* P *is the instantaneous cavity pressure. The units are muscle lengths per second.*

V_{MAX} is V_{CE} extrapolated to zero pressure (Fig. 8.9). Thus V_{MAX} is a measure of the maximum rate of shortening of the unloaded contractile element and is held to be a pure measure of contractility since any change in V_{MAX} can only be due to a change in the peak rate of shortening of the contractile element.

Owing to the large number of assumptions that have to be made there are many theoretical limitations to the use of V_{MAX} as an index of ventricular function.

In fact there are documented changes in fibre length in normal ventricles during the isovolumic contraction phase, [53] the ventricular wall is not of notional thickness and the two element model is a simplistic and possibly inappropriate model [54]. Furthermore the value for κ, the stiffness constant of

the series elastic element, which is commonly taken as 28, is an arbitrary value derived from animal studies [55] and clearly may vary widely in myocardial disease. In fact derived formulae for the calculation of a stiffness constant in the clinical situation suggest mean values of κ for normals, idiopathic hypertrophic subaortic stenosis and congestive cardiomyopathy of 16,26.7 and 20.3 respectively [56]. The difficulties with a stiffness constant can be eliminated by considering the index κV_{MAX} instead of V_{MAX} thus obviating the need to know a value for κ.

There are also practical limitations. There is no consistent mathematical method of extrapolation to zero pressure; consequently the many different methods that may be used cause significant variation in values for V_{MAX} [1, 43] indeed if the force—velocity curve has a truly exponential decay then there can be no value at zero pressure. It was pointed out by Wiggers [5], and it has since been well substantiated, that the gradient of the isometric pressure rise is determined by the initial tension. Thus although all these indices can be considered pure measures of contractility, they are all preload dependent. However this dependence can be minimised by the use of developed ventricular pressure rather than total ventricular pressure [57, 58]:

$$V_{MAX} = \frac{dP/dt}{kDP} \text{ or } kV_{MAX} = \frac{dP/dt}{DP} \qquad (10)$$

Equation for calculation of V_{MAX} *using developed pressure* (DP) *which is the total ventricular pressure minus the EDP.*

Patients with atrioventricular valve regurgitation do not have an isovolumic contraction phase and the use of V_{MAX} in such cases is questionable. Further to these theoretical and practical limitations, clinical comparisons reveal isovolumic indices to be less reliable and less sensitive than ejection phase indices in the detection of myocardial dysfunction [1, 2].

There are also limitations on the value of isovolumic indices of contractility in the assessment of right ventricular function. It is considered that the isovolumic pressure rise of the left ventricle significantly influences that of the right ventricle [59], and consequently pressure-derived indices of right ventricular function are unreliable [60]. Moreover Redington [61] demonstrated a very poorly defined isovolumic contraction period for the normal right ventricle, with ejection starting early during the pressure rise and nearly 40% of ejection occurring before 90% of the peak pressure was achieved.

The problem of inconsistent techniques for extrapolation to zero pressure in order to find V_{MAX} can be overcome by the use of another index, peak measured velocity V_{PM} (Fig. 8.9):

$$V_{PM} = \left[\frac{(dP/dt)}{(\kappa P)} \right]_{MAX} \text{ or } \kappa V_{PM} = \left[\frac{(dP/dt)}{P} \right]_{MAX} \quad (11)$$

This index is probably also more valid than V_{MAX} in patients with atrioventricular valve regurgitation.

Reliable measurement of dP/dt can only be performed with high frequency response manometry and this is best provided by catheter tip micromanometers. The results may be analysed either by differentiating the direct analogue signal or by digital sampling at an optimal rate of 1 millisecond intervals and differentiating a curve fitted to the resulting samples. Averaging of a number of beats is advisable.

Conclusion

These indices are valuable for the assessment of changes in the inotropic state of an individual after certain interventions. For example, the evaluation of a pharmacological agent such as an antiarrhythmic when depression of dP/dt may occur or an inotropic agent when dP/dt should increase. However, such evaluation must be very well controlled since dP/dt is very sensitive to changes in other cardiovascular parameters. It is known to increase with increases in heart rate whether they are physiological, or induced by atrial pacing or anticholinergics. As discussed above it is dependent on changes in preload, increasing with increasing left ventricular EDP, and it is also increased by isometric exercise. With such variability the use of these indices for inter-patient comparison and assessment of left ventricular function in routine clinical practice is limited. For these purposes they have largely been superseded by ejection phase indices and wall motion studies.

DIASTOLIC FUNCTION

Compliance

While systolic ventricular function depends upon mechanical loading, defined in terms of ventricular wall stress, as well as upon intrinsic myocardial contractility, so diastolic performance depends on contractile element relaxation and myocardial compliance (the ability of the myocardium to stretch), as well as overall ventricular distensibility (the ability of the ventricle to fill). There is clearly a difference between the ability of a portion of myocardium to be stretched and the ability of the whole ventricular chamber to be filled. This is exemplified by considering two ventricles one with a small cavity due to secondary ventricular hypertrophy and the other with a dilated cavity due to a cardiomyopathy. The former has a normal myocardium and normal EDV but the ventricular compliance is reduced and filling is slow; the latter, with a large EDV, may fill rapidly despite the diseased myocardium itself being incompliant.

Ventricular compliance

Definition

Compliance is the diastolic increase in ventricular volume per unit intraventricular pressure rise.

The passive elastic properties of the ventricle have been defined in terms of the diastolic pressure–volume relationship. This relationship is assumed to be exponential, as greater pressures cause progressively smaller increases in volume (Fig. 8.10), and takes the form;

$$\ln P = \kappa_p V + \ln c \quad (12)$$

where P is the transmural ventricular pressure, V is the volume, c is the intercept on the pressure axis and κ_p is the slope of the $\ln P/V$ relation commonly considered the stiffness constant.

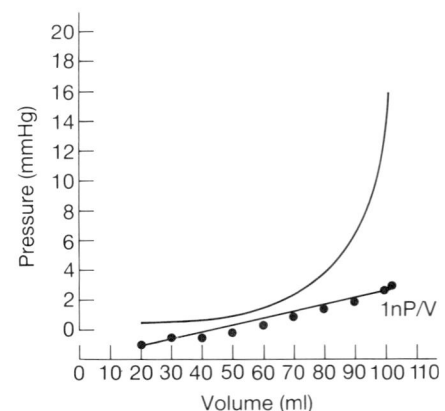

Fig. 8.10 Diastolic pressure/volume relations showing the exponential rise in pressure at the end of diastole and the plot of ln P against volume. The slope of this plot represents ventricular compliance.

The reciprocal of κ_p, $1/\kappa_p$ represents ventricular compliance. If the zero pressure intercept is considered always to be constant then a single measure-of pressure and volume at end-diastole produces a line, the slope of which, dV/dP, represents ventricular distensibility. If this is normalised to EDV, $dV/V \cdot dP$ represents an index of ventricular compliance which can then be used as a comparative index. Using this definition of compliance Gaasch [62] demonstrated a decrease in ventricular compliance in patients with primary and secondary left ventricular hypertrophy, and dilated cardiomyopathy.

There are of course shortcomings to such an approach. The zero pressure intercept c is not constant [63] and values used are based on animal experiment. Compliance varies throughout diastole and a single end-diastolic value may well be unrepresentative. The exponential nature of the pressure—volume relationship is idealised and unlikely to be absolutely true. Indeed at low pressures it is not exponential and the above formula should not be used when pressure is less than 5 mmHg.

Myocardial compliance

Definitions

The compliance of the myocardium as opposed to that of the whole ventricle is defined in terms of its elasticity or stress—strain relationship. Stress is defined as force per unit cross-sectional area. Strain is defined as elongation per unit length.

The simplified formula for the stress—strain relation derived from isolated heart muscle preparations [56] is:

$$d\sigma/d\varepsilon = \kappa\sigma + c \qquad (13)$$

where σ and ε are the Lagrangian stress and strain respectively, κ is the stiffness constant and c is the zero stress intercept.

This calculation again requires that many assumptions be made. For example, that ventricular shape remains the same throughout diastole; that ventricular wall thickness is immaterial; that pressure—volume relations are exponential and that pericardial pressure changes may be ignored. Myocardial strain itself cannot easily be determined for the intact man since the length (c) of the unloaded myocardial fibres is not known. Other formulae have been derived for the stiffness constant in the clinical situation that take account of wall thickness [56].

A simplified measure of compliance was described by Diamond and Forrester [64] when they determined total diastolic $\Delta P/\Delta V$. This is the difference between beginning diastolic pressure and EDP divided by the stroke volume. The slope of $\Delta P/\Delta V$ plotted against mean diastolic pressure represents a passive elastic modulus. Even this simplified index is suspect since stroke volume is not truly representative of ΔV. This is because, as Dodge et al. demonstrated in 1962 [65], there is significant increase in diastolic ventricular volume while intraventricular pressure is still falling. This suggests an active component to early diastolic filling [66—68] which may well be instrumental in determining passive properties in later diastole. The mechanism of this active 'sucking' is uncertain but a substantiated suggestion is that systolic torsion of the ventricle about its long axis results in potential energy being stored in the coiled end-systolic muscle. The energy is released as kinetic energy during early diastolic uncoiling.

The above indices of compliance take no account of the hydraulic effect of coronary artery pressure and flow. Vogel [69] demonstrated in rabbit hearts that compliance is significantly affected by a direct hydraulic effect of coronary artery perfusion, compliance increasing with total ischaemia but decreasing with constant pressure and flow hypoxia. The latter observation supports clinical work demonstrating decreases in ventricular compliance associated with relative ischaemia in coronary artery disease. These may be reversed by successful coronary artery bypass surgery [70].

Conclusion

Although there is increasing awareness of the importance of diastolic dysfunction in ventricular disease difficulties in measurement and the large numbers of assumptions that are required to be made, indices of compliance have a small place in routine clinical practice.

Diastolic volume changes

Rates of change of left ventricular volume have been studied from angiographic images by Hammermeister and Warbasse [71]. They demonstrated that the peak rate of diastolic volume change normalised for EDP,

$$\frac{\mathrm{D}\mathrm{d}V/\mathrm{d}t}{EDV}$$

was significantly decreased in mitral stenosis, coronary artery disease and valvular regurgitation. They also demonstrated that the proportion of the total ventricular filling contributed by atrial contraction (normally 38%) is substantially increased in aortic stenosis, coronary artery disease and valvar regurgitation. This sort of analysis of volume change can readily be derived from digitised M-mode echocardiography without the need for catheterisation and ventriculography. Peak rates of left ventricular wall thinning can also be derived from echocardiographic studies [72, 73].

Isovolumic indices of relaxation

Peak — dP/dt
The time constant of relaxation(T)

The peak rate of decrease of intraventricular pressure during isovolumic relaxation, minimum $\mathrm{d}P/\mathrm{d}t$, has been used as an index of myocardial relaxation but it is very much load dependent. If the decline in pressure following the peak rate of pressure fall during isovolumic relaxation is considered to be mono-exponential, then the rate of ventricular relax-

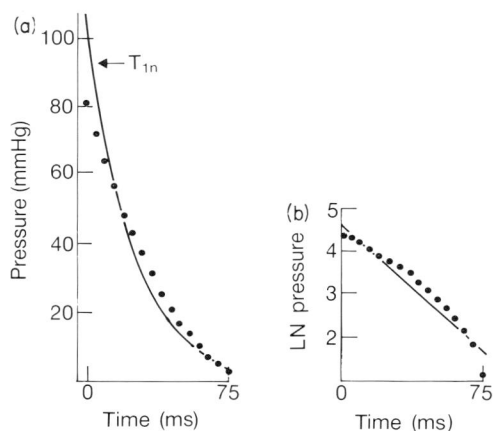

Fig. 8.11 (a) The isovolumic intraventricular pressure fall after the time or peak negative $\mathrm{d}P/\mathrm{d}t$. The points represent the actual pressure recordings, the fitted curve represents the predicted pressure fall using a calculated value for Tau. (b) The semilogarithmic plot of isovolumic intraventricular pressure fall after the time of peak $-\mathrm{d}P/\mathrm{d}t$. Tau the time constant of relaxation, is calculated as the negative reciprocal of the slope of this plot. With kind permission of Dr DS Thompson.

ation can be characterised by a time constant which is load independent (equation 14) [74]. The time constant, Tau (τ), has been used extensively in the study of ventricular relaxation [75–77] and is calculated as the negative reciprocal of the slope of isovolumic ln P plotted against time (Fig. 8.11). It is measured in milliseconds and represents the time taken for pressure to fall by $1/e^{\mathrm{th}}$:

$$\ln P_t = A + bt \qquad \tau = -\frac{1}{b} \qquad (14)$$

where P is instantaneous left ventricular pressure, ln is $\log_e$, t is time after min $\mathrm{d}P/\mathrm{d}t$, and A and b are constants.

As an index of relaxation this time constant is imperfect for a number of reasons. In order for the relationship between ln P and time to be linear, the asymptote of the exponential decline of pressure against time must be assumed to be zero. Calculations that are based on this assumption yield values for τ that are significantly underestimated. If the asymptote is not zero the relationship becomes curvilinear and the value for the slope, derived from either linear regression or exponential analysis [78, 79], depends upon where on the curve it is measured. The slope of ln P against time is dependent on absolute pressure values and is thus not so useful as a comparative index. A modified equation for the calculation of T that takes into account absolute pressure is shown in equation 15:

$$\mathrm{d}P/\mathrm{d}t = \frac{1}{\tau}(P - P_{\mathrm{B}}) \qquad (15)$$

where P_{B} is additional pressure different from zero reference level.

Although in normals the rate of decline of isovolumic pressure after the point of $\mathrm{d}P/\mathrm{d}t_{\mathrm{MIN}}$ can be approximated to an exponential decay, there is no inherent quality of myocardium that dictates that this should be the case. In fact in early diastole it is not exponential, especially in ventricular hypertrophy [77].

The fact is, that although isovolumic relaxation after $\mathrm{d}P/\mathrm{d}t_{\mathrm{MIN}}$ is exponential both the time constant and asymptote are probably variable [80].

As in isovolumic measures of contraction, high fidelity pressure monitoring with catheter tip micromanometers must be used for measurement of these indices of relaxation. Computer facilities are required for the analysis of the data and the determination of τ, although Thompson et al. report [80] a simple programme for the reliable estimation of the time constant 'on-line' on a catheter laboratory computer.

The normal range for the time constant of left ventricular isovolumic pressure fall therefore varies according to which method of calculation is used. Even using the same method there is considerable variation. Employing equation 14 mean values for τ vary from 31 ± 3 to 38 ± 7 [79, 81, 82] and with equation 15 vary from 41 ± 12 [77] to 55 ± 4 msec [79]. However it is accepted that τ increases in ventricular hypertrophy and hypertrophic cardiomyopathy, but, unlike other indices of relaxation (dP/dt_{MIN} peak filling rate and length of isovolumic relaxation time) which are improved by β-blockade or calcium channel blockade [83–85], the time constant is unchanged by either [86]. Indeed nifedipine lengthens the time constant although this mechanism is unclear [82].

Conclusion

There are many variations in the methods of derivation of the time constant of relaxation and great care should be taken when comparing values. Since the peak negative dP/dt is load dependent and the time constant of relaxation varies with wall thickness (hypertrophy) a better comparative index would be peak rate of change of wall stress or the time constant of fall of diastolic wall stress. For routine clinical practice measurements of rates of ventricular filling and wall thinning are more suitable indices of diastolic function providing valve lesions, loading conditions and the state of the pericardium are taken into account.

LEFT AND RIGHT VENTRICULAR INTERACTION AND MUTUAL DEPENDENCE

Since one wall of each ventricular chamber is shared in the form of the interventricular septum, it is not surprising that there is considerable functional interdependence.

Overloading of right ventricular pressure or volume may cause displacement of the interventricular septum towards the left with consequent distortion of left ventricular cavity shape. In patients with pulmonary hypertension, and therefore pressure loading of the right ventricle, diastolic bulging of the interventricular septum has been noted [87]. This diastolic bulging has also been noted in volume loaded right ventricles [88].

Such septal deformation in right ventricular abnormalities is however not confined to diastole. Systolic flattening of the interventricular septum has been reported when the normal right ventricle is loaded, either by the Mueller manoeuvre (inspiration against a closed glottis) [89], or in ventilated patients by the administration of PEEP (positive end expiratory pressure) [90], with resulting decrease in left ventricular cavity size. The changes in septal motion and left ventricular cavity size in right ventricular pressure overload have been confirmed recently but no deleterious effect on left ventricular performance seems to occur [91].

These studies have all been conducted using echocardiography and while there may be some doubt about results derived from M-mode studies because of the restricted sampling site, there seems little doubt about cross-sectional echocardiographic studies. Furthermore there is confirmation of these effects using contrast ventriculography, in dogs with acute pulmonary hypertension — pressure overload [92] — and in humans with right ventricular volume overload [93].

Distortion of the septum can occur in either direction depending on the transseptal pressure gradient [94], the position of the septum in the completely unloaded heart (studied during cardiac arrest on cardiopulmonary bypass) being flat [95]. Thus right ventricular overload causes flattening of the septum or even bulging into the left ventricle while left ventricular overloading results in exaggeration of the normal convexity into the right ventricle.

Haemodynamic studies confirm the ventricular interdependence with increases in right ventricular systolic and diastolic pressures resulting in increases of left ventricular diastolic pressure [96, 97]. Isovolumic pressure studies further confirm the mutual relationship. Oboler's observations in anaesthetised dogs [59], have been confirmed in conscious normal human subjects by Feneley *et al.*, who elegantly showed that left ventricular contraction contributes significantly to the generation of right ventricular systolic pressure [98]. This has implications for right ventricular function either when effective coupling of ventricular contraction is impaired or in left ventricular disease when left ventricular contractility is reduced.

The above effects of one ventricle on the other should be borne in mind when analysing left or right ventricular function.

DERIVATION OF QUANTITATIVE DATA FROM ANGIOGRAPHIC IMAGES

Radiographic images from different projections were originally used to determine the volume of the heart both in postmortem specimens [99, 100] and in live subjects [101, 102]. In these calculations assumptions were made about the similarity of the heart to a particular geometric shape — a parabaloid or an ellipsoid. The advent of cardiac catheterisation, contrast radiography and cine radiography provided the techniques for changes in size and shape of individual cardiac chambers to be examined [103, 104]. Such analysis is now commonplace and although there remain many potential sources of error in the production of angiographic images and many assumptions in their analysis, modern cardiac departments can now employ digital imaging and computer processing to derive automatically accurate measurements of ventricular and coronary arterial morphology.

There are three main problems that need to be overcome in deriving quantitative data from angiographic images:
1 Distortions of the image that are caused by inherent properties of X-ray imaging.
2 An appropriate geometric model for the calculation of volume.
3 A means of calibrating the images so that absolute values can be derived.
Before dealing with these specific problems there are some general points about ventriculography and angiography that require consideration.

General considerations

Position

Cardiac catheterisation and ventriculography are usually performed with the patient recumbent. In this position cardiac size and ventricular stroke volumes are increased as a result of the increased filling pressure.

Stressed state

During catheterisation the patient is considered to be at rest, although the degree of stress produced by the circumstances of the procedure varies, some patients being severely stressed. Such stress results in tachycardia and increases in all measures of cardiac performance. Thus there is no standard basal work load at which to assess cardiac function. On the other hand controlled stress, in the form of physical exercise, is a difficult logistic problem in the cardiac catheter laboratory. Isometric hand exercise is probably the easiest to accomplish although bicycle ergometers for the recumbent position have been used. Atrial pacing can be used to stress the heart in a controlled fashion but it does not simulate all the physiological changes that occur with physical exercise.

Ectopic beats

Intraventricular catheters and the injection of radio-opaque dye are likely to cause ventricular premature beats. This is especially the case if the injection occurs within the first 70% of the R–R interval [105]. Beats that follow such ectopics are subject to 'post-ectopic potentiation' and therefore make the ectopic beat and the one or two beats following it unrepresentative of the normal ventricular function. These should not be included in routine assessment of ejection fraction or wall motion although the degree of potentiation has been used to assess and predict ventricular performance [106].

Effects of contrast on ventricular function and volume estimates

For normal ventriculography 20–40 ml of contrast medium is injected over about 2 seconds. There are many different contrast media available but the standard has been a mixture of sodium diatrixoate and meglumine diatrizoate (urografin, Schering). The rapid injection of contrast media has well recognised physiological effects. The high osmolality, high viscosity and the acidosis it creates on injection combine to cause dramatic shifts in water and electrolytes from the extravascular compartment and blood cells. Plasma sodium, potassium and calcium fall. The circulatory consequences are first a transient improvement in ventricular performance followed by decline.

After the injection of contrast in normals there are significant increases in end-diastolic pressure, end-diastolic volume, stroke volume and cardiac output [107]. There is a fall in arterial pressure and systemic vascular resistance [108] and there is an increase in circulating volume which is directly proportional to the volume of injectate [109]. The hyperosmolarity of the medium is responsible for the fall in vascular resistance and thus in part for the increased cardiac output but dP/dt also increases. The increase in end-diastolic pressure has been shown to be related to an increase in end-diastolic volume rather than as a result of myocardial depression [107]. However the improved performance is short lived and there follows a myocardial depressant effect which can last up to 15−20 minutes [110, 111]. This is likely to be due to contrast medium being delivered to the coronary circulation since depressant effects of intra-coronary injection on contractility are well documented [112, 113]. During ventriculography the depressant effect is more accentuated in patients with coronary artery disease, being more severe the greater the extent of arterial disease and possibly resulting in wall motion abnormalities [107]. This effect has been used to assess ventricular function in patients with coronary artery disease [114].

The peak increase in circulating volume occurs about 2 minutes after injection. The peak effects of contrast on end-diastolic pressure occur approximately 2 to 4 minutes after injection and take approximately 15 minutes to recover. The myocardial depressant effects have been reported as starting on the fourth or fifth postinjection beat [110, 111] suggesting that any comparative study of ventricular volume or function must use the same postinjection beat which should be the third beat, since full opacification is unlikely to have occurred in the first or second.

Newer non-ionic contrast media with low iodination and isotonicity are diminishing the haemodynamic effects of contrast injection [115]. Further improvements may result from slower injection rates of about 10 ml/sec [116].

In order to avoid direct effects of contrast injection the laevo phase of right heart injection has been used [32] but this does not really provide adequate contour delineation [117, 118] and right-sided injection still has systemic haemodynamic effects [108].

Image distortions due to inherent properties of the X-ray imaging system

Distortions caused by the X-ray source

An idealised X-ray beam would have a point source, contain X-rays of equal energy and spread out in a perfect conical distribution. The reality is not so ideal. The large amounts of heat generated in X-ray production prevent the source (focal spot) from being made very small; the larger the focal spot the more X-ray sources there are and as a result the larger the size of the *penumbra* (sometimes called the edge gradient), or fuzziness at the edge of the projected image (Fig. 8.12a). Furthermore the X-rays are polychromatic, i.e. they are of varied photon energy, which gives rise to two effects, *quantum mottle* (see below) and *beam hardening*. The beam is 'hardened' as the X-rays of lower energy are attenuated, thus as the beam passes through the object the mean photon energy of the unattenuated X-rays increases. The distribution of the X-rays depends on accurate collimation of the emitted beam.

Distortions resulting from properties of the object: position, shape, density and motion

Assuming a point source, equal energy X-rays and perfect collimation, the projected image of an object is magnified by the ratio of the source to screen distance and source to object distance (Fig. 8.12b). The equation to correct for magnification caused by non-parallel X-rays is therefore:

$$O_t = \frac{h}{H} O_p \qquad (16)$$

Equation for the correction of magnification caused by non-parallel X-rays where O_t is the true object size, h is the source to object distance, H is the source to screen distance and O_p is the projected object size.

This is acceptable while the object is parallel to the image plane and in the centre of the beam but if the object is angled or eccentric within the beam there will be differential magnification between one end and the other resulting in distortions of size and shape in the projected image (Fig. 8.12c).

The degree of absorption of the X-rays depends on the shape and density of the object. Most absorp-

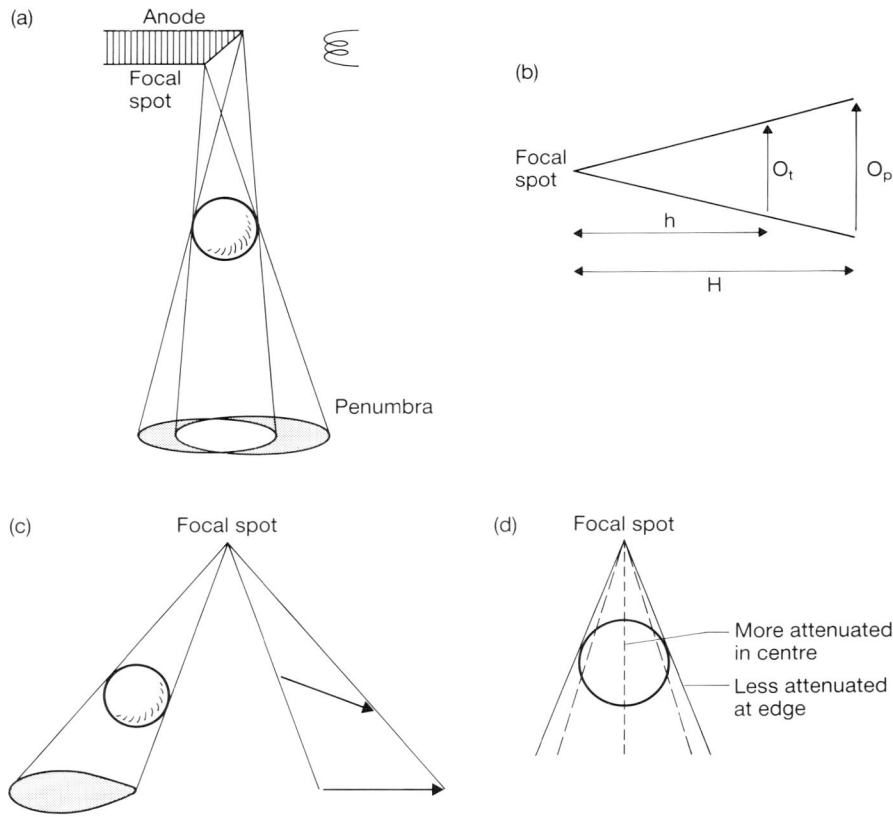

Fig. 8.12 (a) The penumbra results from multiple X-ray sources and causes fuzziness of edges. (b) The magnification effect of non-parallel X-rays. O_t is the object being X-rayed at h distance from the focal spot. O_p is the size of the projected image on the image intensifier at H distance from the focal spot. See equation 16. (c) Distortions of differential magnification for objects eccentric in the X-ray beam and not at right angles to it. (d) There is greater attenuation of X-rays in the centre of objects than at the edges. This may make edges less distinct.

tion occurs with the X-rays that pass through the centre of an object since there is more object through which to pass. There is thus a gradient of absorption decreasing towards the edge of the object, which results in unsharpness of the edges in the X-ray image (Fig. 8.12d). This effect is greatest for round and spherical objects and least for objects whose edges are parallel to the X-rays. It thus has considerable significance for quantitative coronary angiography. The variation in density within the object not only varies the absorption but also affects the degree of scatter of X-rays, adding to decreases in image sharpness.

Motion of the object during exposure causes blurring of the image which is most noticeable as unsharpness of edges. This is obviously of great relevance to cardiac imaging where parts of the ventricular wall and coronary arteries may be moving at 6 to 8 centimetres per second. Motion artefact is minimised by making the exposure times as short as possible.

Distortions introduced by the image intensifier: quantum mottle, pin cushion distortion and vignetting

The number of X-ray photons absorbed by the image intensifier input screen determines the highest possible statistical quality of the system, while the overall statistical quality is determined by that part of the imaging system that most degrades the image. The latter is called the quantum sink and it determines the amount of quantum mottle, recognised as graininess, which is seen in the final image. Increasing the exposure increases the number of X-ray photons absorbed thus decreasing statistical fluctuations in X-ray energy and reducing quantum mottle.

In order to support the high vacuum that is contained within the image intensifier the strength of the glass or metal envelope is increased by making the input screen curved. X-rays impinging upon the caesium iodide of the curved input screen cause

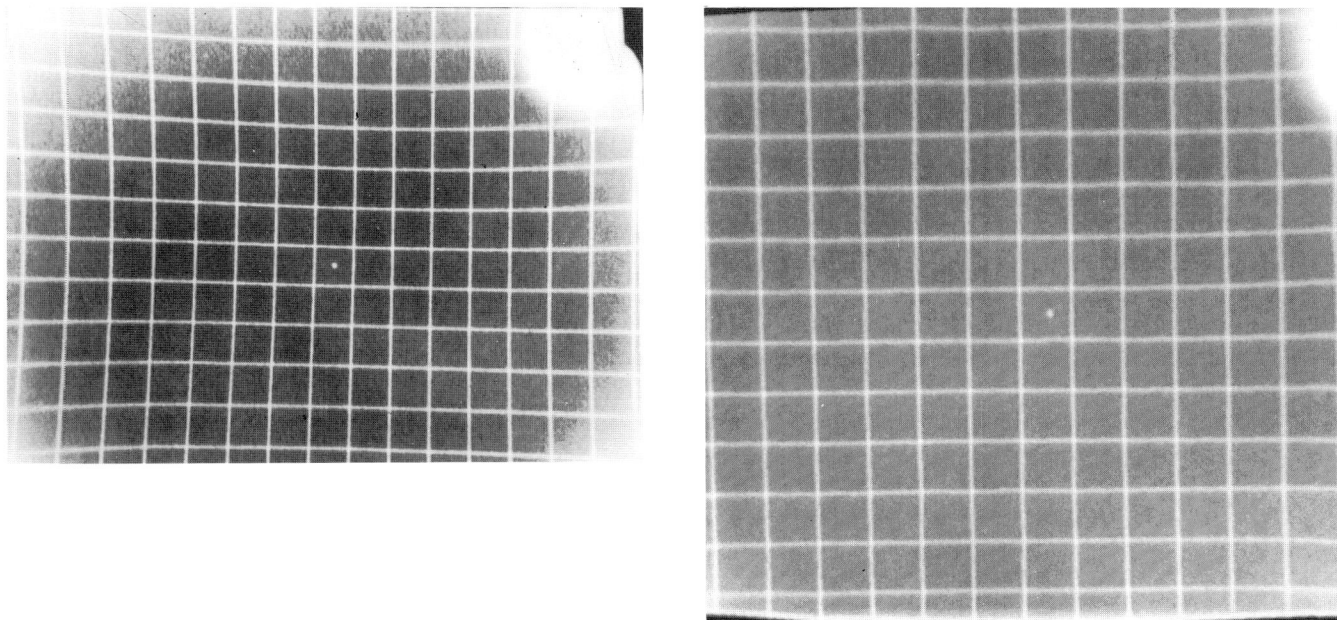

Fig. 8.13 (a) A one centimetre copper wire grid, X-rayed while applied to the image intensifier, showing pincushion distortion. (b) Image after a rubber sheet correction formula has been applied to the digitised image.

electrons to be emitted and these in turn are accelerated towards the smaller output phosphor screen by the accelerating anode. The electron beam is focused by electrostatic lenses. Unfortunately the focusing is not uniform throughout the beam, those electrons in the centre being more accurately focused than those at the periphery. The result is unequal magnification which is worse the larger the image intensifier. This magnification and the convex shape of the input screen combine to produce *pin cushion distortion* in the final image (Fig. 8.13a). Such distortion has implications for quantitative ventriculography and coronary arteriography. For example, using a 9 inch (23 cm) intensifier the periphery of the image in Fig. 8.13a is magnified 15% more than the centre. Digital image processing techniques enable such image distortions to be corrected (Fig. 8.13b).

The same effects also cause unequal illumination so that the image on the output screen is brighter in the centre than at the edge. This is known as *vignetting*. Again this has implications for quantitative digital angiography where pixel intensities may be taken to be representative of radio-opaque dye concentration and thus a measure of the amount of blood in any vessel.

The resolution of the imaging system is dependent on the resolving power of the input screen of the image intensifier. Resolution is the distinction of two objects that are close together and not the quality of sharpness of edges. Thus resolution may be high but edges still fuzzy because of the combination of the above effects of distortion. The resolution of original caesium iodide image intensifier input screens was 4.0 line pairs per millimetre, a dramatic improvement of the 2.5 lp/mm of the zinc cadmium sulphide screens. However, further improvements culminating in metal screens (instead of glass) can now yield a resolution to 7 lp/mm.

Additional distortions may be introduced in the transfer of the image from output screen to film. Camera speeds are often not constant, film quality and responsiveness vary with age, temperature and exposure and the developement of the film is critical in determining the ultimate quality of the image. Finally, distortions can be introduced in the projection of the developed film.

Conclusion

X-ray imaging systems are a compromise, optimising the often conflicting effects of the different component distortions outlined above. Clearly, on the basis of 'rubbish in, rubbish out', it does not matter how sophisticated and accurate the technique for the analysis of the final images, if the images themselves are distorted and full of errors. Further improvements in image quality are required. This brief overview of the problems inherent in cine angiographic image acquisition makes it clear that objective geometric or densitometric quantitation of structures seen in the final image is fraught with potential error and, as has been pointed out before, [120, 121] that subjective quantitative interpretation on anything other than gross scale, may be highly inaccurate. However, quantitative techniques that take account of errors and provide appropriate corrections do produce meaningful, accurate and useful results.

Geometric models and methods for the calculation of ventricular volume

LEFT VENTRICLE

The geometric primitive to which the normal left ventricle most closely approximates is an ellipsoid and a variety of techniques have been described for the calculation of ventricular volume using this model. The different methods summarised below are based on the fact that the projected silhouette of an ellipsoid is an ellipse. The volume of an ellipsoid is calculated as:

$$V = \frac{4}{3} \pi \left(\frac{a}{2}\right)\left(\frac{b}{2}\right)\left(\frac{c}{2}\right) = \frac{\pi}{6} abc \qquad (17)$$

where c is the major axis and a and b are the two minor axes.

The two minor axes of the ventricle can be ascertained from orthogonal biplane ventriculography giving the following equation for ventricular volume:

$$V = \frac{\pi}{6} D_A D_L D_M \qquad (18)$$

where D_A is the minor axis in the anterior view, D_L is the minor axis of the lateral view and D_M is the major axis.

Direct measurement

This method involves the direct measurement of the major and minor axes in each view of the ventriculogram. The major axis is taken as the longer of the two long axes and in each view the long axis is defined either as the line between the apex and the midpoint between the aortic valve leaflet attachments or the longest chord length of the ventricular outline. Originally in the method described by Arvidsson [122] and idealised ellipse was superimposed over the ventricular outline which excluded the left ventricular outflow tract and the area beneath the mitral valve leaflets; axes of the constructed ellipse were then measured. Modifications of this method have included these areas [15, 123, 124]. The minor axes are measured as the maximum chord length perpendicular to the long axis in each view.

This method not only overestimates volume by up to 40% but the high degree of subjectivity involved, especially in irregularly shaped ventricles like those seen in cardiac disease, also increases error. Dodge *et al.* [45] described an area—length method that halved the standard error of the direct measurement technique and overestimated by less than 20%.

Area—length method

Since the area of an ellipse is calculated as $A = \pi DM/4$, where D and M are the minor and major axes of the ellipse, the minor axis is $D = (4A/\pi)M$, and by substituting in equation 18 volume can be calculated as;

$$V = \frac{8}{3} \pi \frac{A_A A_L}{M} \qquad (19)$$

Equation for the calculation of ventricular volume using biplane ventriculography and the area length method where A_A and A_L are the areas of the anterior and lateral projected silhouettes respectively.

The area of each projected ellipse is measured by planimetry. This was originally done by applying the traced outline of the ventricle to 1 mm squared paper or by using a compensated polar planimeter but it is much easier and now commonplace to use a digitising tablet and cursor, like that described by Gibson [125], to draw around the silhouette, and a computer to calculate the area. It is better still if the images are already in digital form as errors resulting from the projection of the image onto the digitising

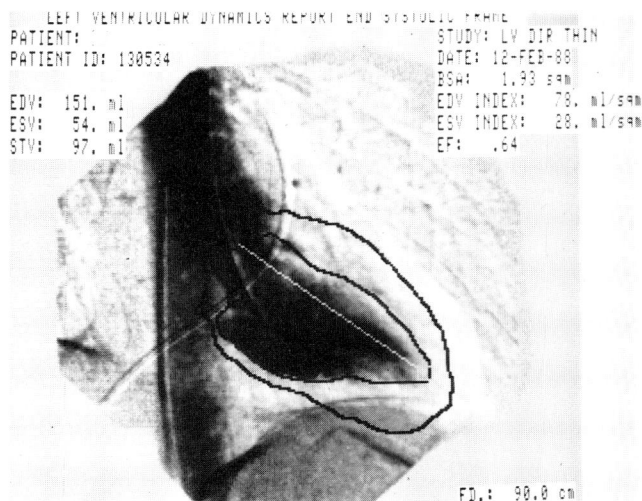

Fig. 8.14 An end-systolic frame of a digital subtraction RAO ventriculogram. The end-diastolic outline, previously taken from the end-diastolic frame, has been superimposed. The long axis is marked as the line from apex to bisected aortic valve, and using the area—length method the chamber volumes and ejection fraction can be calculated and displayed.

tablet are excluded. An example is shown in Fig. 8.14 where the end-systolic frame of a digital subtraction ventriculogram is shown on a video display. The end-systolic outline is drawn and the end-diastolic ventricular outline has been superimposed.

If the ventricle is assumed to approximate to a prolate ellipsoid, i.e. one in which the two minor axes have the same dimensions, the volume of the ventricle can be calculated from a single plane ventriculogram. Analyses by Sandler, Green and Kasser [127—128] have shown that the dimensions are very similar since the direction of the long axis of the ventricle does not change very much through the cardiac cycle. Consequently the volume may be calculated by the following formula:

$$V = \frac{\pi}{6} M \cdot D^2 \tag{20}$$

Equation for the calculation of ventricular volume from single plane ventriculography where M is the maximum chamber length and D is the maximum diameter.

Validation of the area—length method, using postmortem casts of the left ventricle, reveals a systematic overestimate of volume. Provided images have already been corrected for pin cushion distortion there are three further possible causes for this:

1 The ellipsoid may not be such as appropriate model of the left ventricle.

2 The outline of the silhouette, which is drawn by hand, may be inaccurate, including within it the papillary muscles and trabeculae carneae.

3 The angle of projection may distort the shape of the silhouette.

In considering these points the ellipsoid model seems appropriate for the normal ventricle especially at end-diastole. Even as the diseased ventricle dilates and becomes more spherical the equations still hold true since a sphere is a specialised ellipsoid. However any asymmetry resulting from regional wall abnormalities cannot be accounted for with such a model.

Inaccurate or incorrect outlining accounts for a major proportion of the errors. Gault reported that for a true volume of 95 ml an outline drawn concentrically 1 mm larger than the correct outline yields a calculated volume of 105 ml [129], while Gribbe *et al.* demonstrated in dogs, that together the papillary muscles and trabeculae carneae may occupy approximately 30% of the gross ventricular volume [104].

Further errors are derived from the projections, especially in the single plane techniques. Firstly the long axis of the ventricle is not perpendicular to the X-ray beam in any of the above-mentioned views. The 'true' long axis is only seen with angulated views, such as 30° right anterior oblique (RAO) with 10—20° of caudal tilt and 60° left anterior oblique (LAO) with 20—30° of cranial tilt. There have been reports of improvements in accuracy of 10—20% for volume estimation using these biplane views with either the area—length or Simpson's rule methods [130, 131].

Secondly, while single plane methods compare favourably with biplane for normal ventricles there is disparity when diseased hearts are examined, particularly in the presence of asynergy [132].

However this systematic overestimation can be compensated reliably by the application of an appropriate regression equation. Dodge *et al.* use the following regression equations:

$$V_{\text{corrected}} = 0.928V - 3.8 \tag{21a}$$

$$V_{\text{corrected}} = 0.951V - 3.0 \tag{21b}$$

$$V_{\text{corrected}} = 0.81V + 1.9 \tag{21c}$$

Regression equations for the calculation of ventricular volume by the area—length method.

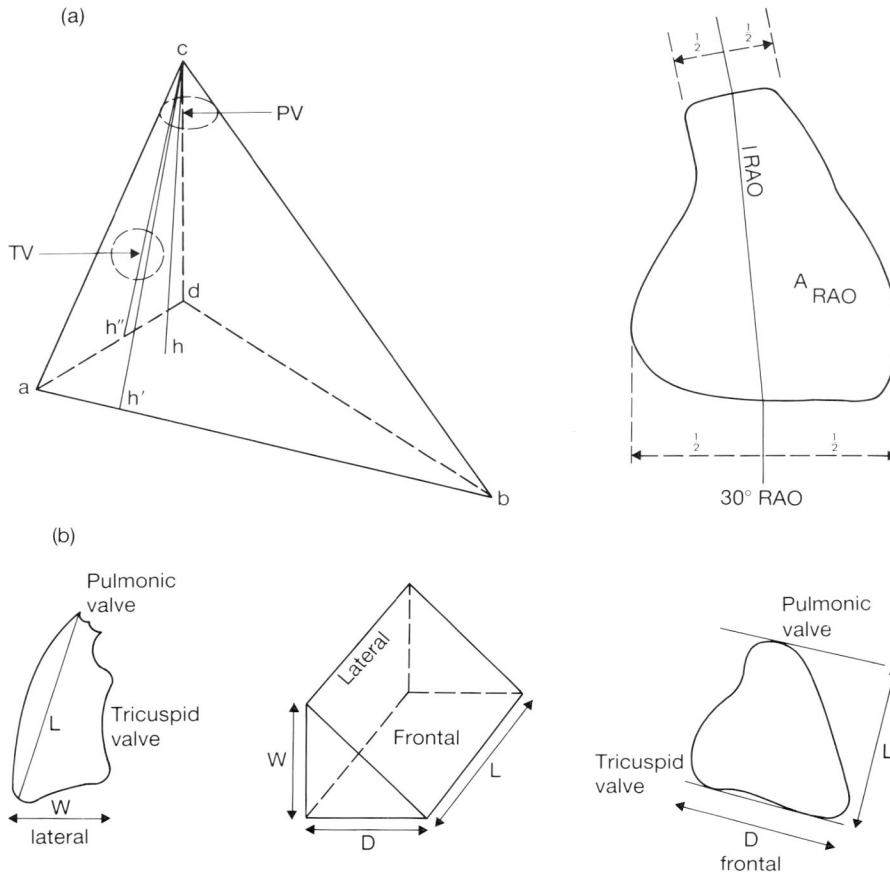

Fig. 8.15 Two methods for the calculation of right ventricular volume from right ventriculograms. In (a) the method based on the pyramid model, PV is the pulmonary valve, TV is the tricuspid valve, and C is the RV apex. Triangles abc and abd are the RAO and LAO silhouettes respectively, and l is the distance from the bisected pulmonary valve to the bisected base; h' and h" are the heights of each silhouette while h is the true height of the pyramid. In (b) the prism method, h is the height of the ventricle and b is the width in the AP view, while l is the maximum dimension in the lateral view.

Equation 21a applies to biplane films using AP and lateral projections, although it can also be applied to 30° RAO and 60° LAO projections [133, 134]. Equation 21b applies to single plane films using the AP projection only. Equation 21c applies to single plane films using the 30° RAO projection.

RIGHT VENTRICLE

While the left ventricular shape lends itself readily to being represented by an ellipsoid, the irregular morphology of the right ventricle defies such obvious geometric representation and there are consequently a number of different methods described. An ellipsoid representation of the right ventricle is inappropriate but two geometric models have been successfully used — the triangular-based pyramid described by Ferlinz *et al.* [12] and the triangular-based prism described by Fisher *et al.* [135] (Fig. 8.15). In the former, biplane 30° RAO and 60° LAO views are used and the resulting images subjected

to area—length analysis using the following formula:

$$V_{RV} = \frac{2}{3} \frac{A_{RAO} \times A_{LAO}}{l_{RAO}} \qquad (22)$$

Equation for the calculation of RV volume using the pyramidal model where A_{RAO} is the area of the RAO projection, A_{LAO} is the area of the LAO projection and l_{RAO} is the distance from the bisected pulmonary valve to the bisected base in the RAO projection.

This method correlates well with postmortem casts but is improved to a correlation coefficient of $r = 0.99$ by means of the following regression equation:

$$V_{RV} = 0.6 \frac{A_{RAO} \times A_{LAO}}{l_{RAO}} + 3.9 \qquad (23)$$

The prism method uses AP and lateral projections from which three dimensions are measured. These are the maximum dimension of the base and the maximum height from the AP projection, and the maximum dimension from the lateral projection. From these a prism can be constructed to represent the volume of the ventricle. The volume is then calculated as:

$$V_{\text{PRISM}} = \frac{A_{\text{AP}} \times A_{\text{LAT}}}{2L} \qquad (24)$$

Equation for the calculation of RV volume using the prism method where A_{AP} is the area of the AP projection, A_{LAT} is the area of the lateral projection and L is the maximum length of the lateral projection.

This method correlates well with volumes derived from the use of Simpson's rule.

Simpson's rule

Irregular shaped ventricles are not well represented by any geometric primitive and their volumes are better calculated by this method. Simpson's rule is a means of calculating the area under a curve defined by equally spaced data points [136] and was first applied to the estimation of ventricular volume by Chapman [103].

The outlines of the biplane projections are divided into a number of slices, normally 1mm thick. The volume of each slice is calculated on the basis that the outline of the slice conforms to a particular shape, most commonly an ellipse but circular or rectangular shapes have been used. The volume of the ventricle is then the sum of the volume of the slices and is given as:

$$V = \frac{\pi h}{3}\left(\sum_{n=1}^{N} DA_n DL_n + \frac{1}{2}\sum_{j=1}^{N} DA_j DL_j\right) \qquad (25)$$

Equation for the calculation of ventricular volume using Simpson's rule where n = odd slices, 1, 3, 5, etc., j = even slices, 2, 4, 6, etc., h = slice thickness, DA = AP slice diameter, DL = LAT slice diameter, N = total number of slices, which should be odd.

The technique is clearly time consuming and tedious to do by hand and lends itself well to computerisation. Even a simple programmable calculator can make using this method a practical proposition [137]. With modifications to Simpson's rule, views other than AP and lateral, including orthogonal oblique projections (RAO and LAO) and non-orthogonal oblique views (with cranial or caudal tilt) can be used with equally good results [131].

Methods of calibration of the images

The projected image is magnified as a result of the non parallel X-rays and the pin cushion distortion effect of the image intersifier (pp. 140 and 141). Both distortions should be corrected if accurate absolute values are required. The best, straightforward method of correction is the use of a 1 cm radio-opaque grid (copper wire) that is filmed at the level of the patients heart, (identified as the apex beat), after ventriculography with the X-ray tube and image intensifier in the same position as it was for the patient. The correction factor is then defined as the ratio of the true grid area, a number of squares, and the planimetered area of the same number of squares in the projected image of the grid. Using the area—length method in single plane RAO projection and including the regression equation (see equations 19 and 21c) the corrected volume is given as:

$$V_{\text{corrected}} = 0.81\left(\frac{8}{3}\pi\,\frac{A^2}{L}\,\text{GR}^3\right) + 1.9 \qquad (26)$$

Equation for the corrected volume of the left ventricle where $V_{\text{corrected}}$ is the corrected volume, A is the planimetered area of the ventricle in the 30° RAO projection, L is the maximum chord length of the projected ventricle and GR is the correction factor derived from the ratio of true grid area/planimetered projected grid area.

The grid technique has the advantage that it accounts for both magnification and pin cushion distortion. Alternative techniques include using the catheter itself as a calibration object or filming a fixed object in the field of view, typically the catheter, in two different positions a known distance apart. Some catheter laboratory tables are designed to include 1 cm calibrations along their length for this purpose, but if not a simple ruler can be fixed to the table. This calibration is particularly useful if analysis of the ventriculograms is done with a digitising tablet and computer. The calibration marks, for example the pigtail catheter tip filmed 6 cm apart, can be entered initially and this calibrates the tablet for the drawing of the ventricular outlines. It should be noted that this method does not account for pin cushion distortion.

The use of the catheter dimension itself is not recommended since the error in determining its edges is considerable and a 0.5 mm error in measurement of a 7F catheter can result in up to 50% error in volume calculation [129].

Conclusion

There are many alternatives to the above methods for the calculation of ventricular volume including the use of implanted radio-opaque metal markers [138, 139], coronary artery bifurcation points [140], digital subtraction video densitometry [141] and impedance catheters [142]. Digital image processing techniques enabling a computer semi-automatically to trace the ventricular contours and calculate volume by whichever formula is favoured, are now available, but good results can be obtained using less sophisticated equipment providing the following appropriate steps are taken.

'How to do it' summary of volume measurement

1 Biplane is preferable to single-plane and should be used if available.
2 The X-ray source and the image intensifier should be as close to the patient as possible. Angulated views, 30° RAO with 20° of caudal tilt and 60° LAO with 25° of cranial tilt, should be used.
3 Adjustable 'fish-mouth'diaphragms which limit the contrast between pulmonary density and the ventricular silhouette should be used. The ventricular outline is thus more accurately delineated.
4 The patient should be still with fixed respiration.
5 To minimise haemodynamic and proarrhythmic effects the injection is best timed towards the end of diastole, and should be of non-ionic, iso-osmolar contrast medium with injection rates of 10—12 ml per second.
6 The image intensifier should be of high resolution phosphor and the camera of constant speed and gated to the electrocardiogram.
7 Digital subtraction angiography is better than film.
8 The images should be calibrated using a grid placed precisely at the position of the patient's heart.
9 The third postinjection beat should be used and ectopics and postectopic beats avoided.
10 The tracing of the outlines is probably best performed with a computerised digitising tablet and cursor attached to a small desk-top computer. End-diastole should be taken as the frame corresponding to the R wave of the ECG, and end-systole as the minimum dimension.
11 The ventricular outlines must include the papillary muscles (especially in the end-systolic frame),

the trabeculae carneae and the part of the inflow tract often obscured by the base of the aortic root. The inclusion of these is taken into account in the regression equations.
12 Simpson's rule is superior to the area—length method if facilities allow. Otherwise use the area—length method with the appropriate regression equation.

Regional wall motion analysis

The segmental nature of coronary artery disease leads to segmental defects in left ventricular function. With frank infarction the ventricular defect may cause a significant change in global ventricular function with a decrease in ejection fraction and a qualitatively obvious angiographic abnormality, but small areas of infarction, peri-infarction tissue and chronically ischaemic myocardium may not have such obvious effects. With the increasing availability of therapeutic intervention in coronary artery disease, whether by surgery, angioplasty or thrombolysis, there is an increasing demand for an accurate and appropriate method of segmental wall motion analysis to provide assessment these affected areas.

The two main difficulties in development of such a method stem from the fact that ventriculography provides a two-dimensional image, lacking discrete features, of a ventricular wall that is a three-dimensional object moving in three-dimensional space. What do we measure? And, with respect to what?

Development has mainly centred on segmental analysis of contrast ventriculograms, the outlines of different frames of a cardiac cycle being divided by some means into an arbitrary number of segments, the motion of which is then studied. Since these are two-dimensional images of a three-dimensional object moving in three space, the true correspondence, (in other words, is it the same piece of myocardium?) between any one segment in one frame and the same segment in another frame, cannot be determined and measures of motion must therefore be approximate. Various methods have been devised to provide discrete markers to overcome this problem [143—146] and recently Slager [147] has described discrete areas of the endocardium identifiable from standard ventriculography.

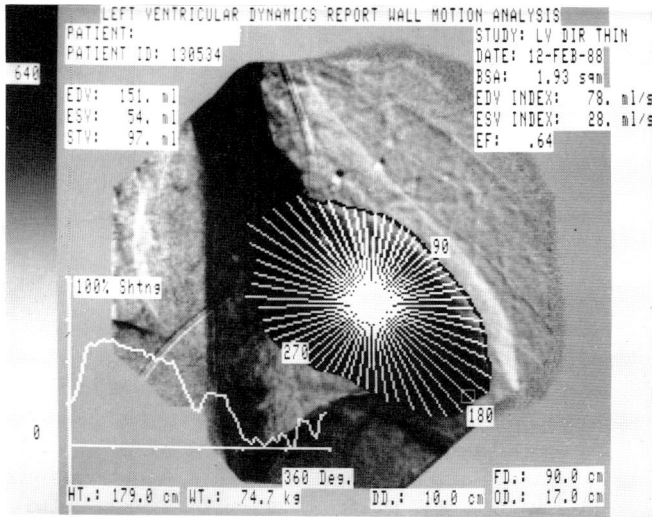

Fig. 8.16 A method for the analysis of left ventricular regional wall motion. The centre point of the long axis is chosen as a reference point towards which each of the regularly spaced radial segments is assumed to move. The degree of shortening of each radial between the end-diastolic frame and the end-systolic frame is measured and displayed in graphic form.

Reference systems

Ventricular motion is complex and, apart from any contracting (radial) motion, involves translation, rotation and torsion. Reference systems have been devised to minimise these effects and so to concentrate on the radial motion. Translation effects are thought to be minimised by superimposing the different frames at the point of the centre of the aortic valve although the apex has also been used. With the contours relatively fixed a reference system for the radial motion can be defined and wall motion measured. Different methods described include:

1 Measurement of motion towards and at right angles to the long axis [148] of the ventricle, although this does not represent apical and basal motion which tends to be along the long axis.

2 Motion towards the geometric centre of gravity [149].

3 Motion towards the centre point of the long axis of the ventricle.

The last method is at present the most commonly used and an example can be seen in Fig. 8.16. It is a single plane 30° RAO, two frame technique using the end-diastolic and end-systolic frames. In each, the long axis of the ventricle is defined as the line between the apex and the bisected aortic valve.

Radials at set intervals, are drawn from the centre point of the long axis to the perimeter of the ventricular silhouette. The aortic valves are superimposed and the degree of shortening of each radial between end-diastole and end-systole is measured. The information can then be displayed graphically as the degree of shortening against radial number or the ventricle can be divided into five or six anatomic segments, for example anterobasal, anterior, apical, infero-apical and mitral, and the shortening values in each segment averaged.

There are limitations to this approach:

1 The apex is not a constant feature especially in distorted diseased ventricles and using it to define a

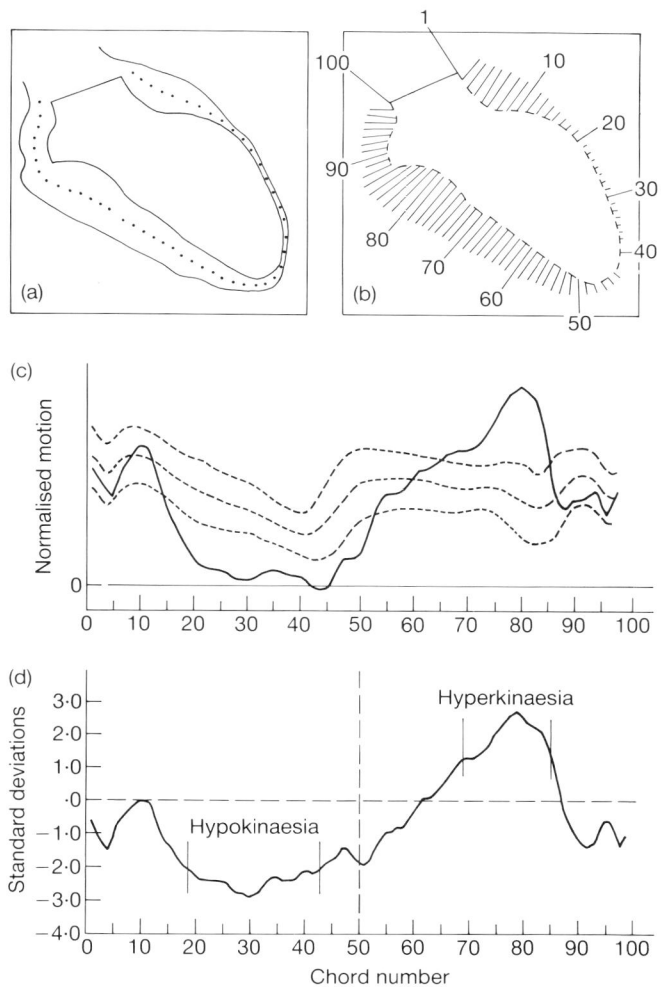

Fig. 8.17 The centreline method of regional wall motion analysis. See text for explanation. With kind permission of Dr FH Sheehan.

long axis is erroneous.

2 While it is obvious from subjective appraisal of the ventriculogram that wall motion tends to be radial it is not directed at a single point, whether it be the centre of the long axis or the centre of gravity. The motion of the wall is in many directions at different times.

3 There is no means by which patients may be compared in terms of th extent of regional wall motion abnormality.

4 It is restricted to use in the RAO view.

5 It is a two-frame technique and therefore measures only the change in position of a segment between those two frames and not true motion.

An improvement on this method has been described by Sheehan *et al.* [150] and is called the centreline method. This is also a two-frame method but the two frames are not superimposed. A centreline, half way between the end-diastolic and end-systolic out lines is generated by a computer (Fig. 8.17a)

and 100 evenly spaced chords perpendicular to the centreline are drawn between the two outlines. (Fig. 8.17b) Motion is normalised by the end-diastolic perimeter to provide a shortening fraction and the normalised chord lengths are then plotted. The plot is compared with that of a group of normals (Fig. 8.17c) and then replotted in units of standard deviations from the normal mean (Fig. 8.17d).

The advantages of this method are that no reference system is required, and that it may be used in any projection, not just the RAO. Also by measuring motion in standard deviations it provides an indication of severity and significance which can be used as a comparative index. This is of great benefit when the effect of some intervention on left ventricular function, for example thrombolysis, is being assessed. However it too does not take account of the artefact introduced by the translation component of ventricular motion and it does only consider two frames.

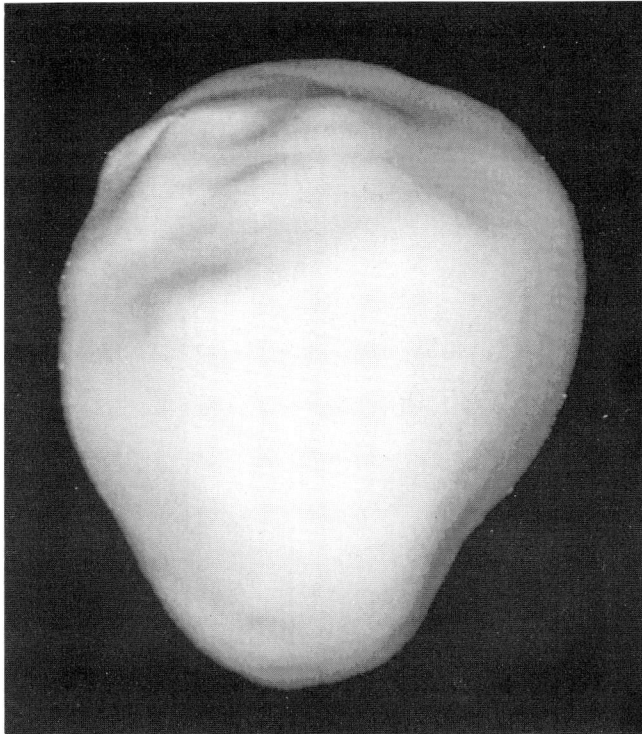

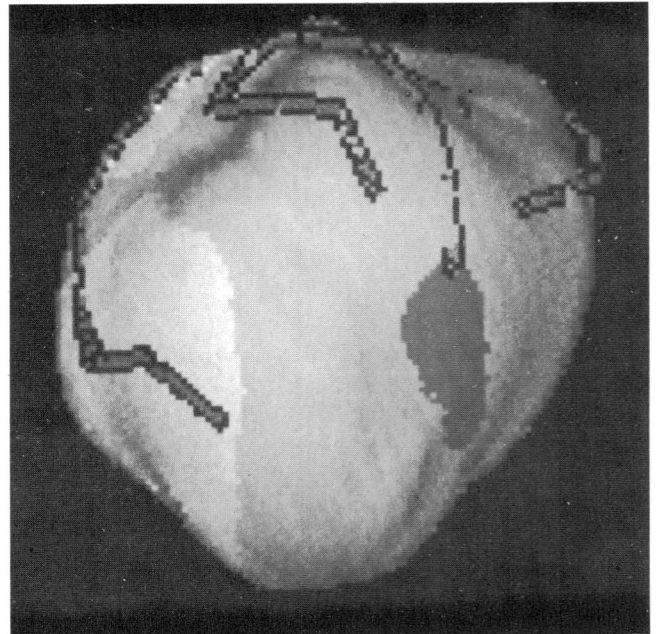

Figs. 8.18 and 8.19 A computer-generated three-dimensional image of the left ventricular epicardial surface of a single frame of the cardiac cycle. It is derived by the interpolation of a surface through the three-dimensional coordinates of coronary artery bifurcation points. Viewing multiple frames in turn gives a qualitative description of motion. Fig. 8.19 shows the same type of image but the quantitative information is coded in the image as different colours (in shades of grey here) representing instantaneous velocity of the wall with respect to a time-dependent centre of contraction.

Errors in volume determination and wall motion analysis may result from using two frames with the end-systolic frame defined as minimum dimension. End ejection has been suggested as a better alternative [151]. The translation component can only be excluded if it can be measured and this is probably only possible with knowledge of three-dimensional motion of discrete points.

Three-dimensional analysis

Clearly a method that could analyse three-dimensional wall motion in an external coordinate system would be of benefit in understanding and measuring segmental wall motion. A number of different approaches to the derivation of three-dimensional data from cardiac angiography have been made. Most require the identification of discrete cardiac markers, whether they are metal markers implanted at surgery [145] or via a catheter tip [147], or endogenous markers such as coronary artery bifurcation points

[140]. Others do not use discrete markers but equally spaced points around the ventricular silhouette [51].

All methods use biplane coronary arteriograms or ventriculograms. For the calibration of images for three-dimensional analysis a three-dimensional reference object must be used that has known dimensions and orientation. Two metal crosses at right angles have been used as have perspex cubes within which are implanted metal markers in known positions.

Computer graphics techniques allow for the display of the large amounts of data that are produced from three-dimensional analysis. Figs 8.18 to 8.21 show two methods each with a qualitative display and a quantitative display.

The computing power necessary to analyse ventricular wall motion in three dimensions precludes such analyses from routine use.

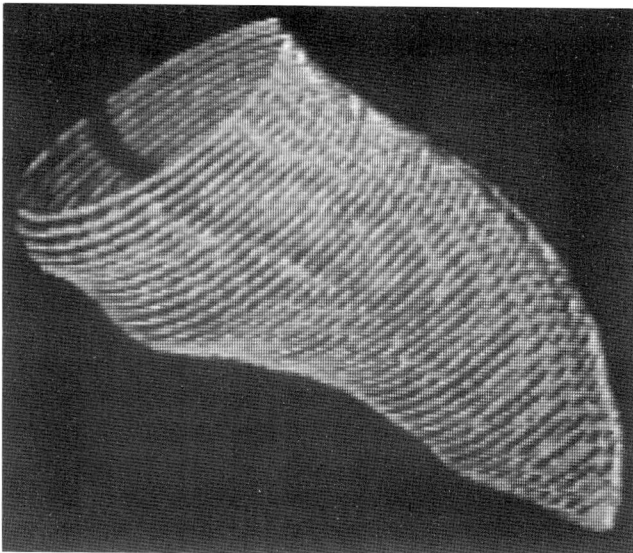

Fig. 8.21 This figure demonstrates the use of computer-generated three-dimensional graphics to display localised wall motion through a single cardiac cycle derived from single-plane ventriculograms of a normal ventricle. Each horizontal line represents wall motion of one site on the perimeter of the ventriculogram out of 40 sites recorded. The diagonal lines are isochrones connecting simultaneous events. The two accentuated isochrones represent the times of minimum volume and mitral valve opening. This representation of the data enables one to see at a glance hypokinesis as well as synchrony. With kind permission of Dr DG Gibson.

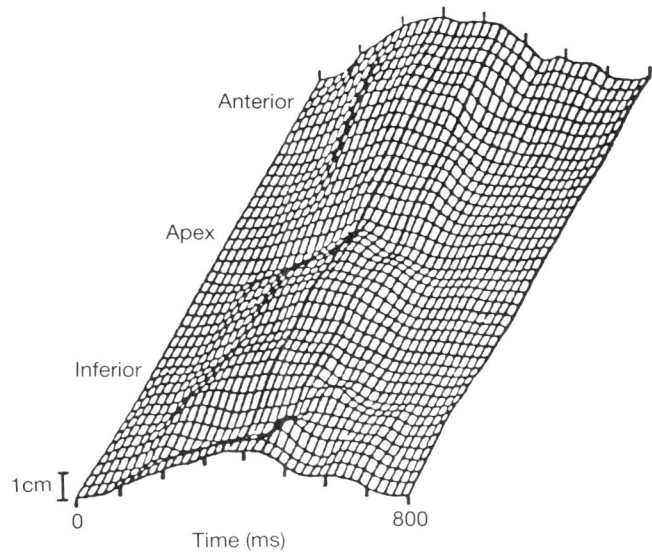

Fig. 8.20 A computer-generated three-dimensional representation of the normal left ventricular endocardial volume. This image has been generated by the analysis of contrast ventriculograms. With kind permission of Dr DG Gibson.

Digital imaging

It is appropriate at this point to provide an introduction to digital imaging and digital image processing as these play an increasingly large part in quantitative angiographic techniques and their application.

The basic stages of digital imaging are:

Sampling. The sampling of continuous image signal at discrete time intervals.
Quantization. The allocation of one of a finite number of amplitude values to each sample (the one to which its amplitude most closely approximates).
Coding. The coding of the discrete signal in binary form.

Either cine film frames or direct video signal output from the image intensifier may provide the continuous source signal for digitising. The finite number of amplitudes is usually 2N. N is normally 8 or 10 thus giving 256 (0−255) or 1024 (0−1023) different amplitudes or grey levels of intensity. In binary coding N bits are required to code the amplitudes. A video frame consists of 5−600 lines output in 30 to 40 ms. If each line is to be sampled 512 times a sampling rate of 10 MHz is required. The result is that for each video frame there are approximately one-quarter million samples (512 × 500) each with its amplitude coded. These samples are picture elements or *pixels*. Every pixel of an image is therefore coded with three values:
• X, the number along the line from 0 to 511;
• Y, the line number;
• grey level, the amplitude value, i.e. the intensity or brightness.

As can be seen from the example above, 10 seconds of video with a frame rate of 25 per second, digitised at 512 samples per line and 512 lines per frame, with an 8 bit grey scale gives $(10 \times 25 \times 512 \times 512)$ 65 536 000 bytes or 65 megabytes, which is a very large amount of data. These huge quantities of data create difficulties in data handling, transfer and storage which to some extent still limit the use of digital radiography. Spatial and temporal resolution may be played off against one another, the same data capacity being utilised if sampling rates are halved and the frame rate is doubled, and vice versa. It is not in the scope of this text to describe in detail the technology of digital angiography, suffice it to say that adequate impetus for further development is provided by the enormous potential advantages of having angiographic data in digital form where it can be easily manipulated to reveal contained information.

Digital image processing uses computers to apply arithmetic functions to the digital data in order to extract particular qualities or features from the image. Functions can be anything from additions or subtractions through simple filters to Fourier analysis and complex convolutions. Consequently feature extractions such as edge detection can be used to make quantitative assessments of ventricular wall position and coronary arterial diameter.

Quantitative coronary arteriography

Subjective analysis of coronary arteriograms is no-

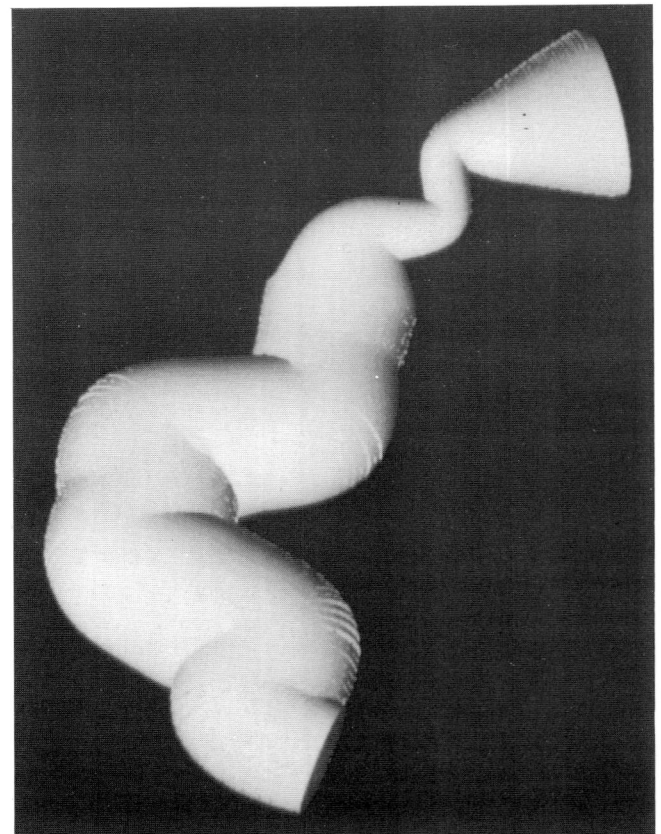

Fig. 8.22 A computer-generated three-dimensional model of a small section of the left-anterior descending artery showing a severe stenosis. The data has been derived semi-automatically from biplane coronary arteriograms. With permission of LDR Smith.

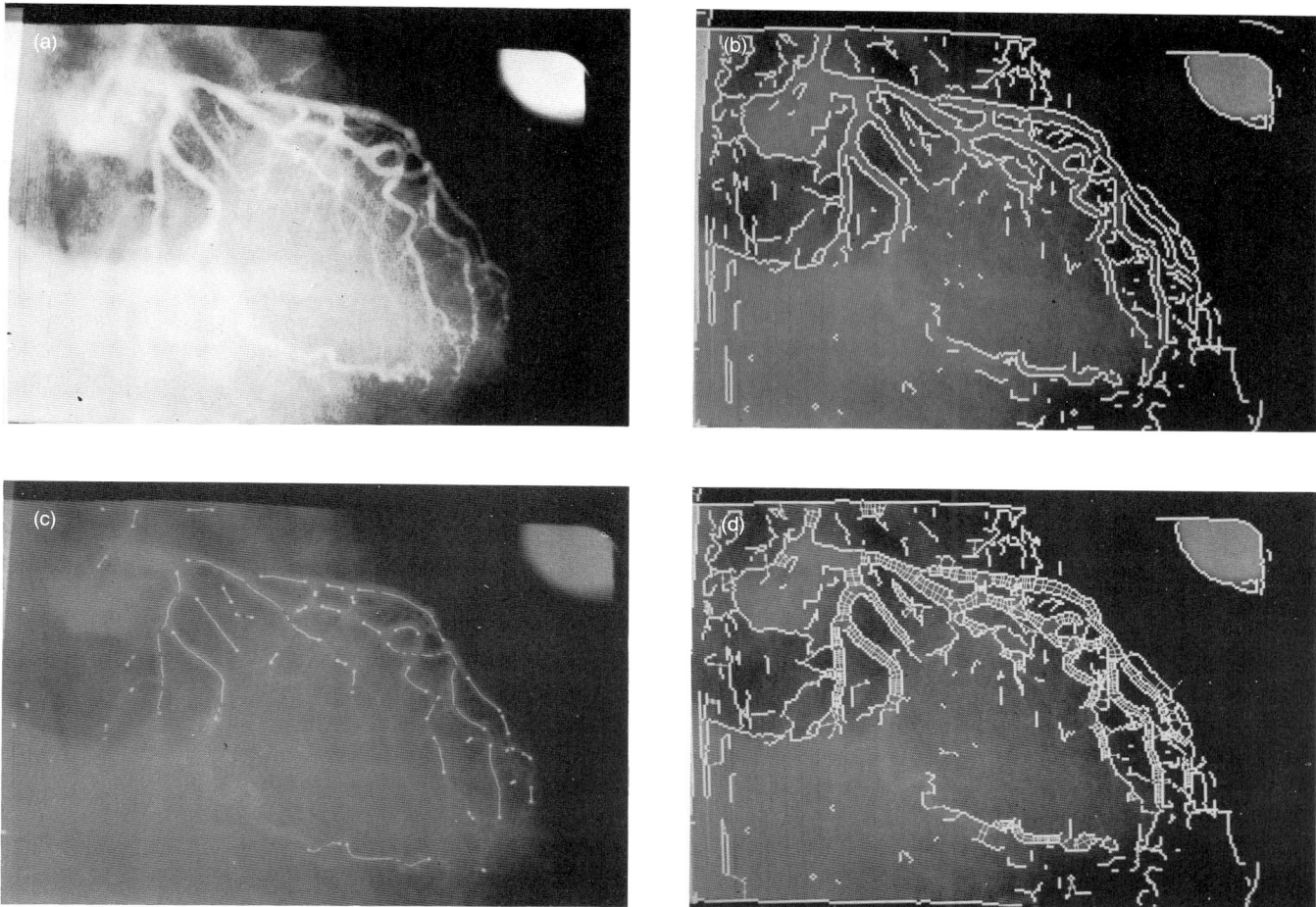

Fig. 8.23 The output of an 'artificial intelligent' vision system for the operator-independent quantitative analysis of arteriograms. The system is relying on higher functions (knowledge sources) that provide descriptions of the appearance of coronary arteries in an arteriogram. (a) Shows the 'raw' arteriogram. (b) All edges are found. (c) Parallel edges are identified and the centrelines constructed. Gaps are filled appropriately. (d) The diameters of the arteries are measured. This type of system may eventually provide 'on-line' quantitative assessment of arterial diameter. With kind permission of ST Rake.

toriously variable especially in the 70–90% stenosis range. Objective quantitation is therefore very attractive and the advent of digital imaging and digital image processing have enabled progress towards achieving this goal.

The prerequisites for successful quantitative arteriography are:
1 High quality X-ray imaging equipment.
2 High spatial resolution digital imaging. This may be direct from video output from the image intensifier or via a plumbicon camera digitising processed cine film.
3 Adequate corrections for image distortions, and accurate calibration of the images, in the same manner as for quantitative ventriculography.

The analysis of these images can then be performed with variable degrees of operator interaction. At its simplest the operator may draw the edges of a segment of a displayed coronary artery and receive a plot of diameter — no more than digital calipers. At the other end of the scale are semi-automatic methods for the production of quantitative three-dimensional arterial models [152] (Fig. 8.22), and computer vision systems that attempt the analysis without any operator intervention at all (Fig. 8.23). The commercially available systems, which are now widespread, fall somewhere between the two with a typical output like that in Fig. 8.24. The processes involved more or less comply with the following description.

A frame of the digitised, calibrated coronary ar-

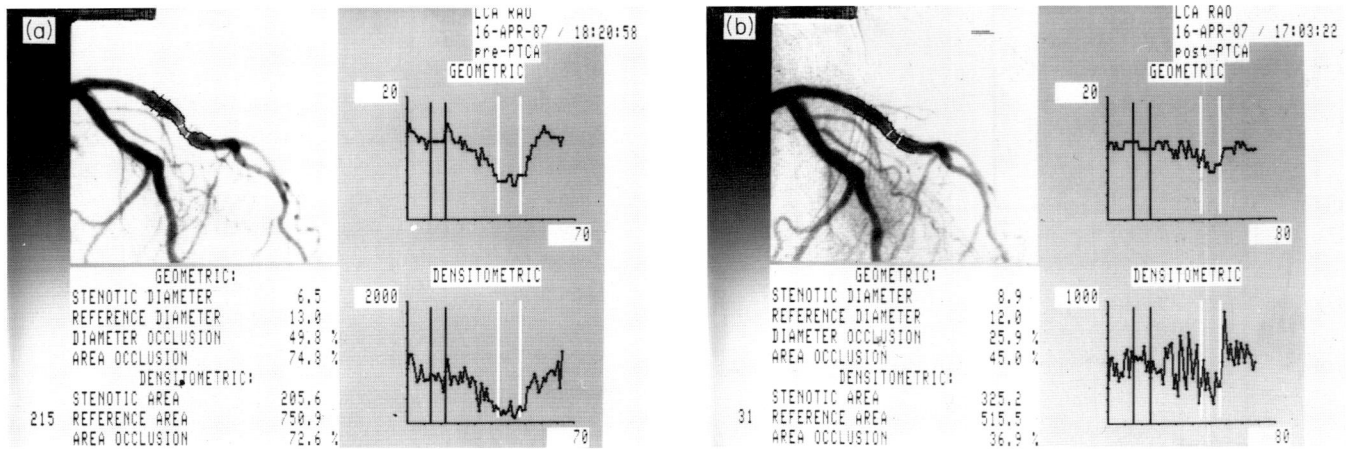

Fig. 8.24 Typical output from commercially available quantitative arteriography systems, showing one of the important functions of quantitative angiography, namely the measurement of the effect of PTCA. (a) Before PTCA (b) after PTCA. This is from the Siemens Digitron II system which uses digital subtraction images.

teriogram is displayed. This is often taken as the end-diastolic frame although there is probably very little change in diameter throughout the cycle. The section of artery of interest is indicated using a light pen or cursor, by marking the beginning and end of the section with points in the approximate centre of the artery. The most accurate measurements will stem from the use of segments that are most closely perpendicular to the X-ray beam.

Some systems require that the operator draws a line along the centre of the arterial segment and the computer can then smooth it using a linear interpolation, other systems are able to 'track' the centreline from the beginning point to the end point. This is effected by algorithms that compare the sum of the pixel values along pairs of orthogonal rays of a certain length radiating from the start point, at regular intervals through 360°. Since the centre of an opacified artery is by definition of high intensity compared with its surroundings, the pair of rays whose summed values differ maximally are probably the pair which has one ray along the centre of the artery and the other perpendicular across the width of the artery. Thus the direction of the centreline can be ascertained and the same procedure iterated at regular increments along the centreline. There are other methods of centreline propagation.

Once a centreline has been constructed whether by hand or computer, and whether straight or following the curves of the arterial segment, the diameter of the artery can be measured at regular intervals along the segment. Most methods of diameter detection are based on the definition of the arterial edge as the second derivative of the intensity profile of the artery. A line orthogonal to the centreline 20 to 40 pixels long is differentiated. The position of the two peaks of the second derivative are taken as the two edges of the artery (Fig. 8.24). This is done all along the segment. This is the most basic form of edge detection and most systems are considerably more sophisticated using correction factors for changes in background intensity and quantum noise.

The results can be displayed as plots of diameter against length, or if a circular or elliptical arterial cross-section is assumed, as plots of cross-sectional area against length. If the operator indicates a section of artery that is normal then percentage stenosis can be calculated and displayed.

Examples of commercial systems that contain such image processing capabilities are the Pye Medical CAAS and the Siemens Digitron system (Fig. 8.24).

SUMMARY

There is a large array of different methods for the evaluation of ventricular function. The following is a list of the most appropriate, in terms of availability and value of the result, for particular purposes.

Routine clinical assessment of global ventricular function: Ejection fraction and end-systolic volume index.

Provided the procedures for limiting errors in measuring volume from the ventriculogram are diligently performed these two indices approach the ideal test outlined in the Introduction.

Regional wall motion: Sheehan's centreline method. Of all the different techniques for analysing two-dimensional wall motion this probably is the most accurate and useful. It does not distort the information by attempts to re-align the image to fit a reference system, it provides a comparative index of wall motion and it can be used in different views for left or right ventricles.

Assessment of effects of drugs: dP/dt, κV_{MAX}, E_{MAX} In research procedures with selected patients to investigate the cardiac effects of drugs or other agents, where the patients may be electively paced, these indices are the most appropriate.

REFERENCES

1 Kreulen TH, Bove AA, McDonough MT, Sands MJ, Spann JF. The evaluation of left ventricular function in man. *Circulation* 1975; **51**:677–88.

2 Peterson KL, Skloven D, Ludbrook P, Uther JB, Ross J Jnr. Comparison of isovolumic and ejection phase indices of myocardial function. *Circulation* 1974;**49**: 1088–101.

3 Sarnoff SJ, Berglund E. Ventricular function. Starling's law of the heart studied by means of simultaneous right and left ventricular function curves in the dog. *Circulation* 1954;**9**:706–17.

4 Bradley RD. *Studies in acute heart failure.* London, Edward Arnold, 1977.

5 Wiggers CJ. The present status of cardiodynamic studies on normal and pathological hearts. *Arch Intern Med* 1920;475–502.

6 Rackley CE, Hood WP, Rolett EC, Young DT. Left ventricular end-diastolic pressure in chronic heart disease. *Am J Med* 1970;**48**(3):310.

7 Rahimtoola SH. Ventricular end-diastolic pressure and filling pressures in the assessment of ventricular function. *Chest* 1973;**63**:858–60.

8 Braunwald E, Ross J Jnr. Editorial: The end diastolic pressure. *Am J Med* 1963;**34**:147–50.

9 Ferlinz J. Right ventricular performance in adult cardiovascular disease. *Prog Cardiovasc Dis* 1982;**25**: 225–67.

10 Moraski RE, Russell RO, Smith M, Rackley CE. Left ventricular function in patients with and without myocardial infarction and one, two, or three vessel coronary artery disease. *Am J Cardiol* 1975;**35**:1–10.

11 Grossman W, McLaurin LP, Saltz SB, Paraskos JA, Dalen JE, Dexter L. Changes in the inotropic state of the left ventricle during isometric exercise. *Br Heart J* 1973;**35**:697–704.

12 Ferlinz J, Bechtel D, Herman MV, Cohn PF, Gorlin R. A new geometric model for right ventricular volume determination. *Circulation* 1974;**50** Suppl III:225 (abs).

13 Sandler H, Dodge HT. Angiographic methods for determination of left ventricular geometry and volume. Mirsky I, Ghista DN, Sandler H (ed.) In: *Cardiac mechanics: physiological, clinical and mathematical considerations.* New York, John Wiley & sons, 1924, 145–70.

14 Arvidsson H, Karnell J. Quantitative assessment of mitral and aortic insufficiency by angiocardiography. *Acta Radiol* 1964;**2**:105–19.

15 Miller GAH, Swan HJC. Effect of chronic pressure and volume overload on left heart volumes in subjects with congenital heart disease. *Circulation* 1964; **30**:205–16.

16 Miller GAH, Kirklin JW, Swan HJC. Myocardial function and left ventricular volumes in acquired valvular insufficiency. *Circulation* 1965;**31**:374–84.

17 Jones JW, Rackley CE, Bruce RA, Dodge HT, Cobb LA, Sandler H. Left ventricular volumes in valvular heart disease. *Circulation* 1964;**29**:887–91.

18 Kennedy JW, Baxley WA, Figley MD, Dodge HT, Blackmon JR. Quantitative angiocardiography. The normal left ventricle in man. *Circulation* 1966;**34**: 272–8.

19 Dodge HT, Baxley WA. Left ventricular volume and mass and their significance in heart disease. *Am J Cardiol* 1966;**23**:528–37.

20 Krayenbuehl HP. Myocardial function. *Eur Heart J* 1985;**6**;(suppl C):33–9.

21 White HD, Norris RM, Brown M, Brandt PWT, Whitlock RML, Wild CJ. Left ventricular end-systolic volume as the major determinant of survival after recovery from myocardial infarction. *Circulation* 1987; **76**:44–51.

22 Grossman W. Cardiac catheterisation and angiography. Philadelphia, Lea and Febiger, 1986;292.

23 Woods RH. A few applications of a physical theorem to membranes in the human body in a state of tension. *J Anat Physiol* 1982;**26**:302–70.

24 Sarnoff SJ, Braunwald E, Welch GH, Case RB, Stainsby WN, Macruz R. Hemodynamic determinants of oxygen consumption of the heart, with special reference to the tension-time index. *Am J Physiol* 1958;**192**:148.

25 Hill AV. The heat of shortening and the dynamic constants of muscle. *Proc Roy Soc* 1938; Series B 126: 136–95.

26 Gorlin R. Recent conceptual advances in congestive heart failure. *J Am Med Ass* 1962;**179** No.6:441−9.

27 Graham TP, Jarmakani JM, Atwood GF, Canent RV. Right ventricular volume determinations in children. Normal value and observations with volume or pressure overload. *Circulation* 1973;**47**:144−53.

28 Gentzler RD, Briseeli MF, Gault JH. Angiographic estimation of right ventricular volume in man. *Circulation* 1974;**50**:324.

29 Ferlinz J. Measurements of right ventricular volumes in man from single plane cineangiograms. A comparison to the bi-plane approach. *Am Heart J* 1977;**94**:87−90.

30 Fernlinz J. Right ventricular performance in essential hypertension. *Circulation* 1980;**61**:156−62.

31 Redington AN, Rigby ML, Oldershaw PJ. Characterisation of the normal right pressure-volume loop using bi-plane ventriculography and simultaneous high fidelity pressure measurements. *Br Heart J* 1986;**55**:525−6 (abs).

32 Carlsson E, Keene RJ, Lee P, Goerke RJ, Angiographic stroke volume correlation of the two cardiac ventricles in man. *Invest Radiol* 1971;**6** No. 1:44−51.

33 Hammermeister KE, Brooks RC, Warbasse JR. The rate of change of left ventricular volume in man. Validation and peak systolic ejection rate in health and disease. *Circulation* 1974;**49**:729−38.

34 Grossman W, Braunwald E, Mann T, McLaurin LP, Green LH. Contractile state of the left ventricle in man as evaluated from end systolic pressure volume relations *Circulation* 1977;**56**:845−52.

35 Borow KM, Green LH, Grossman W, Braunwald E. Left ventricular end systolic stress shortening and stress length relations in human. *Am J Cardiol* 1982;**50**:1301−8.

36 McKay *et al*. Left ventricular pressure-volume diagrams and end systolic pressure-volume relations in human beings. *J Am Coll Cardiol* 1984;**3**;301.

37 Bunnell IL, Grant C, Greene DG. Left ventricular function derived from the pressure-volume diagram. *Am J Med* 1965;**39**:881.

38 Suga H, Sagawa K. Instantaneous pressure-volume relationships and their ratio in the excised, supported canine left ventricle. *Circ Res* 1974;**35**:117.

39 Starling MR, Walsh RA, Dell'italia LJ, Mancini GBJ, Lasher JC, Lancaster JL. The relationship of various measures of end-systole to left ventricular maximum time-varying elastance in man. *Circulation* 1987;**76**:32.

40 Redington AN, Rigby ML, Hodson ME, Oldershaw PJ. Characterisation of the normal right ventricular pressure-volume loop using bi-plane ventriculography and simultaneous high-fidelity pressure measurements. *Br Heart J* 1986;**55**:525−6 (abs).

41 Nivatpumin T, Katz S, Scheuer J. Peak left ventricular systolic pressure/end systolic volume ratio: a sensitive detector of left ventricular disease. *Am J Cardiol* 1979;**43**:969−74.

42 Falsetti HL, Mates RE, Grant C, Greene DG, Bunnell IL. Left ventricular wall stress calculated from one plane cineangiography. *Circ Res* 1970;**26**:71−83.

43 Mirsky I. Review of various theories for the evaluation of left ventricular wall stress. Mirsky I, Ghista DN, Sandler H (eds.) In: *Cardiac mechanics: physiological, clinical and mathematical considerations*. New York, John Wiley & sons, 1974;389.

44 Sandler H, Dodge HT. Left ventricular tension and stress in man. *Circ Res* 1963;**13** No. 2:91−104.

45 Dodge HT, Sandler H, Ballew DW, Lord JD Jnr. The use of bi-plane angiocardiography for the measurement of left ventricular volume in man. *Am Heart J* 1960;**60** No. 5:762−76.

46 Burns JW, Covell JW, Myers R, Ross J Jnr. Comparison of directly measured left ventricular wall stress and stress calculated from geometric reference figures. *Circ Res* 1971;**28**:611−21.

47 Wong AY, Rautaharju PM. Stress distribution within the left ventricular wall approximated as a thick walled ellipsoidal shell. *Am Heart J* 1968;**75**:649−62.

48 Mirsky I. Elastic properties of the myocardium: A quantitative approach with physiological and clinical applications. *Handbook of physiology, Section 2: the cardiovascular system*, American Physiological Society, 497−531.

49 Yin FCP. Ventricular wall stress. *Circ Res* 1981;**49** No. 4:829−42.

50 Gould P, Ghista D, Brombolich L, Mirsky I. In vivo stresses in the human left ventricular wall: Analysis accounting for the irregular three-dimensional geometry and comparison with idealised geometry analyses. *J Biomech* 1972;**5**:521−39.

51 Yettram AL, Vinson CA, Gibson DG. Computer modelling of the human left ventricle. *J Biomech Eng* 1982;**104**:148−52.

52 Mirsky I, Ellison RC Hugenholtz PG. Assessment of myocardial contractility in children and young adults from ventricular pressure recordings. *Am J Cardiol* 1971;**27**:359−67.

53 Karliner JF, Bouchard RJ Gault JH. Dimensional changes of the human left ventricle prior to aortic valve opening: a cineangiographic study in patients with and without left heart disease. *Circulation* 1971;**44**:312−22.

54 Parmley WW, Sonnenblick EH. Re-evaluation of V_{MAX} as an index of contractile state: an analysis of different muscle models. *Circulation* 1970;**41** (suppl III):115 (abs).

55 Parmley WW, Sonnenblick EH. Series elasticity in heart muscle: its relation to contractile element vel-

ocity and proposed muscle models. *Circ Res* 1967;**20**: 112−23.

56 Mirsky I, Parmley WW. Evaluation of passive elastic stiffness for the left ventricle and isolated heart muscle. Mirsky I, Ghista DN, Sandler H (eds) In: *Cardiac mechanics: Physiological, clinical and mathematical considerations.* New York, John Wiley & sons, Chapter 11, 1974;331−58.

57 Urschel CW, Vokonas PS, Henderson AH, Liedke J, Horwitz LD, Sonnenblick EH. A comparison of indices of contractility derived from the isovolumic force-velocity relation. *Circulation* 1970;**41** (suppl II): 115 (abs).

58 Grossman W, Haynes F, Paraskos JA Saltz S, Dalen JE, Dexter L. Alterations in preload and myocardial mechanics in the dog and in man. *Circ Res* 1972;**31**: 83−94.

59 Oboler AA, Keefe JF, Gaasch WH, Benas JS, Levine HJ. Influence of left ventricular isovolumic pressure upon right ventricular pressure transients. *Cardiology* 1973;**58**:32−44.

60 Finnegan P, Forbes MV, Bishop JM. Evaluation of pressure derived indices of right ventricular contractility. *Eur J Cardiol* 1977;**6**:2;139.

61 Redington AN, Rigby ML, Hodson ME, Oldershaw PJ. Characterisation of the normal right ventricular pressure-volume loop using bi-plane ventriculography and simultaneous high-fidelity pressure measurements. *Br Heart J* 1986;**55**:525−6 (abs).

62 Gaasch WH, Battle WE, Oboler AA, Banas JS Jr., Levine HJ. Left ventricular stress and compliance in man: With special reference to normalised ventricular function curves. *Circulation* 1972;**45**:746−62.

63 Gaasch WH, Quinones MA, Waisser E, Thiel HG, Alexander JK. Diastolic compliance of the left ventricle in man. *Am J Cardiol* 1975;**36**:193−201.

64 Diamond G, Forrester JS. Effect of coronary artery disease and acute myocardial infarction on left ventricular compliance in man. *Circulation* 1972;**45**:11−19.

65 Dodge HT, Hay RE, Sandler H. Pressure-volume characteristics of the diastolic left ventricle of man with heart disease. *Am Heart J* 1962;**64**:4,503−11.

66 Brecher GA. Experimental evidence of ventricular diastolic suction. *Circ Res* 1956;**4**:513−22.

67 Katz LN. The role played by the ventricular relaxation in filling the ventricle. *Am J Physiol* 1930;**95**:542.

68 Katz LN. Observations on the external work of the isolated turtle heart. *Am J Physiol* 1932;**99**:579.

69 Vogel JHK, Cornish D, McFadden RB. Underestimation of ejection fraction with single plane angiography in coronary artery disease: role of bi-plane angiography. *Chest* 1973;**64** No. 2:217−21.

70 Miller RR, DeMaria AN, Amsterdam EA *et al.* Improvement of reduced left ventricular diastolic

compliance in ischaemic heart disease after successful coronary artery bypass surgery. *Am J Cardiol* 1975; **35**:11−16.

71 Hammermeister KE, Warbasse JR. The rate of change of left ventricular volume in man. *Circulation* 1974;**49**:739−47.

72 Gibson DG, Traill TA, Brown DJ. Changes in left ventricular free wall thickness in patients with ischaemic heart disease. *Br Heart J* 1977;**39**:1312−18.

73 St John Sutton MG, Tajik AJ, Smith HC, Ritman EL. Angina in idiopathic hypertrophic subaortic stenosis. *Circulation* 1980;**61**:561−8.

74 Weiss JL, Frederiksen JW, Weisfeldt ML. Haemodynamic determinants of the time course of fall in pressure in the canine left ventricle. *J Clin Invest* 1976; **58**:751−60.

75 Fioretti P, Brower RW, Meester GT, Serruys PW. Interaction of left ventricular relaxation and filling during early diastole in human subjects. *Am J Cardiol* 1980;**46**:197−203.

76 Ludbrook PA, Byrne JD, Tiefebrunn AJ. Association of asynchronous protodiastolic segmental wall motion with impaired left ventricular relaxation. *Circulation* 1981;**64**:1201−11.

77 Eichhorn P, Grimm J, Koch R, Hess O, Carrol J, Krayenbuehl HP. Left ventricular relaxation in patients with left ventricular hypertrophy secondary to aortic valve disease. *Circulation* 1982;**65**:1395−404.

78 Thompson DS, Waldron CB, Juul SM, Coltart DJ, Jenkins BS, Webb-Peploe MM. Comparison of two methods of estimating the time constant of left ventricular relaxation. *Br Heart J* 1981;**45**:348 (abs).

79 Thompson DS, Waldron CB, Juul SM, Coltart DJ, Jenkins BS, Webb-Peploe MM. Analysis of left ventricular pressure during isovolumic relaxation in coronary artery disease. *Circulation* 1982;**65**:690−7.

80 Thompson DS, Waldron CB, Coltart DJ, Jenkins BS, Webb-Peploe MM. Estimation of time constant of left ventricular relaxation. *Br Heart J* 1983;**49**:250−8

81 Hirota Y. A clinical study of left ventricular relaxation. *Circulation* 1980;**62**:756−63.

82 Pouleur H, Rousseau MF, Van Eyll C, Brasseur LA, Charlier A. Force-velocity-length relations in hypertrophic cardiomyopathy: Evidence of normal or depressed myocardial contractility. *Am J Cardiol* 1983; **52**:813−17.

83 Swanton RH, Brooksby IAB, Jenkins BS, Webb-Peploe MM. Haemodynamic studies of beta-blockade in patients with hypertrophic obstructive cardiomyopathy. *Eur J Cardiol* 1977;**5**/4:324−41.

84 Hanrath P, Mathey DG, Kremer P, Sonntag F, Bleifield W. Effect of Verapamil on left ventricular isovolumic relaxation time and regional left ventricular filling. *Am J Cardiol* 1980;**45**:1258−64.

85 Webb-Peploe MM, Croxson RS, Oakley CM, Goodwin JF. Cardioselective beta-adrenergic blockade in hypertrophic obstrutive cardiomyopathy. *Postgrad Med J* 1971;**47** (suppl):93–6.

86 Thompson DS, Wilmshurst P, Juul SM, Waldron CB, Coltart DJ, Jenkins BS, Webb-Peploe MM. Pressure-derived indices of left ventricular iso-volumic relaxation in patients with hypertrophic cardiomyopathy. *Br Heart J* 1982a;**49**:259–67.

87 Tanaka H, Tei C, Nakao S, Tahara M, Sakurai S, Kushina T, Kanehisa T. Diastolic bulging of the interventricular septum toward the left ventricle. An echocardiographic manifestation of negative interventricular pressure gradient between left and right ventricles during diastole. *Circulation* 1980;**62**:558–63.

88 Weyman AE, Wann S, Feigenbaum H, Dillon JC. Mechanisms of abnormal septal motion in patients with right ventricular volume overload. An echocardiographic study. *Circulation* 1976;**54**:179–86.

89 Brinker JA, Weiss JL, Lappe DL, Robson JL, Sumner WR, Permutt S, Weisfeldt ML. Leftward septal displacement during right ventricular loading in man. *Circulation* 1980;**61**:626–33.

90 Jardin F, Farcot JC, Boisante L, Margairaz A. Effect of right ventricular loading on left ventricular (LV) performance during respiratory therapy with PEEP. Evaluation by two dimensional echo. *Circulation* 1980;**62** (suppl III):60.

91 Jessup M, St John Sutton M, Weber KT, Janicki JS. The effect of chronic pulmonary hypertension on left ventricular size, function, and interventricular septal motion. *Am Heart J* 1986;**113**:1114–22

92 Stool EW, Mullins CB, Leshin SJ, Mitchell JH. Dimensional changes in the left ventricle during acute pulmonary arterial hypertension in dogs. *Am J Cardiol* 1974;**33**:868–75.

93 Hunter AS, Gentzler JH, Gault WR. Distortion of left ventricular (LV) chamber anatomy by right ventricular (RV) volume overload (VO). (abs) *Am J Cardiol* 1974;**33**:145 (abs).

94 Weber KT, Janicki JS, Shroff S, Fishman AP. Contractile mechanics and interaction of the right and left ventricles. *Am J Cardiol* 1981;**47**:686–95.

95 Lima JAC, Guzman PA, Yin FCP, Brawley RK, Humphrey L, Traill TA, Lima SD, Marino P, Weisfeldt ML, Weiss JL. Septal geometry in the unloaded living human heart. *Circulation* 1986;**74**:463–8.

96 Taquini AC, Fermoso JD, Aramendia P. Behaviour of the right ventricle following acute constriction of the pulmonary artery. *Circ Res* 1960;**8**:315–18.

97 Moulopoulos SD, Sarcas A, Stamateopoulos S, Arealis E. Left ventricular performance during by-pass or distension of the right ventricle. *Circ Res* 1965;**17**:484–91.

98 Feneley MP, Gavaghan TP, Baron dW, Branson JA, Roy PA, Morgan JJ. Contribution of left ventricular contraction to the generation of right ventricular systolic pressure in the human heart. *Circulation* 1985;**71**: 473–80.

99 Rohrer F. Volumbestimmung von Körperhöhlen und Organen auf ortho-diagraphischem Wege. *Forschr Geb Röntgenstr* 1916;**24**;285.

100 Kahlstorf A. Ueber eine orthodiagraphische Herzvolumenbestimmung. *Forschr Geb Röntgenstr* 1932;**45**; 132.

101 Kahlstorf A. Möglichkeiten und Ergebnisse Herzvolumenbestimmung. *Klin Wehnschr* 1938;**17**: 223.

102 Liljestrand G, Lysholm E, Nylin G, Zachrisson CG. The normal heart volume in man. *Am J Cardiol* 1938; **17**:406–15.

103 Chapman CB, Baker O, Reynolds J, Bonte FJ. Use of bi-plane cinefluorography for measurement of ventricular volume. *Circulation* 1958;**18**;1105–17.

104 Gribbe P, Hirvonen L, Lind J, Wegelius C. Cineangiocardiographic recordings of the cyclic changes in volume of the left ventricle. *Cardiologia* 1959;**34** No.6:348–67.

105 Caldwell JL, Kennedy JW. Programmed left ventricular contrast injection. *Am Heart J* 1977;141–6.

106 Hamby RI, Aintablian A, Wisoff BG, Hartstein ML. Response of the left ventricle to postextra-systolic potentiation: Prediction of post-operative ventricular function in coronary artery disease. *Circulation* 1975; **51**;428–35.

107 Hamby RI, Aintablian A, Wisoff BG, Hartstein ML. Effects of contrast medium on the left ventricular pressure and volume with emphasis on coronary artery disease. *Am Heart J* 1977;**93** No. 1:9–18.

108 Friesinger GC, Schaffer J, Criley JM, Gaertner RA, Ross RS. Hemodynamic consequences of the injection of radio-opaque material. *Circulation* 1965;**31**:730–40.

109 Iseri LT, Kaplan MA, Evans MJ, Nockel ED. Effect on concentrated contrast media during angiography on plasma volume and plasma osmolality. *Am Heart J* 1965;**69**;154–8.

110 Carleton RA. Change in left ventricular volume during angiocardiography. *Am J Cardiol* 1971;**27**:460–3.

111 Hammermeister KE, Warbasse JR. Immediate Haemodynamic effects of cardiac angiography in man. *Am Heart J Cardiol* 1973;**31** 307–14.

112 Guzman SV, West JW. Cardiac effects of intracoronary arterial injections of various roentgenographic contrast media. *Am Heart J* 1959;**58** No. 4:597–607.

113 Pijls NHJ, Bos HS, Uijen GJH, Van der Werf T. Nonionic isotonic Iohexol is the contrast agent of choice for quantitative myocardial video-densitometry. *Second International Symposium on Coronary Arteriography* 1987:43 (abs).

114 Brundage BH, Cheitlin MD. Ventricular function curves from the cardiac response to angio graphic contrast: A sensitive indicator of ventricular dysfunction in coronary artery disease. *Am Heart J* 1974;**88**:281–8.

115 Hellige G. Recent developments in contrast media. Just H, Heintzen PH (eds) In: *Angiocardiography — current status and future developments*. Berlin, Springer-Verlag, 1986.

116 Love HG, Brunt JNH, Rowlands DJ. Prompt effects of contrast injection on left ventricular volume. *Clin Sci* 1981;**61**:33.

117 Sandler H. Dimensional analysis of the heart — a review. *Am J Med Sci* 1970;**260**:56–70.

118 Ferlinz J, Herman MV, Cohn PF, Cohn PF, and Gorlin R. Comparison of selective left ventriculograms with levo-phase (forward) ventriculograms in patients with coronary artery disease. *Am Heart J* 1976;**91**:721–5.

119 Bouchard RJ, Gault JH, Ross J Jnr. Evaluation of pulmonary artery end-diastolic pressure as an estimate of left ventricular end diastolic pressure in patients with normal and abnormal left ventricular performance. *Circulation* 1971;**44**:1072–9.

120 De Rouen TA, Murray JA, Owen W. Variability in the analysis of coronary arteriograms. *Circulation* 1977;**55**:324–8.

121 Paulin S. Grading and measuring coronary artery stenoses. *Cathet Cardiovasc Diagn* 1979;**5**:213–18.

122 Arvidsson H. Angiographic observations in mitral valve disease. With special referene to volume variations in the left atrium. *Acta Radiol Suppl* 1958;**158**:1–124.

123 Miller GAH, Brown R, Swan HJC. Isolated congenital mitral insufficiency with particular reference to left heart volumes. *Circulation* 1964;**29**:356.

124 Bunnell IL, Ikkos D, Rudhe UG, Swan HJC. Left heart volumes in coarctation of the aorta. *Am Heart J* 1961;**61**;165.

125 Gibson DG, Prewitt TA, Brown DJ. Analysis of left ventricular wall movement during isovolumic relaxation and its relation to coronary artery disease. *Br Heart J* 1976;**38**:1010–19.

126 Sandler H, Dodge HT. The use of single plane angiocardiograms for the calculation of left ventricular volumes in man. *Am Heart J* 1968;**75**:325.

127 Green DG, Carlisle R, Grant C *et al*. Estimation of left ventricular volume by one plane cine angiography. *Circulation* 1967;**35**:61–9.

128 Kasser IS, Kennedy JW. Measurement of left ventricular volume in man by single plane cineangiocardiography. *J Invest Radiol* 1969;**4**:83–90.

129 Gault JH. Angiographic estimation of left ventricular volume *Cathet Cardiovasc Diagn* 1975;**1**:7–16.

130 Just H. Estimation of left ventricular muscle mass.

Just H, Heintzen PH (eds) In: *Angiocardiography — current status and future developments*. New York, Springer-Verlag, 1986;109–19.

131 Starling MR, Walsh RA. Accuracy of bi-plane axial oblique and oblique cineangiographic left ventricular cast volume determinations using a modification of Simpson's Rule. *Am Heart J* 1985;**110**:1219–25.

132 Cohn PF, Gorlin R, Adams DF, Chahine RA, Vokonas PS, Herman MV. Comparison of bi-plane and single plane left ventriculograms in patients with coronary artery disease. *Am J Cardiol* 1974;**33**:1–6.

133 Wynne J, Green LH, Mann T, Levin D, Grossman W. Estimation of left ventricular volumes in man from bi-plane cineangiograms filmed in oblique projections. *Am J Cardiol* 1978;**41**:726.

134 Kennedy JW, Trenholme SE, Kasser IS. Left ventricular volume and mass from single plane cineangiocardiograms: a comparison of antero-posterior and right anterior oblique methods. *Am Heart J* 1970;**80**:343.

135 Fisher EA, Du Brow RA, Hastreiter AR. Right ventricular volume in congenital heart disease. *Am J Cardiol* 1975;**36**:67–75.

136 James ML, Smith GM, Wolford JC. Applied numerical methods for digital computation with FORTRAN and CSMP. New York, Crowell TY, 1977;328.

137 Pao YC. Measurement of ventricular volume with a programmable calculator. *Comput Biol Med* 1981;**11** No.4:221–9.

138 Caldwell JH, Stewart DK, Dodge HT, Frimer M, Kennedy JW. Left ventricular volume during maximal supine exercise: a study using metallic epicardial markers. *Circulation* 1978;**58**:732–8.

139 Vine DL, Dodge HT, Frimer M, Stewart DK, Caldwell J. Quantitative measurement of left ventricular volumes in man from radio-opaque epicardial markers. *Circulation* 1976;**54**:391–8.

140 Smith LDR, Quarendon P. *Four dimensional cardiac imaging*. SPIE 593 Medical Image Processing; 74–7.

141 Naclioglu O, Seibert JA, Roeck WW, Henry WL, Tobis JM, Johnston WD. Comparison of digital subtraction video densitometry and area-length method in the determination of left ventricular ejection fraction. 1981; SPIE 314 Digital Radiography; 294–298.

142 Baan J, van der Velde ET, de Bruin HG, Smeenk GJ *et al*. Continuous measurement of left ventricular volume in animals and humans by conductance catheter. *Circulation* 1984;**70**:812–23.

143 McDonald IG. Contraction of the hypertophied left ventricle in man studied by cineradiography of epicardial markers. *Am J Cardiol* 1972;**30**:587–93.

144 Daughters GT, Ingels NB, Carrera CJ. Regional myocardial dynamics from single-plane coronary cineangiograms. *J Biomech* 1973;**6**:25–30.

145 Ingels NB, Daughters GT, Stinson EB, Alderman EL.

Measurement of midwall myocardial dynamics in intact man by radiography of surgically implanted markers. *Circulation* 1975;**52**:859.

146 Potel MJ, MacKay SA, Rubin JM, Aisen AM, Sayre RE. Three dimensional left ventricular wall motion in man. *Invest Radiol* 1984;**19**;499−509.

147 Slager CJ, Hooghoudt TEH, Reiber JHC, Schuurbiers JCH, Verdouw PD. Use of endocardial landmarks in the evaluation of left ventricular function: advantages and limitations of automated analysis of the ventriculogram. Just H, Heintzen PH (eds.) In: *Angiocardiography — current status and future developments* New York, Springer-Verlag, 1986;213−26.

148 Harris LD, Clayton PD, Marshall HW. A technique for the detection of asynergistic motion in the left ventricle. *Comput Biomed Res* 1974;**7**:380.

149 Rickards A, Seabra-Gomes R, Thurston P. The assessment of regional abnormalities of the left ventricle by angiography. *Eur J Cardiol* 1977;**5**:167−82.

150 Sheehan FH, Bolson EL, Dodge HT, Mathey D, Schofer J, Hok-Wai Woo MS. Advantages and applications of the centreline method for characterising regional ventricular function. *Circulation* 1986;**74**: 293−305.

151 Marier DL, Gibson DG. Limitations of two frame method for displaying left ventricular wall motion in man. *Br Heart J* 1980;**44**:555−59.

152 Smith LDR, Robinson GR, Burridge JM, Quarendon P. Quantitative moving three dimensional images of the left ventricle and coronary arteries. An automated method or production. *Circulation* 1986;**74** (suppl II) (abs).

CHAPTER 9

Respiratory techniques and the measurement of oxygen consumption

Sometimes in cardiac catheterisation it is helpful to have accurate measurements of pulmonary gas exchange and the gas contents of particular samples of blood, because they allow precise determinations of total, pulmonary and shunt flows. This chapter describes how measurements of respired gas are made and used. Chapters 6 and 11 discuss measurements of gas in blood.

If the body has been at rest or working at a constant level of exertion, for 10 minutes or more, the flow of oxygen ($\dot{V}o_2$) and carbon dioxide ($\dot{V}co_2$) into and out of the tissues, equals the corresponding flows of O_2 and CO_2 at the lips. When this is so, the body is in a respiratory steady state. This is recognised by the stability of expired CO_2 concentrations and of the ratio $\dot{V}co_2/\dot{V}o_2$. The latter is known as the respiratory exchange ratio (R). In steady states it is constant within $\pm$ 0.02 and almost always lies between 0.72 and 1.02. When that is so, measurements of gas flows and blood gas contents can be combined to obtain dependable estimates of blood flows. At other times such calculations are not reliable. Therefore respiratory techniques depend on:

1 Establishing that a respiratory steady-state exists.
2 Measuring gas flows correctly.
3 Taking appropriate blood samples (see Chapter 6).
4 Determining their gas contents (see Chapter 6).
5 Combining the data to estimate blood flows (see Chapter 11).

ESTABLISHING THAT A RESPIRATORY STEADY STATE EXISTS

If a recumbent patient's ventilation and pulse rate have been stable for several minutes, it is reasonable to suppose the patient is in a respiratory steady state. However, wherever possible it is wiser to have objective evidence that this is so, because substantial disturbances of gas exchange are missed on casual observation. Supporting evidence can be obtained at three levels. Firstly if expired or arterial CO_2 tensions have been steady within $\pm$ 2 mmHg and there has been no obvious change in the patients level of exertion, it is very likely a steady state exists. If, in addition, their CO_2 output has been constant over the same period, it is almost definite they are in a steady state. If the ratio $\dot{V}co_2/\dot{V}o_2$ has been constant within ± 0.02 over the gas and blood sampling period, it is absolutely certain the patient's respiration is stable.

Supposing that, from a respiratory point of view, a catheter laboratory is equipped only with a blood gas analyser, and the investigator wishes to calculate shunt flows from blood samples drawn from different sites at times that are close together but not identical. He needs to know that over the total sampling time the respiratory state was steady, so that he can compare the gas contents from different sites with confidence. To do this he should minimise disturbance to the patient for several minutes before, and during the sampling, and obtain evidence that systemic arterial Pco_2 did not change more than 2 mmHg over the time in question. As explained in Chapter 6, to avoid errors associated with fluctuations in gas content with the respiratory cycle, each blood sample should be drawn slowly and evenly over a period of about a minute. Where possible, samples from different sites should be drawn simultaneously.

If the laboratory is equipped with a rapid respired-CO_2 monitor, (90% response time of less than one-fifth the duration of a breath) it is practical to display a continuous trace of respired CO_2, as in Fig. 9.1a, and observe whether the end-tidal tensions are reasonably constant or not. Typical rapid CO_2 meters draw a continuous sample of respired air from a nasal catheter or respiratory mouthpiece at a flow of 20 to 100 ml/minute. Except in expert hands, records from nasal catheters are unreliable as they tend to move in and out of the respired stream unpredictably, so it is usually wiser to put the tip of the sampling catheter perpendicularly into the axis of the respired stream in a mouthpiece, (Fig. 9. lb). This is easily done in adults and children but is not reliable in infants in whom respired flows often fall below the flow demanded by the monitor, so that the device draws gas from elsewhere, contaminating the trace. Also, in infants, the respiratory rate may be too fast for the monitor to respond to, so it will fail to see end-tidal values correctly. In most people, end-tidal $P\text{co}_2$ values are very close to their alveolar and arterial CO_2 tensions. Even when they are not (see later), their stability is good evidence of a respiratory steady state.

With infants, or with slow CO_2 monitors, it is better to use the technique shown in Fig. 9.2. The patient breathes though a mouthpiece, cuffed endotracheal tube, oronasal mask, or ventilated head-box so that all expired air can be collected and ducted through a mixing box. The CO_2 monitor senses the outflow from the box, recording the mixed expired-CO_2 tension continuously. If the patient is at rest and that tension is constant, they are almost certainly in a respiratory steady state. It is a small step from here to the formal measurement of respiratory gas exchange. In the remainder of this chapter, we will go through methods of determining oxygen uptake and CO_2 excretion and then discuss other respiratory techniques that provide information of cardiological value.

MEASURING GAS EXHANGE CORRECTLY

Classically, respiratory gas exchange is measured by collecting all of the expired air while the patient is breathing freely from room air. To do this, expirate is collected for a period of 2 or 3 minutes, so that its composition will not be biased too much by incomplete fractions of the first and last breaths. The collection is made while the patient is demonstrably in a steady state, so that it's composition will not be disturbed by changes in body gas stores. The expirate is usually collected in large 'Douglas' bags that are then pummeled about to ensure good mixing, before the oxygen and CO_2 concentrations of the mixture are determined by suitable analysers. Then the volume of the mixture is measured by slow passage through a wet or dry gas meter. At the end of this procedure, the investigator has nine pieces of information:

1 The patient was inspiring air.
2 The patient was in a respiratory steady state.
3 The collection time was t minutes.
4 The volume of expirate was $\dot{V}\text{E}$ (lATPS).

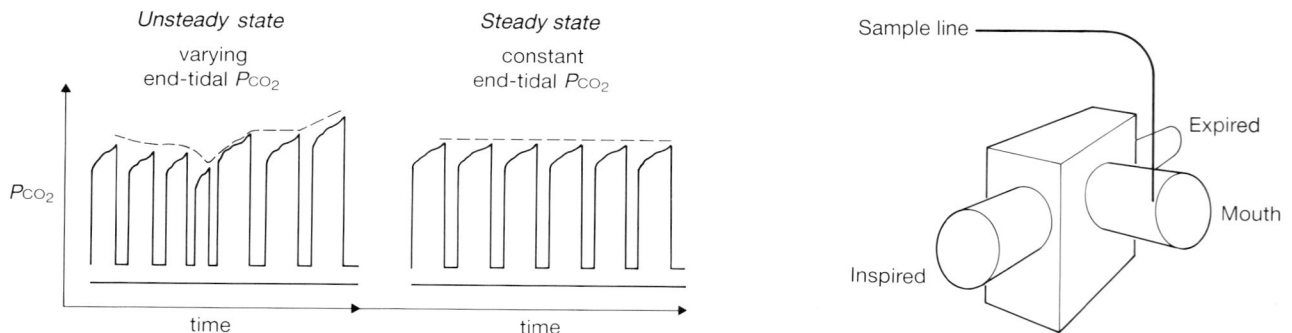

Fig. 9.1 (a) The two traces at the top of the figure contrast respired CO_2 tensions in unsteady and steady respiratory states. In a steady state the end-expiratory (i.e. end-tidal) tensions are constant. (b) To obtain reliable records of respired gas tensions, the sampling probe of the gas analyser should be plumb in the middle of the respired streams. Several phenomena distort the trace if samples are drawn too close to walls or junctions in gas piping.

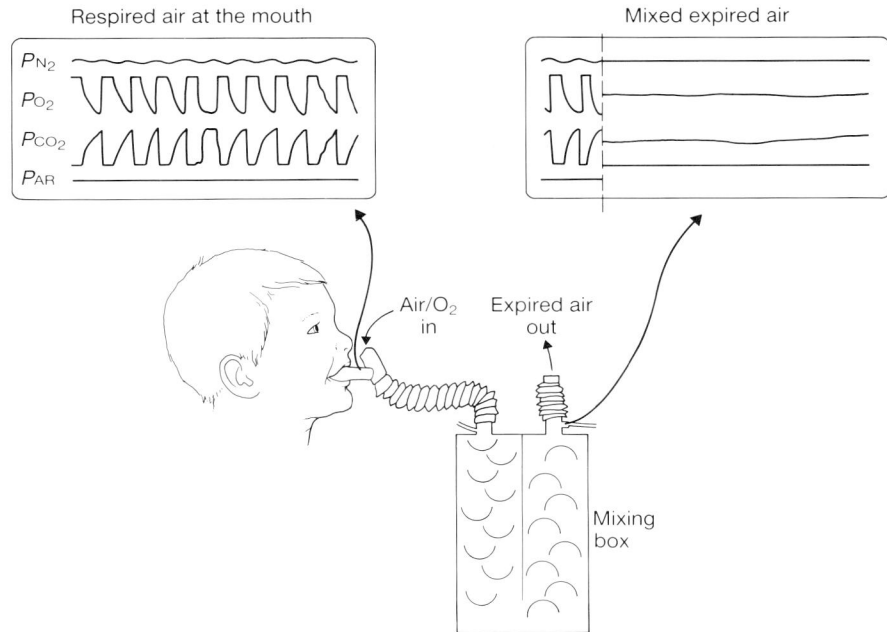

Fig. 9.2 An example of the use of a mixing box to obtain mean expired gas tensions, which can be detectd accurately by relatively slow gas analysers. The panel at the upper left of the figure shows the rapidly changing trace recorded at the mouthpiece as in Fig. 9.1b. The panel at the top right of the figure shows how these rapid changes are smoothed out, and effectively slowed down, by the simple mixing box illustrated in Fig. 9.3.

5 The CO_2 expired/minute was $FEco_2*\dot{V}E/t$ (1 ATPS/minute).

6 The O_2 expired/minute $FEo_2*\dot{V}E/t$ (1ATPS/minute).

7 The ambient pressure was PB mmHg.

8 The ambient temperature was T°C.

9 The saturated water vapour pressure at T°C is W mmHg*.

Firstly it is argued that, for practical purposes, inspired air contains no CO_2, therefore all of the CO_2 in the expirate has come from the patient, so his metabolic CO_2 production ($\dot{V}co_2$) can be calculated, for example in litres STPD i.e. of dry gas at standard temperature (0°C) and pressure (760 mmHg):

$$\dot{V}co_2 = (FEco_2*\dot{V}E/t)*((PB-W)/760)*(273+T))/273$$
$$(1STPD/minute).$$

Next it is argued that, since the patient was in steady state his body nitrogen stores will not have changed, therefore the nitrogen he expired must equal the amount of nitrogen he breathed in over the same period. This allows us to work out how much oxygen he must have breathed in ($\dot{V}_io_2$). Once that is known we can subtract how much he breathed out, to discover how much the he has consumed. These calculations, all in l/minute STPD, are done as follows:

$$\dot{V}En_2 = ((PB - (W + PEo_2 + PEco_2))/760)*(\dot{V}E/t)*$$
$$(273+T)/273$$

$$\dot{V}_io_2 = (0.2093/0.7907)*\dot{V}En_2$$
$$\dot{V}o_2 = \dot{V}_io_2 - \dot{V}Eo_2.$$

Many variants of these formulae can be found, dependent on how many factors have been cancelled out, and the order in which sums have been done, but they should transpose into the ones shown. Corresponding calculations can be done when the inspirate is not air, providing its composition is known accurately. Usually it is slow and impractical to perform classical Douglas bag collections in the catheter laboratory, so other more compact procedures are used instead. It is important to note that any retreat from the classical method involves assumptions that may reduce accuracy, but satisfactory alternatives do exist.

Many laboratories avoid the problems of gas collection, by assuming a resting gas consumption. There is abundant evidence that this is unwise, particularly if the patients are children, [1−6]. Some investigators estimate gas exchange by multiplying the outputs of a polarographic oxygen electrode and a rapidly responding gas flow meter (pneumotachograph). Unfortunately small zero drifts in the latter,

Abbreviations: VE expired volume in litres at ambient pressure and temperature, saturated with water vapour (= 1 ATPS). FEo_2 and $FEco_2$ are the fractional expired concentrations of those gases (range 0 to 1.0).

and differences in time delays between the Po_2 and flow signals, can introduce substantial errors that are difficult to spot. For these reasons we prefer the technique described below, which can also serve several laboratories simultaneously.

The method depends upon a rapidly responding continous gas analyser, the respiratory mass spectrometer, which samples gas through a fine polythene catheter that can be up to 30 metres long [7]. This allows the analyser to be placed outside the catheter room, leaving the investigator unhindered. Continuous data on the patients steady state and metabolic gas exchange, derived from the spectrometer, can be superimposed on the laboratory angiography screen or some other convenient display, at will.

Respiratory mass spectrometers are instruments about the size of domestic washing machines, that draw in a flow of gas of about 20 ml per minute, take a very small fraction of that and subject it to a very hard vacuum (10^{-7} mmHg), ionise it with an electron beam, and then throw the ionised gas particles into an electromagnetic field, where they follow curved trajectories specific to their masses, falling to ground at various points on an electrically scanned landing strip. By measuring how much charge falls where, the composition of the gas can be determined rapidly and accurately. A typical device can follow the concentrations of up to eight components of a gas mixture 'continuously', updating information on each every 25 msec, with an overall 90% response

time of 100 msec and an accuracy of $\pm$ 1 mmHg. This versatility allows it to measure respired volumes as well as composition. To do this, the patient's expirate is ducted through a mixing box strapped to the head of the catheter table, (Fig. 9.3a). Immediately upstream of the box, a fixed flow (about 100 ml per minute) of argon is injected into the expirate via another 30 metre fine polythene catheter. The argon and the expirate mix in the box, and the spectrometer samples the well-stirred expirate that

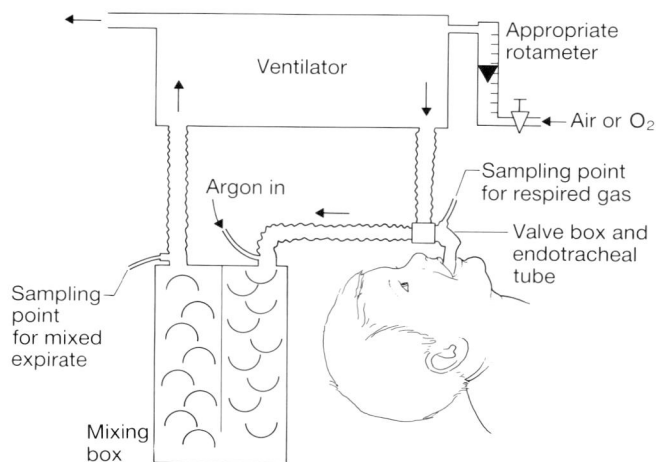

Fig. 9.3 (a) A sketch of the set-up used in artificially-ventilated children. A constant low flow of argon is injected into the expiratory airstream immediately proximal to a mixing box. The argon content of the mixture leaving the box gives an accurate measure of respired flow.

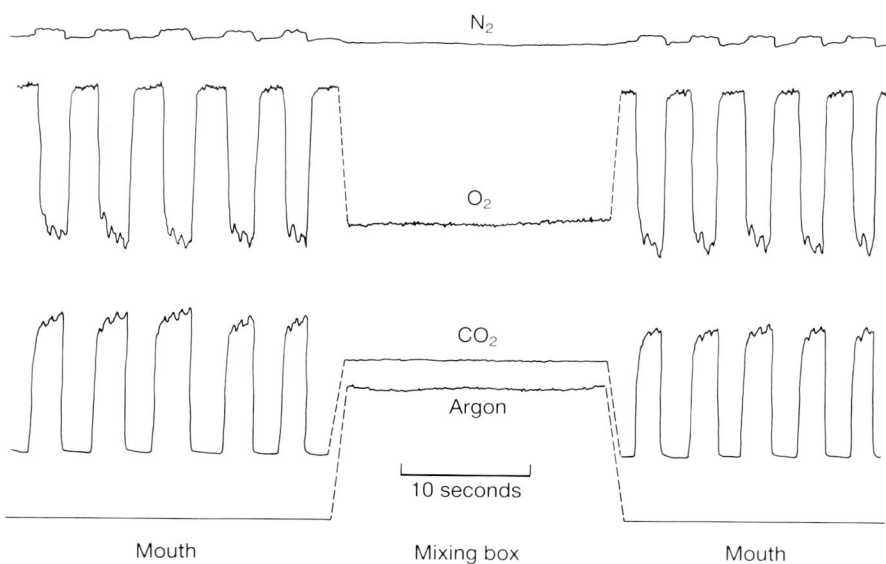

(b) A typical trace of respired nitrogen, oxygen carbon dioxide and argon tensions, during steady state respiration, as seen at the mouth, downstream of the mixing box, and at the mouth again. Tensions were measured by respiratory mass spectrometry.

emerges (Fig. 9.3b). The argon content of the mixture betrays the total gas flow (since the inflow of additional argon is known), and the exchange of oxygen and CO_2 can be calculated as before, by mass spectrometry alone, [8]. This system only requires two polythene tubes and a mixing box, in the laboratory. Evidence of its accuracy is shown in Fig. 9.4.

There are several other respiratory techniques that can sometimes be of help in cardiology. These are discussed below.

OXYGEN AS A TEST OF 'REVERSIBILITY'

The precapillary vessels of the healthy lung are under a small degree of resting tone, which can be slightly reduced by the administration of oxygen. When a segment of lung becomes hypoxic, blood is diverted elsewhere, supposedly by 'hypoxic vasoconstriction'. When the hypoxia is widespread, whether from a gaseous or circulatory cause, the resistance to flow is generalised and pulmonary arterial pressure rises. If in these circumstances or in the presence of some other reason for pulmonary hypertension, oxygen is administered, the pulmonary vascular resistance may go down substantially. If so, the pulmonary vascular component of the disorder is said to be reversible, which may be a good prognostic sign. Thus it is common practice to give oxygen to patients with pulmonary hypertension to discover whether this is so. The aim of the test is to measure the patient's pulmonary vascular resistance while breathing air, switch them to breathe oxygen, ensure the oxygenation is as complete as possible, and measure vascular resistance again. This implies some test of the completeness of oxygenation, and two measurements of pulmonary pressure and pulmonary flow.

It is not sufficient to measure pulmonary arterial pressure and see whether it falls. In many situations oxygenation leads to a rise in pulmonary blood flow rather than a fall in pulmonary arterial pressure, therefore flow has to be measured and vascular resistance calculated [5, 9]. Usually 'reversibility' is assessed by a brief exposure to oxygen (10 minutes or less). However recent experience suggests pulmonary hypertension, due to congenital cardiac defects in children or chronic lung disease in adults, can be reduced by exposure to domiciliary oxygen over several weeks or months [10, 11]. The prognostic and therapeutic implications of this finding are not yet clear.

We assess oxygen-induced reversibility, taking particular care that the patient is in a well-established respiratory steady state. Then we measure oxygen consumption while the patient breathes air, using the mass spectrometric technique described earlier. Slowly drawn samples of pulmonary and systemic arterial blood are taken simultaneously. The pulmonary arterial and wedge pressures are noted immediately before and after. The patient is then switched to breathing oxygen for 5–10 minutes, without disturbing the respiratory steady state. Then metabolic gas exchange, blood samples and vascular pressures are noted again. As there is no nitrogen in the expirate the volume of oxygen inspired during the second collection cannot

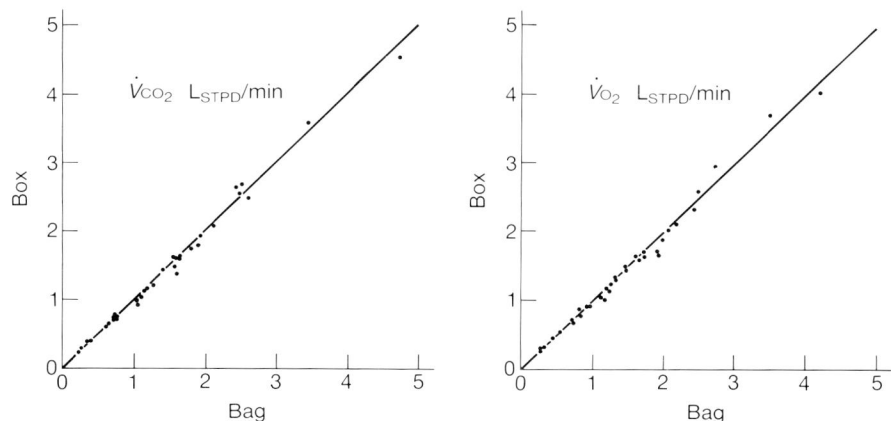

Fig. 9.4 Comparisons of measurements of respiratory gas exchange made by the argon dilution (box) technique and classical Douglas bag collections in various subjects ranging from a resting infant to an Olympic athlete exercising maximally (litre STPD; V_{O_2}).

be calculated. However, if the respiratory steady state has been preserved it is reasonable to assume that the relation of $\dot{V}co_2$ to $\dot{V}o_2$, is unchanged, therefore $\dot{V}o_2$ can be calculated from $\dot{V}co_2$, using the $\dot{V}co_2/\dot{V}o_2$ ratio of the air-breathing period studied immediately before. This can only be justified if the end-tidal CO_2 tensions are constant throughout both periods.

The test supposes that oxygen reaches the part of the pulmonary vascular bed causing some of the hypertension. This is not easy to check. If a substantial part of the bed is very constricted, almost all of the flow will be going through the remainder of the bed, which may not have a particularly high tone. Nevertheless, because the flow through the remainder is disproportional, its upstream pressure will be high, and it will dominate measurements of resistance. Similarly, a high oxygen pressure in pulmonary venous blood is poor evidence that the majority of vessels in its drainage are well oxygenated, because flow through the most constricted part of the bed will be small, leaving little mark on the venous mixture downstream. A steady high oxygen pressure in expired air implies that oxygen has been thoroughly washed into the well-ventilated parts of the lung. It can say little about the oxygen content of vessels in poorly ventilated spaces. In addition, two recent papers [12, 13] suggest that a substantial part of the hypoxic pressor response in the lungs is due to a change in red cell deformability, rather than alterations in the vessel walls. Therefore, for all these reasons, the results of oxygenation tests must be interpreted cautiously. In principle, if a fall in vascular resistance occurs it is significant, but the absence of a fall may simply be due to failure of oxygen to reach the vessels concerned.

OXYGENATION TO MEASURE ANATOMIC SHUNT

As haemoglobin is normally fully saturated at oxygen tensions above 100 mmHg, it is supposed that if the lung is ventilated with 100% O_2 this will completely oxygenate any blood within sight of alveoli, thus any desaturation in systemic arterial blood must be due to some right-to-left shunt that has bypassed the lungs entirely. If that is so, and the oxygen

content of pulmonary artery blood can be measured, then the shunt fraction (Q_s/Q_{tot}) can be calculated as described in Chapter 11. To do this, the patient breathes 100% oxygen through a mouthpiece or endotracheal tube, for 10 minutes, which ensures that almost every ventilated alveolus has an oxygen tension above 100 mmHg. At the end of that time, while still breathing oxygen, a reliable sample of systemic arterial blood is drawn, and its oxygen tension is measured. Where possible, a sample of mixed venous (ideally pulmonary arterial) blood is also drawn and analysed. Otherwise, some value for its oxygen content is assumed. Again, where possible, the haemoglobin content of the samples is measured; otherwise, that too is assumed. The anatomical shunt is then calculated, as described in Chapter 11.

It is important to note that assumptions of haemoglobin content, mixed venous and systemic venous blood compositions, and haemoglobin dissociation characteristics are most likely to be wrong in patients with cardiac and vascular abnormalities, i.e. in those where shunt measurements are most needed. As a rough guide, in a patient at rest with a normal cardiac output, each 1% shunt flow will drop systemic arterial Po_2 by 20 mmHg. If the cardiac output at rest is high, the drop will be less. If the cardiac output is low, or metabolic rate is increased, it will be greater. Thus if, in any patient, there is no evidence of a high-output state and the systemic arterial Po_2 is above 500 mmHg, it is reasonable to calculate the shunt from an arterial blood sample alone. Otherwise, it is wiser to measure all of the variables necessary. In healthy people anatomical shunt flow, measured in this way, is approximately 5%. When it is found to be significantly greater (say, above 7.5%), the results must be interpreted with caution. Undoubtedly, they represent an abnormal finding, but they may still be in error because breathing oxygen reduces the resistance of the pulmonary vascular bed, particularly in patients with hypoxic pulmonary arterial blood. Therefore, the procedure is likely to underestimate the shunt that exists when breathing air. To determine this it is better to collect pulmonary and systemic arterial blood samples, measure or assume a respiratory exchange ratio (R, which equals $\dot{V}co_2/\dot{V}o_2$), and use the alveolar air equation (Fig. 9.5) to estimate pulmonary venous Po_2, when the patient is actually breathing air (see Chapters 6 and 11 for further details).

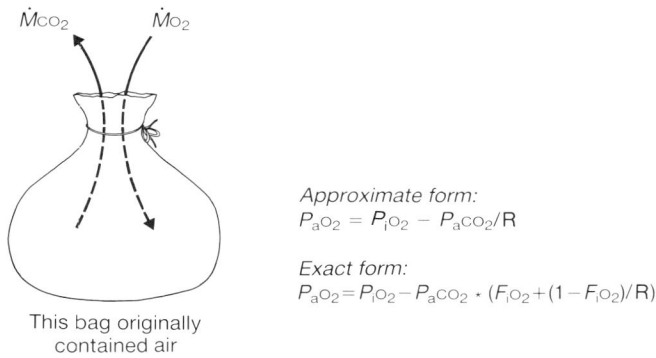

Approximate form:
$$P_aO_2 = P_iO_2 - P_aCO_2/R$$

Exact form:
$$P_aO_2 = P_iO_2 - P_aCO_2 \cdot (F_iO_2 + (1 - F_iO_2)/R)$$

This bag originally contained air

Fig. 9.5 The alveolar air equation is based on a simple idea, namely that you can treat expired air as if it has always been contained in a floppy bag. As oxygen is removed the bag gets smaller and its oxygen tension falls. As CO_2 is added the bag gets bigger and its CO_2 tension rises. The outcome of the two processes depends on the ratio (R) of CO_2 output to oxygen uptake. (See text for further details).

SOLUBLE GAS MEASUREMENTS OF EFFECTIVE PULMONARY BLOOD FLOW

All gases entering the lung are subject to the same physicochemical rules summarised in Fig. 9.6a, and are taken up by passing blood in a roughly exponential way, at a rate proportional to blood flow and their solubility in blood. For the great majority of gases, equilibration between capillary blood and alveolar gas is complete. Therefore if a novel gas such as acetylene, nitrous oxide or Freon 22 is introduced in the lung, the blood flow removing it can be measured non-invasively by observing the falling alveolar tension during a single breath or rebreathing manoeuvre (Fig. 9.6b). Such measures have a long history, dating from Humphrey Davy in 1802, and in experienced hands give highly reproducible results that allow blood flow to be monitored easily and painlessly between invasive studies [14]. They can be used at rest and during exercise, and can also be recorded from subdivisions of the lung during fibre-optic bronchoscopy [15, 16] (Fig. 9.6c). They do not measure cardiac output. They measure that part of cardiac output which is effective in exchanging gas in the lung, (effective pulmonary blood flow). In patients who do not have significant lung disease, they measure cardiac output minus anatomical shunt. In patients with lung disease they measure the fraction of non-shunt flow that is active in gas exchange.

These measurements are easy to make, and are highly reliable providing they are done with care. We use a single-breath technique in adults, and a rebreathing method in children. Both can also be done on anaesthetised patients, whether they are on or off a ventilator. In the single-breath technique, the patient expires to residual volume, sharply inspires test gas to total lung capacity, breath-holds for a couple of seconds and then breathes out slowly and evenly back to residual volume. The test gas is oxygen-enriched air marked with low concentrations of an insoluble gas (helium or argon) and one of the soluble gases mentioned previously. We prefer Freon 22 because it is easily measured by respiratory mass spectrometry. The exponential fall in expired soluble gas tension is recorded together with the initial fall in insoluble gas tension. Blood flow is derived simply and rapidly from the two traces [17]. The measurement can be performed every 3 or so minutes and becomes repeatable after the second exposure. Children under 8 years old have difficulty performing this manoeuvre reproducibly, but easily manage a rebreathing procedure [11, 18]. For this they expire to residual volume and are turned to rebreathe the test gas from an balloon for 5 to 20 seconds. The traces are treated as before.

CARBON MONOXIDE TRANSFER AND PULMONARY CAPILLARY BLOOD VOLUME

At rest, a red cell takes about 1 second to traverse a pulmonary capillary. During this passage, inert gases such as nitrogen, helium and argon, that are equally soluble in blood and water, only require one-fortieth of a second for complete equilibration. Oxygen and carbon dioxide, which are substantially more soluble in blood than water, need about one-third of a second. Carbon monoxide is many times more soluble in blood than water, and so requires much longer. Consequently its uptake is limited by diffusion rather than blood flow. For a long time it was thought that there were two roughly equal obstacles it had to traverse (the alveolar membrane and the red cell interior). Nowadays the resistance of the alveolar membrane is regarded as less important [19], and so for practical purposes, the uptake of carbon monoxide has become a measure of the ac-

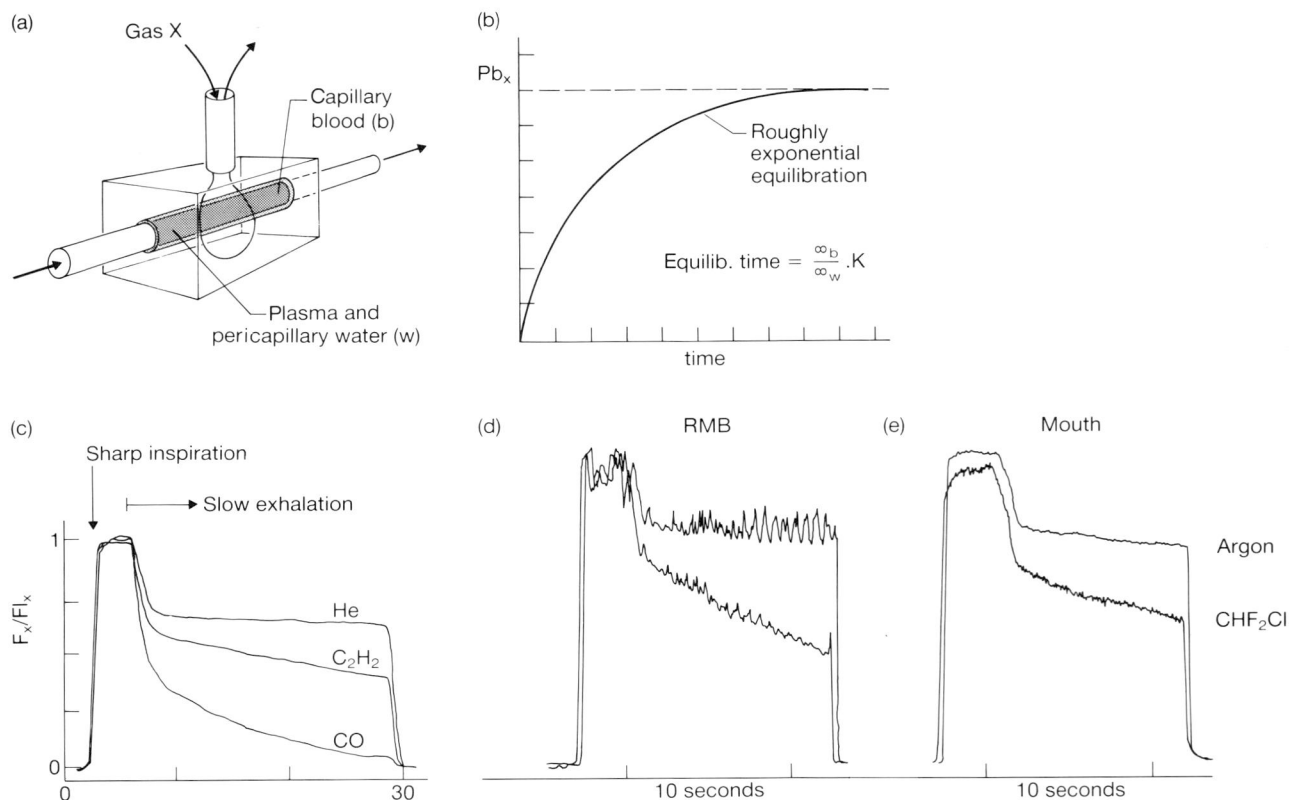

Fig. 9.6 (a) The sketch at the top left shows a useful model of inert gas exchange in the lung. A single capillary traverses the alveolar space. Its red cells are surrounded by plasma and water. Gases have to dissolve in this layer on their way to and from blood. The time constant of their exponential uptake or excretion is set by the ratio of the gas's solubility in blood and water, as indicated in the graph (b) A respiratory mass spectrometry trace (c) of a single slow exhalation of breath marked with low concentrations of very poorly blood-soluble helium, moderately blood-soluble acetylene and very blood-soluble carbon monoxide. (d) Similar traces of a single breath marked with poorly blood-soluble argon and moderately blood-soluble Freon 22, as seen in the right main bronchus (RMB) (d) and at the mouth (e), during fibre-optic bronchoscopy. The oscillations in the endobronchial trace are caused by the massaging action of the heart on adjacent well-perfused lungs. The difference between the helium and Freon 22 traces is a measure of effective total or regional blood flow.

cessible haemoglobin content of the lung, or effective pulmonary capillary blood volume. In people who do not have *obstructive* airways disease it measures total pulmonary capillary blood volume. In those with airway obstruction it only sees those capillaries active in gas exchange. It is a very easy measurement to make, and can be used to predict how much arterial desaturation can be attributed to capillary damage in the lung [20].

This test is very similar to the previous one. There are single-breath and rebreathing versions, and the single-breath version is practised in many hospitals. The patient expires to residual volume, rapidly inhales a vital capacity of test gas, breath-holds for exactly 10 seconds, and then sharply exhales to residual volume. Concentrations of an insoluble

marker (helium) and carbon monoxide are compared, and the whole lung carbon monoxide transfer factor (TLCO) obtained directly. The degree of dilution of helium measures the accessible lung volume (VA) and the ratio TLCO/VA measures carbon monoxide uptake per litre of accessible gas volume (KCO). The latter can be taken as the pulmonary capillary blood volume per litre of useable lung. Some children, and adults who are very breathless, cannot manage the 10-second breath-hold and are asked to do a rebreathing procedure instead. Both forms of the test can also be done on subdivisions of the lung during fibre-optic bronchoscopy and can also be combined with measurements of metabolic gas exchange and effective blood flow, (as in Fig. 9.6b), in a single manoeuvre [21].

CHARACTERISING THE LUNG BY INERT GAS ELIMINATION

In healthy people there are several-fold variations of blood flow and ventilation between alveoli at the top and the bottom of the lung. Weak bronchial and stronger vascular reflexes minimise random variations of the two to preserve an approximately $1:1$ ratio of blood flow to gas flow in each small unit of lung (ventilation/perfusion matching). This is necessary for efficient gas exchange. If matching is disturbed by vascular or airway disease, equilibration of gas overall becomes inefficient although it is complete in each alveolus; so pulmonary venous Po_2 falls. This condition, of ventilation/perfusion inequality, is the commonest respiratory cause of central cyanosis. Sometimes, in patients with combined heart and lung disease, it is necessary to know the pulmonary contribution. The best test for predicting the mismatch component is the multiple inert gas elimination technique ('MIDGET') developed by Wagner and West [22, 23]. Saline saturated with six inert gases of widely different gas/water partition coefficients, is infused into a vein, and the elimination of each gas in the lung and the retention of each in arterial blood is noted, by gas chromatography. The data is then subjected to a formidable but well-tested mathematical transformation which produces a statistical description of the distribution of ventilation/perfusion ratios throughout the lung. The fall in Po_2 in pulmonary venous blood due to mismatch can be predicted from this distribution.

This test can now be run on a personal computer, but does need gas chromatographic and equilibration apparatus that are not usually available. It has proved to be a very valuable research and assessment tool, and has been insufficiently applied to the problems of assessing combined heart and lung disease in cardiology.

SUMMARY

Modern analysers allow respiratory gas exchange to be measured accurately and unobtrusively in the cardiac catheter laboratory. The measurements are not worth interpreting unless the patient is in a cardiorespiratory steady state and associated blood samples are drawn slowly and simultaneously. If these conditions are met, it is possible to obtain precise and reliable measures of cardiac output, right-to-left shunt, effective pulmonary blood flow, and effective pulmonary capillary blood volume. It is also possible to measure the drop in pulmonary vascular resistance on oxygen administration. If this occurs it implies the pulmonary vascular component of the disorder is reversible. If it does not occur, it may simply be because the oxygen did not reach its target.

REFERENCES

1 Baum D, Brown AC, Church SC. Effect of sedation on oxygen consumption of children undergoing cardiac catheterisation. *Pediatrics* 1967;**39**:891−5.

2 Owen-Thomas JB, Meade F, Jones RS, Jackson-Rees G. The measurement of oxygen uptake in infants with congenital disease of the heart during general anaesthesia and intermittant positive pressure ventilation. *Br J Anaesth* 1971;**43**:746−52.

3 Kappagoda CT, Greenwood P, Macartney FJ, Linden RJ. Oxygen consumption in children with congenital diseases of the heart. *Clin Sci Mol Med* 1973;**45**:107−14.

4 Fixler DE, Carrell T, Browne R, Willis K, Miller WW. Oxygen consumption in children during cardiac catheterisation under different sedation routines. *Circulation* 1974;**50**:788−94.

5 Davies NJH, Shinebourne EA, Scallan MJ, Sopwith TA, Denison DM. Pulmonary vascular resistance in children with congenital heart disease. *Thorax* 1984;**39**:895−900.

6 Kendrick AH, West J, Papouchado M, Rozcovec A. Direct Fick cardiac output: Are assumed values of oxygen consumption acceptable? *Eur Heart J* 1988;**9**:337−42.

7 Davies NJH, Denison DM. The use of long probes in respiratory mass spectrometry. *Respir Physiol* 1979;**37**:335−46.

8 Davies NJH, Denison DM. The measurement of metabolic gas exchange and minute volume by mass spectrometry alone. *Respir Physiol* 1979;**36**:261−7.

9 Honey M, Cotter L, Davies NJH, Denison DM. Clinical and haemodynamic effects of diazoxide in primary pulmonary hypertension. *Thorax* 1980;**35**:269−76.

10 Timms RM, Khaja FU, Williams GW and the Nocturnal Oxygen Therapy Trial Group. Hemodynamic response to oxygen therapy in chronic obstructive pulmonary disease. *Ann Int Med* 1985;**102**:29−36.

11 Bowyer JJ, Busst C, Denison DM, Shinebourne EA. Effect of long term oxygen treatment at home in children with pulmonary vascular disease. *Br Heart J* 1986;**55**:385−90.

12 Hakim TS, Malik AB. Hypoxic vasoconstriction in blood and plasma perfused lungs. *Respir Physiol* 1988; **72**:109−122.

13 Hakim TS, Macek AS. Role of erythrocyte deformability in the acute hypoxic pressor response in the pulmonary vasculature. *Respir Physiol* 1988;**72**:95−108.

14 Sackner MA. Measurement of cardiac output by alveolar gas exchange. In: Farhi LE, Tenney SM (eds) *Handbook of physiology*. Section 3, Vol 4 'Gas exchange'. American Physiological Society. Bethesda Ma, 1987; 233−55.

15 Denison DM, Davies NJH, Meyer M, Pierce RJ, Scheid P. Single exhalation method for study of lobar and segmental lung function by mass spectrometry in man. *Respir Physiol* 1980;**42**:87−99.

16 Denison DM, Waller JF. Studies of regional lung function by mass spectrometry. *Prog Resp Res* 1981; **16**:232−40.

17 Denison DM, Waller JF. Interpreting the results of regional single-breath studies from the patient's point of view. *Bull Eur Physiopathol Respir* 1982;**18**: 339−51.

18 Bowyer JJ, Warner JO, Denison DM. Effective pulmonary blood flow in normal children at rest. *Thorax* 1988. (In press).

19 Forster RE. Diffusion of gases across the alveolar membrane. In: Farhi LE, Tenney SM (eds) *Handbook of physiology*. Section 3, Vol. 4 'Gas exchange'. American Physiological Society, Bethesda Ma, 1987; 77−88.

20 Denison DM, Al-Hillawi H, Turton C. Lung function in interstitial lung disease. *Semin Respir Med* 1984;**6**:40−54.

21 Bush A, Busst CM, Johnson S, Denison DM. Rebreathing method for the simultaneous measurement of oxygen consumption and effective pulmonary blood flow during exercise. *Thorax* 1988;**43**: 268−75.

22 Wagner PD, Saltzman HA, West JB. Measurement of continuous distributions of ventilation-perfusion ratios: theory. *J Appl Physiol* 1974;**36**:588−99.

23 Wagner PD, Naumann PF, Laravuso RB. Simultaneous measurement of eight foreign gases in blood by gas chromatography. *J Appl Physiol* 1974;**36**:600−5.

CHAPTER 10

Diagnostic applications of indicator dilution techniques

An indicator dilution curve is a time/concentration curve; a plot in which the vertical axis records the concentration of indicator at the sampling site (mg/l) and the horizontal axis represents time (in seconds). Such curves are obtained when a suitable indicator (indocyanine green or cold saline) is injected into the circulation and detected downstream by some device — a densitometer in the case of indocyanine green, a thermistor when the indicator is cold saline. Where dye is used as an indicator it must be non-toxic and its detection must not be influenced by the relative amounts of oxy- and reduced haemoglobin in the blood at the sampling site. Indocyanine green is rapidly removed from the circulation but is still present during recirculation and background dye causes a base-line shift if several curves are performed. The presence of recirculating indicator can help in providing diagnostic information but is troublesome when the indicator dilution technique is used to estimate cardiac output. Cold (saline) has the advantage that it 'disappears' during passage through the body (by being warmed) and is the indicator of choice for cardiac output determination.

A typical indicator dilution curve has a number of components (Fig. 10.1):

1 Appearance time (*ta*). The time taken for the fastest travelling particles of indicator to reach the sampling site from the point of injection, i.e. until the beginning of the initial deflection.

2 The build-up phase from the beginning of the initial deflection to its peak concentration (*Cp*). The time this takes is the 'build-up time' (*tb*).

3 The disappearance phase which is an exponential decay in concentration until interrupted by the fastest travelling particles which have reappeared at the sampling site as a result of recirculation.

4 There may be one or more recirculation (reappearance) curves which become progessively reduced in amplitude and spread out in duration as indicator is dispersed in the circulation.

Indicator dilution techniques have found many applications in the past and some are still of use in the catheterisation laboratory. Those that will be discussed here are:

1 Determination of cardiac output.

2 Detection and quantitation of left-to-right intracardiac shunts.

3 Detection and quantitation of right-to-left shunts.

4 Detection and quantitation of valve regurgitation.

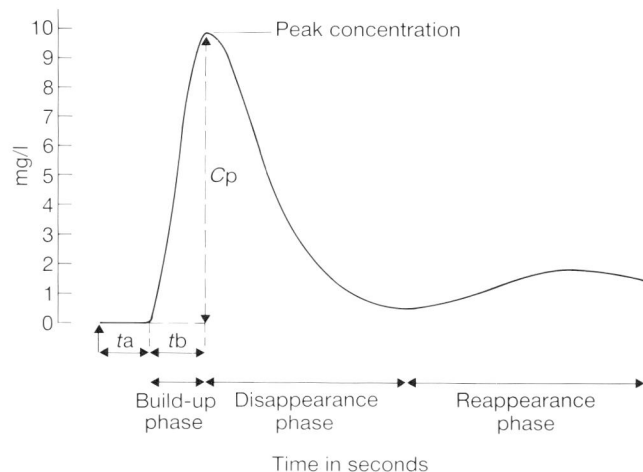

Fig. 10.1 A typical indicator dilution curve.

DETERMINATION OF CARDIAC OUTPUT BY INDICATOR DILUTION

Indocyanine green: Stewart–Hamilton method [1]

If a known quantity of indicator, I, is injected into the blood stream and the mean concentration (c) of indicator in downstream blood estimated until, at time t, the concentration is zero then the amount of blood (Q) which has mixed with indicator is given by:

$$Q = I/ct$$

Since cardiac output is expressed in l/minute and indicator concentration was measured in mg/l while time was recorded in seconds the cardiac output (CO) will be:

$$CO = I \times 60/ct$$

The product, ct, is the area under the primary curve — excluding recirculation. Unfortunately the disappearance phase will be interrupted by recirculating indicator so that we cannot directly measure concentration over the whole length of the disappearance phase. However since the disappearance phase of the primary curve should be exponential we can make use of a trick to estimate what the curve would have been if not interrupted by recirculating indicator [2].

The trick is to plot the disappearance phase on semi-logarithmic paper (vertical axis logarithmic for plotting concentration, horizontal axis linear for plotting time) on which an exponential decay will produce a straight line. It is then easy to see the point at which the straight line is broken by recirculation and to extrapolate the straight line to zero concentration (in practice to 1% of peak concentration). The steps involved are:

1 Measure the height of the curve in centimetres at 1 second intervals from the beginning of the curve to the lowest point of the disappearance phase.
2 Convert centimetre deflection into concentration of dye in mg/l from previous calibration of the densitometer.
3 Plot the descending limb of the curve (in mg/l) on semi-logarithmic paper.
4 Draw a straight line including the earliest part of the descending limb and extrapolate to zero past the point at which the plot breaks from the straight line (this point is te — the point of extrapolation).

5 After te recalculate values for dye concentration by reading values from the straight line plot down to 1% of peak concentration.
6 Add all the values for concentration from the start of the curve to te, plus the values obtained from the extrapolated curve after te.
7 Divide the amount of dye injected (mg) $\times$ 60 by the sum obtained in step (6) to give the cardiac output in l/minute.

Indocyanine green: forward triangle method [3]

There are simpler methods of calculating cardiac output from curves obtained using indocyanine green; they can be used when intracardiac shunts or valve regurgitation so distort the disappearance phase that the primary curve cannot be separated by semi-logarithmic plotting. These methods depend on the fact that dilution curves show a degree of consistency of contour which allows prediction of one part of the curve from another. In the forward triangle method the initial part of the curve (if undistorted by a right-to-left shunt) is used to predict what the total curve would have been if undistorted — and therefore to obtain a measure of cardiac output (Fig. 10.2):

$$CO \text{ (l/min)} = \frac{60 \times I}{0.5 \times tb \times Cp} \times 0.37$$

where I is the amount of dye injected in mg, tb is the build-up time in seconds and Cp is the peak concentration in mg/l, and 0.37 is an empirical constant.

Classically indocyanine green indicator dilution curves for calculation of cardiac output are performed

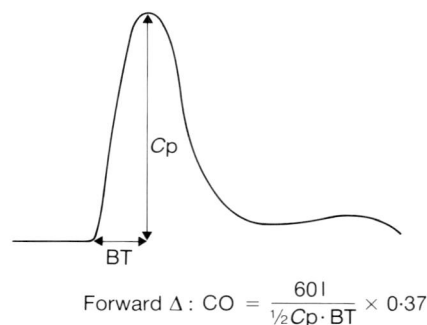

Forward Δ : $CO = \dfrac{60I}{\frac{1}{2}Cp \cdot BT} \times 0.37$

Fig. 10.2 Calculation of cardiac output by the 'forward triangle' method.

with injection into the right heart. It is possible to obtain reasonably accurate curves if the injection is made into the left ventricle (sampling in a systemic artery) thus obviating the need for right heart catheterisation for this purpose [4, 5].

Thermodilution technique [6, 7]

Indocyanine green is not the ideal indicator for measuring cardiac output; apart from the cost of the dye and the need to sample from an arterial puncture the chief drawback is the unavoidable presence of recirculating indicator. As we have seen recirculating indicator distorts the disappearance phase of the primary curve necessitating semi-logarithmic plotting and extrapolation in order to display the primary curve. Thus the ideal indicator is one which is lost from the circulation after inscription of the primary curve. This is precisely what happens if cold saline or dextrose is injected into the right atrium — the cold indicator solution is warmed during passage through the systemic circulation and there is no recirculation curve. This allows simple computer calculation of the area under the primary curve without the need for extrapolation and recalculation and is the basis of the widely used thermodilution technique for measuring cardiac output. In order to calculate cardiac output by this technique we need to know the amount of indicator injected — just as we did when indocyanine green was the indicator. Here the indicator is 'cold' and the amount of 'cold' given supplies the numerator, I, in the basic formula:

$$CO = I/ct$$

In practice commercially available thermodilution cardiac output computers are used; a thermistor in the injectate and another at the catheter tip (positioned in the pulmonary artery) continuously record the temperature of the injectate and the blood. The area under the curve is integrated by the computer and the actual performance of the determination merely requires a constant to be dialed in followed by the rapid injection of a suitable volume of indicator — usually 10 cc of ice-cold 5% dextrose. Multilumen catheters are used which have an injection port 30 cm from the catheter tip (for adult use) so that the cold dextrose is injected in the right atrium. There is an additional lumen to the catheter tip for recording pressure and the catheter incorpor-

ates a thermistor at the tip and its electrical leads. Several patterns of catheter are available suitable for adult and paediatric use and incorporating other features for specific purposes (Fig. 10.3).

The advantages of the thermodilution technique are:

1 It is almost infinitely (and rapidly) repeatable.
2 It does not require the removal of blood or an indwelling arterial 'needle'.
3 The indicator is harmless and cheap.
4 There is effectively no recirculation of indicator.
The technique is most accurate when the cardiac output is normal or high. When cardiac output is low (<2.5 l/min) there is loss of 'cold' during the slow passage of indicator through the right heart chambers with a resulting tendency for the technique to overestimate cardiac output — by as much as 35%. In general, however, thermodilution estimates of output have an error of less than 10% and agree well with estimates by the Fick method. Accuracy is greatest if ice-cold indicator is used (by immersing syringes of 10 cc 5% dextrose in a basin of crushed ice) but the temperature of the injectate can be anything from 0 to 25°C.

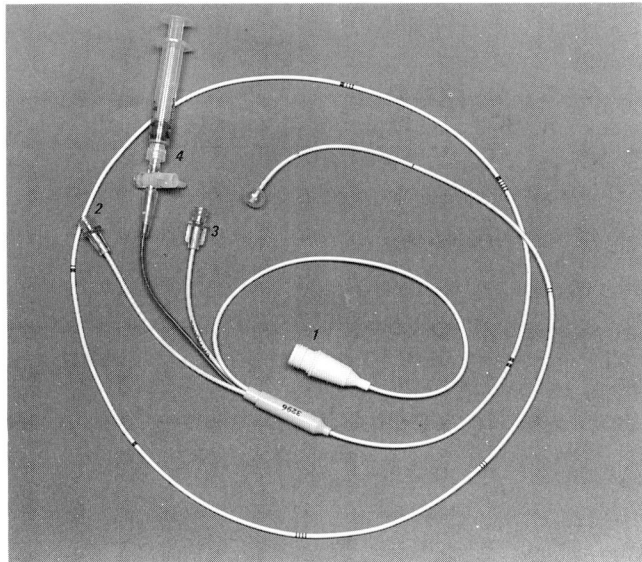

Fig. 10.3 Multi-lumen balloon-tipped thermistor catheter used for determination of cardiac output by thermodilution. (1) Electrical connection to thermistor. (2) Connection to distal lumen — pressure measurement pulmonary artery or wedge pressure). (3) Connection to proximal lumen — pressure measurement (central venous right atrial pressure) and injection of cold indicator. (4) Connection to balloon — inflation/deflation.

Problems (for example, unexplained variations in calculated output) can be minimised by attention to detail: the syringe must be filled to precisely the same volume each time and injections should be made at regular intervals and at the same time in the respiratory cycle. The syringe must not be held by the barrel or the injectate will be warned by the heat of the hand. The proximal (injection) port must be flushed with injectate prior to making the first injection (or the first reading discarded). Very high and erratic readings may be due to the thermistor bead contacting the wall of the pulmonary artery; reposition the catheter in the main pulmonary artery.

DETECTION AND QUANTITATION OF LEFT-TO-RIGHT SHUNTS

Carter formula

When a left-to-right intracardiac shunt is present, a very short pathway is available for indicator to re-enter the pulmonary circulation (bypassing the systemic circulation). As a result recirculating particles will continually appear at the arterial sampling site with resulting distortion and prolongation of the disappearance phase (Fig. 10.4.) The amount by which the disappearance phase is distorted has been used to estimate the percentage left-to-right shunt [8]. This method is illustrated in Fig. 10.4.

$$A = 141 \, [C(p + BT)/Cp] - 42$$
$$B = 135 \, [C(p + 2BT)/Cp] - 14$$
$$\text{Percent L}-\text{R shunt} = A + B/2$$

where Cp is the peak concentration (measured as centimetres deflection), and BT is the build-up time. $C(p + BT)$ and $C(p + 2BT)$ are the concentrations at twice and three times the build-up time respectively.

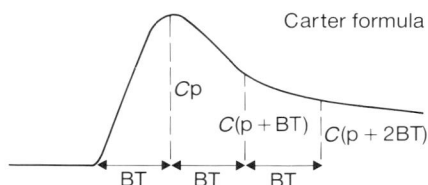

Fig. 10.4 Quantitation of left-to-right intracardiac shunt by the Carter formula.

Central sampling techniques

If indicator is injected into, for example, the distal pulmonary artery, and sampling is from a catheter in the right ventricle then, if there is a ventricular septal defect, indicator will appear in the right ventricle *before* being detected at a peripheral arterial sampling site. If the sampling catheter is now withdrawn to the right atrium and the injection repeated this early appearing dye will no longer be detected. Thus the presence of a left-to-right shunt at ventricular level is established. The permutations on this basic principle are, obviously, numerous. The technique has drawbacks; not only are two catheters required but allowance has to be made for the time that it takes for blood to be withdrawn through the long sampling catheter to the densitometer. We need to know the volume of the blood in the catheter and the rate of withdrawal. Having thus 'calibrated the system' further sampling must be at exactly the same rate. Cine angiography has rendered this type of study obsolete.

DETECTION AND QUANTITATION OF RIGHT-TO-LEFT SHUNTS

The effect of a right-to-left intracardiac shunt is to provide a short pathway whereby particles of indicator injected into the right heart proximal to the shunt may enter the left heart and be detected at an arterial sampling site before the arrival of indicator which has traversed the pulmonary circulation. The effect is to distort the build-up phase of the primary curve producing a small, early curve superimposed on the main curve (Fig. 10.5). The 'forward triangle' method has been applied to quantitate the percent right-to-left shunt by relating the size of the early to the primary curve [9].

$$\triangle'' = Cp'' \times tb''$$
$$\triangle' = Cp' \times tpc' \times 0.44$$
$$\text{Percent R}-\text{L shunt} = \triangle''/\triangle' + \triangle'' \times 100$$

Triangle $\triangle''$ is easily seen to be given by the peak concentration of the early appearing dye (Cp'') and the time (tb'') from the beginning of the deflection to Cp''. While Cp', the peak concentration of the primary curve is easily detected the build-up time of the primary curve cannot be read directly as the beginning of the primary deflection is obscured by the deflection due to early-appearing dye. Thus use is made of the constant relationship which was found (in patients without shunts) between the time from injection of indicator to peak concentration ($t$pc') and the appearance time for the same curve. From these measurements it was possible to calculate the theoretical build-up time of the primary curve as 0.44 $t$pc' and the area of the primary triangle can be calculated Cp'× ($t$pc' × 0.44).

When the right-to-left shunt is small there will not be a clearly defined 'hump' due to early-appearing dye. Instead there will be an indentation on the build-up phase of the primary curve; Cp" and tb" are measured at this indentation. There is no need to convert deflection into mg/l or time into seconds, all measurements can be in centimetres on the recording paper.

If the indicator is injected distal to the site of right-to-left shunting the early curve will no longer be seen at the arterial sampling site. Thus selective injections of indicator at different points in the right heart can serve to localise the site of right-to-left shunting.

It is possible to use such indicator dilution techniques to provide a great deal of diagnostic information in cases of congenital heart disease. Although providing a stimulating intellectual exercise such techniques are time consuming and unlikely to be used today. The same information (and more) is provided by modern, high quality, cine angiocardi-

ography. It is worth pointing out that a cine angiocardiogram is also an indicator dilution technique. When we see contrast appearing early in the left heart following a right heart injection we are seeing early-appearing dye; the indicator is radio-opaque contrast medium and the sampling device is X-ray film and the viewer's eye.

DETECTION AND QUANTITATION OF VALVE REGURGITATION

CL/CR ratio

Valve regurgitation has an effect similar to that of a left-to-right shunt; thus in mitral regurgitation fractions of the dye entering the left ventricle return to the left atrium to reappear later at the downstream sampling site. The result is again distortion and prolongation of the disappearance phase together with a reduction in the peak concentration. The degree of prolongation has been employed as a measure of the severity of mitral regurgitation [10]. The CL/CR ratio is illustrated in Fig. 10.6.

CL is the concentration (measured as centimetres deflection) at the lowest point of the primary curve (least concentration) and CR the concentration at the peak of the recirculation curve. A value for CL/CR greater than 0.65 is said to indicate significant mitral regurgitation and a lower value to exclude significant regurgitation.

Regurgitant index

A 'central sampling technique' can be used to quantitate valve regurgitation. Thus in mitral regurgitation indicator is injected into the left ventricle and sampling is from the left atrium by means of transseptal catheterisation [11]. The relationship between the curve obtained at a downstream sampling site (e.g. femoral artery) and that obtained from the left atrium can be used to provide a regurgitant index. This is illustrated in Fig. 10.7. Triangle A is

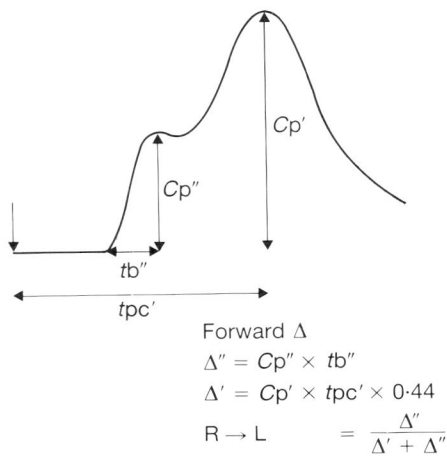

Forward Δ
$$\Delta'' = Cp'' \times tb''$$
$$\Delta' = Cp' \times tpc' \times 0.44$$
$$R \rightarrow L \quad = \frac{\Delta''}{\Delta' + \Delta''}$$

Fig. 10.5 Quantitation of right-to-left shunt by the 'forward triangle' method.

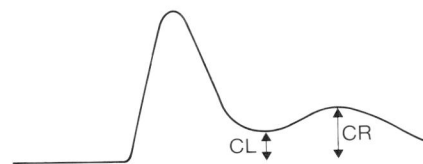

Fig. 10.6 Quantitation of mitral regurgitation by indicator dilution — CL/CR ratio.

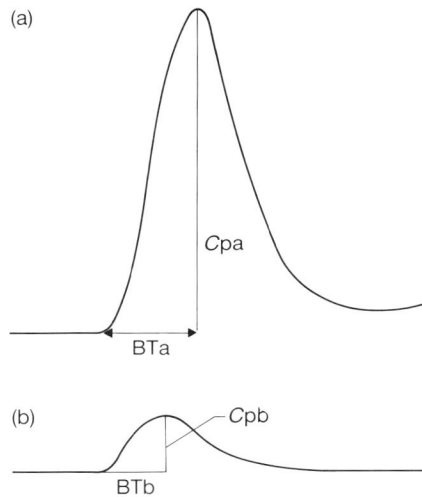

Fig. 10.7 (a) Equals forward curve-sampling from systemic artery. (b) Equals regurgitation curve-sampling from left atrium:

$$\text{Regurgitation index} = \frac{Cpb \times BTb \times 100}{Cpa \times BTa}$$

given by the peak concentration multiplied by the build-up time for the curve obtained from the systemic arterial sampling site and triangle B is given by the same two measurements made from the curve obtained when sampling from the left atrial catheter. The regurgitant index is given by B/A × 100.

REFERENCES

1 Stewart GN. Researches on the circulation time and on the influences which affect it. IV: The output of the heart. *J Physiol* 1897;**22**:159.

2 Kinsman JM, Moore JW, Hamilton WF. Human studies on the circulation. 1: Injection method. Physical and mathematical considerations. *Am J Physiol* 1929;**89**:322.

3 Hetzel PS, Swan HJC, de Arellano AAR, Wood EH. Estimation of cardiac output from first pass of arterial dye dilution curve. *J Appl Physiol* 1958;**13**:92.

4 Sanders M *et al*. Single catheter technique for accurate cardiac outputs from left ventricle. *Cathet Cardiovasc Diagn* 1983;**9**:97.

5 Van den Berg E *et al*. Measurement of cardiac output without right heart catheterisation. Reliability, advantages and limitations of a left sided indicator dilution technique. *Cathet Cardiovasc Diagn* 1986;**12**:205.

6 Branthwaite MA, Bradley RD. Measurement of cardiac output by thermodilution in man. *J Appl Physiol* 1968;**24**:434.

7 Ganz W *et al*. A new technique for measurement of cardiac output by thermodilution in man. *Am J Cardiol* 1971;**27**:392.

8 Carter SA, Bajec DF, Yannicelli E, Wood EH. Estimation of left-to-right shunt from arterial dilution curves. *J Lab Clin Med* 1960;**55**:77.

9 Swan HJC, Zapata-Diaz J, Wood EH. Dye dilution curves in congenital cyanotic heart disease. *Circulation* 1953;**8**:70.

10 Wood EH, Woodward E Jr. A simple method for differentiating mitral regurgitation from mitral stenosis by means of indicator-dilution curves. *Proc Mayo Clin* 1957;**32**:536.

11 Gorelick MM, Leukei SCM, Heinbecker RO, Gunton RW. Estimation of mitral regurgitation by injection of dye into left ventricle with simultaneous left atrial sampling; a clinical study of 60 confirmed cases. *Am J Cardiol* 1962;**10**:62.

12 Weisel RD, Berger RL, Hechtman HB. *New Engl J Med* 1975;**292**:682.

CHAPTER 11

Calculations used in cardiac catheterisation

Cardiac catheterisation produces *numbers* making it possible to test the accuracy of a clinical diagnosis and to quantitate severity. Inevitably, therefore, much effort has gone into deriving various *indices* from the numeric data obtained at catheterisation. Some of these indices have stood the test of time, others have not. It must always be remembered that most of the commonly produced data is liable to error; over- or under-damping or errors of baseline determination can produce errors even in straightforward pressure measurements. In particular the measurement of oxygen consumption, basic to the determination of flow and to many calculations derived therefrom, is liable to error. Even if measurements are accurate the derived data reflect only the situation at the time of measurement, influenced by the patient's anxiety or the effects of sedation or anaesthesia, and certainly does not reflect the situation during exercise. In recognition of this many laboratories employ an intervention, such as exercise, to obtain at least two points on a plot relating the haemodynamic state to the cardiac output, heart rate and so on. What needs to be emphasised is that most measurements, and certainly most derived indices, are only approximations; calculations to two decimal points represent self-delusion.

With the above caution, this chapter describes the calculations of flow, shunt size and resistance commonly used in the presentation of the findings at catheterisation. These measurements and indices are:

Name	Units
Systemic flow index (QS)	l/min/m^2
Pulmonary flow index (QP)	l/min/m^2
Pulmonary-to-systemic flow ratio (QP/QS)	
Left-to-right shunt	%
Right-to-left shunt	%
Effective pulmonary flow index	l/min/m^2
Total pulmonary resistance (Rp)	units × m^2
Pulmonary 'arteriolar' resistance (Rpa)	units × m^2
Total systemic resistance (Rs)	units × m^2
Pulmonary-to-systemic resistance ratio (Rp/Rs)	

Methods of calculating the area of stenotic cardiac valves are described in Chapter 15. The calculation of cardiac output by indicator dilution and thermodilution techniques and indices derived from indicator dilution curves have been described in Chapter 10. The measurement of ventricular volumes and of indices of ventricular performance are described in Chapter 8.

SYSTEMIC AND PULMONARY FLOW — THE FICK PRINCIPLE

The general form of the Fick principle [1] is that the uptake or release of a substance by an organ is the product of the blood flow through that organ and the difference in concentration of the substance between blood flowing into and out of the organ. Thus if we know the arteriovenous difference of the substance and also the amount of substance released from the organ (or taken up by the organ) we can calculate the blood flow through it. The same principle underlies the indicator dilution technique for measuring cardiac output (Chapter 10). In what is usually meant by the Fick method of measuring cardiac output the indicator substance is oxygen and the organ is the lung. The principle can be understood by reference to a simple analogy (Fig. 11.1). In this analogy we imagine a number of customers

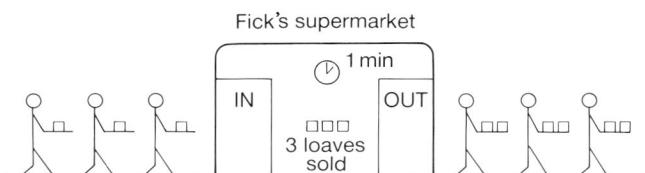

Fig. 11.1 The Fick principle.

passing through a supermarket. As they enter the supermarket it is observed that each customer is already carrying one loaf of bread and it is also observed that each is carrying two loaves as he leaves. If we know the number of loaves that have been sold in unit time we can calculate how many customers passed through in that time. Thus if three loaves were sold in one minute and each customer added one loaf to his shopping basket, three customers must have passed through in that minute. In this analogy each customer represents a unit of blood, each loaf being carried represents a unit of oxygen contained in a unit of blood, each loaf sold represents a unit of oxygen taken up in the lungs and the supermarket represents the lung.

Bearing this analogy in mind we see that pulmonary flow index (QP) can be calculated provided we know (1) the oxygen content of blood flowing into (pulmonary arterial blood) and out of (pulmonary vein blood) the pulmonary circulation, and (2) the oxygen consumption. Thus:

$$Qp = \frac{\text{Oxygen consumption/m}^2}{\underset{\text{O}_2 \text{ content}}{\text{Pulmonary vein}} - \underset{\text{O}_2 \text{ content}}{\text{Pulmonary artery}}}$$

In practice pulmonary vein blood is usually assumed to be 97% saturated as direct sampling from pulmonary vein is not usually possible. Pulmonary vein saturation must always be at least as high as any systemic arterial sample and is usually 1 or 2 percentage points higher as Thebesian veins contribute some desaturated blood to the blood in the left ventricle. Pulmonary vein saturation may be significantly less than 97% if there is intrapulmonary right-to-left shunting or impaired gas transfer across the alveolar membrane (e.g. pulmonary AV fistula, parenchymal lung disease), under these circumstances pulmonary flow cannot be measured without a pulmonary vein sample.

To calculate systemic flow we make the assumption that, over the period of measurement, the amount of oxygen taken up by the lungs is in balance with the amount consumed by the body for metabolic processes. Thus the systemic flow index is given by:

$$QS = \frac{\text{Oxygen consumption/m}^2}{\underset{\text{O}_2 \text{ content}}{\text{Systemic arterial}} - \underset{\text{O}_2 \text{ content}}{\text{'Mixed venous'}}}$$

Note that in the denominator of each equation a value is needed for oxygen *content*. Before describing how this value is obtained it is appropriate to define some of the terms that will be used.

Definitions

OXYGEN CONSUMPTION

This is the amount of oxygen taken up by blood passing through the lungs in unit time and is reported ml/min STPD (standard temperature and pressure, dry). Oxygen consumption may be obtained (1) by measurement (see Chapter 9), or (2) from tables of normal values (see below). Oxygen consumption and cardiac output are obviously related to body size and it is conventional to normalise values by correction for *body surface area in m²*. Resting oxygen consumption is normally between 100 and 150 ml/min/m². Oxygen consumption per m² (and cardiac output) is highest in infants and children and thereafter falls with increasing age [2]. It is slightly higher in males than in females.

BODY SURFACE AREA

This is expressed in m² and is conventionally obtained from nomograms or tables constructed according to the formula of Dubois [3]. These tables will be found in the Appendix at the end of this chapter (p. 180).

OXYGEN CONTENT

This is the amount of oxygen present (in ml/l blood) in a sample of blood. It includes both oxygen present as oxyhaemoglobin and any oxygen present in physical solution in the plasma. Classically the oxygen content of a sample of blood is determined by the manometric method of Van Slyke and Neill [4] but the method is too time consuming for routine use. In practice the content is obtained by multiplying the *oxygen capacity* (see below) of the patient's blood by the percentage saturation obtained by reflection oximetry [5]. If calculated in this way the value obtained does not include oxygen in physical solution. Below a saturation of 75% there is very little oxygen in solution, as almost all is bound to haemoglobin; above 75% an allowance can be made for oxygen in solution by adding 1.0 ml/l where the saturation is between 75 and 84%, 2.0 ml/l where the saturation is between 85 and 94% and 3.0 ml/l where the saturation is 95% or more.

OXYGEN CAPACITY

This is the amount of oxygen which can combine (as oxyhaemoglobin) with 100 ml of the subject's blood when that blood is fully saturated and depends on the haemoglobin level. Oxygen capacity is reported in ml/l. The oxygen capacity does not include oxygen which is in physical solution in the plasma. The oxygen capacity is obtained by multiplying the value for haemoglobin of the subject's blood (gm/100 ml, gm%) by a constant, 1.36 (x 10 to obtain the value in ml/l).

OXYGEN SATURATION (%)

This is the amount of oxygen bound to haemoglobin in relation to the capacity. It does not include oxygen in physical solution so that:

% saturation = (content − dissolved oxygen)
× 100/capacity

Percent saturation is usually measured by reflection oximetry and this, together with the value for haemoglobin are the only *measurements* involved in obtaining the oxygen content which is then calculated as described above.

We are now in a position to summarise the calculation of arteriovenous oxygen difference — the denominator in the Fick equation for calculating cardiac output.
1 Calculate the oxygen capacity of the patient's blood:

Hb (gm %) × 1.36 × 10 − ml/l blood

2 Calculate the oxygen content of arterial blood:

Capacity × % saturation arterial blood — ml/l blood

3 If arterial saturation >75% add value for dissolved oxygen to step (2) above (1.0, 2.0 or 3.0 ml/l according to % saturation). This step is often omitted from the calculation.
4 Repeat calculation (step 2 above) for oxygen content of mixed venous blood — ml/l blood.
5 Subtract (4) from (3) = AV O_2 difference ml/l.

Example

Hb = 14.0 gm%
Arterial saturation = 97%
Mixed venous saturation = 70%
Calculation:
Capacity = 1.36 × 14 × 10 = 190.4 ml/l
Arterial O_2 content = 190.4 × 97/100 = 184.7 ml/l
Add 3.0 ml/l for dissolved O_2 = 187.7 ml/l
Mixed venous O_2 content = 190.4 × 70/100
= 133.3
AV O_2 difference = 187.7 − 133.3 = 54.4 ml/l
Assuming the oxygen consumption was known to be (say) 120 ml/min/m^2 then the cardiac output corrected for body surface area (cardiac index) will be:
120/54.4 = 2.2 l/min/m^2

Notes

1 The use of tables of normal values for deriving oxygen consumption is a potential source of major error [6]. This is well recognised and where accurate estimation of systemic or pulmonary flow is required either the true oxygen consumption must be *measured* (as detailed in Chapter 9) or an alternative technique, such as thermodilution, must be used.
2 Over the normal range of arterial and venous saturation found when the patient is breathing room air reflection oximetry provides better discrimination than do measurements of oxygen *tension*. Reflection oximetry is accurate to 1 or 2%. Under these conditions the amount of oxygen in solution is small in relation to the total oxygen content and can be ignored. This is not true if inspired oxygen tension is high or if the AV difference is small (as occurs when breathing high inspired O_2 concentrations or when there is a large left-to-right shunt). Under these circumstances oxygen content must be measured (e.g. by oxygen cell 'Lex-O_2-Con' Lexington Instruments, for address see Appendix 2) or derived from measurements of oxygen tension — PO_2.

3 'Mixed venous' saturation. This term refers to the saturation that would be found if all systemic venous blood returning to the heart were completely mixed. Where there is no left-to-right shunt pulmonary arterial blood provides the best mixed venous sample; the right ventricle and pulmonary valve having done the mixing. Pulmonary arterial blood cannot be used as mixed venous when there is a left-to-right shunt, instead samples taken proximal to the shunt must be used. Unfortunately several streams of blood of differing saturation combine to form mixed venous blood in the right ventricle. The saturation of superior caval blood is usually a few percentage points lower than the true mixed venous saturation while inferior caval blood contains highly saturated blood from the renal veins ('low IVC') and blood of low saturation from the hepatic veins ('high IVC'). The lowest saturation of all is found in coronary sinus blood. All these streams combine to form mixed venous blood and if right ventricular or pulmonary artery samples cannot be used due to a left-to-right shunt some formula has to be derived to average the caval samples. A number of formulae have been proposed [7, 8] of which either:

$$(SVC + High\ IVC + Low\ IVC)/3 \qquad (1)$$

or

$$[(3 \times SVC) + IVC]/4 \qquad (2)$$

are probably the most satisfactory.

4 Finally note that if the value for oxygen consumption that is used has been corrected for body surface area (ml/min/m^2) no further correction is needed and the calculations will produce the systemic (or pulmonary) flow *index*.

INTRACARDIAC SHUNTS

So far pulmonary and systemic flow calculations have been described as though they are interchangable, and in the patient without a shunt they are; the two circulations are in series and pulmonary flow (QP) = systemic flow (QS) = cardiac output. The ratio between the two is unity (QP/QS = 1). This is not so when there is an intracardiac shunt; when the shunt is a pure left-to-right one the pulmonary flow will be higher than systemic flow. When the shunt is a pure right-to-left one the reverse is true. Since pulmonary and systemic flow can be

separately calculated it is possible to quantitate pure left-to-right shunts as:

$$L{-}R\ shunt = QP - QS\ (l/min/m^2)$$

and pure right-to-left shunts as:

$$R{-}L\ shunt = QS - QP\ (l/min/m^2)$$

Unfortunately there are many congenital cardiac anomalies which produce *bidirectional* shunting (right-to-left and left-to-right) so that this simple calculation of shunt size is not possible. If, under these circumstances, the relative magnitudes of the right-to-left and left-to-right shunts need expression, this can be done from saturation data alone:

$$L{-}R\ shunt = \left[\frac{PA\ sat - MV\ sat}{PV\ sat - MV\ sat}\right] \times \frac{100}{1}$$

$$R{-}L\ shunt = \left[\frac{PV\ sat - SA\ sat}{PV\ sat - MV\ sat}\right] \times \frac{100}{1}$$

Note that a left-to-right shunt (%) is the amount of pulmonary flow derived directly from pulmonary veins (i.e. bypassing the systemic circulation) and a right-to-left shunt (%) is the amount of systemic flow derived directly from systemic veins (bypassing the lungs).

The pulmonary-to-systemic flow ratio (QP/QS)

In practice the fact that there is bidirectional shunting will be obvious (from saturation data) and a record of the magnitude of the pulmonary and of the systemic flows provides the important information. A simple expression of the *relative* magnitudes of the two flows is the pulmonary-to-systemic flow ratio (QP/QS). This expression has the advantage that it is valid even if the value taken for oxygen consumption (and therefore the absolute values for QP and QS) was in error. Indeed the QP/QS ratio can be derived from saturation data alone:

$$QP/QS = (SA\ O^2\ sat - MV\ O^2\ sat)/(PV\ O_2\ sat - PA\ O_2\ sat)$$

Where SA, MV, PV and PA sat are the % saturations of systemic arterial, mixed venous, pulmonary vein and pulmonary arterial blood respectively.

One final flow calculation that is sometimes performed is the *effective pulmonary flow index*. This is the amount of blood to which oxygen can be added during its passage through the lungs, in other words it excludes left-to-right shunting blood which is already fully saturated and 'ineffective' for oxygen uptake.

$$\text{Effective QP} = \frac{\text{Oxygen consumption ml/min/m}^2}{\underset{\text{O}_2\text{ content}}{\text{Pulmonary vein}} - \underset{\text{O}_2\text{ content}}{\text{Mixed venous}}}$$

'RESISTANCES'

Ohms law states that the relationship between (electrical) resistance (R), current flow (I) and voltage (V, 'pressure') is given by:

$$R = V/I$$

The same relationship holds for haemodynamics:

$$R\text{(esistance)} = P \text{ (mean pressure)}/Q \text{ (flow)}$$

Thus the resistance to flow through the pulmonary circulation (Rp) is:

$$Rp = P\text{pa}/QP$$

where Ppa is the mean pulmonary artery pressure and QP the pulmonary flow. The resistance to flow through the systemic circulation (Rs) is:

$$Rs = P\text{sa}/Qs$$

Part of the resistance to flow through the pulmonary circulation is provided by the downstream (left atrial) pressure (so too does right atrial pressure contribute to systemic resistance). If we wish to investigate that part of the pulmonary resistance due to the pulmonary vasculature and exclude the left atrial, contribution the above expression for *total* pulmonary resistance (Rp) is modified:

$$Rpa = P\text{pa} - P\text{la}/QP$$

where Rpa is the so-called 'pulmonary arteriolar resistance' (since the arterioles are the main resistance vessels) and Pla is the mean left atrial (or wedge) pressure.

The correct units for expressing resistance are dynes sec/cm^5 but are never used. Resistance is expressed in Wood units obtained when mean pressure is measured in mmHg and flow as l/min. If flow is expressed as an index (l/min/m^2) then resistance measurements (units $\times$ m^2) are normalised. Units of resistance can be converted to dynes sec/cm^5 by

multiplying by 80. The upper limit of normal pulmonary arteriolar resistance is 2.0–3.0 units $\times$ m^2.

As with flow *ratios* resistance ratios are often used to remove the inaccuracies resulting from errors in oxygen consumption measurement. The 'pulmonary-to-systemic resistance ratio' usually given is between the *total* resistances — Rp/Rs.

The above calculations complete the list of those usually recorded at the completion of a diagnostic study. The descriptions given are often simplifications of a complex subject and that there are inherent inaccuracies is always recognised. Where greater accuracy is required special measurement techniques must be used; catheter-tip micro-manometry for the measurement of pressure and accurate measurement of oxygen consumption and A–V difference (Chapter 9) for instance. Other specialised measurements of valve area or ventricular performance are detailed elsewhere (Chapter 8 and 15). To complete the description of the commonly reported calculations the following example — a patient with congenital heart disease and bidirectional shunting due to 'mixing' may be helpful:

1 *Data*

Site	Pressure (syst. diast. mean)	Saturation (%)
SVC	—	60
RA	—	70
High IVC	—	57
Low IVC	—	66
Ventricle	100/1–10	87
PA	50/25 mean 33	86
PV	—	97
LA	mean 10	96
Ao	100/75 mean 83	86
Hb	16.0 gm%	
O$_2$ consumption	160 ml/min/m^2	

2 *Calculations*

O$_2$ capacity = $16.0 \times 1.36 \times 10 = 217.6$ ml/l

Mixed venous saturation = $(60 + 57 + 66)/3 = 61\%$

Mixed venous O$_2$ content = $217.6 \times 61/100 = 132.7$ ml/l

Pulmonary artery O$_2$ content = $217.6 \times 86/100 = 187.1$ ml/l

(add 2.0 ml/l for dissolved O$_2$ = 189.1 ml/l)

Pulmonary vein O$_2$ content = $217.6 \times 97/100 = 211.1$ ml/l

(add 3.0 ml/l for dissolved O_2 = 214.1 ml/l)
Aortic O_2 content = 217.6 × 86/100 = 187.1 ml/l
  (add 2.0 ml/l for dissolved O_2 = 189.1 ml/l)
QP = 160/(214.1 − 189.1) = 160/25 = 6.4 l/min/m²
QS = 160/(189.1 − 132.7) = 160/56.4 = 2.8 l/min/m²
'Effective' QP = 160/(214.1 − 132.7) = 160/81.4 = 1.9 l/min/m²
QP/QS = 6.4/2.8 = 2.3 : 1
Rp = 33/6.4 = 5.2 units × m²
Rpa = (33 − 10)/6.4 = 3.6 units × m²
Rs = 83/2.8 = 29.6 units × m²
Rp/Rs = 5.2/29.6 = 0.2 : 1
L−R shunt = (86 − 61) × 100/(97 − 61) = 2500/36 = 69%
R−L shunt = (97 − 86) × 100/(97 − 61) = 1100/36 = 30%

APPENDIX

Table 11.1a Body surface area can be calculated from the height and weight of the patient using the nomogram below constructed according to the formula of Dubois [3].

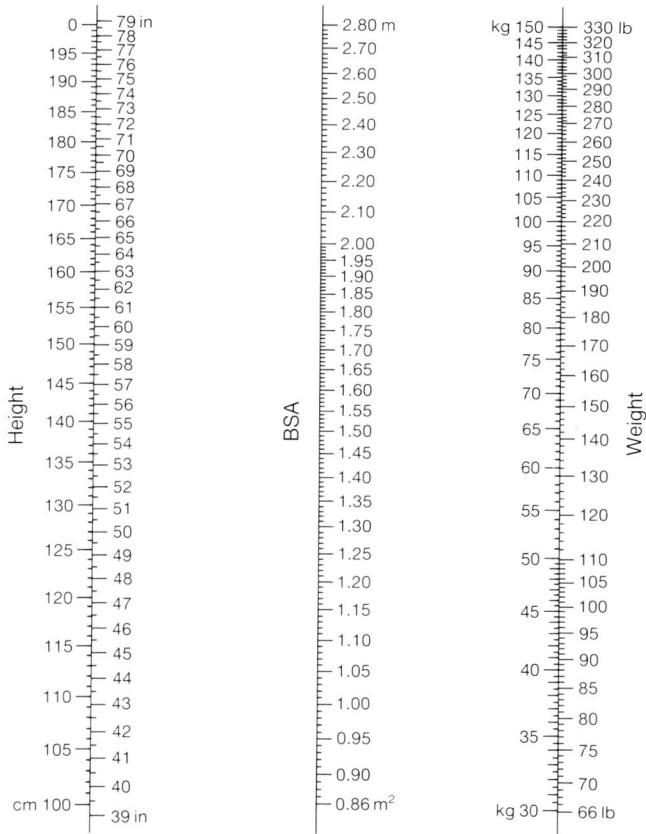

Table 11.1b If only weight is known an approximate estimate of body surface area can be obtained from this table.

Weight (kg)	BSA (m²)	Weight (kg)	BSA (m²)
1.0	0.10	20.0	0.82
1.5	0.12	21.0	0.85
2.0	0.15	22.0	0.87
2.5	0.18	23.0	0.90
3.0	0.20	24.0	0.93
4.0	0.25	25.0	0.95
5.0	0.29	26.0	1.00
6.0	0.33	27.0	1.03
7.0	0.38	28.0	1.06
8.0	0.42	29.0	1.08
9.0	0.45	30.0	1.11
10.0	0.49	31.0	1.13
11.0	0.52	32.0	1.15
12.0	0.55	33.0	1.18
13.0	0.58	34.0	1.20
14.0	0.61	35.0	1.23
15.0	0.64	36.0	1.25
16.0	0.71	37.0	1.27
17.0	0.74	38.0	1.30
18.0	0.76	39.0	1.32
19.0	0.79	40.0	1.34

Table 11.2 *Oxygen consumption*. For children below 3 years of age oxygen consumption is very variable but this table, based on data from Cayler *et al.* [9], can be used to give an approximation.

BSA (m²)	Resting O_2 consumption (ml/min/m²)
0.225−0.275	140
0.275−0.325	150
0.325−0.375	172
0.375−0.425	175
0.425−0.475	179
0.475−1.0	174
1.0−1.5	150

Table 11.3 *Cardiac output*. These normal values for resting cardiac output and stroke volume for patients over the age of 20 are taken from the data of Brandfonbrener *et al.* [2].

Age	Cardiac index (l/min/m²) Mean	SD	Stroke index (ml/min/m²) Mean	SD
20−30	3.72	0.28	48.9	3.1
30−40	3.57	0.3	49.4	3.8
40−50	2.96	0.17	43.3	2.5
50−60	2.78	0.13	40.3	2.2
60−70	2.58	0.15	41.5	2.4
70−80	2.54	0.18	39.3	3.2
80+	2.36	0.23	36.5	3.3

Table 11.4 For children above 3 years of age and for adults this table from LaFarge and Miettenen [10], can be used to obtain resting oxygen consumption at varying ages and heart rates.

Age (year)	Heart rate (beats per min)												
	50	60	70	80	90	100	110	120	130	140	150	160	170
Male patients													
3			155	159	163	167	171	175	178	182	186	190	
4		149	152	156	160	163	168	171	175	179	182	186	
6		141	144	148	151	155	159	162	167	171	179	182	186
8		136	141	145	148	152	156	159	163	167	171	175	178
10	130	134	139	142	146	149	153	157	160	165	169	172	176
12	128	132	136	140	144	147	151	155	158	162	167	170	174
14	127	130	134	137	142	146	149	153	157	160	165	169	172
16	125	129	132	136	141	144	148	152	155	159	162	167	
18	124	127	131	135	139	143	147	150	154	157	161	166	
20	123	126	130	134	137	142	145	149	153	156	160	165	
25	120	124	127	131	135	139	143	147	150	154	157		
30	118	122	125	129	133	136	141	145	148	152	155		
35	116	120	124	127	131	135	139	143	147	150			
40	115	119	122	126	130	133	137	141	145	149			
Female patients													
3				150	153	157	161	165	169	172	176	180	183
4			141	145	149	152	156	159	163	168	171	175	179
6		130	134	137	142	146	149	153	156	160	165	168	172
8		125	129	133	136	141	144	148	152	155	159	163	167
10	118	122	125	129	133	136	141	144	148	152	155	159	163
12	115	119	122	126	130	133	137	141	145	149	152	156	160
14	112	116	120	123	127	131	134	139	143	146	150	153	157
16	109	114	118	121	125	128	132	136	140	144	148	151	
18	107	111	116	119	123	127	130	134	137	142	146	149	
20	106	109	114	118	121	125	128	132	136	140	144	148	
25	102	106	109	114	118	121	125	128	132	136	140		
30	99	103	106	110	115	118	122	125	129	133	136		
35	97	100	104	107	111	116	119	123	127	130			
50	94	98	102	105	109	112	117	121	124	128			

GENERAL READING

1 Grossman W (ed.). *Cardiac catheterisation and angiography*. 3rd edn. Philadelphia, Lea & Febiger, 1986.
2 Yang SS *et al. From cardiac catheterization data to hemodynamic parameters*. Philadelphia, FA Davis, 1978.

REFERENCES

1 Fick A. *Über die Messung des Blutquantums in den Hertzventrikeln*. Sitzungsberichte der physikalisch-medicinischen Gesellschaft zu Wurtzberg. **XVI**;1870.
2 Brandfonbrener M, Landowne M, Schock NW. Changes in cardiac output with age. *Circulation* 1955; **12**:556.
3 Dubois EF. *Basal metabolism in health and disease*. Philadelphia, Lea & Febiger, 1936.
4 Van Slyke DD, Neill JM. The determination of gases in blood and other solutions by vacuum extraction and manometric measurements. *J Biol Chem* 1924;**61**:523.
5 Zijlstra WG, Mook GA. *Medical reflection photometry*. Assen, Netherlands, Van Gorcum, 1962.
6 Dehmer GJ, Firth BG, Hillis LD. Oxygen consumption in adult patients during cardiac catheterization. *Clin Cardiol* 1982;**5**:438.
7 Flamm MD, Cohn KE, Hancock EW. Measurement of systemic cardiac output at rest and exercise in patients with atrial septal defect. *Am J Cardiol* 1969;**23**:258.
8 Miller HC, Brown DJ, Miller GAH. Comparison of formulae used to estimate oxygen saturation of mixed venous blood from caval samples. *Br Heart J* 1974;**36**:446.
9 Cayler GG, Rudolph AM, Nadas AS. Systemic blood flow in infants and children with and without heart disease. *Pediatrics* 1963;**32**:186.
10 LaFarge CG, Miettinen OS. The estimation of oxygen consumption. *Cardiovasc Res* 1970;**4**:23.

Complications of cardiac catheterisation

Many studies of the complications of cardiac catheterisation have been reported — with widely varying results. It is not surprising that reported complication rates differ since the incidence of complications varies with the experience of the operator or the unit, with the ages and types of patients being studied and with the definitions used and adequacy of the reporting system. A meaningful figure can only be obtained from studies involving a large number of patients. Two such large multicentre studies have been reported. The first was reported in 1968 and is now of historical interest in that the complication rates experienced reflected lack of experience of what were then relatively new techniques [1]. In 1979 the Society for Cardiac Angiography instituted a registry of the complications experienced in 65 laboratories over a 14 month period. A total of 53 581 patients were studied in this time and details of the complications experienced were reported in 1982 [2]. A third study used data derived from the multicentre, prospective study of the results of coronary artery surgery (the CASS study) to provide data relating to the complications of coronary arteriography [3]. An earlier study of the complications of coronary arteriography is of particular interest in demonstrating the effect of experience in reducing the complication rates. For centres performing less than 100 studies per year the mortality was eight times as high as in centres performing more than 400 studies per year [4]. At the Brompton Hospital a computer-based data logging and retrieval system has been in existence since 1970 and between then and mid-1986, details of 17 582 catheterisation procedures have been entered allowing a similar analysis of the complications of catheterisation.

MORTALITY

Table 12.1 The results of the study of the mortality rate from the Registry study (October 1979 to December 1980) and the study of the Brompton Hospital (1970 to 1986).

Age	No. of deaths	No. of studies	Mortality rate
Registry study			
<1 year	8	457	1.75%
1 to 60 years	24	34 966	0.07%
>60 years	43	16 712	0.25%
Total	75	53 581	0.14%
Brompton Hospital			
<1 year	16	2 509	0.64%
1 to 60 years	13	12 444	0.10%
>60 years	7	2 628	0.27%
Total	36	17 582	0.20%

The two sets of figures are remarkably similar and demonstrate that the overall mortality associated with cardiac catheterisation should be 0.2%, or less and that the highest mortality occurs in infants and neonates and is higher in those over 60 than in younger patients. The relatively high risk when neonates and infants are being studied highlights the importance of the case mix in determining mortality; a laboratory studying a high proportion of such cases will inevitably have a higher mortality than one concerned largely with adult cardiac disease. The figures also demonstrate the benefit of experience; laboratories participating in the Registry study had a small experience in patients under 1 year of age (457 cases) and a mortality two and a half times as great as our own laboratory where the experience in this age group was much larger (2509 cases). The higher mortality in neonates and infants is partly due to the more demanding nature of studies in small infants with low tolerance to blood loss, hypothermia and so on but also reflects the serious nature of the disease in many such patients. It is often difficult to decide to what extent the procedure was responsible for a death and how much it was the inevitable result of the disease itself. It is not surprising that the mortality is highest among those with the most severe disease; Table 12.2 taken from the Registry report demonstrates the increased risk in relation to the severity of disease.

Table 12.2 Mortality rate by functional class (Registry Study).

Functional class	No. of deaths	No. of studies	Mortality rate
I	1	6 356	0.02%
II	3	13 692	0.02%
III	13	12 032	0.12%
IV	40	5 999	0.67%

The left ventricular ejection fraction is another measure of the severity of disease and patients with an ejection fraction <30% have a catheter-associated mortality some ten times higher than those with a normal ejection fraction (see Table 12.3).

Table 12.3 Mortality related to left ventricular ejection fraction.

Ejection fraction(%)	Mortality(%) Registry study	CASS study
>50	0.05	0.07
30 to 49	0.23	0.46
<30	0.76	1.2

Similarly the Registry study found an overall mortality rate for studies in valvular heart disease of 0.28% as compared with the lower figure of 0.11% for coronary arteriography in a group of patients 20% of whom had no organic heart disease. In coronary arteriography the increased risk associated with disease of the left main stem is well known (Table 12.4).

Again the close similarity of the figures is of interest and, though the mortality associated with left main stem disease is some ten times as high as for other coronary artery disease, neither figure approaches the 15% mortality which has been

Table 12.4 Mortality associated with coronary arteriography.

	No. of deaths	No. of studies	Mortality(%)
Registry study			
All cases	47	41 204	0.11%
Left main stem	22	2 452	0.86%
Brompton series			
All cases	12	7 607	0.16%
Left main stem	5	468	1.07%
CASS study			
All cases	15	7 553	0.19%
Left main stem	5	657	0.76%

reported as associated with left main stem disease in earlier studies [5].

Table 12.5 summarises those factors which have been shown to be associated with an increased risk of death as a consequence of cardiac catheterisation.

Table 12.5 Factors associated with increased mortality.

Factor	Increased risk
1 Age less than 1 year	Risk approximately three times population as a whole (Brompton figures)
2 Age > 60 years	Risk approximately two times higher than in younger adults
3 Functional class	Risk approximately ten times as great for class IV as compared with class I–II
4 Left main stem disease	Risk more than ten times as high as for other coronary artery disease
5 Valvular heart disease	Risk two to three times as high as risk for coronary arteriography alone

OTHER COMPLICATIONS

The incidence of complications other than death will again be determined by the case mix. Thus the Registry study, concerned largely with coronary arteriography and including 20% of patients with no cardiac abnormality, reported a low complication rate (excluding death) of 1.6%. A more realistic figure for a laboratory studying all forms of adult and congenital heart disease is our own overall complication rate (from 1970) of 2.6%. Just as the mortality is higher in neonates and infants so too is the complication rate (Table 12.6).

Table 12.6 Complication rate related to age (Brompton figures).

Age	Complications (excluding death) %
<1 year	4.6
1 to 60 years	2.2
>60 years	2.5
All cases	2.6

The following is a description of the more frequently encountered complications of catheterisation, their prevention and treatment.

Arrhythmias

The arrhythmias that are likely to be encountered as a complication of cardiac catheterisation are:
1 Sinus bradycardia.
2 AV dissociation — partial or complete.
3 Atrial fibrillation/flutter.
4 Ventricular tachycardia.

SINUS BRADYCARDIA

This is most likely to occur as part of a *vasovagal reaction* and is the most common arrhythmia encountered. Vasovagal reactions are most likely to occur when the patient is apprehensive and when poor operative technique has caused him pain. The onset of a reaction is heralded by restlessness accompanied by a slowing heart rate and peripheral vasoconstriction with nausea and sweating. These signs demand the prompt intravenous (or intra-arterial if there is no immediate venous access) administration of 0.6 mg of atropine sulphate which can be repeated once if there is not an almost immediate response. Vasovagal reactions with the associated hypotension and bradycardia require immediate treatment since they can lead to impaired coronary perfusion and a cycle of events which, especially in patients with poor cardiac reserve, can lead to death. Fortunately the response to atropine is almost always rapid and dramatic.

Profound sinus bradycardia is a fairly common event immediately following the injection of contrast medium in the coronary arteries — particularly the right. It is almost invariably of brief duration but return to sinus rhythm can be hastened by asking the patient to cough.

AV DISSOCIATION

A prolonged P-R interval leading to complete heart block can occur during a vasovagal attack, can be the result of catheter manipulation in the region of the AV node, can follow the injection of contrast medium (e.g. during coronary arteriography) or may be the first sign of under-ventilation in an anaesthetised or oversedated infant. In all these situations spontaneous recovery usually follows cessation of catheter manipulation or improved ventilation. Right heart catheter manipulation may provoke right bundle branch block; in patients with pre-existing left bundle branch block this can result in complete AV dissociation. It may be wise to insert a temporary transvenous pacemaker catheter in such patients before starting the study; certainly a pacemaker and transvenous wire should be instantly available.

ATRIAL FIBRILLATION/FLUTTER

These arrhythmias are most likely to occur as a result of prolonged catheter manipulation within the right atrium but can, occasionally, be precipitated the moment the catheter enters the atrium. Unless the ventricular rate is very rapid the arrhythmias are unlikely to be life-threatening. Spontaneous reversion to sinus rhythm is likely to occur once atrial manipulation has ceased but the arrhythmias can often be 'broken' if the catheter is manipulated in the right (or left) ventricle so as to provoke a ventricular ectopic beat. If the arrhythmia cannot be aborted in this way and is having an adverse haemodynamic effect DC cardioversion should be employed after sedation with intravenous Diazepam 10 to 20 mg.

VENTRICULAR TACHYCARDIA

Short salvos of ventricular ectopic beats often accompany catheter manipulation within the right or left ventricle but sustained ventricular tachycardia, though uncommon, may follow catheter manipulation or the intracoronary injection of contrast medium. Sustained ventricular tachycardia requires immediate DC cardioversion together with the intravenous administration of 75 to 100 mg (1.0 to 1.5 mg/kg) lidocaine.

EMBOLISM, MYOCARDIAL INFARCTION AND CEREBROVASCULAR ACCIDENTS

The incidence of these complications from the Registry and our own figures is shown below (Table 12.7).

Table 12.7 Incidence of embolism, myocardial infarction and cerebrovascular accidents.

	Registry study	Brompton Hospital
Myocardial infarction	0.07%	0.04%
Cerebrovascular accident	0.07%	0.03%

Systemic embolism during catheterisation can be from air or blood clot. Air embolism is always due to careless technique; the flushing system should always be purged of air as should the catheter before being connected. This is particularly important whenever the catheter has been disconnected from the system — as for angiocardiography or a scout injection. Air embolism can result from failure to purge a long sheath before introducing a tightly fitting catheter and from rupture of the balloon of a flow-guided catheter. The balloon of such catheters should not be inflated beyond the maximum volume recommended by the manufacturer and carbon dioxide should be used if such catheters are used on the left side of the heart or anywhere in the heart of a patient with a right-to-left shunt. Embolisation by mural thrombus has occurred as a result of catheter manipulation or ventriculography in patients with prior myocardial infarction and aneurysm formation. In such patients the catheter should not be advanced as far as the apex so as to minimise the risk of this, rare, complication. Embolism by blood clot can most easily occur when clots and fibrin thrombi form on guide wires and within catheters. In coronary arteriography it is possible that fibrin formed on a guide wire may be deposited at the catheter tip as the guide wire is removed; subsequent coronary arteriography may result in this material being injected into the coronary artery. It is for this reason that whole-body heparinisation (1 mg/kg) is almost universally employed before coronary arteriography; and it is why guide wires and catheters are treated (heparin bonded, Teflon coating) to minimise clot formation and why they are 'for one use only'. Clot formation within a catheter is signalled by a damped pressure record and difficulty in withdrawing blood

samples. Such a catheter should be removed and flushed clear or discarded and heparin given if the patient has not already been heparinised.

Myocardial infarction is almost exclusively a complication of coronary arteriography (and PTCA). It may result from embolism by blood clot but is probably more often the result of coronary dissection. The forceful injection of contrast medium through an end-hole catheter when the end-hole is lodged beneath an atheromatous plaque is the most likely cause — and a reason for advocating additional side holes for coronary catheters so that there is an alternative escape route for the contrast medium. Coronary air embolism may lead to transient ECG, changes but is unlikely to cause infarction. The Registry study, concerned almost entirely with coronary arteriography, reported a 0.07% incidence of myocardial infarction and an identical incidence of cerebrovascular accidents (0.07%).

While the incidence of myocardial infarction is likely to be overestimated in studies which include a high proportion of coronary arteriograms, the risk of a *cerebrovascular accident* is probably greater in studies of congenital heart disease when right-to-left shunting puts the cerebral circulation at risk from any right-sided emboli. One risk in particular is the occurrence of cerebral venous thrombosis in cyanotic, polycythaemic infants. The probable cause is dehydration in an already polycythaemic patient and the effect of contrast media leading to deformation of red cells. Hydration by intravenous drip must be maintained during *and after* the study in such patients.

In adults transient cortical blindness or field defects are occasionally reported and are presumably the result of micro-emboli [6]. Alarming cortical blindness of some 12 hours duration has followed repeated attempts to opacify an internal mammary graft and results from contrast medium spilling into the vertebral artery.

LOCAL ARTERIAL COMPLICATIONS

The incidence of local arterial complications is dramatically influenced by the experience of the unit or operator with figures ranging from 28% in a study involving 96 procedures [7] to 0.57% in the Registry study involving 53 581 procedures. In a recent study from the Brompton Hospital [8] the local arterial complication rate over a 10 year period for patients aged 20 and over was 0.69% (55 of 7926). The rate for the brachial artery approach was 0.8% and for the percutaneous, transfemoral approach was 0.45%. For one experienced operator the local complication rate for brachial arteriotomy was 0.5% while for all other operators, including physicians in training, it was 0.9%.

Brachial arteriotomy

The commonest complication of this technique is loss of the radial pulse; in the extreme situation this could lead to loss of the limb or, more likely, claudication of the forearm during activities involving raising the arm such as hair brushing. In fact in the study referred to above [8] only one patient (0.01%) had any residual disability — mild claudication of the forearm. Loss of the radial pulse is invariably due to poor operative technique. Good technique includes (1) use of a horizontal (not vertical) incision, (2) repair by interrupted (not purse-string) sutures — 6/0 or finer, (3) use of angled arterial clamps during the repair (not traction by arterial tapes), and (4) whole-body heparinisation — 1 mg/kg (not merely the local instillation of heparin). Most importantly the patient should not be allowed to leave the laboratory without an adequate radial pulse. Spasm must not be invoked as an excuse for an absent pulse in the hope that the pulse will return. Spasm can occur, always as a result of challenging the artery with a catheter that is too big, but the subsequent lost pulse is the result of consequent trauma to the artery or a poor repair. Thrombus formation is not the immediate cause of a lost pulse in a heparinised patient though it can occur later due to stasis following a poor technical repair. When thrombus formation has occurred it can usually be dealt with by gentle use of a no. 4 or 5 Fogarty embolectomy catheter. Re-repair of the arteriotomy in the laboratory by the most experienced operator available is at least as successful as referral to the surgical team for a formal repair in theatre though this must be done if all else fails to restore the pulse. Conservative management with a heparin drip is associated with more failures than is an aggressive policy of immediate re-exploration.

Other complication of this technique are rare and include late bleeding with haematoma or false aneurysm formation and damage (usually temporary) to the median nerve.

Percutaneous transfemoral (Seldinger) approach

The local arterial complications that can result from this technique include (1) haematoma formation with considerable loss of blood into the tissues, (2) false aneurysm, or (3) arteriovenous fistula formation at the puncture site, (4) trauma to the artery or dissection of the artery leading to ischaemia of the leg, and (5) iliofemoral venous thrombosis as a result of the above or from prolonged compression and this in turn has lead to pulmonary embolism. All these complications require urgent surgical intervention.

Delayed haemorrhage at the puncture site can also occur; it is usually the result of inadequate compression of the puncture site at the end of the procedure but may be due to too early ambulation. Patients who have had a percutaneous transfemoral study should remain in bed for at least 6 hours after the procedure and some laboratories insist on a longer period — 12 to 18 hours. Delayed haemorrhage is more likely when there is a coagulation defect or the patient is receiving anticoagulants. Most laboratories employ whole-body heparinisation to prevent both local and systemic or coronary thrombosis/embolism and this may increase the risk of local haemorrhage. Our practice is to give 0.5 mg/kg of heparin when the percutaneous approach is used. Although the action of 1 mg (100 units) of heparin can be reversed by the slow intravenous infusion of 1 mg of protamine sulphate we do not use protamine as heparin is rapidly excreted and 'protamine reactions' can occur and can be life threatening. Protamine reactions resemble anaphylactic shock with hypotension, bronchospasm and circulatory collapse. They occur immediately following the intravenous injection of protamine and require immediate treatment with hydrocortisone sodium succinate 100–500 mg i.v. and adrenaline 0.5–1.0 mg i.m. together with general resuscitative measures — raising the legs, oxygen by face mask or endotracheal intubation, etc. There is an increased risk of protamine reactions in diabetic patients being treated with protamine zinc insulin.

PERFORATION OF THE HEART OR GREAT VESSELS

For a catheter actually to perforate a vessel or myocardium is rare. More commonly a minor dissection of a vessel can result when a catheter is advanced against resistance or when attempts are made to traverse a tortuous and atheromatous artery. The junction between the right subclavian artery and the innominate is a point of particular danger as is the iliac artery in patients with aorto-iliac disease. These complications will be avoided if a number of rules are followed:

1 Never advance a catheter against undue resistance.
2 Avoid the transfemoral approach in any patient with suspected aorto-iliac disease (reduced femoral pulses, history of claudication).
3 Always lead an end-hole catheter past these danger points with a guide wire — preferably one with a J-tip.
4 Always use the softest and smallest catheter compatible with the aims of the study.
5 Never persist with attempts to manipulate a catheter through a vessel if the patient complains of pain.
6 If a scout injection is used to elucidate the problem with a tortuous vessel inject only a very small quantity initially and do so very slowly; the catheter tip may be under the intima or beneath a plaque and the injection of contrast medium may cause the subintimal dissection to spread.
7 Plan the study so as to reduce the amount of catheter manipulation to a minimum.

Teflon catheters and the Lehman ventriculography catheter are more likely to cause damage than others such as the pigtail ventriculography catheter. The pigtail catheter is particularly suitable for traversing, atraumatically, the subclavian/innominate junction. It is our practice to explore the heart with a thin-walled Goodale—Lubin catheter and to reserve the stiffer angiographic catheters for the angiographic part of the study so as to minimise intracardiac manipulation with the larger, stiffer catheter. The transseptal technique carries a significant risk of perforation of a vessel or cardiac chamber.

As a rule, minor catheter-induced dissections cause no problems but may occasionally spread and result in occlusion of the vessel or in the formation of a large haematoma which might require surgical evacuation.

TAMPONADE

Perforation of a cardiac chamber is itself very rare and it is even rarer for this to lead to tamponade. There is always a small risk of tamponade following percutaneous, transapical puncture of the left ventricle; for this reason we do not perform this procedure on anticoagulated patients until the prothrombin time has been reduced to less than twice the normal value. Routine postcatheterisation monitoring includes recordings every 15 minutes of pulse and blood pressure and a portable chest X-ray. Should the signs indicate developing tamponade immediate pericardial drainage and blood replacement is needed. Fortunately many of the patients who require a transapical puncture have had previous cardiac surgery with an open (or adherent) pericardium so that the risk is more of a haemothorax than of tamponade.

PULMONARY OEDEMA, INTRAPULMONARY HAEMORRHAGE

The incidence of pulmonary oedema as a complication of cardiac catheterisation is 0.06% (Brompton series). There is always a risk of pulmonary oedema occurring in patients with a high left atrial pressure (e.g. severe mitral stenosis) when they are required to lie flat for the duration of the study. Additional precipitating factors include the effect of contrast media in increasing the blood volume and causing depression of left ventricular function, tachycardia due to anxiety, increased cardiac output (for the same reason) and catheter-induced arrhythmias. Ideally studies are delayed in such high risk patients until the maximal benefit has been obtained from medical therapy. Diuretics must not be witheld prior to the study and the study should be completed as rapidly as possible; it should be possible to perform a complete right and left heart study in less than 20 minutes. The patient should be propped up on as many pillows as is possible while still allowing fluoroscopy. If, despite these precautions, the patients develop a cough one can be sure that frank pulmonary oedema will ensue within minutes. A fast-acting diuretic, e.g. frusemide 20—50 mg, should be given intravenously and the study terminated as rapidly as possible.

Fatal intrapulmonary haemorrhage/infarction has been reported as a complication of flow-guided catheterisation with balloon-tipped catheters [9]. The balloon should never be inflated in a peripheral pulmonary artery but allowed to be carried there from a more central position. An inflated balloon, recording the wedge pressure, should not remain inflated for more than 5 minutes.

INFECTION, INFECTIVE ENDOCARDITIS AND 'PYROGENIC REACTIONS'

Local infection at a cut-down site should not occur if correct sterile procedures have been followed. Rarely such local infection can result in thrombophlebitis in which case the appropriate antibiotic should be given. Perhaps surprisingly infective endocarditis attributable to catheterisation is almost unknown and most laboratories have long abandoned routine pre- or postcatheter antibiotic prophylaxis. Much more important is the risk of transmitting viral hepatitis from one patient to another or to the operator or assistant. For this reason no patient should undergo routine catheterisation until he has been screened and shown to be negative for hepatitis B surface antigen (HBsAg — Australia antigen). Exceptions to this rule depend on local laboratory regulations but may include emergency studies and infants of Caucasian origin under the age of 1 year. Where a study has to be performed on a patient who is HBsAg positive, stringent precautions must be taken against infection and all catheters, etc. destroyed after use. As a guide the following are the precautions adopted in our laboratory:

1 No personnel are allowed in laboratory if they have cuts or abrasions; only essential personnel are allowed in laboratory.
2 Disposable gowns, drapes, etc. used and all non-essential equipment are covered with plastic sheeting.
3 Laboratory staff wear disposable gowns, overshoes and gloves and operator(s) wear double gloves and masks and disposable plastic aprons.
4 Any blood spilled is immediately mopped with 10% hypochlorite solution.
5 All catheters, manometer tubing, syringes, swabs, etc. used are placed in infection risk bags for destruction by incineration.
6 Any non-disposable instruments used are im-

mersed in activated Cidex for 3 hours before cleaning and subsequent sterilisation, (non-metallic instruments in 10% hypochlorite).
7 All contaminated surfaces (e.g. floor) are swabbed with 10% hypochlorite using a disposable mop and are left wet. The laboratory is not to be re-occupied for 3 hours.

Pyrogenic reactions, common before the days of disposable catheters and equipment, are rarely seen today. They are due to foreign protein or endotoxin adherent within the lumen of the catheter or within the flush system; angiography or flushing the catheter introduces this material to the patient's circulation. A typical pyrogenic reaction occurs during or soon after the study and consists of a high fever with rigors. The use of disposable catheters and other equipment and meticulous cleaning and sterilisation techniques should prevent their occurrence.

POSTCATHETER HYPOTENSION

Occasionally a patient may become profoundly hypotensive for some hours following catheterisation without any obvious cause. Grossman [10] has suggested that postcatheter hypotension is due to the effect of contrast medium in causing an osmotic diuresis which, together with continuing vasodilatation, results in hypovolaemia and has noted that such patients are hypotensive with a *warm* skin. The patients respond to fluid replacement or plasma expansion with dextran and elevation of the foot of the bed.

COMPLICATIONS DUE TO ANGIOGRAPHY

These are discussed in Chapter 7.

COMPLICATIONS IN NEONATES AND INFANTS

A number of complications are peculiar to this group of patients, they include hypothemia, hypoglycaemia, disturbed acid-base balance, significant blood loss, worsening heart failure as a result of giving excessive amounts of contrast medium and hypercyanotic attacks due to provoked infundibular spasm. The prevention of these complications is discussed in the chapter devoted to the techniques of catheterisation in infants and children with congenital heart disease.

CATHETER 'KNOTTING'

Occasionally trouble will be experienced when manipulation of a catheter results in it assuming a conformation which makes further manipulation impossible or which makes it impossible to withdraw the catheter from the vessel. The fluoroscopic appearance may resemble a knot though it is unusual for a true knot to form. None the less it may be very difficult to restore the catheter to a straight configuration; no detailed description of how this may be done is possible but some tricks may be found useful;

1 An intra-arterial catheter may have become bent back on itself forming a loop which is too long to be straightened within the vessel or chamber. Attempt to engage the tip in an aortic arch vessel (if the approach was from the arm) or the contralateral iliac artery (if from the leg); if the catheter is now withdrawn while the tip remains in place the loop can be straightened. The aortic bifurcation can often be used in this way to straighten a bent catheter. A similar technique is to pass an overlong loop into the left ventricle where the tip can be trapped while the loop is straightened by traction.

2 A guide-wire, perhaps with the rigid end leading, can sometimes be used to push a knot or large loop towards the tip of the catheter and help to undo it.

3 Some catheters are particularly liable to form unmanageable loops or knots during manipulation. The so-called 'head-hunter' catheter, the left Judkins and some graft-seeking catheters may do this if the guide wire is removed prematurely.

If all attempts to disentangle the catheter fail then the catheter may have to be removed by force and the resulting damage to the vessel repaired. Alternatively surgical exploration may be needed.

Very rarely a catheter may fracture or an introducing sheath allowed to escape into the vessel. Surgical removal may be needed but various catheter-snare techniques have been described for removing intravascular foreign bodies (see Chapter 5).

AVOIDING COMPLICATIONS — GENERAL PRINCIPLES

It is probable, but unproven, that a speedily completed study is less likely to result in complications than one which is prolonged and trying for both patient and operator. It is certain that a short study is appreciated by the patient. The experience of the operator is one factor which determines the length of the study but we have to accept that operators have to be trained and not all studies can be performed by experts. However we can ensure that the laboratory is equipped and organised in such a way as to impose no needless delays or risks. The X-ray equipment must be capable of providing all the required views in rapid succession without having to move the patient — modern U-arm and parallellogram tube suspensions do this. The fluoroscopic image must be of high quality so that the operator never has any difficulty in seeing the catheter or guide wire anywhere in the heart. The operator needs to have all essential information — pressure, ECG, etc. — displayed in a single, convenient position but must not be so overloaded with information that he is distracted. Finally the patient needs to be reassured that the procedure is routine, safe and painless. How this is done is the concern of the laboratory director and cannot be detailed here but attention to these aspects of cardiac catheterisation make a very important contribution to reducing the risks of catheterisation. The procedure should be swift, safe and free of stress for both patient and staff.

REFERENCES

1 Braunwald E, Swan HJC (eds). Cooperative study on cardiac catheterisation. *Circulation* 1968;**37** (suppl 3):1.

2 Kennedy JW *et al*. Complications associated with cardiac catheterization and angiography. *Cathet Cardiovasc Diagn* 1982;**8**:5.

3 Davis K *et al*. Complications of coronary arteriography from the collaborative study of coronary artery surgery (CASS). *Circulation* 1979;**59**:1105.

4 Adams DF, Fraser DB, Abrams HL. The complications of coronary arteriography. *Circulation* 1973;**48**:609.

5 Cohen MV, Cohn PF, Hermann MV, Gorlin R. Diagnosis and prognosis of left main coronary artery obstruction. *Circulation* 1972;**46** (suppl 1):57.

6 Vik-Mo H, Todnem K, Følling M, Rosland G. Transient visual disturbance during cardiac catheterisation with angioplasty. *Cathet Cardiovasc Diagn* 1986;**12**:1.

7 Brener BJ, Couch NP. Peripheral arterial complications of left heart catheterization and their management. *Am J Surg* 1973;**125**:521.

8 Miller GAH. Local arterial complications of left heart catheterisation. *J Royal Coll Phys* 1986;**20**:288.

9 Haapaniemi J *et al*. Massive haemoptysis secondary to flow-directed thermodilution catheters. *Cathet Cardiovasc Diagn* 1979;**5**:151.

10 Grossman W. *Cardiac catheterization and angiography*. Philadelphia, Lea & Febiger, 3rd edn 1986;37.

PART 2
Catheterisation
in specific disorders

CHAPTER 13

Coronary arteriography — coronary artery disease

THE NORMAL CORONARY CIRCULATION [1, 2]

Two coronary arteries supply the normal coronary circulation. The left coronary artery arises from the left sinus of Valsalva at an angle of 25° posterior to the frontal plane. The right coronary artery arises from the right sinus at an angle of 35° to the right of the sagittal plane (Fig. 13.1). In some 50% of subjects the right coronary artery supplies the whole of the right ventricle and through left ventricular and posterior descending branches, the posterior half of the interventricular septum and a large part of the posterior wall of the left ventricle. This pattern of coronary arterial distribution is termed *right dominant* (Fig. 13.2). In 15 to 20% of subjects a *left dominant*

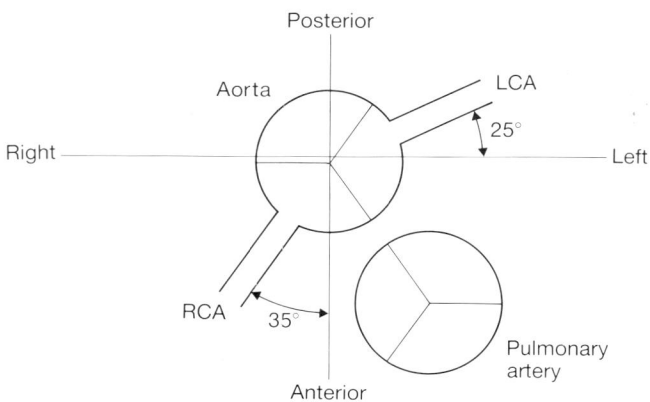

(a)

(b)

Cx

Fig. 13.2 Right dominance. (a) Right dominance — right coronary artery. The posterior descending coronary artery is a branch of the right coronary artery. The right coronary artery supplies the posterior half of the interventricular septum and part of the posterior wall of the left ventricle as well as the right ventricle. (b) Right dominance — left coronary artery. The circumflex left coronary artery (Cx) is a small vessel in 'right dominant' circulations.

Fig. 13.1 Orientation of the origins of the right and left coronary arteries.

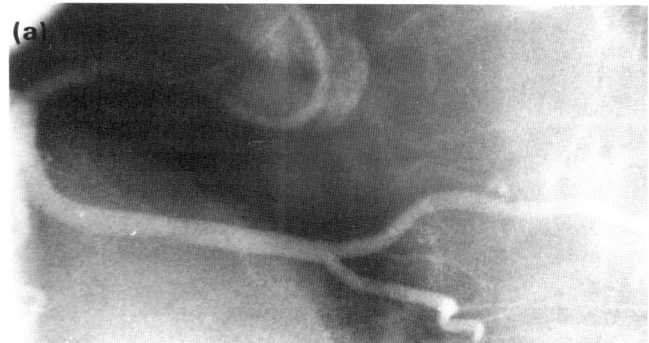

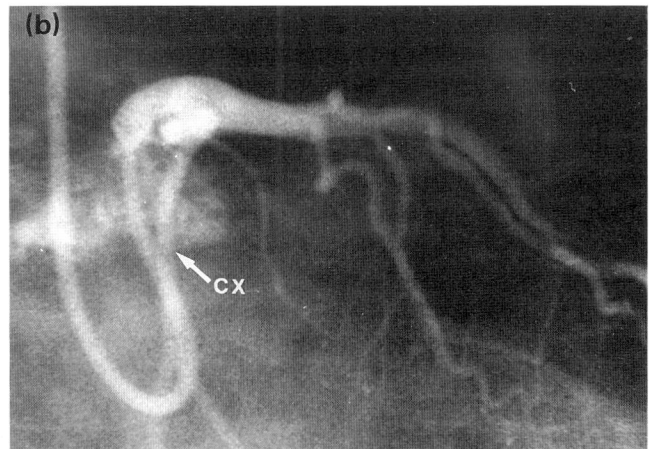

distribution is found (Fig. 13.3). In these the posterior descending coronary artery is a branch of the circumflex left coronary artery and the left coronary supplies the whole of the left ventricle and interventricular septum together with a small part of the right ventricle posteriorly and in the region of the pulmonary conus. In such subjects the right coronary artery is a small vessel supplying only the right ventricle. In the remaining 30 to 35% of the population the circulation is *balanced* with the right coronary supplying the right ventricle and posterior third of the septum while the left coronary supplies the left ventricular free wall and the anterior two-thirds of the septum.

The left coronary artery (Fig. 13.4)

The main left coronary ('left main stem') varies between a few millimetres and a centimetre or so in length. Orientated backwards and to the left at its origin it curves anteriorly beneath the left atrial appendage and to the left of the pulmonary trunk before dividing into its circumflex and anterior descending branches. The anterior descending branch is a direct continuation of the left main stem and lies to left of the pulmonary conus before entering the anterior interventricular groove between the two ventricles. The anterior descending branch runs the length of the interventricular groove to reach the cardiac apex where it turns round to the diaphragmatic surface to terminate in two small branches (Fig. 13.5). The anterior descending left coronary artery (LAD) gives rise to (1) vertically directed branches which supply the interventricular septum, and (2) epicardial branches to the anterolateral free wall of the left ventricle — the so-called *diagonal* branches. Of the former, *septal* branches the first, arising close to the bifurcation of the main stem, is usually a relatively large branch ('the first septal branch') which may divide into two or more subdivisions. The downward course of the septal branches paralleling each other to form a 'pallisade' appearance is characteristic and helps the angiographer identify the anterior descending artery from which the septal branches arise (Fig. 13.5a). The anterior descending is also identified as it is usually the only vessel to reach the cardiac apex. The diagonal branches are variable in number; sometimes there is

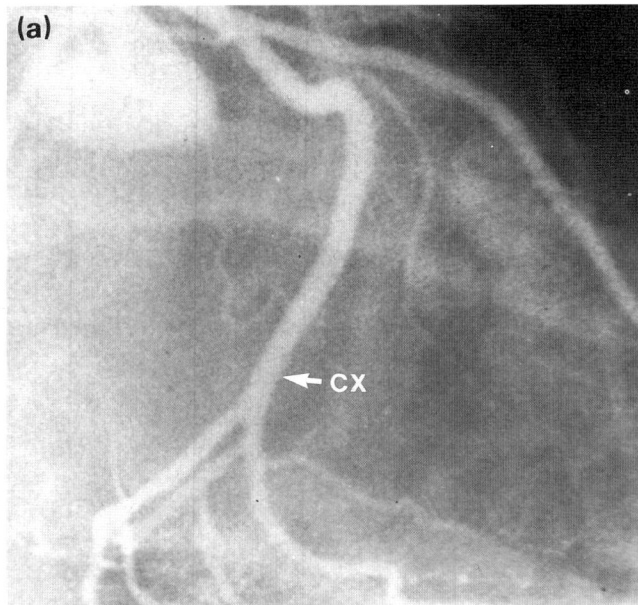

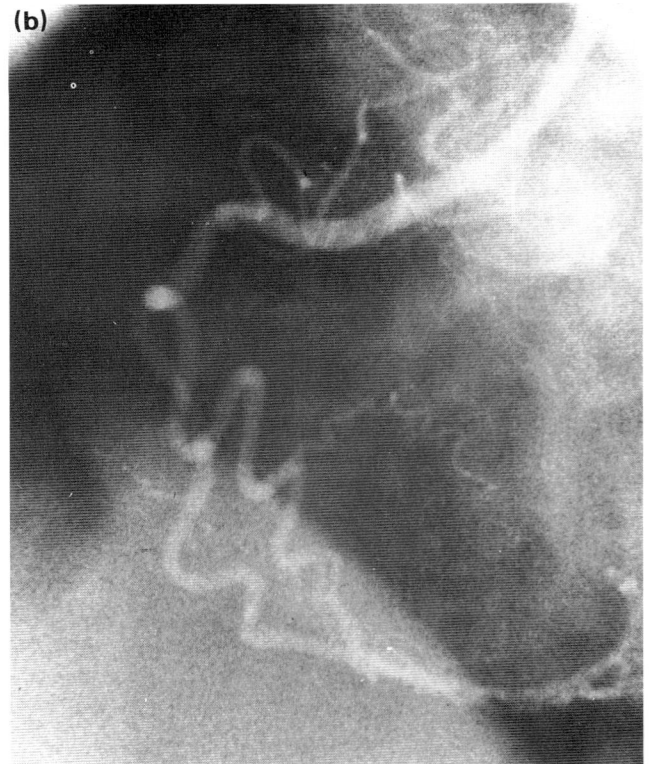

Fig. 13.3 Left dominance. (a) Left dominance — left coronary artery. The left circumflex (Cx) is a large vessel and supplies the posterior descending branch. (b) Left dominance — right coronary artery. The right coronary artery is a small vessel in a 'left dominant' circulation and supplies the right ventricle only.

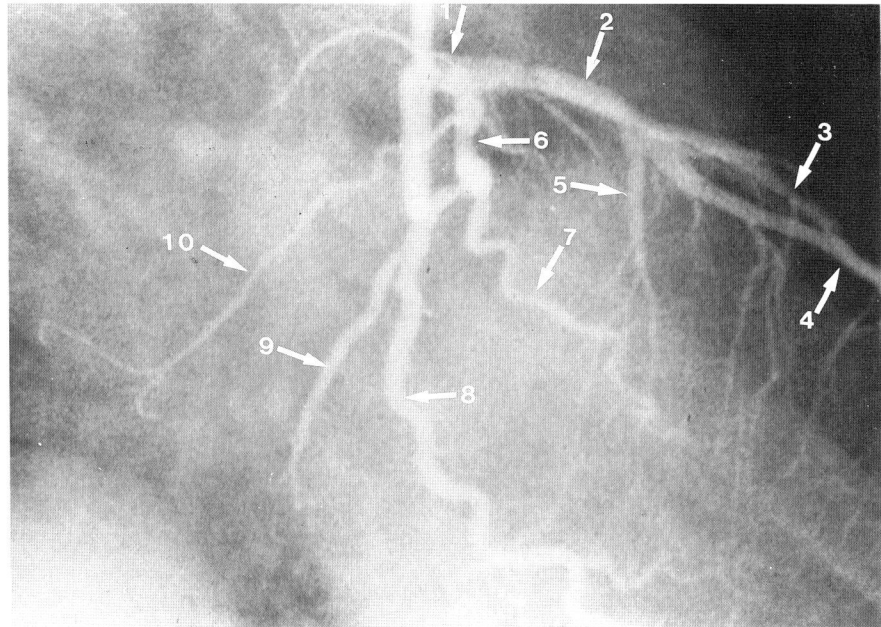

Fig. 13.4 The branches of the left coronary artery as seen in the right oblique projection. (1) Left main stem, (2) left anterior descending branch (LAD), (3) diagonal branch of LAD, (4) distal or apical LAD, (5) 1st septal branch of LAD, (6) main left circumflex (Cx), (7) anterolateral branch of Cx, (8) obtuse marginal branch of Cx, (9) Posterolateral branch of Cx, (10) left atrial circumflex.

one large branch which parallels the anterior descending and may be mistaken for it; particularly if the anterior descending is occluded at its origin. Some branches of the anterior descending course towards the right ventricle and of these one, running towards the pulmonary conus, is relatively constant and may provide an anastomotic supply with the conus branch of the right coronary when either the anterior descending or the right coronary artery are occluded.

The *circumflex* branch of the left coronary artery arises at almost right angles to the main stem and courses posteriorly in the atrioventricular groove (sulcus) towards the crux of the heart. The circumflex left coronary artery gives off a variable (two to four) number of branches which supply the posterolateral aspect of the left ventricular free wall and are termed *obtuse marginal branches*. The first of these is usually a large vessel (sometimes called the *lateral circumflex*) after which there is marked reduction in the calibre

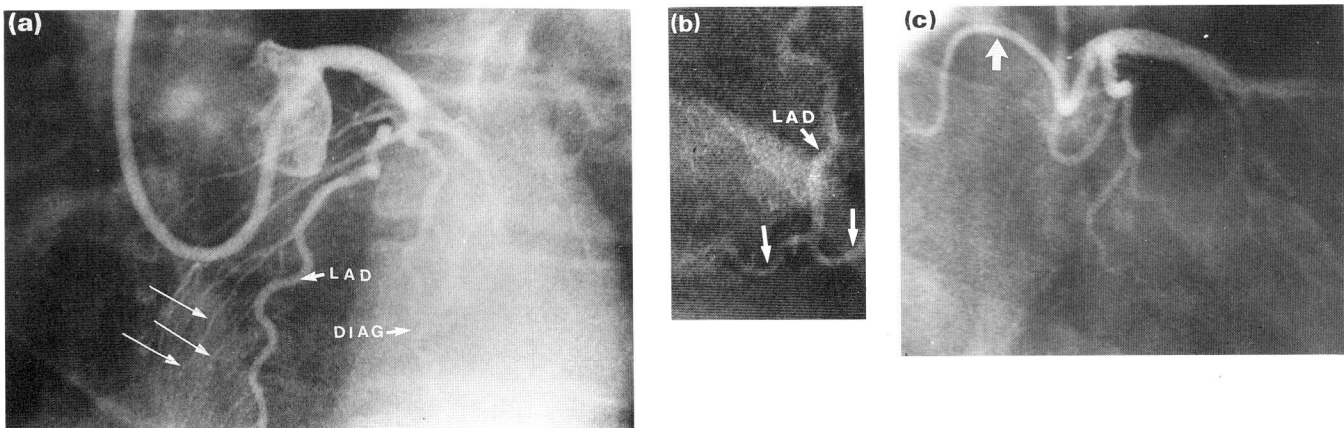

Fig. 13.5 Identification of the left anterior descending (LAD). (a) Septal branches of the LAD (long arrows) forming a 'pallisade' in the LAO projection. (DIAG — diagonal branch of LAD). (b) The distal LAD reaches the apex of the heart and terminates in two small branches (arrows). (c) The sinus node branch (arrow) may be a branch of the right coronary artery (see Fig. 13.6) or, as here, of the circumflex left coronary artery.

of the rest of the circumflex in the atrioventricular groove (Fig. 13.4). In those 15% or so of subjects with a left dominant circulation the circumflex continues as a large vessel in the atrioventricular groove until it reaches the crux of the heart where it turns to run in the posterior interventricular groove as the *posterior descending* coronary artery. In some hearts a large *intermediate artery* arises at the bifurcation of the left coronary artery and supplies territory between the circumflex and anterior descending branches ('trifurcation pattern'). The circumflex also gives off atrial branches and, in some 25 to 30% of hearts, one of these courses over the atrium to reach and encircle the right atrial/superior caval junction to supply the sino-atrial node — the *sinus node branch* [3]. Finally a large atrial branch — the *left atrial circumflex* — may arise from the circumflex and run parallel and superior to it in the atrioventricular groove to supply most of the atrium.

The right coronary artery (Fig. 13.6)

The right coronary artery arises from the right sinus of Valsalva at an angle of 35° to the right of the sagittal plane and runs down the right atrioventricular groove to reach the inferior surface at the

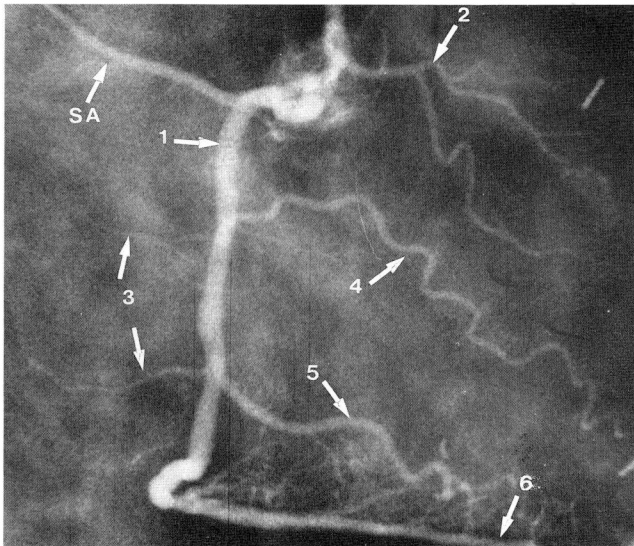

Fig. 13.6 The branches of the right coronary artery as seen in the right oblique projection. (1) Main right coronary artery (RCA), (2) conus branch of RCA, (3) atrial branches: anterior — branch to SA node (SA); intermediate and posterior, (4) right ventricular branch(es), (5) acute marginal branch, (6) posterior descending branch.

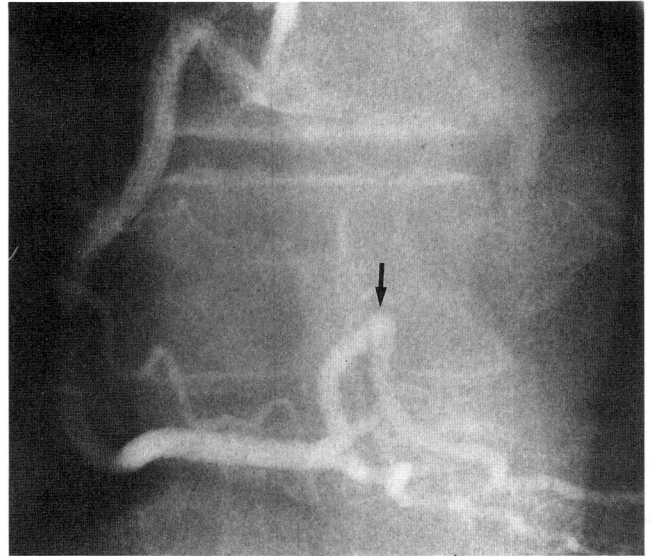

Fig. 13.7 The U-bend (arrow) taken by the left ventricular branch of the right coronary artery.

crux of the heart. The first branch to originate from the right coronary is the *conus branch* running anteriorly to supply the right ventricular outflow tract. In some 40% of subjects the conus branch has a separate origin a millimetre or so anterior to the main ostium of the right coronary. The conus branch is a common source of anastomosis with the left coronary in cases of coronary artery disease. Arising from the right coronary and running in an opposite direction are several atrial branches (*anterior, intermediate and posterior atrial branches*). In approximately 70% of subjects the first of these supplies the sino-atrial node and is seen to encircle the superior vena cava/right atrial junction [3]. Other branches arise at a near right angle and pass forwards and to the left to supply the free wall of the right ventricle. Commonly there is a relatively large right ventricular branch at the acute margin of the heart which runs towards the cardiac apex and may supply some of the posterior part of the interventricular septum. The termination of the right coronary artery depends on whether the circulation is 'right-dominant' or 'left-dominant.' When, as in some 50% of subjects, the right coronary artery is dominant, the vessel continues past the crux to form the posterior descending coronary artery in the posterior interventricular groove. When this is the pattern the artery usually bifurcates just before the crux and a second branch (*left ventricular branch*) enters the myocardium

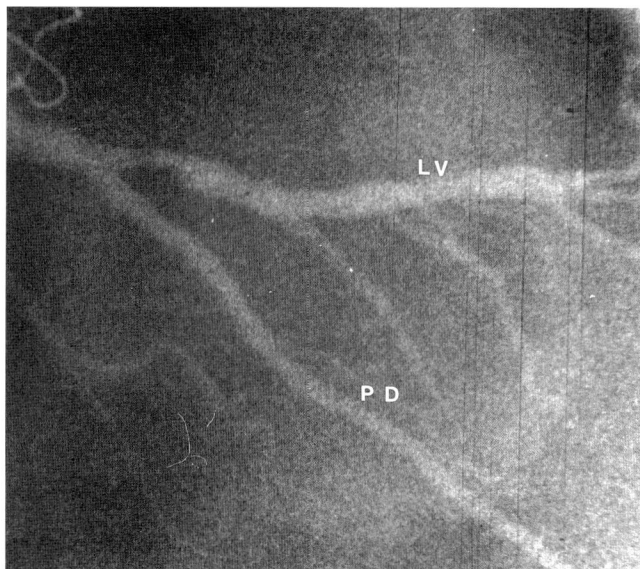

Fig. 13.8 Dominant right coronary artery. This left oblique cranial view displays the distal branches of the right coronary artery — the posterior descending branch (PD) and left ventricular branches (LV).

with a pronounced U-bend to emerge to the left of the posterior descending branch and supply a part of the posterior aspect of the left ventricle in parallel with (small) terminal branches of the circumflex (Figs 13.7 and 13.8). The right dominant pattern with the right coronary artery supplying the posterior descending is, in reality, part of a spectrum in which there is a reciprocal balance between the circumflex and right coronary arteries. In left-dominant circulation the right coronary is a small vessel supplying the right ventricle only. Between these extremes about 30% of subjects have a balanced circulation in which the right coronary only extends a short way beyond the crux and into the posterior interventricular groove.

CORONARY ARTERIOGRAPHY — TECHNIQUES

Two techniques will be described; the Judkins technique of percutaneous transfemoral coronary arteriography and a transbrachial technique using a preformed (Castillo) catheter. Other techniques using other catheters are in use — notably the Sones technique [4, 5] — but the two techniques described

here are both excellent and provide examples of the two main options: percutaneous transfemoral and transbrachial by arteriotomy. The catheters used for the two techniques have been described in Chapter 3 and the techniques of percutaneous entry and arteriotomy in Chapter 4.

Judkins technique (Fig. 13.9) [6, 7]

Percutaneous transfemoral coronary arteriography can be performed using the traditional Seldinger technique but is probably best done using an introducing sheath fitted with a haemostatic valve. A pigtail catheter which has been straightened with a guide wire is introduced first and advanced to the thoracic aorta when the guide wire can be removed. The guide wire should be used to lead the catheter through the tortuous femoral and iliac arteries. It may be wise to use a guide wire with a J-tip to guard against the danger of lodging the guide beneath an atheromatous plaque and thus causing an intimal dissection. Certainly such a wire should be used if there is any difficulty in advancing the wire and catheter; alternative 'movable core' or 'tapered core' guide wires should be available in case of any continuing difficulty. Neither guide wires nor catheters should ever be advanced against resistance.

Whole body heparinisation is advisable during coronary arteriography to guard against the danger of thrombus formation on the guide wire or catheter tip resulting in coronary (or cerebral) embolisation. Heparin in a dose of 0.5 mg/kg (e.g. 3000–5000 units in an adult male) should be given through the pigtail catheter at this stage. The catheter is then advanced around the aortic arch and across the aortic valve to enter the left ventricle. This manoeuvre is described in Chapter 5. The catheter tip should be positioned in the inlet or mid-cavity of the ventricle and in a position which does not generate ectopic beats. A left ventriculogram is performed using 30–50 ml of contrast medium injected at no more than 15 ml/second. If single plane angiography is to be used a 45° right oblique projection is preferred. Biplane angiography is best performed by adding a 60° left oblique projection with 25° of cranial angulation. Left ventriculography is more fully described in Chapter 6. Left ventricular systolic and diastolic pressures should be recorded before angiography is performed since the introduction of contrast medium can affect, particularly, the diastolic pressures.

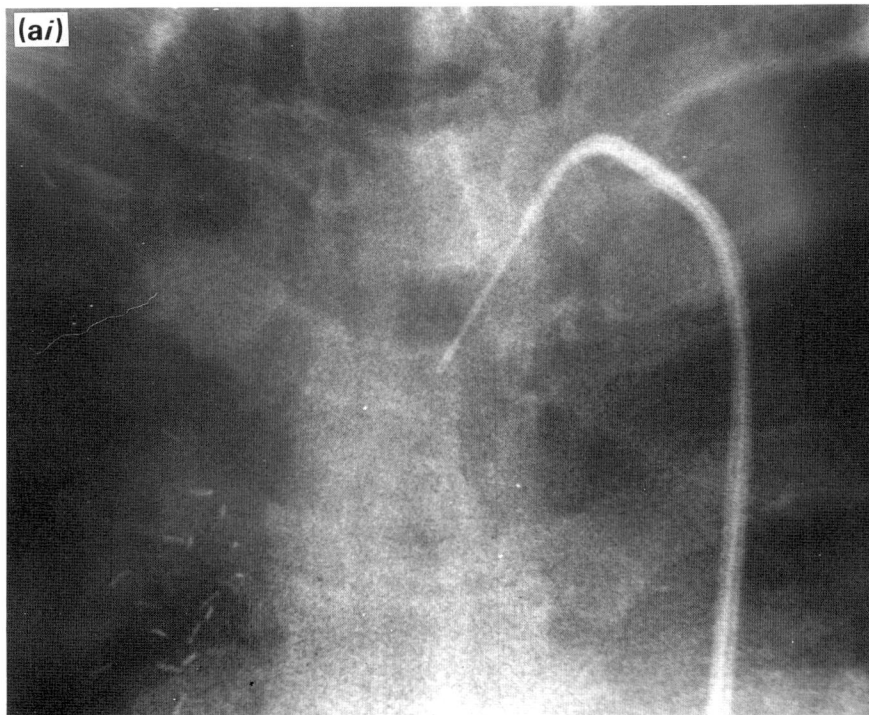

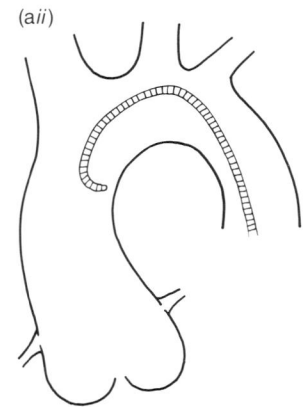

Fig. 13.9 The Judkins technique of coronary arteriography. Cannulation of the left coronary artery, left oblique projection. (a*i* and *ii*) Do not remove the guide wire until the catheter is in this position — around the aortic arch.

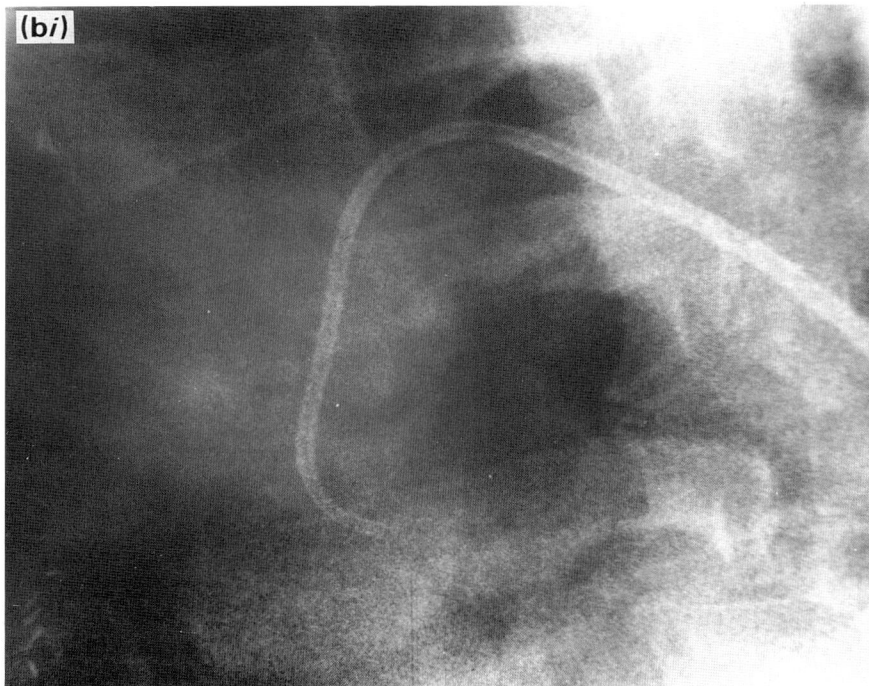

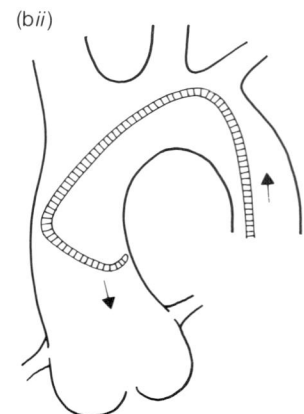

(b*i* and *ii*) Advance the catheter *slowly*; the tip moves down the aortic wall until it engages the left coronary as in (c).

(ci)

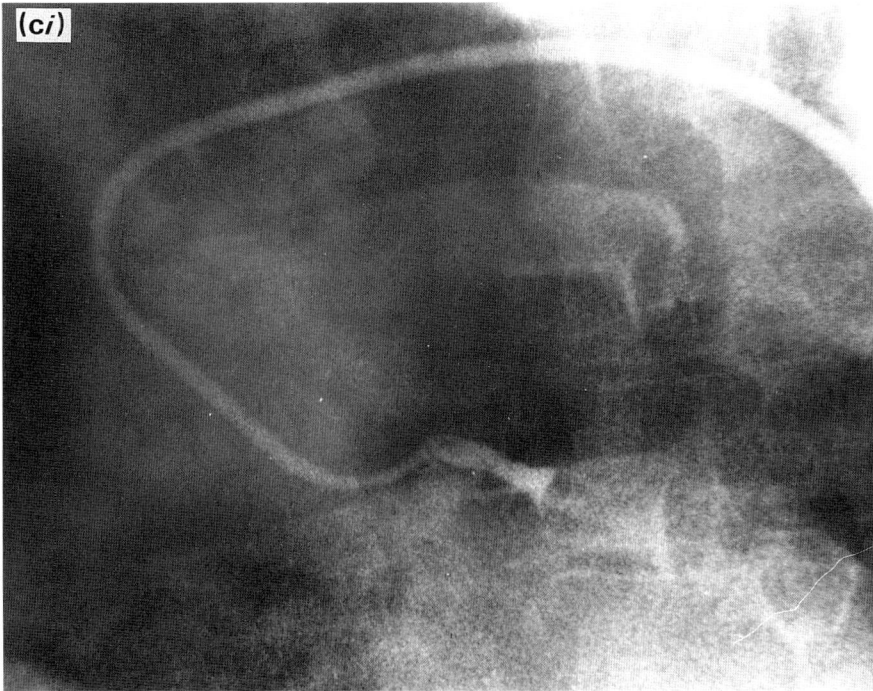

(cii)

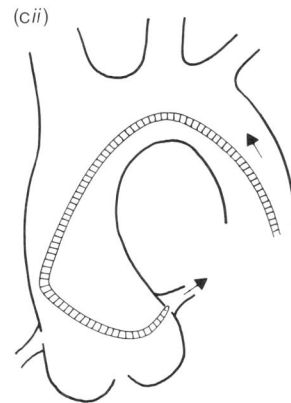

(*ci* and *ii*) The left coronary is engaged. The tip will move slightly to the left at this moment.

(di)

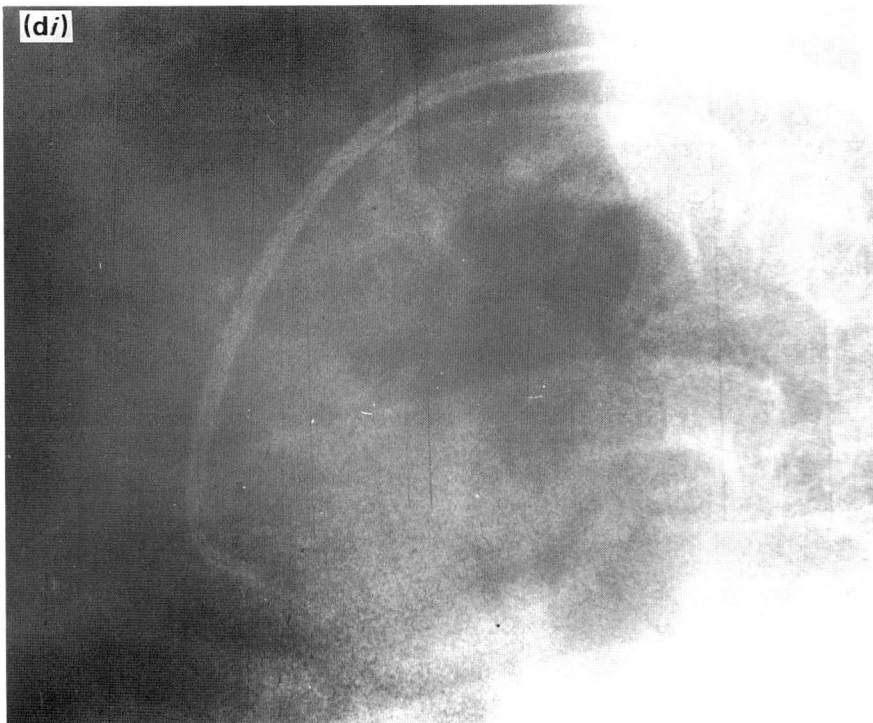

(dii)

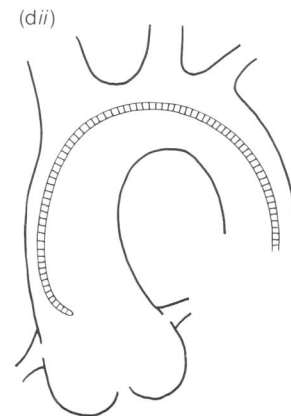

(*di* and *ii*) Judkins technique — Right coronary artery. Advance the catheter until its tip is 2–4 cm above the aortic valve. Rotate the catheter *very slowly* clockwise. The catheter will advance, of its own accord, towards the aortic valve and the right sinus.

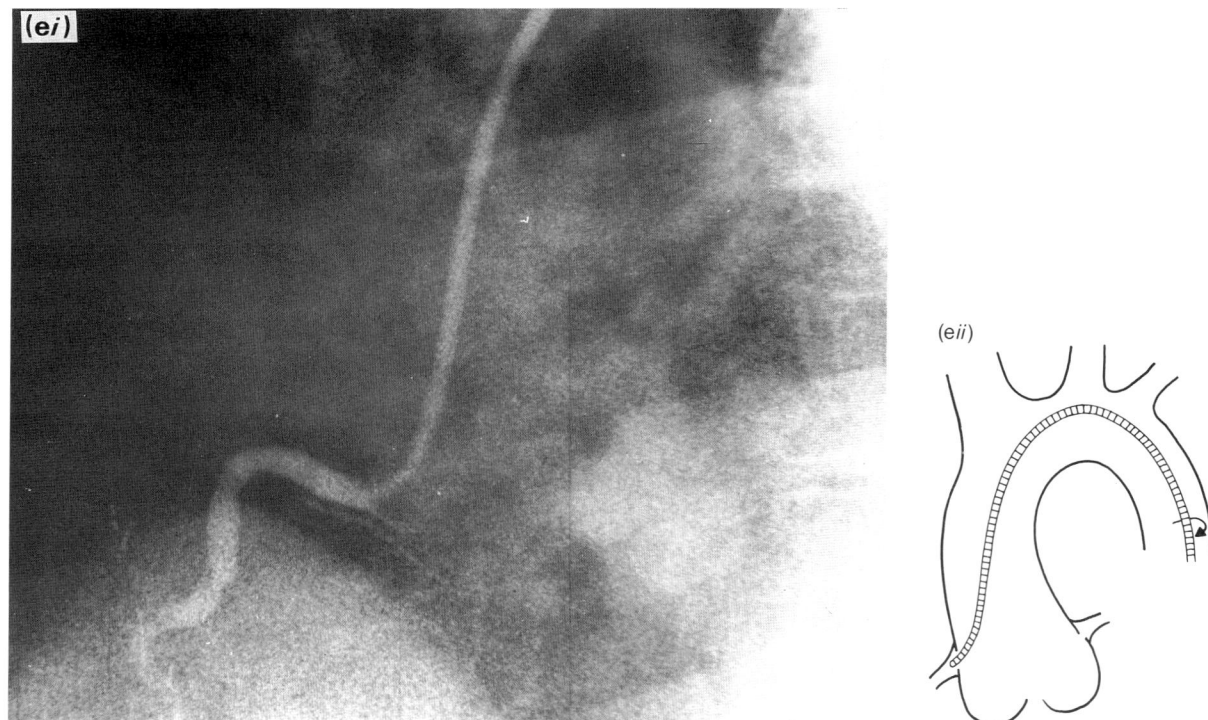

Fig. 13.9 *cont.* (e*i* and *ii*) Continue slow rotation until the tip moves slightly to the right as it engages the ostium. An alternative technique is to advance the catheter to the aortic valve and to withdraw the catheter 2–4 cm during the slow clockwise rotation.

Glyceryl trinitrate: in many laboratories, and in ours, it is routine to administer sublingual glyceryl trinitrate 500 μg immediately before performing coronary arteriography as this will protect against catheter-induced coronary arterial spasm. Any stenotic lesions that are seen can then be assumed to be due to atherosclerotic lesions and not spasm. It is impossible to demonstrate that this practice increases the safety of the procedure but it is with the feeling that it does that we have adopted this policy. The only exception to this practice occurs if a patient is being studied in whom the referring diagnosis includes the possibility of spasm (Prinzmetal angina) as a cause of symptoms.

The pigtail catheter is now removed and replaced by a *left Judkins catheter*. These catheters are available in several sizes designated according to the length of the secondary arm (i.e. from the apex of the 180° curve to the beginning of the final curved tip). For most patients a 4 cm left Judkins is appropriate but in patients with an elongated or dilated ascending aorta left coronary cannulation may require a 5 or even 6 cm left Judkins catheter. As with the pigtail the left Judkins catheter must be straightened with a

guide wire before insertion and this guide wire must lead the catheter through the iliac artery and aorta. The guide wire must not be withdrawn until the catheter has traversed the aortic arch; premature removal of the guide wire will result in the catheter adopting its 180° curve within the descending thoracic aorta and it may then be difficult to restraighten the catheter. If this does happen it may be necessary to withdraw the catheter to the level of the iliac bifurcation so as to engage the tip in the left internal iliac artery. Further withdrawal will then straighten the catheter and permit the guide wire to be re-advanced beyond the catheter tip and into the thoracic aorta. With the catheter tip in the ascending aorta fluoroscopy is changed to a 25° LAO projection and the catheter advanced further until a sharp leftward movement indicates that the tip has engaged the left coronary ostium. During this manoeuvre it is important that the curve of the catheter is seen in profile; any departure from this appearance indicates that the catheter is rotated and must be corrected by gentle counter-rotation. A 25° LAO projection is selected as this places the first part of the left coronary at right angles to the X-ray beam. The pressure at the catheter tip must be constantly monitored and displayed throughout this final manoeuvre and at all times during coronary arteriography except when contrast medium is being injected through the catheter. A damped pressure may be due to ostial or left main stem stenosis and the catheter should be withdrawn and a semi-selective (sinus of Valsalva) injection performed to elucidate this.

When left coronary arteriography is complete the catheter is withdrawn a centimetre or so and the guide wire re-inserted as far as the tip to allow the catheter to be withdrawn and replaced by a right Judkins catheter.

The *right Judkins catheter* is also available in 4, 5 and 6 cm sizes and again the 4 cm is the most generally useful with longer secondary arms being suitable for patients with a dilated ascending aorta. Again the catheter is straightened and lead through the vessels by the guide wire though this can be removed somewhat earlier — in the thoracic aorta or aortic arch. Cannulation of the right coronary artery is slightly more difficult than the left. The first step is to advance the catheter tip to a position just above the aortic valve; at this stage, with fluoroscopy in a slightly steeper (55°) LAO projection, the catheter tip will point to the left. The catheter is now *slowly* rotated in a clockwise direction. This clockwise rotation will result in the catheter straightening and advancing itself so that at the same time it must be *slowly* withdrawn a centimetre or so. An alternative technique is to start by positioning the catheter tip 2–3 cm above the level of the aortic valve; as the catheter advances itself during *slow* clockwise rotation the tip will move down the aortic wall and engage the right coronary ostium. If these manoeuvres are successful a slight rightward movement of the catheter tip will announce engagement in the right coronary ostium. Usually the position has to be held by the operator as residual torque would otherwise cause the catheter to disengage. Pressure must be continuously monitored; a damped pressure record may indicate that the catheter tip (which is no. 5F) is occluding a small (non-dominant) right coronary or has entered a separate origin of a conus branch. Alternatively the catheter may be seen to have advanced itself a long way down the right coronary and should be withdrawn, slowly, until it is engaged within the ostium only. Cautious infusion of contrast medium will clarify the situation. It should be remembered that these catheters have no side

holes to relieve pressure or allow antegrade flow through an occluding catheter.

Following right coronary arteriography the catheter may be withdrawn (without the need for a guide wire) and the procedure is completed by manual compression of the femoral artery for 10 minutes (or as long as is necessary to obtain haemostasis). Ideally compression should be firm enough to prevent haematoma formation while still allowing the foot pulses to be felt.

In the vast majority of cases the Judkins technique allows successful completion of coronary arteriography without difficulty and in a very short time — less than 10 minutes.

Occasionally cannulation of one to other coronary artery will be found or be impossible despite using different sizes of Judkins catheters. If this happens there is a need for an alternative technique which will still utilise the transfemoral entry site. An alternative which will almost always succeed if the Judkins technique had failed is to employ the Amplatz technique [8]. Amplatz catheters resemble very closely the catheters used for the Castillo technique described below but are available for both the transfemoral and transbrachial approach. Used from the femoral artery a left Amplatz catheter is introduced over a guide wire until the tip lies just above the aortic valve when its position resembles that adopted by a right Judkins catheter — that is the tip will point to the left. The guide wire is removed and further advancement of the catheter (25° LAO projection) will cause the secondary curve to rest on the right aortic cusp while the tip advances to, and engages in, the left coronary ostium. For this manoeuvre to be successful it is essential to have the correct radius curve; Amplatz catheters are available in three sizes suitable for small, normal or large aortic roots. Cannulation of the right coronary artery by the Amplatz technique is achieved in much the same way as with the right Judkins catheter; slow clockwise rotation accompanied by slow withdrawal of a centimetre or so.

Transbrachial coronary arteriography — Castillo technique (Fig. 13.10) [9, 10]

The advantage of a cut-down, as distinct from a percutaneous technique, it that reliable haemostasis

Fig. 13.10 The Castillo technique of coronary arteriography (brachial approach). Left coronary artery: (a*i* and *ii*) Initial catheter position, tip in right or non-coronary sinus.

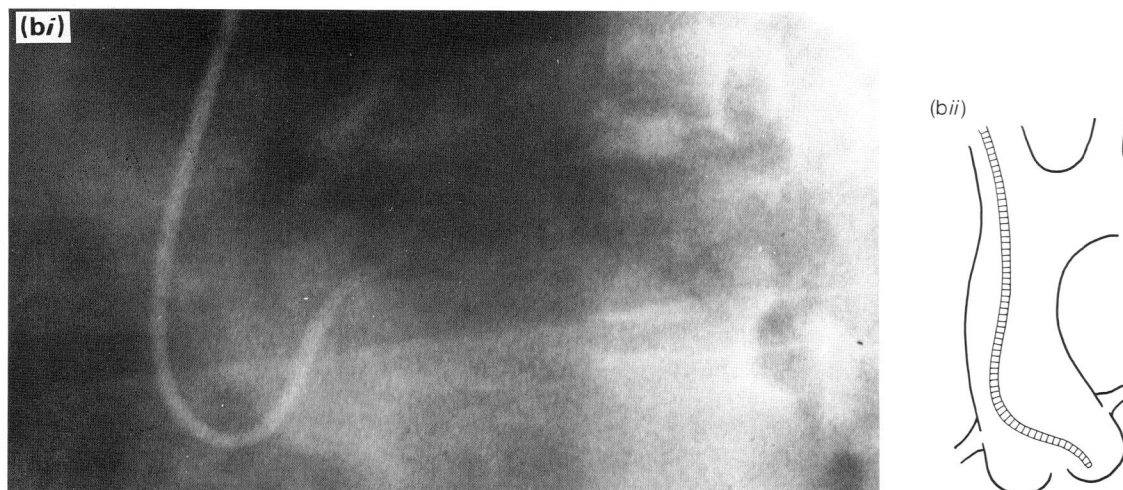

(b*i* and *ii*) 'Lift' the tip over the aortic cusps until it moves to the left into the left sinus.

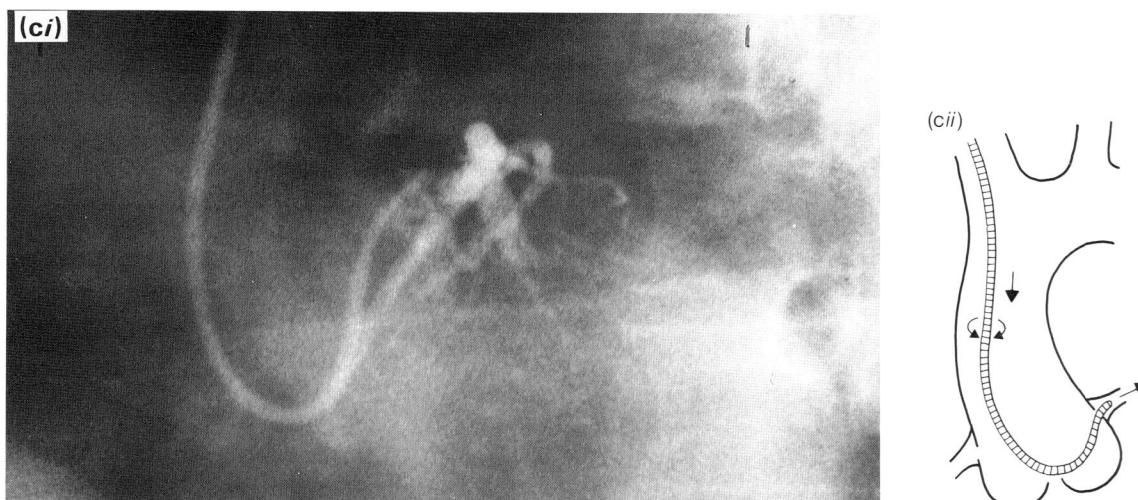

(c*i* and *ii*) Advance the catheter so that its tip moves upwards to engage the left coronary ostium when it will move slightly to the left. A few degrees of clockwise or anti-clockwise rotation may be needed during this manoeuvre.

(d*i*)

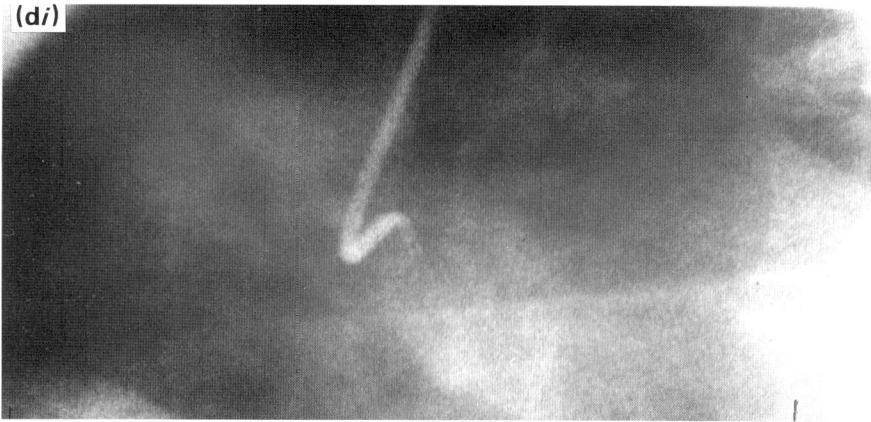

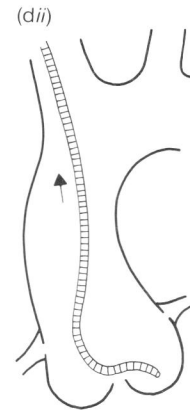

Right coronary artery: (d*i* and *ii*) Disengage the catheter from the left coronary (or advance to this position in the left sinus if the right coronary is to be cannulated first).

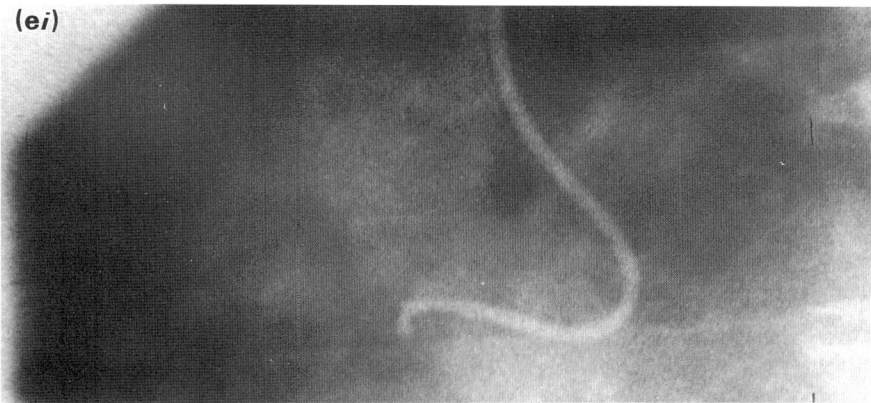

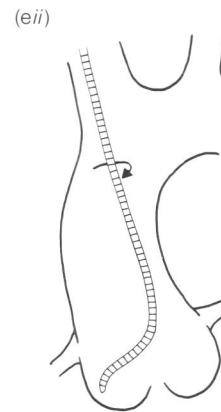

(e*i*)

(e*ii*)

(e*i* and *ii*) *Slowly* rotate anti-clockwise to this position with the tip of the catheter in the right sinus.

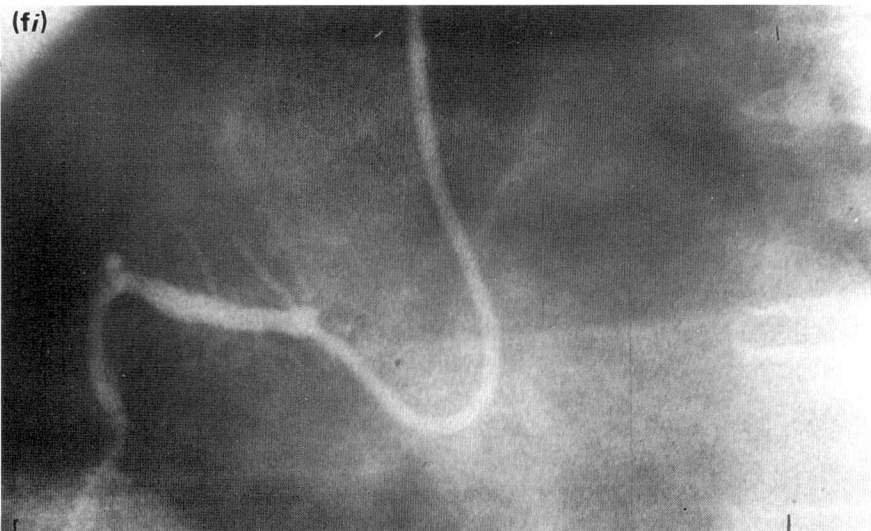

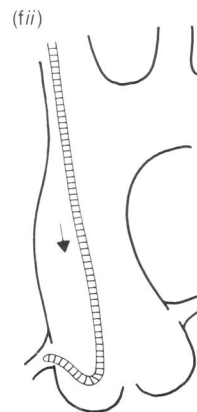

(f*i*)

(f*ii*)

(f*i* and *ii*) *Slowly* advance the catheter until the tip engages the right coronary ostium.

(g*ii*)

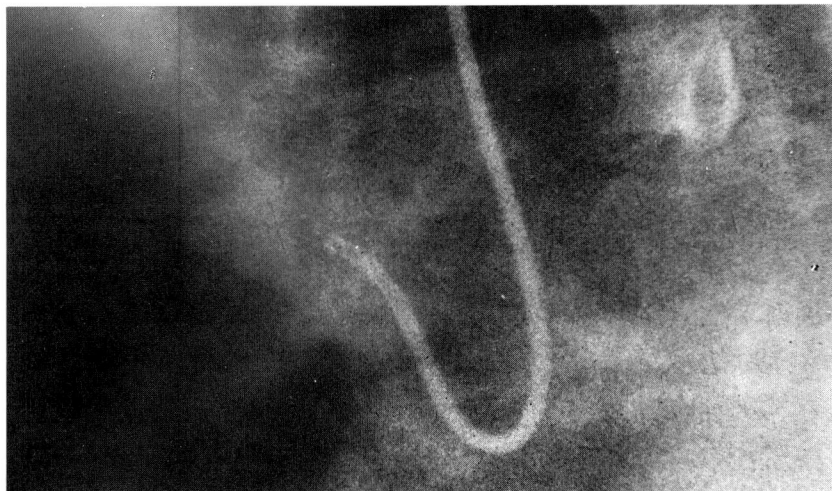

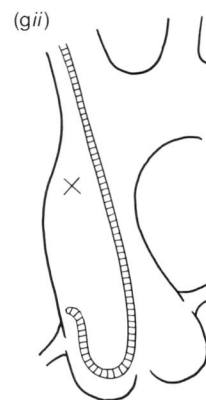

Do not allow a 'loop' to form as in (g*i* and *ii*) — but this position, with the tip exploring the anterior aortic wall, is the starting position for graft cannulation.

is obtained immediately the artery has been repaired so that patients studied in this way can be discharged from hospital the same day. This has attractions for the patients, most of whom would prefer to be admitted as day cases rather than having to remain in hospital overnight. It also means that the cost of the investigation is less. Most investigators are reluctant to discharge a patient on the same day that a percutaneous arterial puncture has been performed; there is always the danger of late bleeding from the puncture site.

One reason why the Judkins percutaneous approach has found so much favour is that cannulation of the coronary arteries with preshaped catheters is much easier than with the original, transbrachial, Sones catheter. The situation has been transformed by the development of preshaped catheters designed to be inserted from the arm by a brachial arteriotomy. The Castillo brachial coronary catheter is such a catheter.

The technique involves a cut-down on the brachial artery. A pigtail catheter is lead into the artery by a guide wire and advanced to the ascending aorta. Heparin is then given through this catheter at a dose of 1.0 mg/kg (e.g. 7000 units for a 70 kg man) and, after recording aortic pressure, is advanced to the left ventricle for ventriculography. This catheter is then replaced with a Castillo coronary arteriography catheter and sublingual glyceryl trinitrate given in preparation for coronary arteriography. Castillo coronary arteriography catheters are available

in three sizes of which the smallest is of use in patients of slender build and the largest in those with a dilated aortic root. The standard Castillo catheters have no side-holes but are much improved by the addition of four side-holes — a modification readily available from the manufacturers (Cordis Corporation). The catheter is advanced until its tip lies in the left sinus of Valsalva. At this stage the tip will be pointing inferiorly and to the left. The catheter must not be allowed to form a loop during its passage down the ascending aorta and may need to be rotated slightly during this manoeuvre so that this does not happen. It is often found that the catheter tip engages the right (or possibly the non-coronary) sinus. Minimal withdrawal and slight rotation followed by further advancement will result in the catheter tip being seen to move sharply to the left as it rides over the aortic cusps and comes to rest in the left coronary sinus. Once the catheter tip is in the left coronary sinus it can be further advanced so that the secondary curve presses against the right coronary cusp while the tip moves superiorly and to the left to engage the ostium of the left coronary artery. The moment of engagement is usually signalled by a sudden further leftward and superior movement of the catheter tip. If the ostium is not immediately engaged small clockwise or anticlockwise rotations, short of reversing the orientation of the tip, will usually succeed. In patients with a dilated aortic root or a high take-off of the left coronary the catheter tip will not reach the ostium; the catheter must be changed to the large size (no. III). In some patients with a small aortic root there is not enough room to accommodate the curve of the catheter which will have to be changed to the smaller size (no. I). In 90% of patients success will be achieved with the standard size (no. II).

Following left coronary arteriography the catheter is removed from the left coronary ostium, rotated so that the tip points inferiorly and to the right and lies in the right coronary sinus. If, at this stage, the catheter is advanced slightly it will engage the right coronary ostium and allow a right coronary arteriogram to be performed with the same catheter. Again small clockwise or anticlockwise rotations may help at this stage. The catheter must not be allowed to form a loop in the ascending aorta; if it does it will have to be withdrawn to the aortic arch until it is straight and then carefully re-advanced to the left coronary sinus when rotation to the right can be repeated. Cannulation of the right coronary artery is marginally more difficult than of the left. If the right coronary cannot be entered the catheter should be changed to a right Judkins catheter (introduced through the arteriotomy) which will almost always overcome the problem.

Other popular techniques of coronary arteriography include the multipurpose transfemoral technique, which does away with the need for multiple catheter changes [11], and the El Gamal modification of the multipurpose catheter which is used for coronary arteriography but not for ventriculography [12].

AORTOCORONARY GRAFTS

Saphenous vein coronary bypass grafts are inserted into the anterolateral surface of the ascending aorta. As a rule grafts to the right coronary are inserted close to the aortic valve (2—3 cm above the native right coronary ostium) and in the most lateral position. Grafts to the circumflex and diagonal branches of the left coronary artery are the most distal (cephalad) and anterior in origin while grafts to the anterior descending branch take origin from an intermediate position (Figs 13.11 to 13.14). Occasionally grafts are inserted in a very anterior and leftward position so that they appear to take origin from the lesser curve of the aorta — cannulation of such grafts can be difficult. Some surgeons place radio-opaque markers at

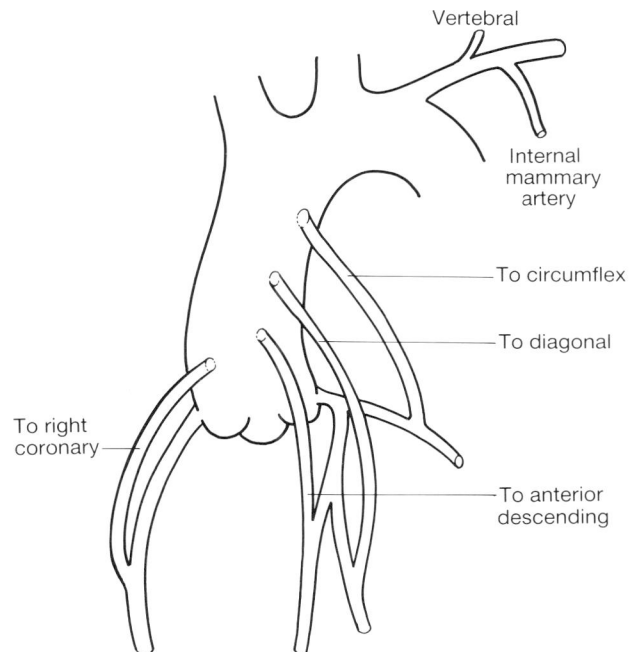

Fig. 13.11 The usual arrangement of saphenous vein graft attachments to the ascending aorta.

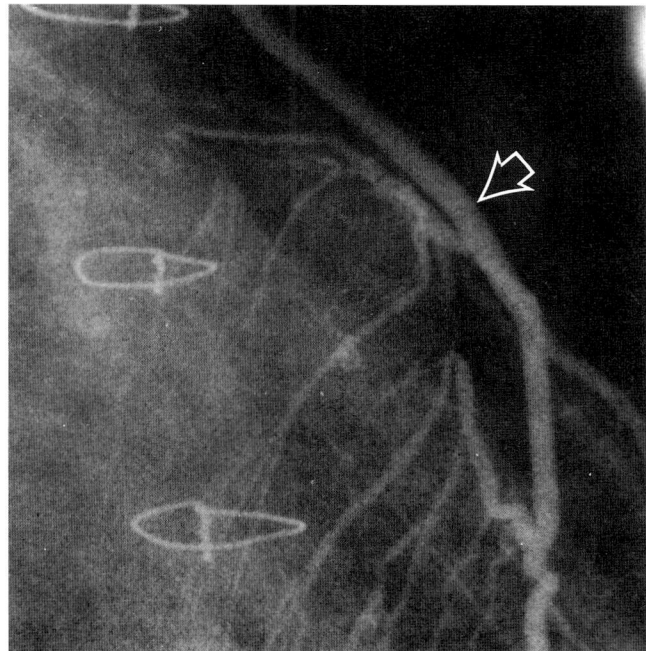

Fig. 13.12 Saphenous vein bypass graft (arrow) to diagonal and distal branches of the left anterior descending. Side-to-side anastomosis to the diagonal, end-to-side to distal LAD; a 'jump' graft.

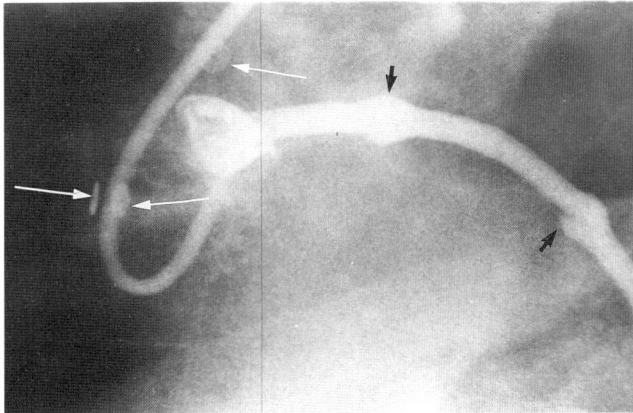

Fig. 13.13 Vein graft with venous valves clearly seen (black arrows). The points of aortic anastomosis have been marked, at the time of operation, with radio-opaque 'sequins' (white arrows).

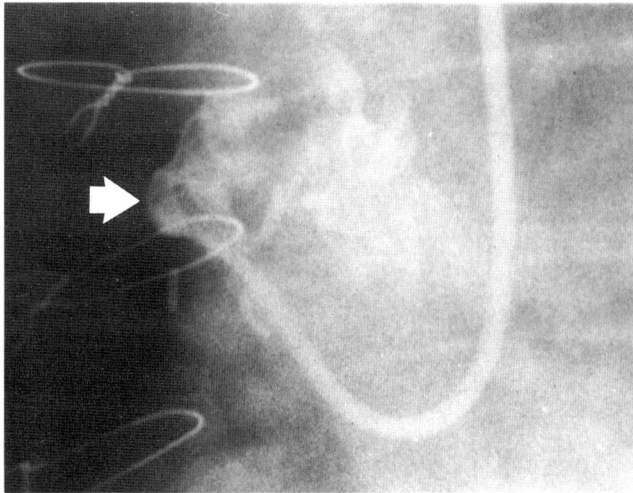

Fig. 13.14 The appearances of an occluded vein graft leaving a 'nipple' on the anterior aortic wall (arrow). There is faint filling of another (patent) graft arising just above the origin of the occluded graft.

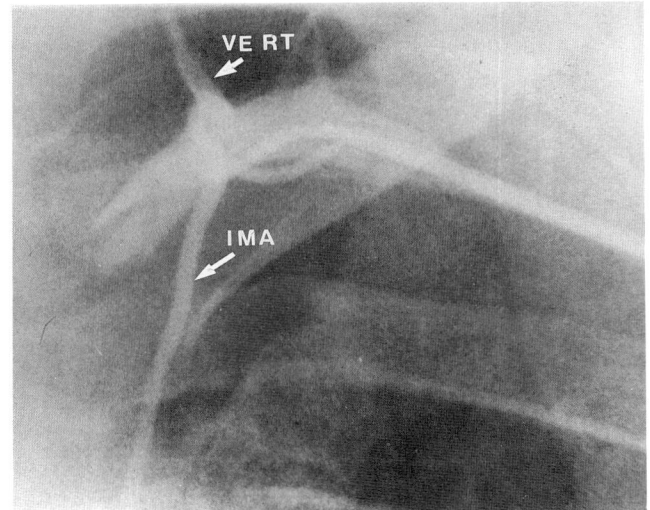

Fig. 13.15 The origin of the internal mammary artery (IMA) is close to the origin of the vertebral artery (VERT). In this example catheterisation has been from the left arm.

Technique of graft catheterisation

FEMORAL APPROACH

A right Judkins catheter frequently allows cannulation of *right coronary grafts* and may allow cannulation of left coronary grafts; since postoperative studies require restudy of the native coronary circulation as well as the grafts catheter changes may be minimised of this catheter is used in the first instance. The technique of cannulation is as follows. With fluoroscopy in a 60° left oblique projection the catheter is positioned just above the right coronary ostium (slow clockwise rotation and withdrawal from the leftward starting position). Further slow withdrawal with slight variations in rotation will allow the operator to explore the lateral and anterior wall of the aorta and, hopefully, to engage the graft ostium. The reverse procedure, advancing the catheter from a position cephalad to the graft ostium while still maintaining rightward and anterior orientation of the tip, is equally appropriate. If neither approach is successful the catheter is changed to one of several alternative patterns. The femoral-right coronary by-pass catheter is very similar to the right Judkins catheter except that the primary curve (the curve at the tip) is 110 to 120° instead of 90°. In fact this catheter can be used for cannulating the native right coronary just as the right coronary catheter can be

the anastomotic sites; these may be helpful but may also migrate and provide an unreliable guide to the position of the graft ostia.

Internal mammary artery grafts as illustrated in Fig. 13.15 (usually to the anterior descending branch of the left coronary artery) arise from the antero-inferior aspect of the left subclavian artery just distal to the origin of the vertebral artery. Occasionally the right internal mammary artery is used and will be found to originate just distal to the origin of the common carotid artery.

used to cannulate grafts. A standard (II) Amplatz right coronary catheter is an excellent alternative; the object is always to use a configuration that will allow the tip of the catheter to press against the anterior surface of the aorta during exploration. Another catheter which will do this is a modification of the Sidewinder catheter originally used for carotid cannulation; graft cannulation has been reported to be easy and quick when this catheter is used [13].

Left coronary grafts are best cannulated using a special femoral left coronary bypass catheter which differs from the right bypass catheter in having a more pronounced (70°) secondary curve. Cannulation is achieved by positioning the tip at a level which is slightly higher than the origin of a right graft and then rotating the tip anteriorly until it points slightly to the left of the mid-point. Fluoroscopy in the right oblique projection may be preferable to the left oblique in some instances.

Internal mammary artery cannulation requires the use of yet another special catheter. The important difference between this and right coronary and graft catheters is that the tip points backwards on itself; the primary curve is less than 90°. Without this backwards-pointing tip it would be difficult to engage the sharp take-off of the internal mammary artery from the subclavian. The tip is also slightly longer so that it is pressed against the antero-inferior surface of the subclavian artery. The backwards-pointing tip makes initial cannulation of the subclavian slightly more difficult than it would be with a straighter catheter. Clockwise rotation to explore the anterior and superior aspect of the aortic arch and the use of a straight guide wire to straighten the catheter may be helpful. The guide wire is removed after the catheter has been advanced beyond the origin of the internal mammary artery; slow withdrawal of the catheter while maintaining an antero-inferior orientation of the tip should now allow its engagement in the acutely angled origin of the internal mammary artery.

Attempts at internal mammary artery catheterisation can be uncomfortable for the patient. Test injections of contrast medium into the subclavian artery and branches supplying the chest wall cause an unpleasant burning sensation; the patient needs to be warned of this and it may be wise to use 50% dilutions of contrast until the internal mammary artery has been satisfactorily engaged. Cortical blindness (which resolves in 12–4 hours) is a possible complication if excessive amounts of contrast have been injected close to the vertebral artery.

BRACHIAL APPROACH

The Castillo technique of transbrachial coronary arteriography has been described previously and the Castillo catheter has proved an excellent catheter for graft cannulation. Using a left oblique projection the anterior and lateral wall of the ascending aorta is explored cephalad to the origin of the native right coronary artery. Whenever the tip of the catheter is felt, and seen, to engage in a structure a test injection is made and will usually demonstrate a saphenous vein bypass graft.

Internal mammary artery: while cannulation of the ipsilateral internal mammary artery is easily achieved from the brachial approach access to the contralateral subclavian and internal mammary artery is difficult. As a result the transfemoral approach may be selected in patients with a left internal mammary graft. However Singh [14] has reported successful selective cannulation of the contralateral internal mammary in 78% of attempts by using a specially designed catheter (Cordis Corporation). The catheter has two preformed curves; an 80° curve 7.5 cm from the tip and smaller (1 cm) curve at the tip which is orientated in the opposite direction (Fig. 2.8). A loop is formed by pushing the catheter tip against the aortic valve and the looped catheter pulled back into the ascending aorta where a sudden pull will recover the primary curve with the tip directed towards the left part of the aortic arch. Further manipulation will engage the origin of the contralateral subclavian whereupon pulling on the catheter will cause the tip to advance towards the orifice of the internal mammary.

CORONARY ARTERIOGRAPHY — GENERAL REMARKS

It is important to monitor continuously the pressure at the catheter tip throughout the procedure; only when contrast medium is actually being injected is this pressure record momentarily lost. This requires a manifold with two or three side-arms. One side-arm is connected to a reservoir containing contrast medium and the other to the manometer/flush.

Contrast is drawn into a 10 ml syringe from the side-arm at every opportunity without loss of the pressure record. Approximately 6 to 8 ml of contrast medium will be required for satisfactory opacification of the left coronary; 3 to 4 ml are usually adequate for the right coronary. The amount of contrast needed is assessed visually and not by a rigid protocol. The pressure record should display an undamped arterial (aortic) waveform. A low pressure or damped record may indicate that the catheter tip has traversed a proximal (e.g. left main stem) stenosis, is in a small branch (e.g. conus branch of the right coronary) or has advanced itself some way beyond the ostium (particularly liable to occur during right coronary cannulation). On occasion the pressure record will change to one that has a low diastolic pressure resembling a ventricular pressure. Such 'ventricularised' records have much the same significance as a damped record; in all cases the catheter should be withdrawn while the operator assesses the situation. A left main stem or ostial stenosis requires a semi-selective (sinus) injection for safe visualisation. On occasion a damped or ventricularised record may have to be accepted — as when the catheter will only remain in the right coronary artery when it has advanced some way down the vessel — but extreme caution and speed in completing the investigation is then indicated.

RADIOLOGICAL PROJECTIONS

It is conventional to describe projections used in radiology according to the direction to the X-ray beam; thus a chest X-ray obtained with the tube behind the patient and the film in front is termed a 'PA' (postero-anterior) film. A different convention is used to describe the projections employed in the catheterisation laboratory. The projections are named according to the position of the image intensifier. Thus the view obtained is that which an observer would have of the heart and coronary arteries if his face were in the same position as the intensifier. An anterior view is that obtained with the intensifier vertically above the patient's chest (and the X-ray tube below the table); if the intensifier is now rotated 45° to the left the view obtained is a left anterior oblique (LAO). If, from this position, the intensifier is now tilted towards the patient's head so as to lie above his left shoulder the view is termed 'LAO cranial'; tilted towards the patients feet the view would be 'LAO caudal'. Greater precision is provided if the degree of rotation and the degree of tilt is specified; thus we can define a view as, for example, 45° LAO, 30° cranial.

In order to visualise three-dimensional structures such as the coronary arteries it is necessary to obtain two views at roughly right angles to each other and

Table 13.1   Suggested sequence of angiographic projections for coronary arteriography.

View no.	Projection	Vessels well seen	Foreshortened/ overlapped vessels
1	25° LAO Cannulate LCA	Ostium. Distal LAD	Prox. Cx
		Mid. Cx	Lt. main stem
		Distal RCA (if filling from LCA)	Diagonal
2	10° RAO	Lt. main stem	
3	30° RAO	Most of LCA	Overlap mid. LAD and diagonal. Prox. Cx. foreshortened
4	30° RAO, 15° caudal	Mid. LAD. Diagonal. Prox.Cx.	
5	15° RAO, 30° cranial	Mid. LAD. Diagonal. Prox.Cx.	
6	45° LAO, 30° cranial	Lt. main stem. Prox. Cx.	
7	Cannulate RCA	Rt. ostium. Prox. RCA Post. desc. RCA and LV brs	
8	45° LAO	Most of RCA Post. desc. RCA and LV brs	
9	30° RAO	Most of RCA	

with the X-ray beam perpendicular to the vessel. Since the orientation of the coronary arteries is continuously changing as they pass over the surface of the heart it is clear that multiple views will be needed to visualise each segment of a given vessel; in any one view some segments will be well seen while others are foreshortened or overlapped by other vessels. In order to complete an examination as expeditiously as possible it is wise to adopt a sequence of views which will achieve optimal visualisation of the whole of the coronary arterial tree with the least possible movement from projection to projection. A suggested sequence is outlined in Table 13.1. This sequence is only intended as a guide, individual cases may require different projections for proper visualisation of problem areas. The left coronary artery arises from the left coronary sinus at an angle of about 25° posterior to the frontal plane; it follows that the first part of the left coronary and its ostium will be perpendicular to the X-ray beam in a 25° LAO projection; this projection is employed for the initial cannulation of the left coronary. The right coronary artery arises from the right coronary sinus at an angle of about 35° to the right of the sagittal plane and a 55° LAO projection will provide a perpendicular projection for cannulation. In practice a 45° LAO projection is equally satisfactory. The scheme outlined below provides a sequence of projections which allow, firstly, cannulation of the left coronary artery followed by six views of this vessel before the right coronary is cannulated in 45° LAO, 30° cranial projection and three views of this vessel are obtained.

TRAPS FOR THE UNWARY AND CLUES TO THEIR PRESENCE

In any laboratory a proportion of patients thought to have coronary artery disease will be found to have a normal coronary arterial supply. Indeed a study which yields such a result is often of great value. However it is important that this is genuinely the situation and not the result of error leading to lesions being overlooked. It is of equal importance that coronary artery disease is not diagnosed when it is absent or that the severity of disease is over- or underestimated. In the past the poor quality of angiographic equipment and in particular the unavailability of angulated views resulted in many diagnostic errors. Such errors should not occur today

but there are still a number of situations which, unless recognised by the angiographer, can lead to diagnostic errors. These errors will be considered under four headings: (1) failing to recognise that a vessel is absent, (2) concluding that a vessel is absent when it is not, (3) underestimating, and (4) overestimating the severity of disease.

Failing to recognise an absent vessel

LEFT ANTERIOR DESCENDING

The absence of a vessel may be missed when it is occluded at its origin so that no 'stump' is visible and when another vessel is mistaken for the one that is missing. The diagonal branches of the anterior descending are often large and supply much the same territory as the distal anterior descending. They may therefore be mistaken for the anterior descending when that vessel is occluded at the origin of a diagonal branch. A number of clues should help the angiographer to avoid this mistake. Firstly the anterior descending gives rise to a number of parallel and vertically directed septal branches; only rarely do such branches arise from the diagonal branches. Secondly, the anterior descending almost always reaches the apex of the heart and curves round it; the diagonal branches do not. Finally occlusion of the anterior descending will almost certainly result in a significant area of akinesis/dyskinesis involving the anterior free wall and apex of the left ventricle which could not be explained if the anterior descending was free of disease. If there is such a dyskinetic area the angiographer must seek the cause and a further clue may be delayed filling of an occluded vessel via collaterals; either from other branches of the left coronary artery or via conus, right ventricular or terminal branches of the right coronary artery. In general the presence of a dykinetic area and delayed filling of distal vessels should alert the angiographer to search for occluded vessels.

On occasion a large first septal branch may be mistaken for the anterior descending when that vessel is occluded immediately beyond the origin of the first septal branch. In the left oblique projection the two vessels run in much the same direction but the right oblique view should clarify the situation when the first septal will be seen to run more vertically and to end short of the apex (Fig. 13.16).

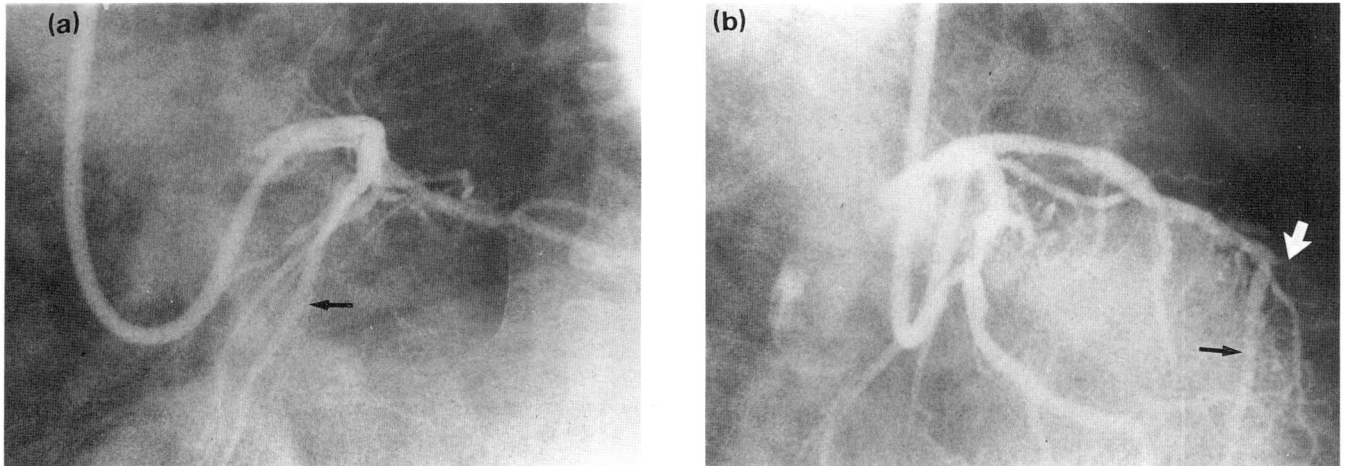

Fig. 13.16 Coronary artery disease. *Traps for the unwary.* (a) 'Missing an absent vessel': in this left oblique projection the anterior descending appears to be present (arrow). (b) But in the right oblique projection it is apparent that the anterior descending branch is occluded (white arrow) just beyond the origin of a large septal branch. It is this large septal branch (black arrow) which mimicked the distal anterior descending branch in the left oblique projection.

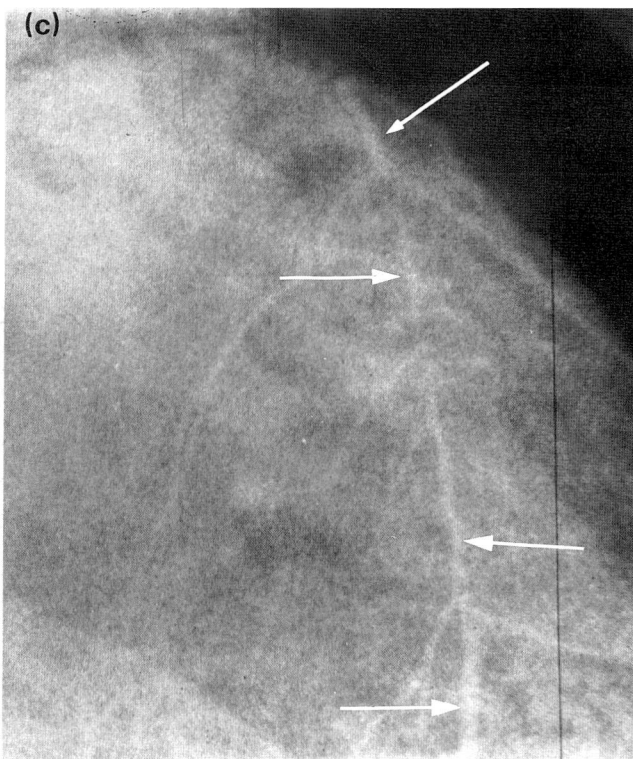

(c) The clue to a missing vessel is often that it is seen to fill late (via collaterals). In this example faint, delayed filling of the distal anterior descending and diagonal branches is seen (arrows) and confirms proximal occlusion of the vessel seen in Fig. 13.16b.

RIGHT CORONARY, CONUS BRANCH AND CIRCUMFLEX

When the right coronary artery is very dominant the circumflex will be a small vessel; when both are diseased it may be difficult to detect occlusion of distal branches of the circumflex. Delayed filling of these branches may be noted but the vessels wrongly interpreted as distal branches of a diseased right coronary artery. This mistake is avoided by studying multiple projections, in the left oblique projection distal circumflex branches are seen to be directed superiorly and to the left in the left atrioventricular groove. Distal branches of the right coronary artery are seen to originate more horizontally and to the right. Only in right oblique projections are the left and right atrioventricular grooves superimposed (Figs 13.17 and 13.18).

Confusion can also arise when the left coronary is dominant; the right coronary is small and occluded branches may be missed. This is particularly liable to happen if the conus branch is selectively cannulated and mistaken for a non-dominant right coronary which has not, in fact, been visualised. Selective cannulation of the conus branch (Fig. 13.19), which has a separate origin in about 50% of cases, is also responsible for the second category of error; assuming a vessel (the right coronary) to be absent when it is not.

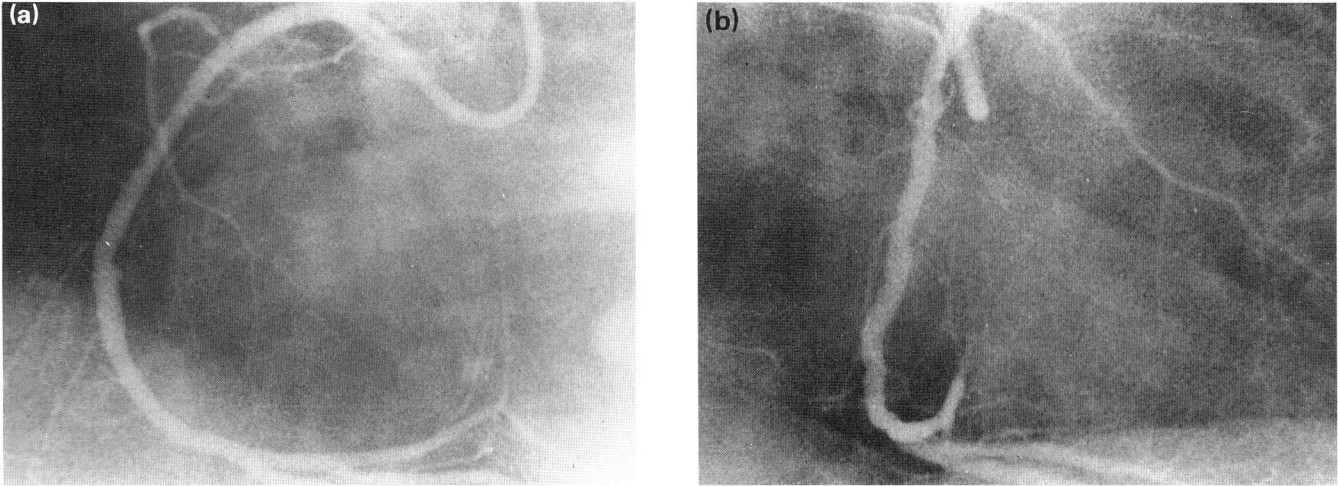

Fig. 13.17 The orientation of the coronary arteries. (a) The coronary arteries are so called because they can be seen as forming a ring (in the atrioventricular groove) from which branches arise at more or less of a right angle thus suggesting a 'crown'. The ring is made by the right and left circumflex coronary arteries which meet in the region of the posterior interventricular groove. In this *left oblique projection* the right coronary artery is seen forming a semicircle. (b) In the *right oblique projection* the ring formed by the right and circumflex coronary arteries is seen on edge with the two vessels more or less superimposed. The branches of the ring are well seen — in this case right ventricular and posterior descending branches of the right coronary artery.

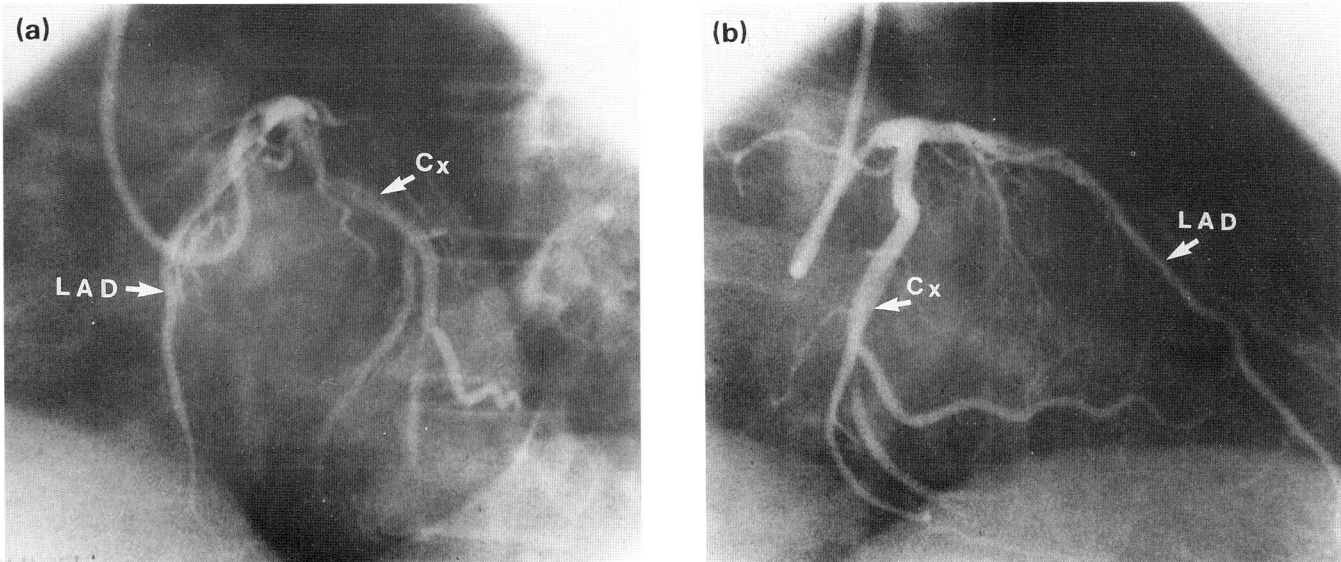

Fig. 13.18 Orientation of the coronary arteries. (a) The left coronary artery in the *left oblique projection*. The circumflex branch (Cx) forms the left half of the 'ring'. The anterior descending branch (LAD) is directed downwards and slightly to the right as seen in this projection. (b) The left coronary artery in the *right oblique projection*.

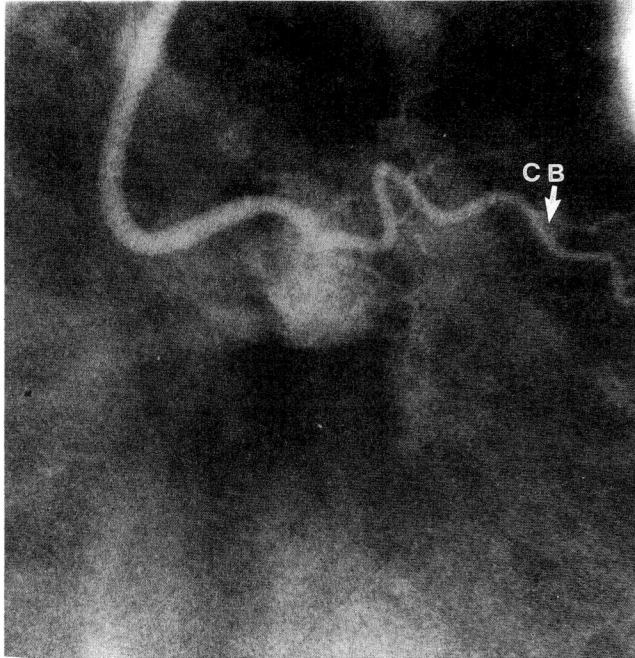

Fig. 13.19 *Traps for the unwary* — 'assuming a vessel to be absent when it is not'. Selective injection of the conus branch (CB) of the right coronary artery which has a separate ostium. It might have been assumed that the main right coronary artery was occluded. In fact when separately cannulated it was found to be large and free of disease.

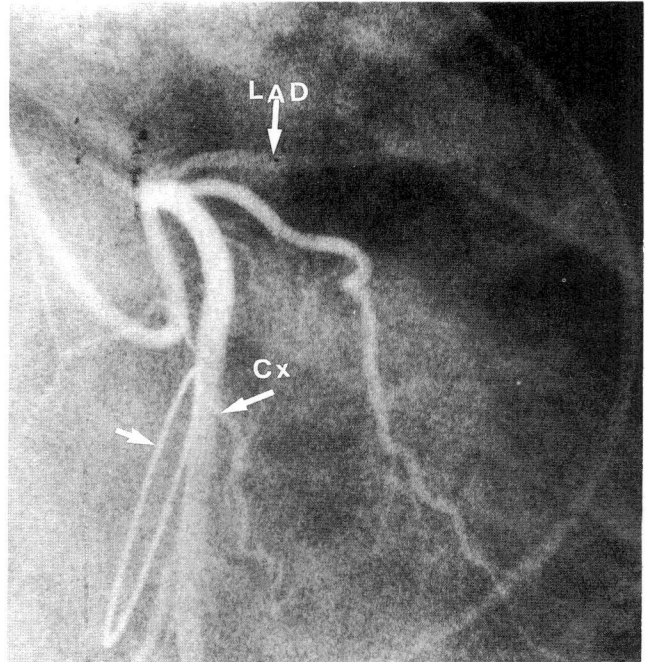

Fig. 13.20 Coronary artery disease. *Traps for the unwary* — 'assuming a vessel to be missing when it is not'. Virtual absence of the left main stem ('double orifice left coronary'). Contrast medium has been injected selectively into the circumflex branch (Cx). Only faint filling of the anterior descending (LAD) has occurred as a result of spill-over of contrast medium into the left sinus. The anterior descending branch was later selectively cannulated and shown to be free of disease. (In this patient it is also possible to see the base ring of a Hancock xenograft in the mitral position — arrow.)

SMALL BRANCHES

Small branches of the right and left coronary are often occluded or stenosed at their origins. These vessels may be overlapped in some views and the disease overlooked. Overlap is a common cause of error and is avoided by careful inspection of multiple projections. Again it is often delayed filling from collaterals that reveals an occluded vessel; filming should continue into the venous phase and an adequate field size (15 cm or 6 in) selected so that extensive panning does not result in late-filling vessels being overlooked.

Concluding that a vessel is absent when it is not

This error is liable to occur when there is an anomalous origin of a coronary artery or when there is absence of the left main stem with resulting double orifice left coronary artery. The varieties of anomalous origin are discussed below. The commonest is anomalous origin of the circumflex from the right

coronary sinus (Fig. 13.33). In this condition cannulation of the left ostium will opacify the anterior descending only (Fig. 13.33a*iii*); cannulation of the right coronary will only result in opacification of the circumflex if there is some spill-back into the sinus. That the circumflex is present and not occluded at its origin is suggested by lack of a corresponding area of dyskinesis and absence of collateral filling of the distal vessel. An even more common potential source of error results from selective cannulation of either the circumflex or the anterior descending with failure to opacify the other vessel (Fig. 13.20). This occurs when there is a very short left main stem or when it is absent and there are separate, side by side, ostia of the circumflex and anterior descending branches of the left coronary artery (double orifice LCA). The clue is again that there is no dyskinetic area corresponding to the vessel presumed to be absent and no collateral filling of its distal branches. The catheter should be withdrawn and repositioned in the 'missing' branch. If this is difficult a forceful, semi-selective, sinus injection may provide at least faint filling of the 'missing' vessel.

The conus branch of the right coronary artery has a separate origin in some 50% of cases. If this is selectively cannulated it may be wrongly identified as a small, non-dominant, right coronary or it may be thought that the main right coronary artery is occluded when, in reality, it has not been cannulated (Fig. 13.19). The conus branch passing anteriorly and to the left in the right oblique view should not be mistaken even for a non-dominant right coronary which has a more vertical direction in this view. Selective injections in the conus branch frequently result in capillary filling as a forceful injection over-fills a vessel with limited run-off; the appearance has been termed a 'myocardial blush'. It is important to remember that the conus branch is a potential channel for collateral supply to an occluded anterior descending. When proximal occlusion of the anterior descending is detected or suspected but no collateral filling can be seen it may be that the conus branch has not been opacified; either because it has a separate origin or because the catheter has been advanced down the right coronary beyond the origin of the conus branch.

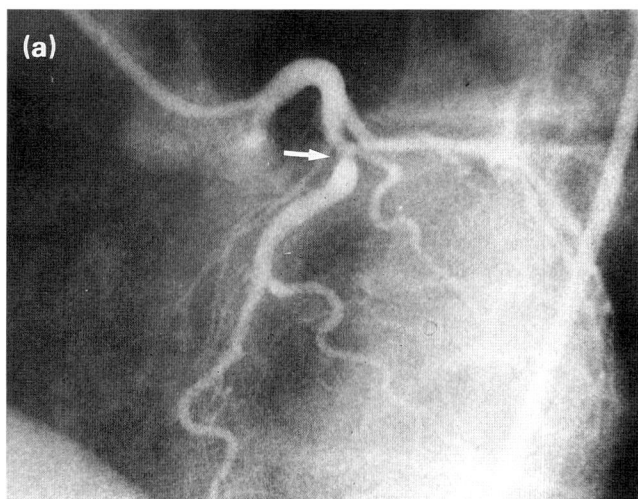

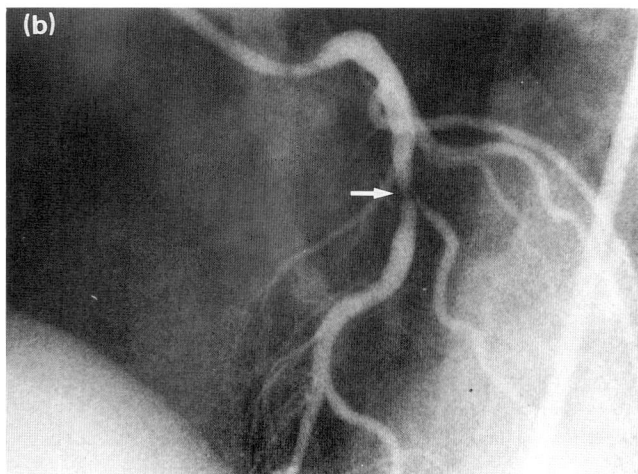

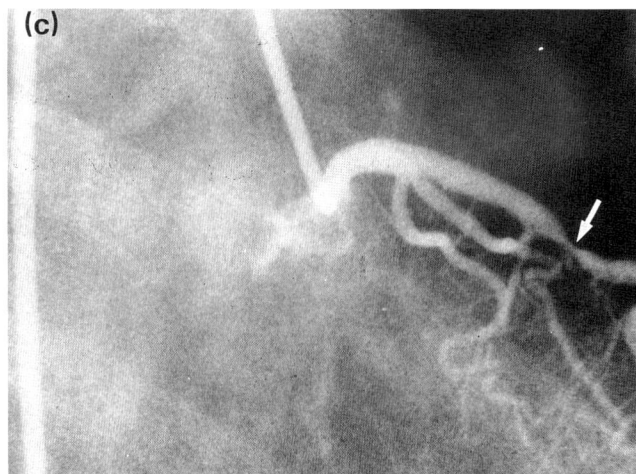

Underestimating the severity of disease

Coronary artery stenoses need not be circumferential; they are frequently eliptical in cross-section so that what may appear a mild degree of narrowing in one projection will be seen to be severe when a second view is obtained at right angles to the first. Provided multiple views are obtained this error should not occur (Fig. 13.21), but the possibility of such 'mis-estimate' of severity should always be born in mind. On occasion the true severity of what appears to be a mild lesion is suggested by the presence of marked collateral filling of the distal vessel. Collateral filling

Fig. 13.21 Coronary artery disease. Underestimating the severity of stenosis; the effect of projection. In (a) the appearances suggest a mild stenosis of the left anterior descending (LAD) branch (arrow). The projection is a left oblique, however, and the vessel is foreshortened in this view. Adding cranial angulation (b) removes this foreshortening and shows the stenosis (arrow) to be severe; as does the right oblique projection in (c).

only occurs when antegrade flow is severely reduced by a proximal stenosis or occlusion. It is always, of course, possible to overlook a localised lesion if it is obscured by overlapping vessels and such overlap is a second cause of the mis-estimate of severity of disease. There are two other, closely similar, situations in which severity of disease may be underestimated: *left main stem stenosis* and *ostial stenosis* (Fig. 13.22). When there is a proximal stenosis of the left main stem the catheter tip may be beyond the narrowed segment which is not, therefore, opacified. Clues to this situation are provided by the pressure record which may show either a damped or a ventricularised waveform (low diastolic pressure). The risks of coronary arteriography are significantly increased when there is a main stem stenosis as the catheter tip may dislodge or damage the atheromatous plaque. Main stem stenosis may be suspected when symptoms are severe and when S-T depression on exercise exceeds 2 mm or is seen at a low level of exercise. In all these circumstances a semi-selective (sinus) injection is indicated which may reveal the true situation.

Coronary ostial stenosis is a feature of syphilitic aortitis, of Takayasu aortitis (Fig. 20.45) and of familial hypercholesterolaemia. It may also occur as part of generalised coronary atherosclerosis [15]. Recently it has become apparent that ostial stenosis, sometimes without evidence of any other coronary disease, is particularly liable to occur in females and at a younger age than is the rule for atherosclerotic coronary disease [16]. As with main stem stenosis the lesion may easily be missed as the catheter tip will be beyond the stenosis. When catheters without end-holes are used the appearances may be interpreted as being due to the narrow jet of contrast medium emerging from the catheter tip before spreading to opacify the width of the vessel. Clues to the presence of ostial stenosis are, again, damping or ventricularisation of the pressure record and lack of spill-back of contrast medium into the sinus. Semi-selective (sinus) injections in a 10° right oblique (for the left ostium) or a 45° left oblique projection (for the right ostium) are indicated.

Overestimating the severity of disease

There is evidence that coronary arteriography tends to underestimate the real degree of coronary artery narrowing and that an overestimate of severity is an

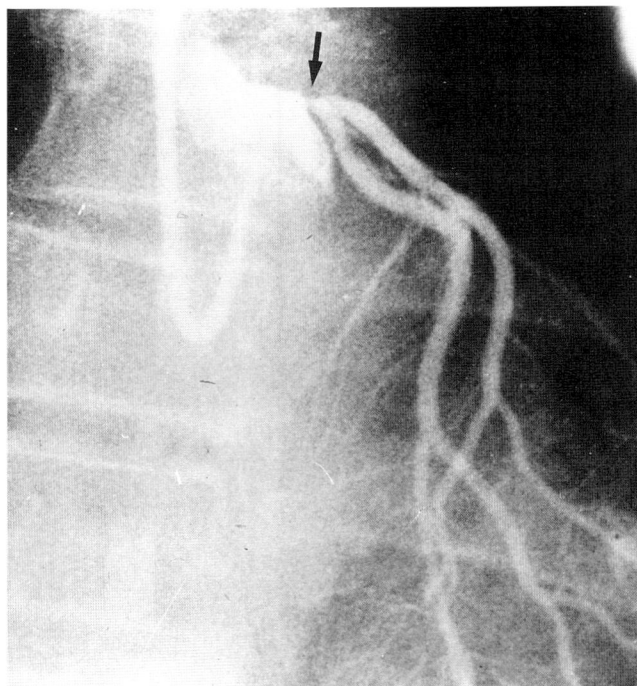

Fig. 13.22 *Traps for the unwary.* Coronary ostial stenosis (arrow) in a middle-aged female with otherwise normal coronary arteries. This lesion is easily missed unless specifically sought (see text).

uncommon error. However, two conditions may lead to this error; *myocardial bridging* and *coronary spasm*. In some subjects a coronary artery, particularly the distal anterior descending branch, may tunnel beneath epicardial muscle for a short distance. During ventricular systole the vessel lumen is compressed by the contracting fibres; giving an appearance of a smooth stenosis at this point. The true cause is apparent if it is observed that the narrowing disappears during diastole. Since coronary flow is largely diastolic it is probable that myocardial bridges are benign though in a few cases they have been thought to be the cause of symptoms.

Coronary spasm can be induced by the catheter tip. This iatrogenic spasm is particularly likely to occur in the proximal right coronary and is rare in the left. A smoothly tapering stenosis of the right coronary beginning at the catheter tip suggests the possibility of catheter-induced spasm. The routine administration of glyceryl trinitrate before performing coronary arteriography should prevent this complication. If this is not routine glyceryl trinitrate should be given and the arteriogram repeated.

There is good evidence that spontaneously occurring spasm is the cause of Prinzmetal variant angina; angina which is not related to exercise and is accompanied by S-T elevation [17]. Spontaneously occurring spasm is usually seen in association with an atheromatous lesion but may occur in an otherwise normal vessel. As a result many centres employ the 'ergonovine test' in an attempt to provoke spasm — in patients with chest pain and angiographically normal coronaries, for example. Prinzmetal angina is recognisable clinically when attacks are accompanied by S-T segment shift or T-wave changes — at lesser risk than by provocation testing. The justification for ergonovine testing is controversial and the case against has been lucidly expressed by Fester [18]. The test is uncomfortable for the patient, prolongs the procedure and is not without risk [19]. Both false positive and false negative findings occur [20]; it is not our practice to perform the test except in very exceptional circumstances. Guidelines for performing the ergonovine provocation test have been published by Pepine [21]:

1 Exclude patients with:
  Uncontrolled chest pain or ventricular arrhythmias.
  Acute myocardial infarction (<6 weeks).
  Severe aortic stenosis or hypertension.
  Premenopausal amenorrhea.
2 No premedication (sedatives, atropine, long-acting nitrates).
3 In catheterisation laboratory with prepared nitroglycerin solution available for intravenous or intracoronary use. Intravenous nitroprusside available.
4 Record 12-lead ECG, LV pressure and right and left coronary arteriograms.
5 Ergonovine maleate given as 0.05 mg bolus through a right atrial catheter containing pacing electrodes.
6 Record heart rate, blood pressure, ECG and observe for symptoms for 3—5 minutes.
7 If chest pain or ECG/LV pressure changes occur, repeat step 4 and give nitroglycerin 0.4—0.8 mg sublingually. Repeat sublingual nitroglycerin in 3—5 minutes if evidence that ischaemic episode is beginning to regress. If spasm and/or ischaemia persist or worsen or patient becomes hypotensive intracoronary nitroglycerin 100 μg is given.
8 If no ECG changes or chest pain repeat step 5 (i.v. ergonovine 0.05 mg) up to a total cumulative dose of 0.2 mg.
9 Repeat step 4 even if ECG changes or chest pain do not occur.

CORONARY ARTERY DISEASE: ATHEROSCLEROSIS

In a description of the arteriographic findings that may be present in patients with coronary artery disease some simplification is unavoidable; the possible combinations of findings are almost as numerous as the patients themselves. As a first step we can attempt to describe, firstly, the abnormalities that may be present in the coronary arteries and, secondly, the possible consequences — impaired ventricular function, ventricular aneurysm and so on. No attempt will be made to discuss clinical aspects of coronary artery disease such as the indications for coronary arteriography, the mortality associated with various patterns of disease and so on.

The coronary arteries in coronary heart disease

IRREGULARITY OF THE LUMEN

The earliest sign of coronary atherosclerosis is irregularity of the lumen of a vessel. Clearly this appearance, due as it is to atheroma of the vessel wall, is only one end of a spectrum of disease which runs through stenoses of varying degree to complete occlusion of the vessel. By itself, vessel irregularity without significant narrowing is neither a cause of symptoms nor an indication for treatment. Progression to frank stenosis or occlusion is likely but the time course of such progression is unpredictable. There are three other manifestations of coronary artery disease that need not be associated with localised stenosis; they are ectasia (Fig. 13.23) and aneursym formation), (Fig. 13.24), calcification in the vessel wall and generalised narrowing of the vessel. Dilated and irregular (ectatic) vessels with, sometimes, aneurysms of the vessels are the result of widespread coronary atherosclerosis. These appearances are usually associated with stenotic lesions elsewhere. Coronary calcification is also most commonly associated with widespread coronary artery disease in the elderly though localised calcification is frequently seen at the site of a discrete stenosis where there has been haemorrhage into an atheromatous plaque. Generalised narrowing of a vessel, if associated with irregularity of the vessel wall, is also a feature of widespread coronary artery disease and often associated with diabetes or hypercholesterolaemia. The significance of narrow but smooth

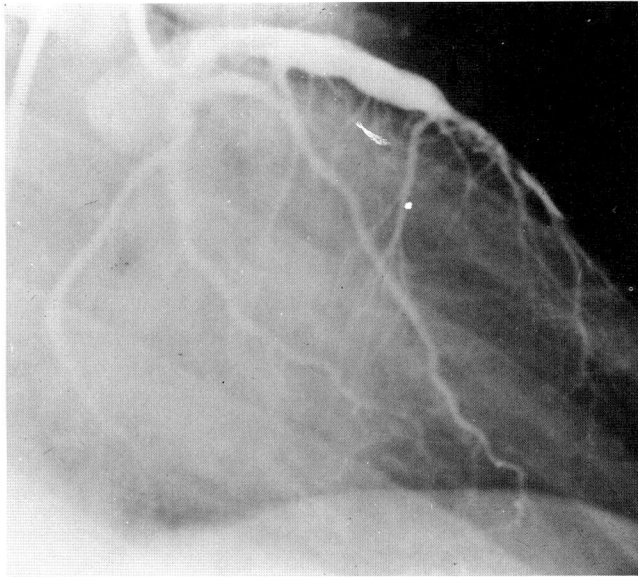

Fig. 13.23 Coronary atherosclerosis: coronary ectasia.

vessels is uncertain. Spasm is a possibility and is a reason for recommending the routine administration of glyceryl trinitrate before performing coronary arteriography; any persisting narrowing will then be more easily seen against a background of dilated vessels. It must be remembered that vessels tend to be smaller in females. Large dilated vessels are found when there is ventricular hypertrophy; as in hypertrophic cardiomyopathy or when there is aortic stenosis or systemic hypertension.

STENOSES (Figs 13.24 and 13.25)
AND FILLING DEFECTS

The arteriographer is concerned with the severity, distribution and morphology of coronary stenoses.

Severity

Coronary stenoses need not be concentric, they are often eliptical or D-shaped in cross section [22, 23]. For this reason the severity of a lesion cannot be assessed from a single X-ray projection; what may appear to be a mild stenosis in one view may be seen to be severe in another. Indeed a lesion may be entirely overlooked in all but one projection. Thomas *et al.* [22] have shown that, for an eliptical lesion with a ratio between long and short axes of 4 : 1, an overestimate of stenosis (by area) of 19% and an underestimate of 68% can occur according to the angle of the X-ray beam. In general coronary arteriography tends to underestimate the severity of stenoses. It is important to remember that a given percentage narrowing of the *diameter* of a vessel will, for a circular lesion, result in a reduction of the *area* of the orifice greater by up to 25% (Table 13.2).

Finally we must not delude ourselves that we can measure even the diameter of a vessel with any great accuracy. Bjork and O'Keefe [24] have shown that measurement errors of at least 15% occur when the diameter of a barium-filled tube 1.5 mm wide is measured from radiographs. Errors at least as large

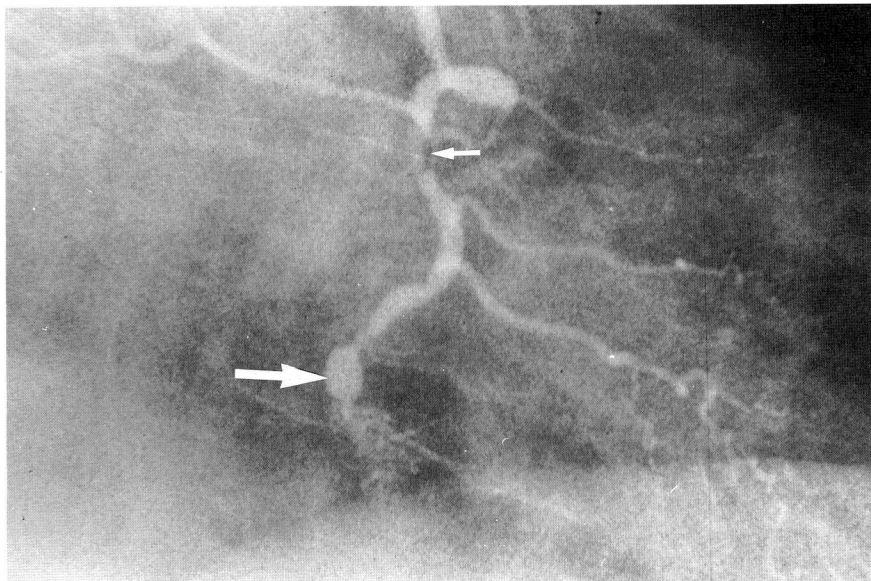

Fig. 13.24 Coronary atherosclerosis. A plaque (small arrow) and an aneurysm (large arrow).

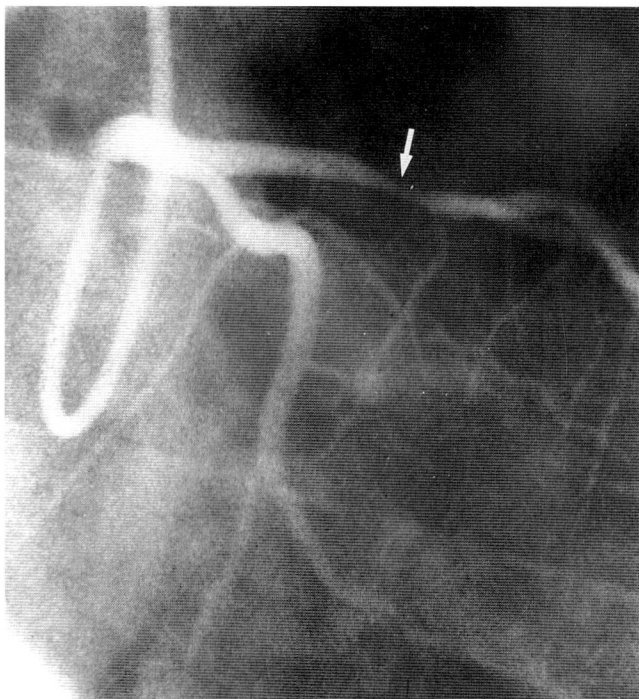

Fig. 13.25 Coronary atherosclerosis: circumferential stenosis of the proximal left anterior descending branch (arrow).

Table 13.2 Percentage reductions in the area of the orifice of circular lesions.

Reduction in diameter (%)	Reduction in area (%)
15	28
25	44
35	58
45	70
55	80
65	88
75	94
85	98

are to be expected when still frames of coronary arteriograms are measured. Many studies have shown wide inter- and intra-observer variations in duplicate measurements of vessel diameter.

For all these reasons it is suggested that a simple grading of severity as *mild, moderate* or *severe* will avoid self delusion. A 50% reduction in diameter represents a 75% reduction in area and is the level at which flow begins to be reduced. Anything less than a 50% reduction in diameter may therefore be regarded as mild. A reduction in diameter of two-thirds (66%) represents an 88% reduction in area and anything above this must be regarded as a severe stenosis. If an attempt is made to report stenosis in terms of percentage narrowing then it is essential that it is made clear whether the narrowing is assessed by diameter or by area.

Even if we were able to assess accurately the reduction in lumen caused by each stenosis we would still be far from reporting the severity of coronary artery disease as it affects myocardial blood supply. It is not only the severity of a lesion but its location that is important. Clearly a severe stenosis of the left main stem is of much more importance than a lesion of similar severity far down the distal anterior descending branch. It is also probable that a number of lesions in series have a greater effect in reducing flow than a single lesion of the same severity. In recognition of these problems a number of systems have been proposed for grading the severity of coronary artery disease. Such schemes include that proposed by the American Heart Association [25] (see Appendix) and that employed by Brandt *et al.* [26]. No universally accepted scheme exists, however the above formalised proformas, though essential in any comparative or multicentre trial, are often of great complexity and inappropriate for day to day clinical use.

There are indications of severity other than the degree of narrowing caused by a lesion. In particular delayed filling of a vessel beyond a stenosis is a clear indication that the stenosis is severe; indeed this may indicate complete occlusion with distal filling via collaterals. The presence of collaterals is another indication that perfusion pressure is severely reduced.

Distribution of lesions

The majority of coronary arterial lesions are found in the proximal segments of the major coronary arteries. The commonest site is in the conduit portion of the right coronary followed, in order, by the anterior descending before and after the first septal or first diagonal branch. When only a single vessel is diseased the disease is found in the anterior descending with slightly greater frequency than the right coronary artery. The most proximal site at which narrowing can occur is at the coronary ostia. Ostial stenosis may be due to syphilitic aortitis or aortitis of the Takayasu type and ostial stenosis is a feature of familial hypercholesterolaemia. In the majority of instances, however, ostial stenosis is due to atherosclerosis and is accompanied by other artherosclerotic lesions of the coronary arteries [15]. Ostial stenosis appears to occur with a higher frequency in females than males; the right coronary ostium is more frequently affected than the left. Occasionally disease is confined to the ostia (isolated ostial stenosis); a condition which appears to be peculiarly liable to affect middle-aged females [16]. Ostial stenosis is easily overlooked for reasons which are described elsewhere (see the section on Traps for the unwary); particularly when there is no other coronary artery disease.

Ostial stenosis merges into stenosis of the left main stem and it is probable that both are associated with a relatively worse prognosis and higher risk both at catheterisation and at surgery; this is certainly true of left main stem stenosis. The mortality associated with catheterisation when left main stem disease is present has been variously assessed but is probably at least 3%. It is not surprising that a lesion at this site has a high associated mortality since the whole of the left ventricular blood supply is jeopardised; of almost equal importance are lesions of the anterior descending before the origin of the first septal branch; the lesion has been called 'the widow maker'.

Stenotic lesions may occur anywhere in the major coronary arteries and their large branches; where branches are affected the stenosis is often found at the origin of the branch from the parent vessel. It is the function of the physician performing coronary arteriography to describe the position and severity of all lesions revealed by the study.

Morphology

Distinction has been made between stenoses and filling defects. But both are due to deposits of atheroma and both cause coronary artery narrowing though it is true that some lesions project into the lumen in a way that suggests the presence of a plaque of atheroma as distinct from an hour-glass constriction due to an endothelialised fatty or fibrous plaque. Of more importance are what have been termed 'complicated stenoses'. Complicated stenoses are characterised by having irregular borders and intraluminal translucencies and are distinguished

from those with smooth borders and an hour-glass configuration. There is now good evidence of a significant association between complicated stenoses and pathological findings of plaque rupture, haemorrhage and ulceration and associated thrombus deposition. Complicated stenoses are associated with a higher risk of myocardial infarction and sudden death [27]. The complicated stenosis with a rather poorly defined vessel wall and evidence of recanalisation is often, in my experience, found in patients studied shortly after suffering a myocardial infarct.

OCCLUSIONS (Fig. 13.26)

It is not usually difficult to identify vessel occlusion but problems can occur and these have been discussed in the section on Traps for the unwary. Among changes responsible for difficulties in interpretation is the tendency for thrombus formation to extend back to the origin of the nearest proximal branch so that a visible stump becomes obliterated. Most coronary occlusions are the end result of thrombosis on an atheromatous lesion but some are due to emboli. On occasion a convexity of the filling defect may suggest such an embolic cause.

The development of a collateral circulation is intimately linked with vessel occlusion; whenever a collateral circulation has developed it means that the perfusing pressure of the vessel supplied is low — because of a proximal occlusion or severe stenosis. Collaterals are of three types; some connect branches of one coronary artery to another (intercoronary collaterals — Figs 13.27 and 13.28) while others connect one branch of a coronary to another branch of the same vessel (intracoronary collaterals) (Fig. 13.29). The third type bridge an occluded segment ('bridge collaterals'); such vessels may not be true collaterals but may be dilated vasavasorum or adventitial vessels. Depending on the point of anastomosis collaterals may result in either retrograde filling of the vessel beyond the occlusion or in antegrade filling when the collateral connects with the occluded vessel close to the point of occlusion. An example of retrograde filling is seen when branches of the circumflex or right coronary anastomose with distal branches of an anterior descending artery which is occluded near its origin. Antegrade filling of, for example, the anterior descending is seen when conus branches of the right coronary anastomose with the anterior descending close to the point of a

(a)

(b)

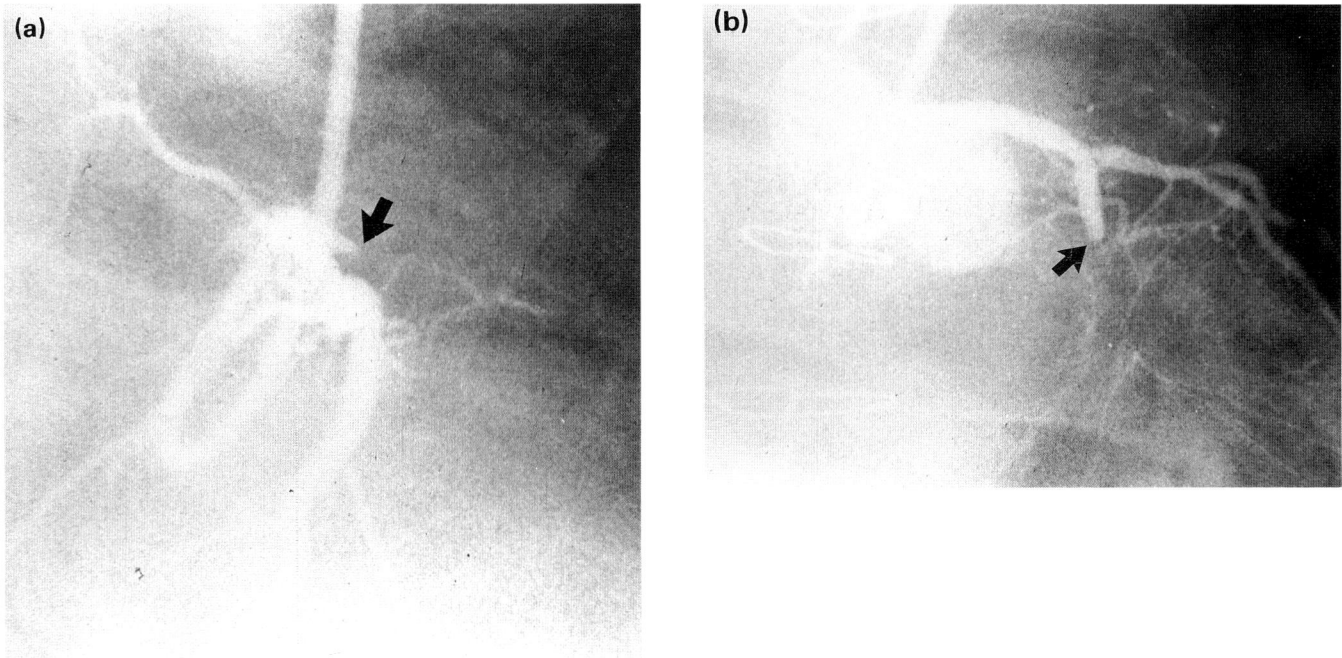

Fig. 13.26 Coronary atherosclerosis: vessel occlusion. (a) The 'stump' (arrow) of an occluded proximal left anterior descending, and (b) of an occluded circumflex branch.

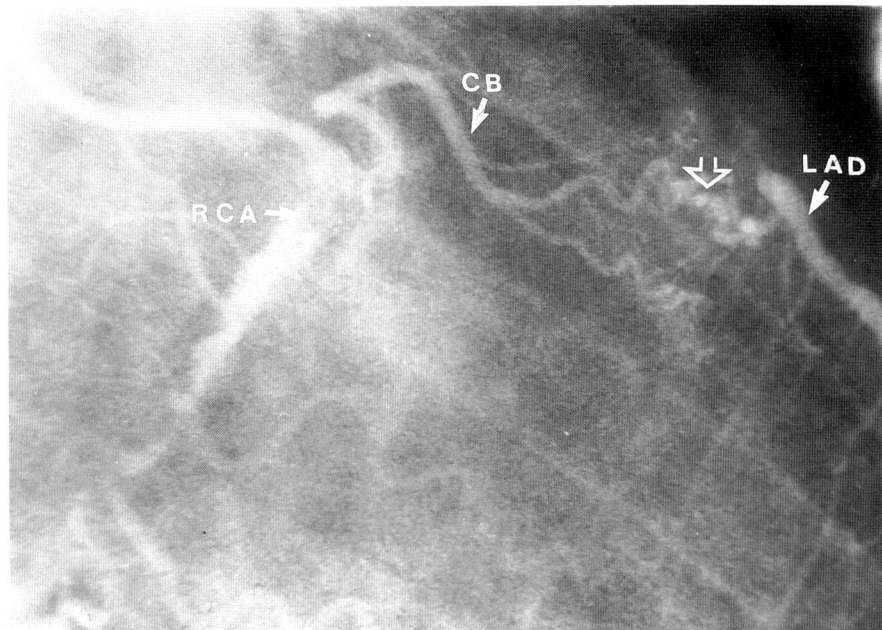

Fig. 13.27 Coronary atherosclerosis. *Intercoronary* anastomoses. A large conus branch (CB) of the right coronary artery anastomoses with branches of the left anterior descending (LAD) which fills antegradely as a result although occluded proximal to the site of anastomosis. Typical tortuous anastomotic vessels are seen (open arrow).

proximal occlusion. Common sites for the development of a collateral circulation are:

1 The interventricular septum, where anastomoses may develop between the anterior descending and posterior descending arteries.

2 At the apex of the heart where distal branches of the anterior descending may also anastomose with the posterior descending.

3 At the posterior interventricular groove near the crux where distal branches of the right coronary and

(a)

(b)

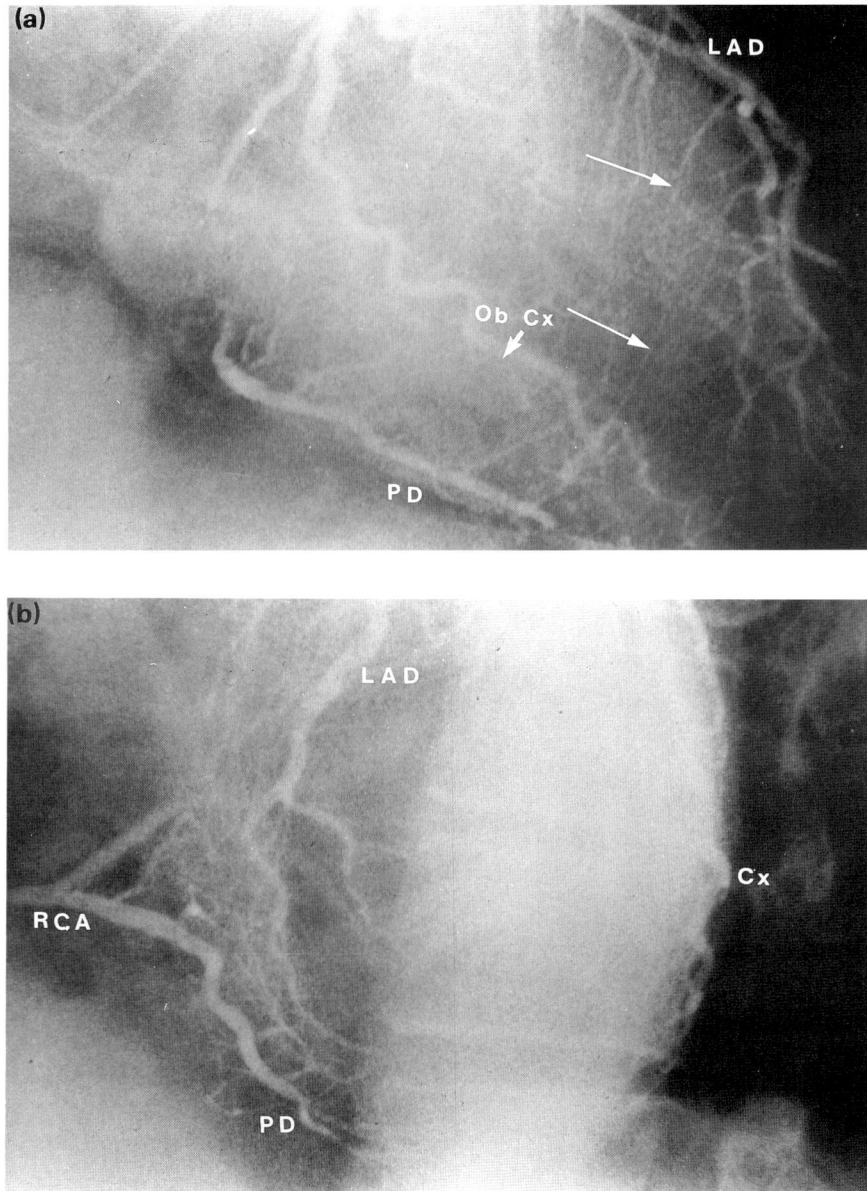

Fig. 13.28 Coronary atherosclerosis. *Intercoronary* anastomoses. (a) The posterior descending branch (PD) is filling via collaterals from the obtuse marginal branch of the circumflex left coronary artery (ObCx) and, via a number of fine septal collateral vessels (long arrows), from the left anterior descending branch (LAD). In this right oblique view it would be difficult to determine if the posterior descending artery was a branch of the circumflex or of the right coronary artery. (b) In the same patient the right oblique view makes it clear that the posterior descending was a branch of the right coronary artery (directed towards the right) which is filling retrogradely from the left coronary artery. In this view the circumflex is widely separated from the right coronary artery.

circumflex left coronary approach each other.

4 On the epicardial surface of the right and left ventricular free walls where right ventricular branches, conus branch and acute marginal branches can anastomose with branches of the anterior descending or posterolaterally where diagonal branches of the anterior descending can anastomose with obtuse marginal branches of the circumflex.

5 Between right and left atrial branches.

Collateral filling of an occluded vessel is usually delayed and slow and is unlikely to provide a normal amount of blood supply to the occluded or stenosed vessel. Nonetheless remarkably dense filling of the diseased vessel is often seen angiographically. Although there is controversy about the protective role of collaterals there can be little doubt that they can play such a role; every angiographer has encountered cases of complete occlusion of the anterior descending, or even of the left main stem, in whom there has been almost complete preservation of left

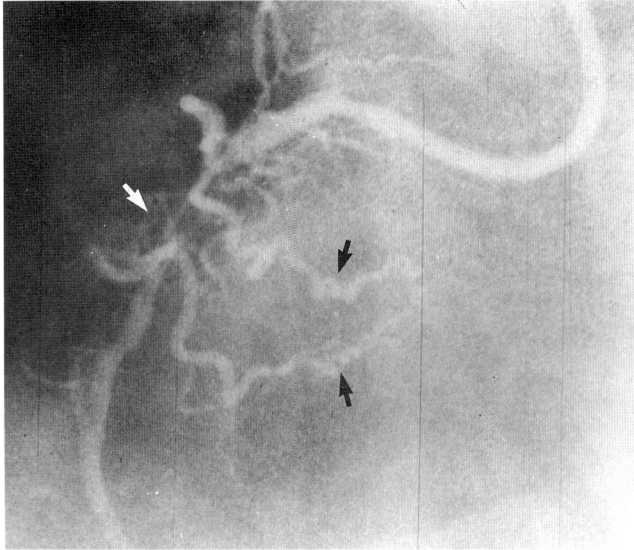

Fig. 13.29 Coronary atherosclerosis. *Intracoronary* anastomoses. The right coronary artery is occluded at the point indicated by the white arrow but the distal vessel fills antegradely via anastomoses between right ventricular branches (black arrows).

ventricular function and in whom there is invariably a rich collateral supply. At the other extreme the same lesion, without collaterals, may result in left ventricular aneurysm formation. Left ventricular aneurysm, with avascular fibrous replacement of myocardium, is one situation in which collaterals are absent despite severe disease. Collaterals take time to develop and their, presence indicates relatively long standing and progressive disease. Collaterals are absent when vessel occlusion has been sudden and recent.

Recanalisation of occluded vessels undoubtedly occurs and may be so complete as to leave no trace of disease — at least this is one possible explanation of the well recognised syndrome of myocardial infarction (perhaps with aneurysm formation) and a normal coronary arteriogram. Spasm and blunt chest trauma are alternative explanations. Recanalisation is more usually seen as a rather long, narrow vessel in the area of prior occlusion; an appearance similar to 'bridge collaterals' and possibly being, in fact, an enlarged vasa vasorum.

Consequences of coronary artery disease

Myocardial ischaemia resulting from coronary stenosis or occlusions may affect myocardial function in a number or ways that can be detected and assessed at cardiac catheterisation. These are:

1 Localised abnormalities of systolic and diastolic left ventricular function.
2 Left ventricular aneurysm formation.
3 Papillary muscle dysfunction or rupture.
4 Rupture of the interventricular septum.
5 Formation of mural thrombus.
6 Generalised left ventricular dysfunction (ischaemic cardiomyopathy).

Cardiac rupture and tamponade is another (rare) complication of myocardial infarction but the patient is unlikely to survive or be referred for catheterisation. Other consequences such as the development of collaterals have already been discussed.

LOCALISED LEFT VENTRICULAR DYSFUNCTION

The characteristic feature of ventricular dysfunction resulting from ischaemia is that only some areas of myocardium are involved while others, whose arterial supply is normal, are spared. This finding, while characteristic, is not specific and is sometimes observed in patients with congestive cardiomyopathy and normal coronaries. Sophisticated analyses of systolic and diastolic dysfunction are possible but for routine clinical purposes it is sufficient to describe dysfunction under three headings:

1 Asychronous contraction/relaxation (dyskinesis).
2 Reduced amplitude of movement (hypokinesis).
3 Absence of movement (akinesis).

To these we can add (4) aneurysm formation — discussed below. These abnormalities should be revealed by left ventriculography which is usually performed in the right oblique projection. The segments displaying abnormal movement should be identified and the nomenclature proposed by the AHA grading committee is one that is widely adopted. The segments are named, in counterclockwise direction from the aortic valve, as (1) anterobasal, (2) anterolateral, (3) apical, (4) diaphragmatic, and (5) posterobasal.

If biplane left ventriculography is performed the second projection is likely to be a left oblique in which case it will be possible to identify two further segments; the septal wall anteriorly and the posterolateral segment posteriorly.

In addition to the angiographic appearances the height of the left ventricular end-diastolic pressure provides some measure of ventricular performance. This measurement should be obtained *before* any contrast medium has been injected and before performing coronary arteriography since these interventions alter left ventricular dynamics in a somewhat inconstant way and cause end-diastolic pressure to rise.

LEFT VENTRICULAR ANEURYSM (Fig. 13.30)

The distinction between an akinetic segment and an aneurysm is somewhat artificial. Paradoxical movement (outward movement during ventricular systole) often turns out to be an illusion due to inward movement of adjacent segments contrasting with lack of movement of an akinetic segment. Most angiographers reserve the term 'aneurysm' to describe a sharply demarcated segment(s) which is not merely akinetic but which bulges outward forming a discontinuity in the outline of the ventricular cavity.

PAPILLARY MUSCLE DYSFUNCTION/RUPTURE AND RUPTURED INTERVENTRICULAR SEPTUM

These two conditions are considered together since clinical distinction between them is often impossible and catheterisation is undertaken in order to deter-

mine which is present. The setting is of a patient who, a few days following a myocardial infarct, suddenly develops acute cardiogenic shock and what appears to be pulmonary oedema. A systolic murmur suggests acute mitral insufficiency or an acquired ventricular septal defect as the cause. In these circumstances bedside, flow-guided, cardiac catheterisation (Swan–Ganz) can provide the answer; though the two conditions can coexist. A (usually) large increase in oxygen saturation at right ventricular level establishes the diagnosis of ruptured ventricular septum (VSD). When no such 'step-up' is found and there are giant v-waves in the wedge pressure tracing the diagnosis is of papillary muscle dysfunction or rupture. In both cases the cause is myocardial necrosis following infarction. Although the left-to-right shunt is usually large (Qp/Qs of as much as 4:1) right ventricular pressure is seldom more than half of the systemic pressure. Rupture of the ventricular septum occurs with approximately equal frequency following anterior or inferior infarction. If formal catheterisation and angiography is undertaken the defect will be seen to be in the muscular septum towards the apex. At surgery the defect will be in the anterior portion of the muscular septum when there has been anterior infarction and in the posterior part after inferior infarction. Papillary muscle dys-

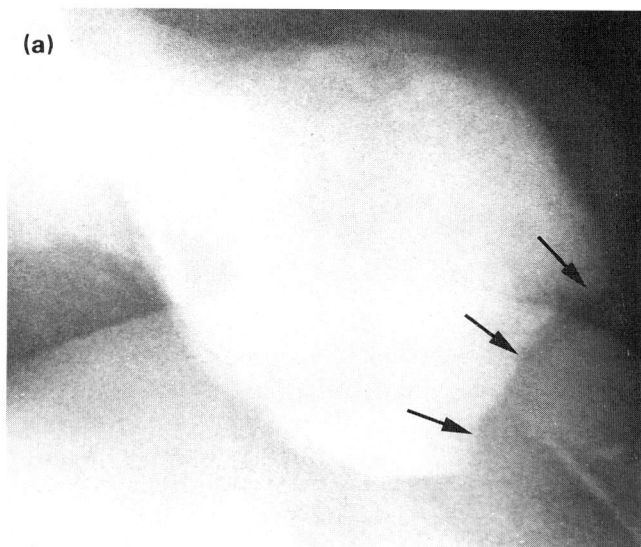

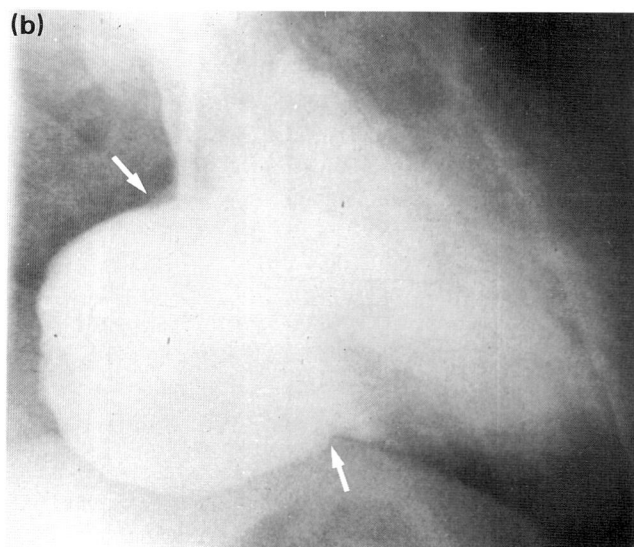

Fig. 13.30 The consequences of myocardial infarction — ventricular aneurysm. (a) Large aneurysm of the left ventricle involving the apex and most of the anterior and inferior surfaces of the ventricle. There is also mural thrombus at the apex (arrows). (b) Unusually large posterior left ventricular aneurysm between the two arrows.

function or rupture leading to acute mitral insufficiency is more common following inferior than anterior infarction. In both conditions there is likely to be severe myocardial dysfunction with possible aneurysm formation since infarction tends to be massive.

MURAL THROMBUS

Thrombus formation is a common accompaniment of extensive infarction and aneurysm formation. Angiographically thrombus may be detected as a frank filling defect extending into the ventricular cavity or as a flattening of the smooth curve of the outline of the ventricular cavity. Calcification may occur. Occasionally a free-floating pedunculated filling defect is seen and such thrombi may be especially liable to embolise.

GENERALISED LEFT VENTRICULAR DYSFUNCTION

Although ischaemic myocardial dysfunction is typically patchy there are many patients in whom there is generalised dysfunction affecting all segments so that the ischaemic aetiology is uncertain until coronary arteriography, by demonstrating widespread coronary artery disease, leads to a diagnosis of 'ischaemic cardiomyopathy'. The severity of ventricular dysfunction can be categorised by measuring the 'ejection fraction'. Although frequently measured in patients with more localised dysfunction the ejection fraction, a measure of overall ventricular performance, seems a less appropriate index in those with localised dysfunction than in those with generalised ischaemic cardiomyopathy. The various indices of ventricular performance are discussed in Chapter 8.

CONGENITAL ANOMALIES OF THE CORONARY ARTERIES

Congenital coronary anomalies may be divided into (1) anomalous origin from the pulmonary artery, (2) anomalous aortic origin of the coronary arteries, and (3) abnormalities of coronaries which have a normal origin (e.g. fistulae) (see Table 13.3).

Table 13.3 Classification of congenital coronary anomalies [28]

1 Anomalous origin of one or both coronary arteries from the pulmonary artery:
    Left coronary from PA
    Right coronary from PA
    Right and left coronary from PA
    Left anterior descending from PA
    Circumflex left coronary from PA

2 Anomalous origin from the aorta:
    Origin of the left coronary or its branches from the right sinus:
        Circumflex from right sinus — posterior to PA
        Left anterior descending (LAD) from right sinus:
            anterior to PA
            between PA and aorta
        Left main from right sinus:
            anterior to PA
            between PA and aorta
            posterior to PA
    Right coronary from left sinus — between PA and aorta
    Single aortic ostium ('single coronary artery')
    'Double orifice' left coronary
    Right coronary from posterior sinus
    High origin

3 Anomalous aortic origin in association with other congenital cardiac anomalies:
    Tetralogy of Fallot
    Complete transposition
    'Univentricular hearts'
    'Corrected transposition'
    Double outlet right ventricle with L-malposition

4 Anomalies with normal aortic origin:
    Coronary-cameral fistulae
    Sinusoids communicating with left coronary in pulmonary atresia with intact ventricular septum
    Coronary artery aneurysms

Anomalous origin of one or both coronary arteries from the pulmonary artery

Anomalous origin of the left coronary artery from the pulmonary artery (Fig. 13.32) occurs in about 0.25% of cases of congenital heart disease. Patients with this anomaly usually present in the neonatal period with severe heart failure and an electrocardiographic pattern of anterior myocardial infarction. Left ventriculography demonstrates considerable enlargement of the left ventricular cavity with anterior and apical akinesis/aneurysm formation. Aortography and selective right coronary arteriography demonstrate a single right coronary artery arising from the aorta followed by retrograde opacification of the whole of the left coronary circulation through collateral channels. Contrast medium will be seen to escape from the left coronary into the pulmonary trunk.

Anomalous origin of the right coronary from the pulmonary artery has an incidence one-tenth that of anomalous origin of the left coronary. All other varieties are exceedingly rare and the subject of isolated case reports only.

Anomalous aortic origin of the coronary arteries [29]

A large number of anomalies have been described under this heading; most are very rare occurring in less than 0.1% of subjects. The anomalies can be classified under three main headings: (1) anomalous origin of the circumflex, anterior descending or main left coronary arteries from the right sinus of Valsalva; (2) anomalous origin of the right coronary artery from the left sinus; and (3) various forms of 'single coronary artery' (since there are actually three coronaries in many of the forms of 'single coronary' a better term is 'single aortic ostium').

In addition the coronary ostia may arise from above the sinuses — posing a problem for the angiographer attempting to cannulate them.

ANOMALOUS ORIGIN OF THE LEFT CORONARY OR ITS BRANCHES FROM THE RIGHT SINUS

Origin of the circumflex from the right sinus

The commonest of these anomalies, and the commonest of all abnormally arising coronaries, is origin of the circumflex from the right sinus (Fig. 13.33). The reported incidence is between 0.3 and 0.6% of all coronary arteriograms. In this anomaly the circumflex branch of left the coronary artery arises from the right sinus posterior to the right coronary ostium (or sometimes from the proximal part of the right coronary artery) and courses behind the aortic root to reach the left atrioventricular groove from which point it follows the normal course of the left circumflex. The anterior descending branch arises as a single vessel from the left sinus. The anomaly should be suspected when only the anterior descending can be opacified from the left ostium; a separate circumflex origin from the right sinus must then be sought. A clue to this anomaly is the so-called 'aortic root sign'; following left ventriculography in the right oblique projection the contrast-filled circumflex is seen end on forming a small, circular opacity behind the aortic root.

Origin of the left anterior descending from the right sinus (Fig. 13.33)

This anomaly is rare, occurring in 0.04 to 0.2% of coronary arteriograms. The vessel arises from the right sinus anterior to the right coronary ostium (or from the proximal right coronary) and passes anterior to the pulmonary conus to reach the anterior interventricular groove whence it follows the usual course to the apex of the heart. The anomaly occurs in 2 to 7% of patients with tetralogy of Fallot and is then of importance as the vessel may be damaged during reconstruction of the right ventricular outflow tract. Rarely the anomalous vessel may pass between the aorta and pulmonary trunk.

Origin of the main left coronary from the right sinus

This is another rare anomaly with an incidence of less than 0.02 to 0.04%. The vessel arises from the right sinus anterior to the right ostium and passes between the pulmonary trunk and the aortic root. The anomaly is of importance having been reported as being associated with sudden death: presumably as a result of compression of the vessel as it passes between the two great arteries. Rarely the anomalous left main coronary artery may pass anteriorly to the pulmonary artery or even behind the aortic root.

ANOMALOUS ORIGIN OF THE RIGHT CORONARY ARTERY FROM THE LEFT SINUS (Fig. 13.33)

In this rare anomaly the right coronary arises from the left sinus anterior to the left coronary ostium and passes between the pulmonary artery and the aortic root to reach the right atrioventricular groove whence it follows the normal course or the right coronary artery. Reports suggest that this anomaly may be associated with sudden death.

SINGLE AORTIC OSTIUM ('SINGLE CORONARY ARTERY')

A number of variants of this anomaly have been described; they have been classified by Lipton *et al.*

[30]. This classification is based on (1) whether the single ostium is from the right or the left sinus, and (2) whether there is a single vessel which provides the entire coronary supply (group I) or whether there is a single ostium but a 'joining' vessel linking the right and left coronary circulations (group II). This group is subdivided into three subgroups depending on the course of the 'joining' vessel; in front of the pulmonary artery (anterior), between the two great vessels (between), or behind the aortic root (posterior). Finally group III anomalies are single right coronary arteries in which the circumflex courses posterior to the aortic root and the anterior descending branch passes either in front of the pulmonary artery (group IIIA) or between the aorta and pulmonary artery (group IIIB). In the last variety there is a possibility of compression of the anterior descending leading to ischaemia or sudden death.

Finally, among anomalous aortic origins of the coronaries, there are patients with virtual absence of the left main stem so that the left coronary appears to have two separate ostia ('double orifice left coronary'). In such patients selective cannulation of one or other of the ostia may result in apparent absence of one of the two main branches of the left coronary artery. The catheter must be repositioned in order to differentiate this condition from occlusion of a branch at its origin.

A high origin above the sinus causes difficulties in cannulation and is particularly associated with a bicuspid aortic valve.

Anomalous aortic origin associated with other congenital heart disease

Anomalous aortic origin is of importance in certain forms of congenital heart disease since the anomalous vessel, if not recognised, may be injured during corrective surgery. These conditions are:
1 Tetralogy of Fallot. In 4 to 7% of cases the anterior descending (or left main) arises from the right sinus and courses over the right ventricular outflow tract.
2 Complete transposition. In 60% of cases the right coronary arises from the posterior sinus. In 25% of cases both the right and circumflex arise fron the posterior sinus (circumflex posterior to the pulmonary artery). Other patterns occur.
3 'Corrected transposition'. The anterior sinus of the anterior, left sided, aorta is the non-coronary sinus and the course of the vessels is reversed with the left coronary passing to the right to supply the right sided morphologic left ventricle.
4 'Univentricular hearts'. Most cases have right and left 'delimiting arteries' (Fig. 13.36) outlining the margins of the outlet chamber and right sided parallel delimiting branches which may be injured during surgery [31]. Other patterns occur.
5 Double outlet right ventricle with L-malposition. In this rare anomaly the right coronary always courses from the left sided aorta to the right across the subpulmonary conus.

ATLAS-CONGENITAL CORONARY ANOMALIES

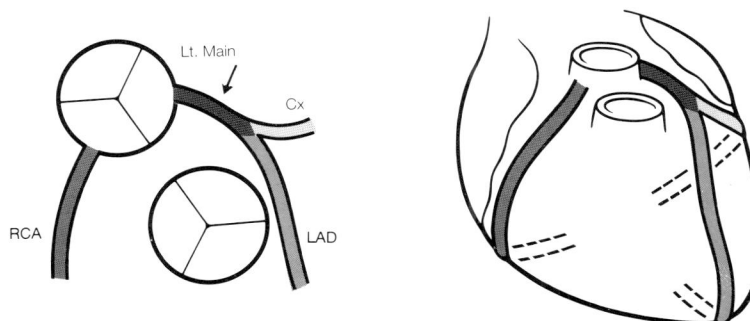

Fig. 13.31 Normal coronary arterial origin and distribution.

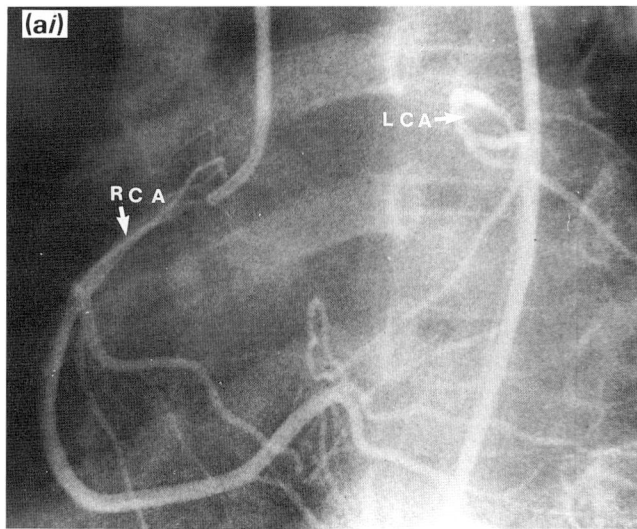

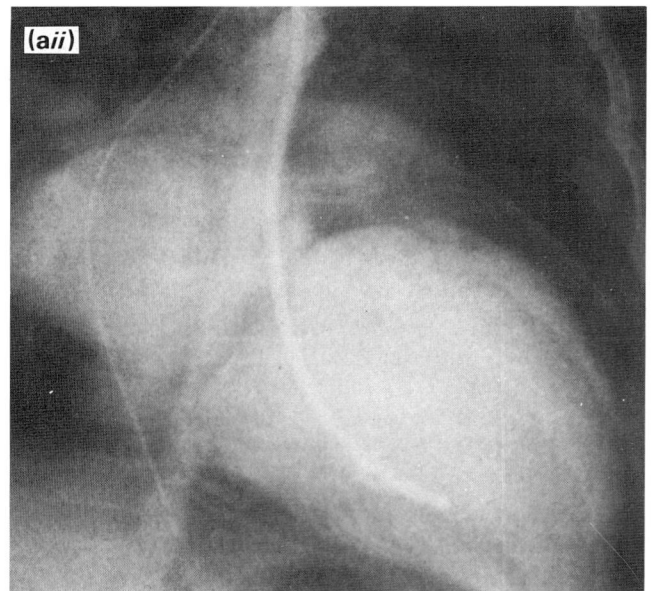

Fig. 13.32 (a–f) Anomalous origin of one or both coronary
arteries from the pulmonary artery.

(ai) Origin of the left coronary artery from the pulmonary artery. The origin of the left coronary has been ligated in this patient
(postoperative study) but an injection of contrast medium into the right coronary artery fills the whole of the coronary arterial circulation
bia collaterals. (aii) Large poorly functioning left ventricle and mitral regurgitation in an infant with anomalous origin of the left coronary
from the pulmonary artery.

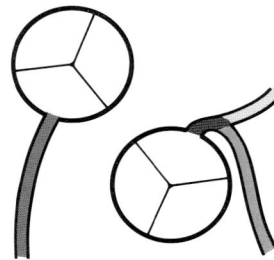

(b) Left coronary from PA (see Fig.
13.32a).

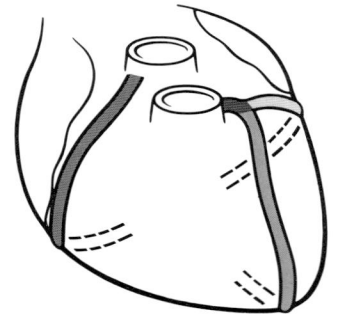

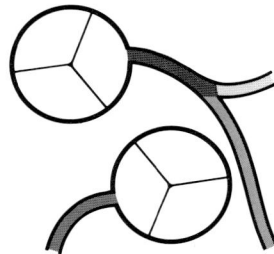

(c) Right coronary from PA.

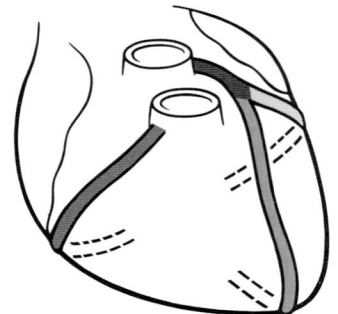

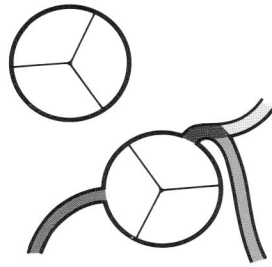

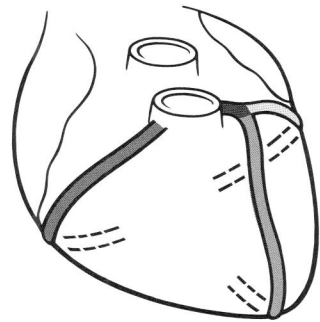

(d) Right and left coronaries from PA.

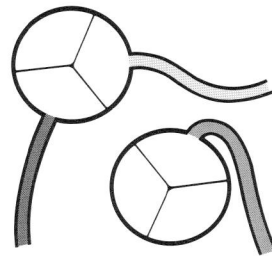

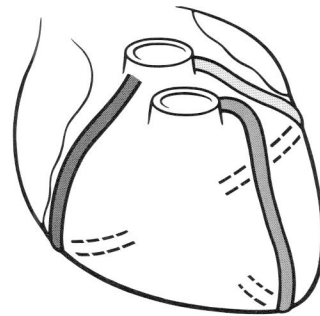

(e) Left anterior descending from PA.

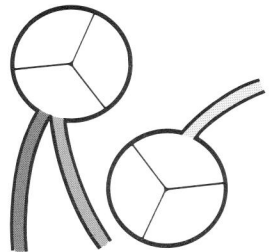

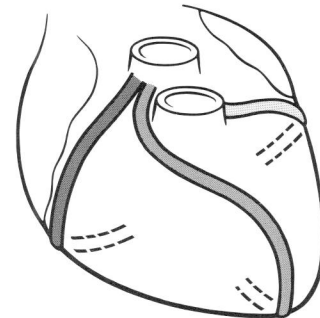

(f) Left circumflex from PA.

(ai)

Rt→

Cx↗

(aii)

Cx→

Rt→

(aiii)

LAD

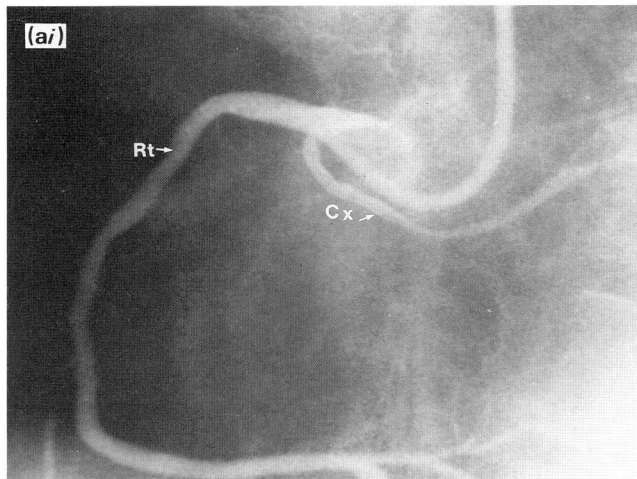

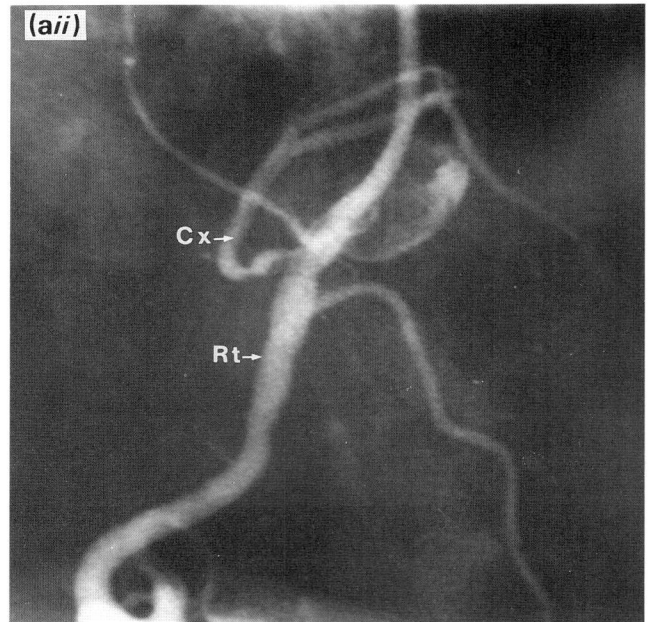

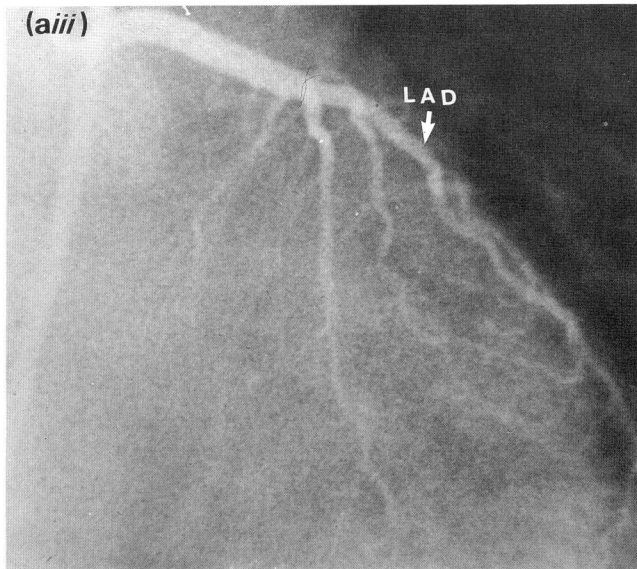

Fig. 13.33 (a−e) Anomalous origin from the aorta.

(a) Origin of the circumflex left coronary artery from the right coronary artery. Both figures show an injection into the right coronary artery and the characteristic course of the circumflex behind the aorta. (ai) Left oblique and (aii) right oblique projections. This is the most frequently encountered anomalous aortic origin of a coronary artery.

In (aiii) an injection into the left coronary artery fills the anterior descending branch only. This appearance, unaccompanied by any other sign of circumflex occlusion must prompt a search for an anomalous origin of the missing vessel.

(b) Left circumflex from right sinus — posterior to aorta.

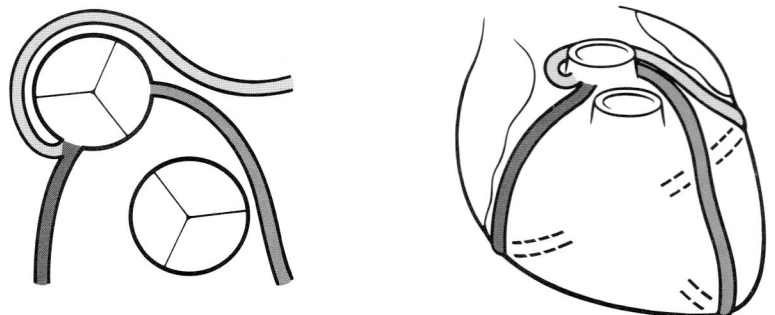

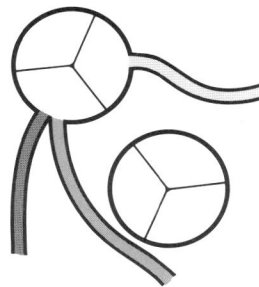

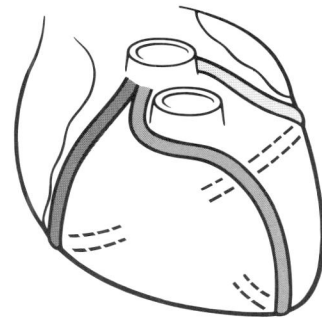

(*ci*) Left anterior descending from right sinus anterior to PA.

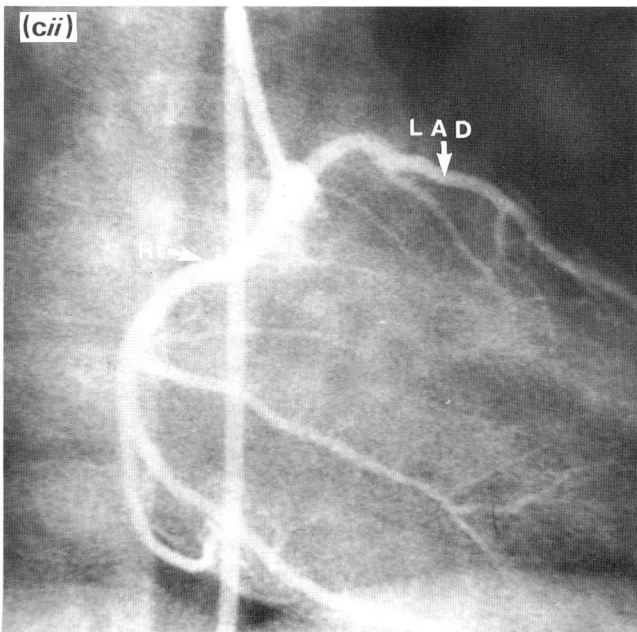

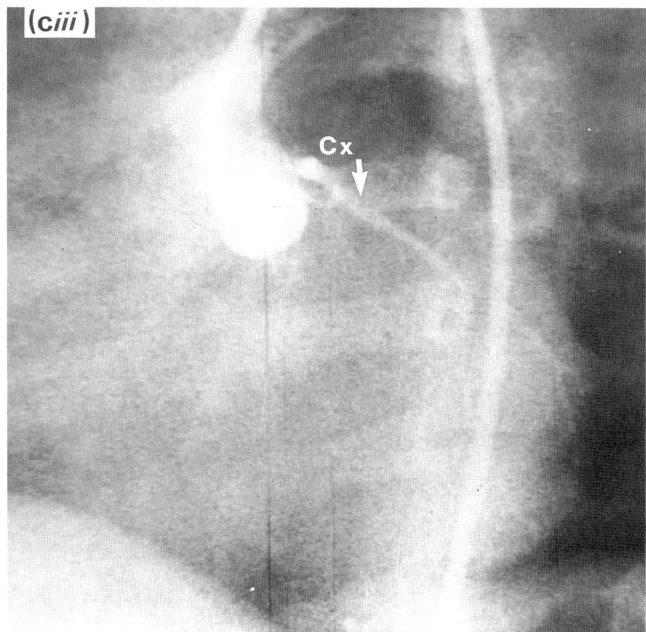

(*cii*) Origin of the anterior descending branch from the right coronary artery (between the aorta and pulmonary artery). Injection into the right coronary artery in the right oblique projection. Both the right coronary and the interior descending (LAD) fill with contrast medium. (*ciii*) In the same patient an injection into the left sinus of Valsalva (left oblique projection) fills the circumflex branch only.

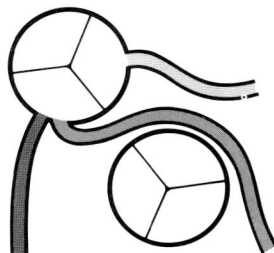

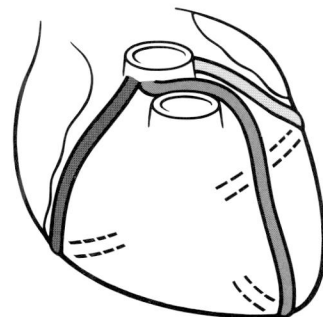

(*civ*) Left anterior descending from right sinus between PA and aorta.

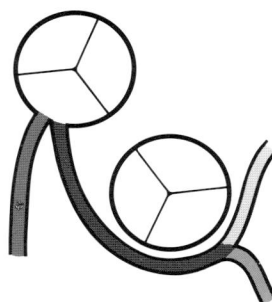

(d*i*) Left main from the right sinus anterior to PA.

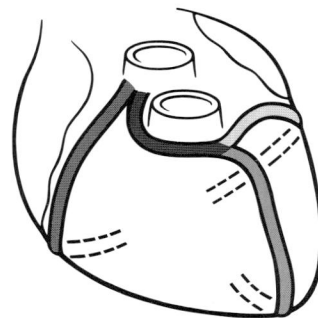

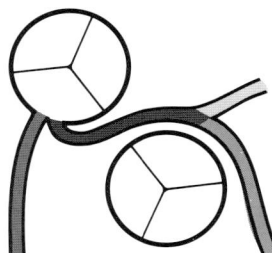

(d*ii*) Left main from right sinus between PA and aorta.

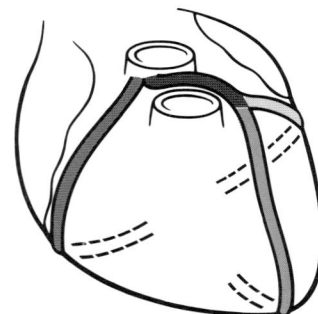

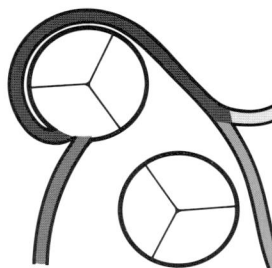

(d*iii*) Left main from right sinus posterior to aorta.

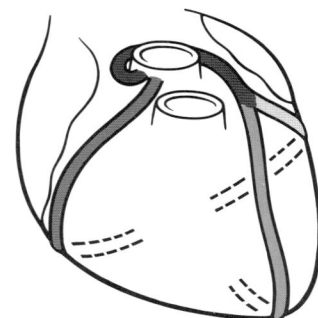

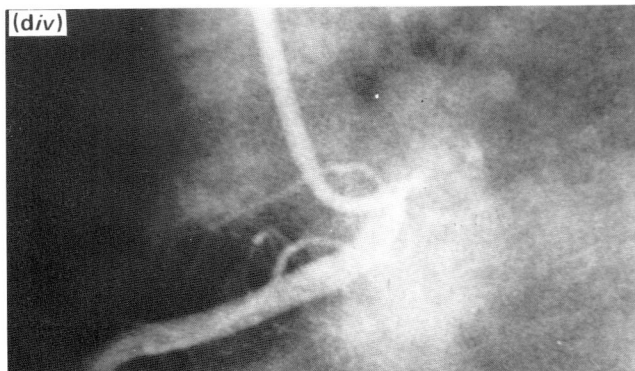

(d*iv*) Origin of the right coronary artery from the left sinus of Valsalva.

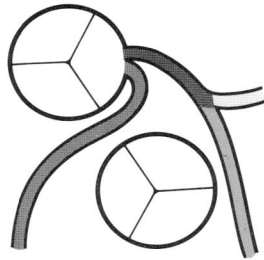

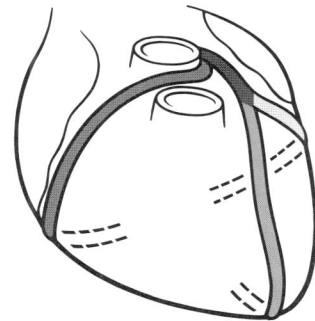

(d*v*) Right coronary from left sinus between PA and aorta.

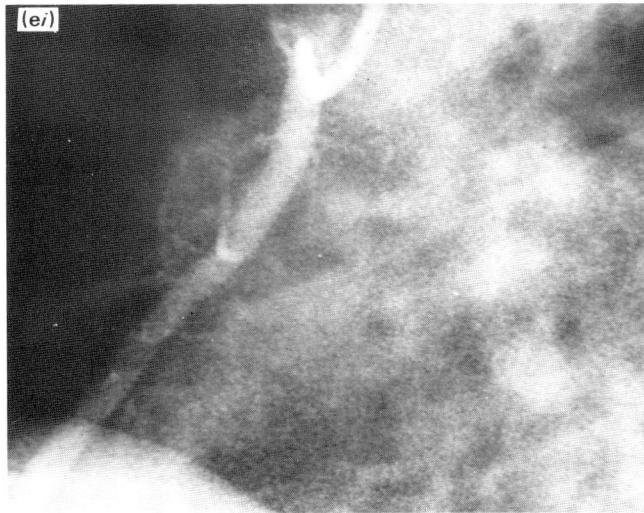

(e*i*) Origin of the right coronary artery from the non-coronary sinus (compare with Fig. 13.33d*iv*).

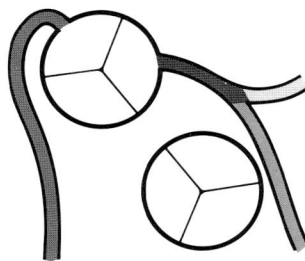

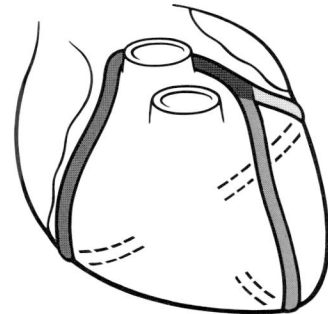

(e*ii*) Right coronary from posterior (non-coronary) sinus.

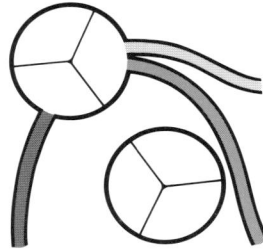
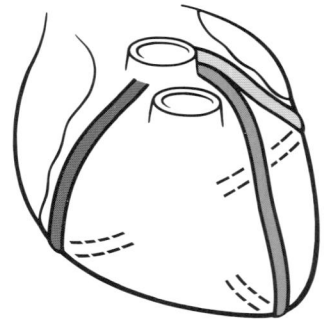

Fig. 13.34 'Double orifice' left coronary.

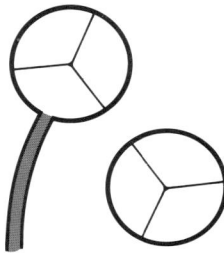
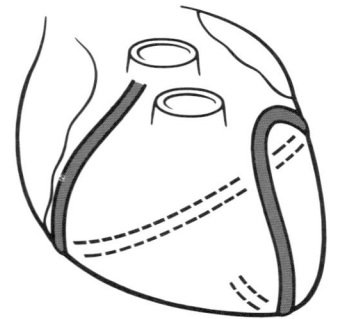

Fig. 13.35 (a–q) Single aortic ostium
('single coronary artery') — classification
according to Lipton *et al.* [30].

(a) Right I.

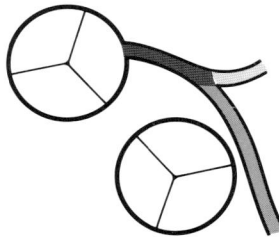
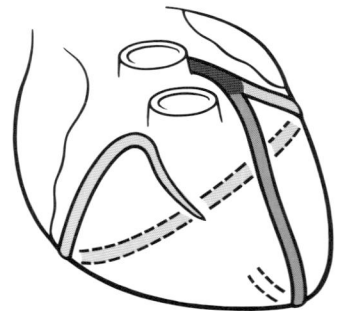

(b) L(eft) I.

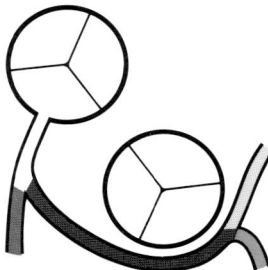
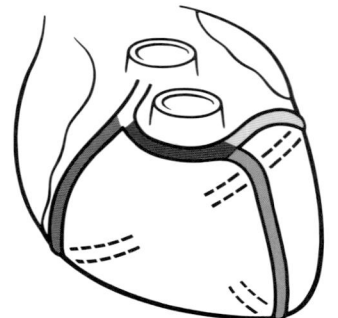

(c) R(ight) II A(nterior).

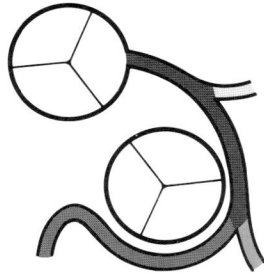

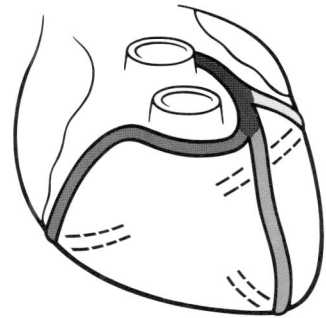

(d) L(eft) II A(nterior).

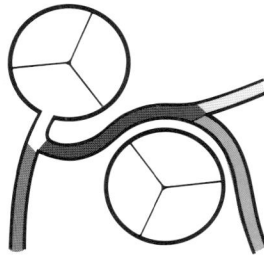

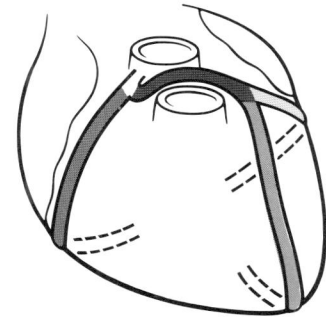

(e) R(ight) II B(etween).

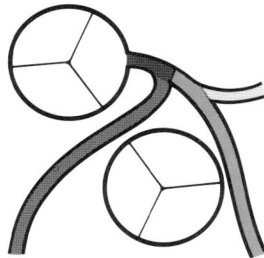

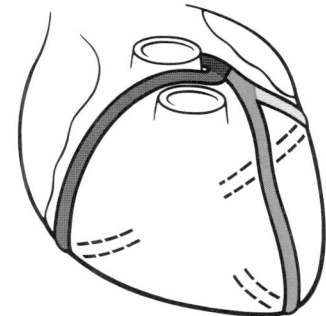

(f) L(eft) II B(etween).

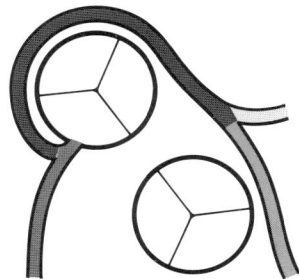

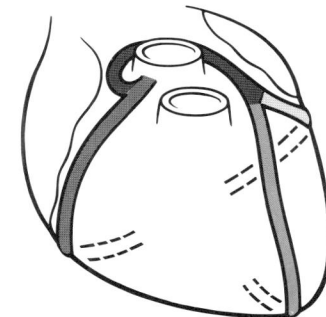

(g) R(ight) II P(osterior).

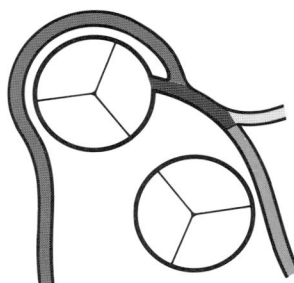

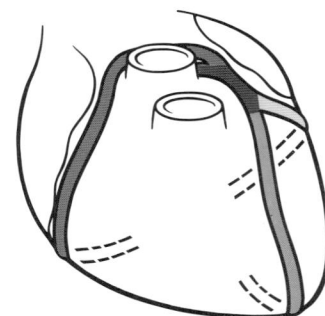

(h) L(eft) II P(osterior).

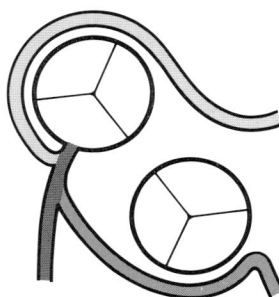

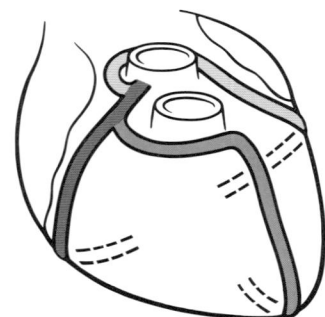

(j) R(ight) III A(nterior).

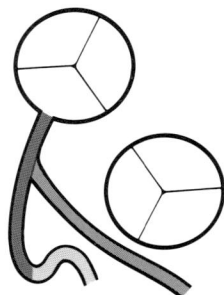

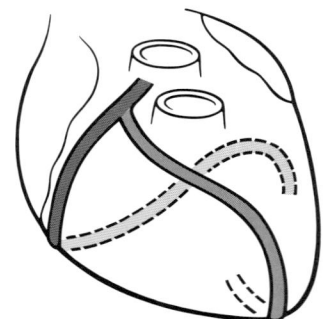

(k) R(ight) III A(nterior).

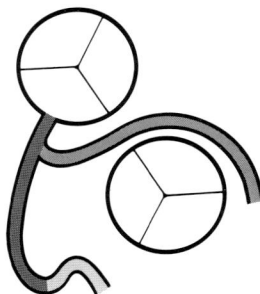

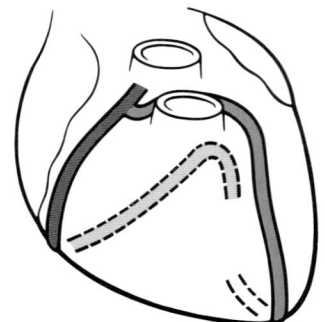

(m) R(ight) III B(etween) — variant (Cx continuation of RCA).

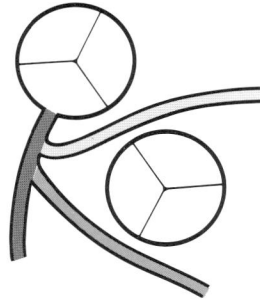

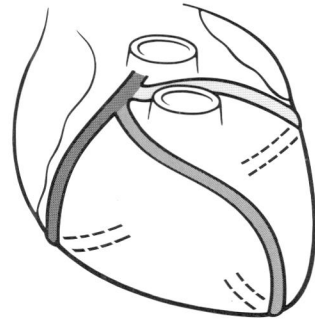

(n) R(ight) III A(nterior) — variant Cx
between PA and aorta.

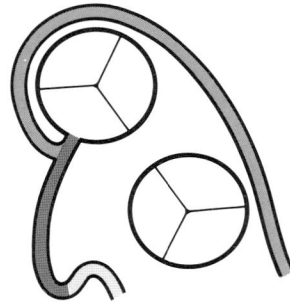

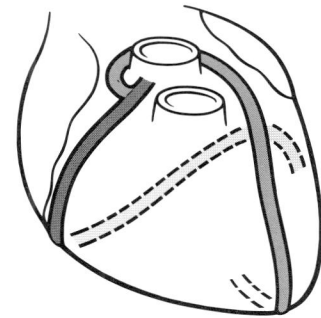

(p) R(ight) III P(osterior) — variant Cx
continuation of RCA, LAD posterior.

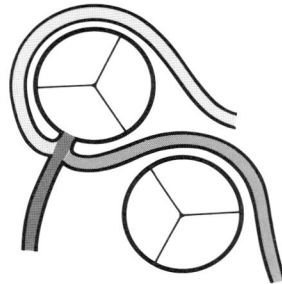

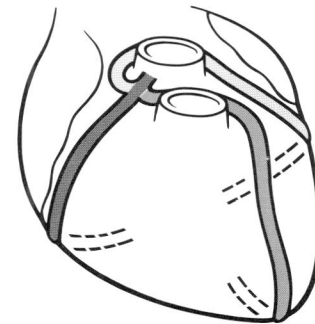

(q) R(ight) III B(etween).

Fig. 13.36 (a–d) Anomalous aortic origin in association with other CHD.

(a) Tetralogy of Fallot.

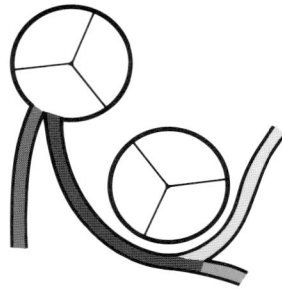

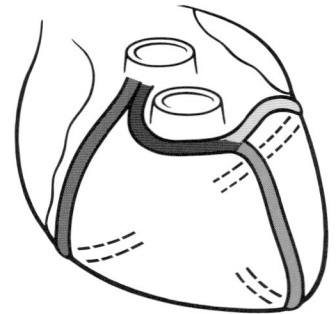

(b) 'Corrected transposition'.

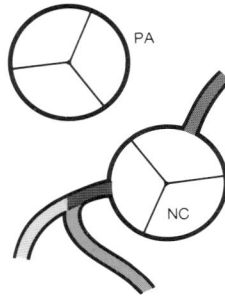

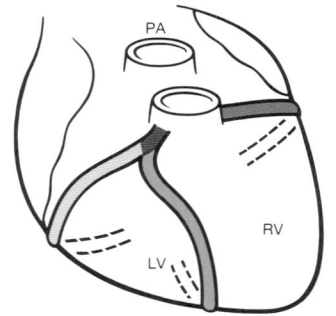

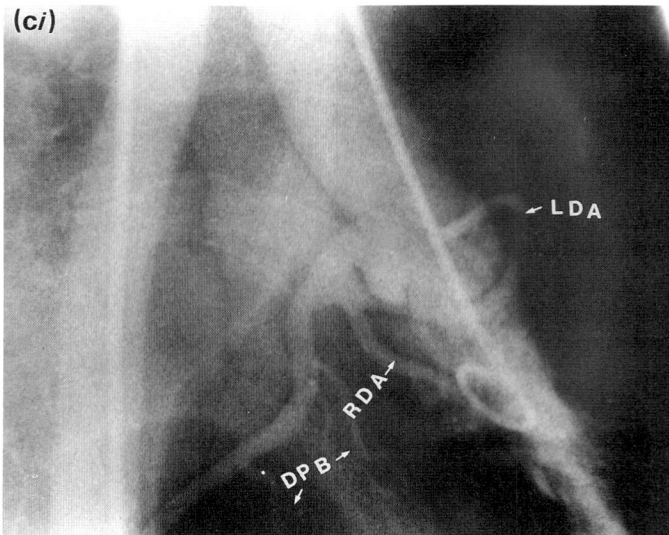

(c) 'Univentricular hearts': left delimiting artery (LDA), right delimiting artery (RDA), delimiting parallel branches (DPB), and outlet chamber (OC).

(ci) The coronary arteries in 'univentricular heart'. The injection has been made into a left-sided subaortic outflow chamber. Left (LDA) and right (RDA) delimiting parallel branches (DPB) are seen.

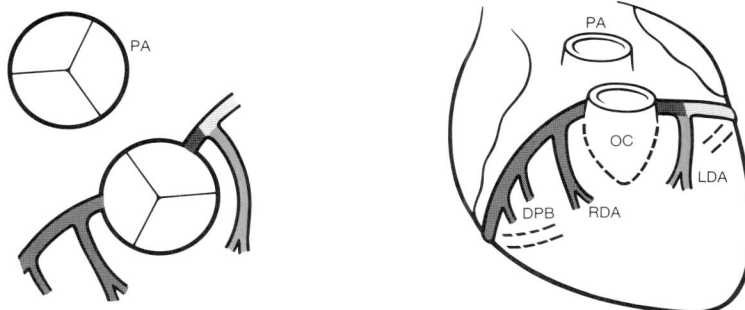

(cii) 'Typical pattern'.

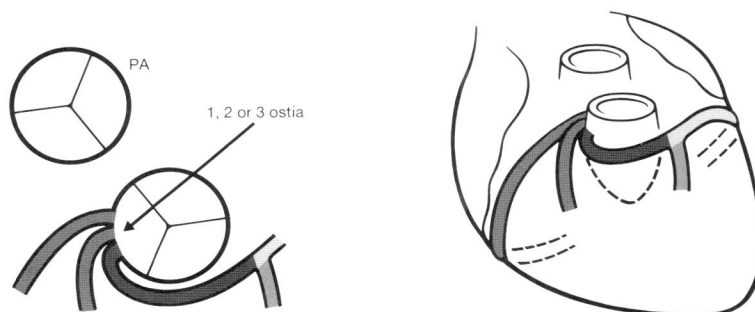

(ciii) Alternative typical pattern.

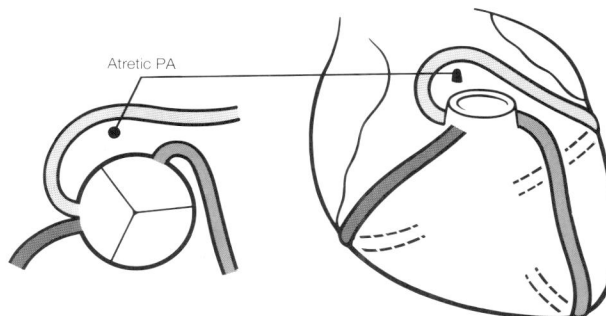

(civ) Alternative typical pattern.

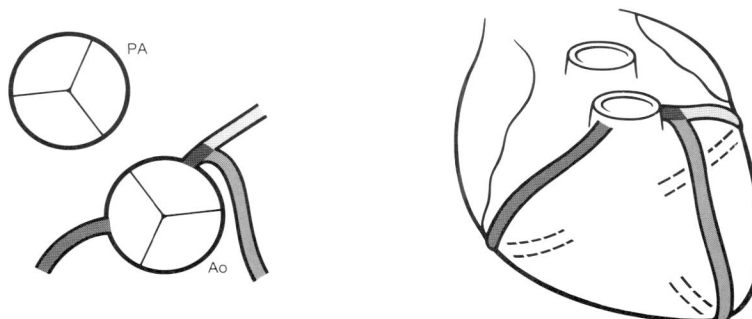

(d) Double outlet right ventricle with 'L' malposition.

(a)

(b)

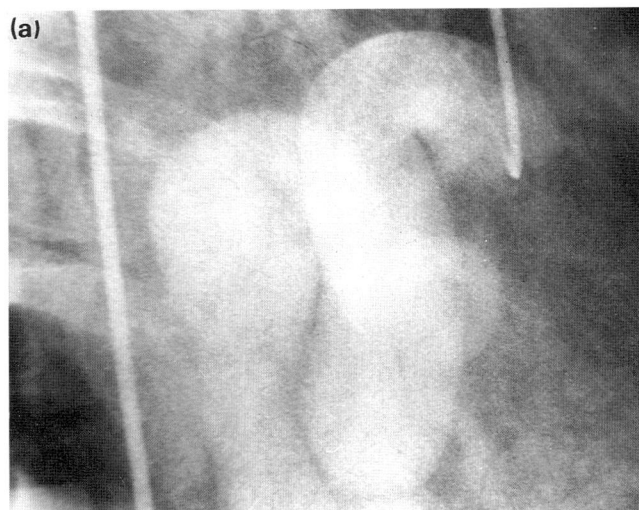

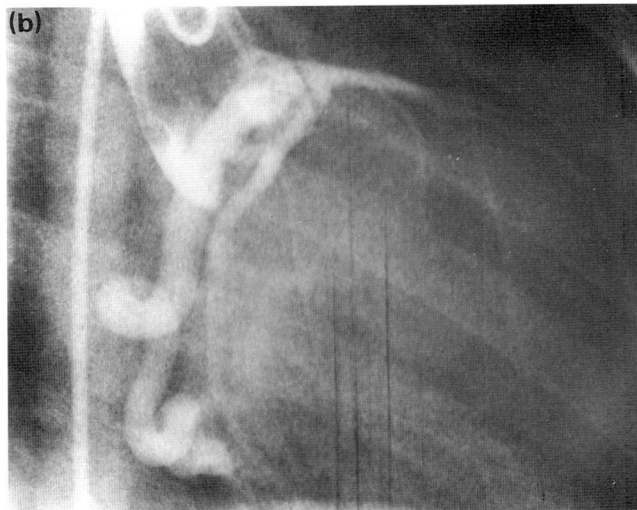

Fig. 13.37 (a and b) Two examples of 'coronary-cameral fistula'. The coronary artery is enormously dilated as a consequence of high flow. The communication is to the right atrium.

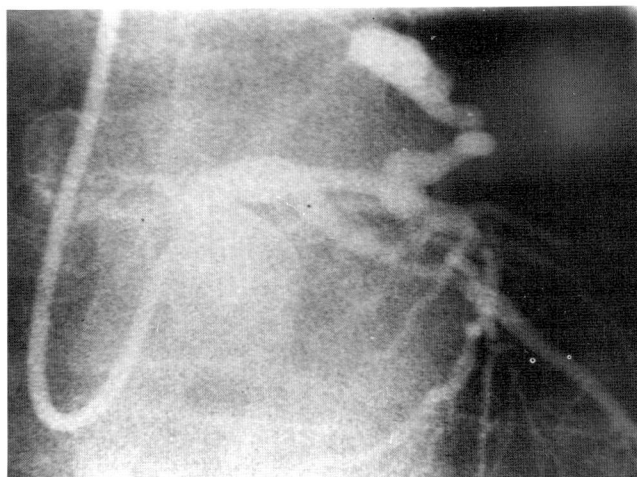

Fig. 13.38 Fistula between the left coronary artery and the pulmonary artery. Such fistulae may be small and may in some instances be acquired in association, for example, with bronchiectasis.

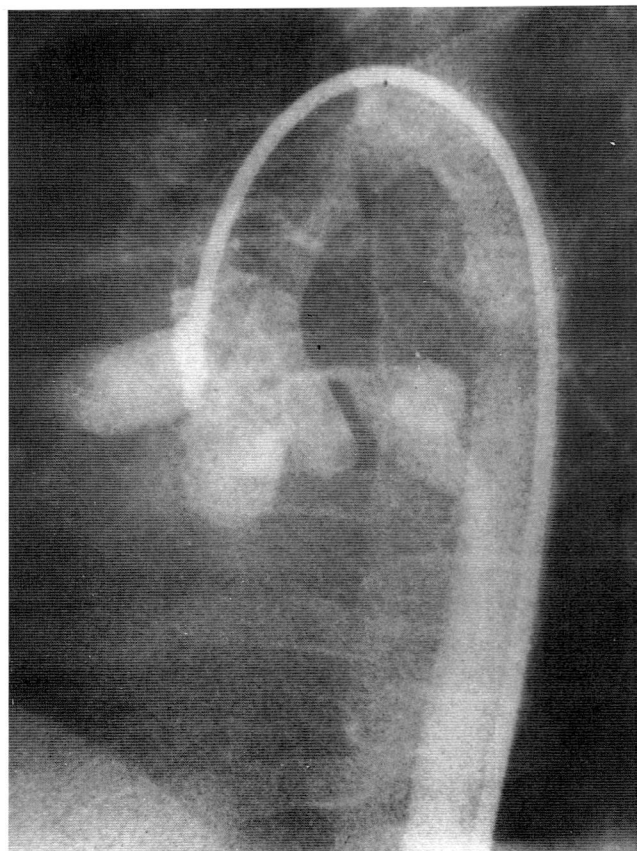

Fig. 13.39 Congenital coronary anomalies: coronary artery aneurysms due to Kawasaki disease.

Anomalies with normal aortic origin

1 Coronary-cameral fistulae (Fig. 13.37). The right coronary artery is involved in slightly more cases than the left. Both coronaries are involved in 5% of cases. The most common drainage site is to the right ventricle (approximately half of the cases) followed, in order of frequency, by the right atrium, the pulmonary artery (Fig. 13.38), the coronary sinus, the left atrium, the left ventricle and the superior vena cava. Drainage is to the right heart in 90% of cases. Where drainage is to a right sided structure there is a potential for a left-to-right shunt. The fistulous communication is usually large with a high flow so that the vessel is enormously dilated and tortuous. The large shunt may lead to congestive heart failure or the 'coronary steal' may lead to myocardial ischaemia and angina. Other complications include infective endocarditis and rupture of the fistulous vessel. Selective injections into the abnormal vessel in multiple projections are needed to delineate the site of drainage.

2 Sinusoids communicate between the right ventricle and the left coronary in infants with pulmonary atresia and intact ventricular septum (Fig. 17.60).

3 Coronary artery aneurysms occur in Kawasaki disease and it is possible that those labelled 'congenital' are also due to unrecognised episodes of this disease (Fig. 13.39).

AMERICAN HEART ASSOCIATION — CORONARY ARTERY DISEASE REPORTING SYSTEM

LEFT VENTRICULOGRAM (LVG)

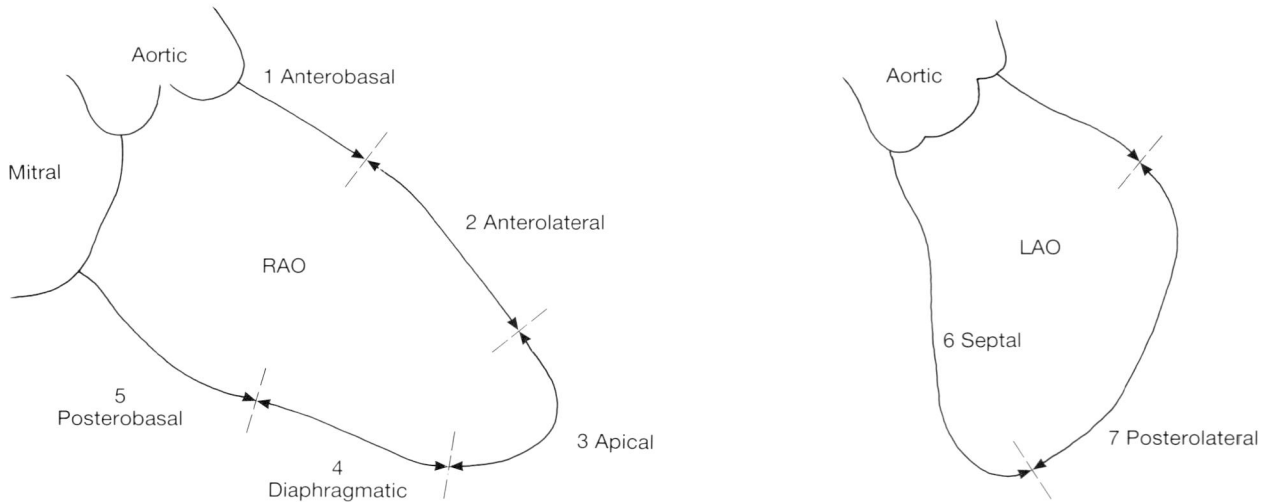

Normal	Normal wall motion of indicated ventricular segment
Reduced	Velocity and/or amplitude of indicated wall ventricular segment motion are/is reduced.
None	Absence of appropriate wall motion of indicated ventricular segment.
Dyskinetic	Paradoxical wall motion of indicated ventricular segment.
Aneurysmal	Aneurysmal bulging with sharply defined margins of indicated ventricular segment.
Undefined	Status of indicated ventricular wall segment cannot be described because of improper visualisation or omission of appropriate views.

CORONARY ARTERIOGRAM

Note: Record the most severe narrowing of the indicated coronary arterial segment if more than one narrowing is present in a particular segment.

Records as follows:

Normal	Indicated segment is entirely within normal limits.
Gives collateral	Indicated segment is *giving* collaterals to some other vessel or branch.
Small	Indicated vessel or segment of vessel is small throughout either because of anatomic variation or diffuse narrowing. Score both 'normal' and 'small' if normal *and* small; score both 'small' and degree of narrowing if disease is diffuse.
25%	Lumen diameter reduction up to but not exceeding 25%.
50%	Lumen diameter reduction from 26% up to but not exceeding 50%.
75%	Lumen diameter reduction from 51% up to but not exceeding 75%.
90%	Lumen diameter reduction from 76% up to but not exceeding 90%.

Filled by collaterals	Indicated vessel or segment of vessel is being opacified by collateral channels.
99%	Lumen appears nearly obliterated or reduced to hair-width (greater than 90% narrowing) but some contrast still passes by this narrowing.
100%	Complete occlusion of indicated branch or segment of vessel.
Graftable	Segment of vessel that either appears angiographically suitable for graft anastomosis (when arteriogram is a preoperative study) or where graft was placed (if arteriogram is a postoperative study).
Absent	Indicated segment is absent due to *unquestionable* anatomic variation. *Note*: 1 Not to be checked when vessel may be absent because of proximal occlusion.
	2 This should also be checked for the first segment of a major artery when there is ectopic origin of that artery (e.g., origin of circumflex from right coronary artery). Site of anomalous origin of artery should also be written in.

RIGHT CORONARY ARTERY (RCA)

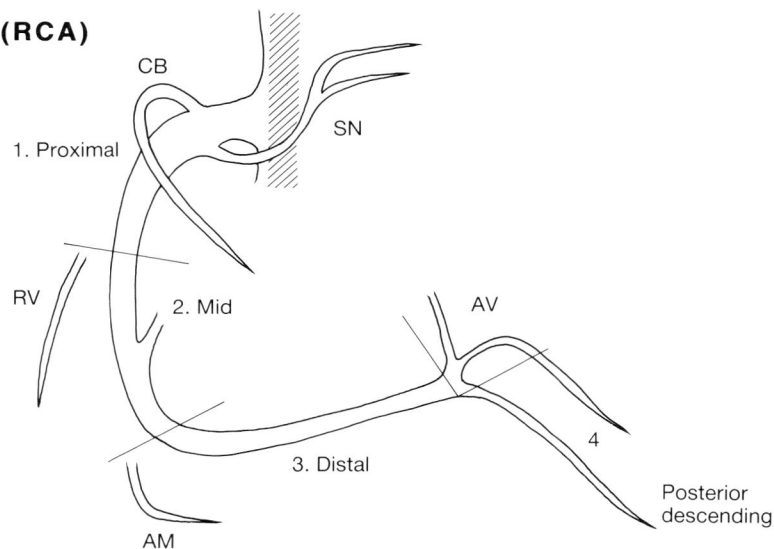

1 Proximal	RCA from ostium to one-half the distance to the acute margin of heart. *Note*: Distal portion of this coronary segment may coincide with origin of one of the large right ventricular branches (RV).
2 Mid	RCA from end of above segment to acute margin of heart. *Note*: Distal portion of this segment *usually* (but not always) coincides with origin of the acute marginal branch (AM).
3 Distal	RCA running along the posterior right atrioventricular groove, from the acute margin of heart to the origin of the posterior descending branch. *Note*: In the 'predominant' left coronary pattern (posterior descending from left circumflex), this segment may be very small.
4 Posterior descending	Posterior descending branch, when present. *Note*: Minor branches such as the conus (CB); sinus node (SN); right ventricular (RV); acute marginal (AM); and AV node (AV) branches are indicated in diagram only for general orientation. These branches may or may not be visualised in the individual patient. Those that are highly variable as to their origins are shown unattached to parent artery.

MAIN LEFT CORONARY ARTERY (LCA)

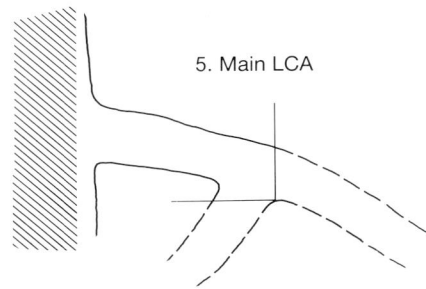

5 Main left   LCA extends from the ostium of LCA through bifurcation into left anterior descending and left circumflex branches.

LEFT ANTERIOR DESCENDING ARTERY (LAD)

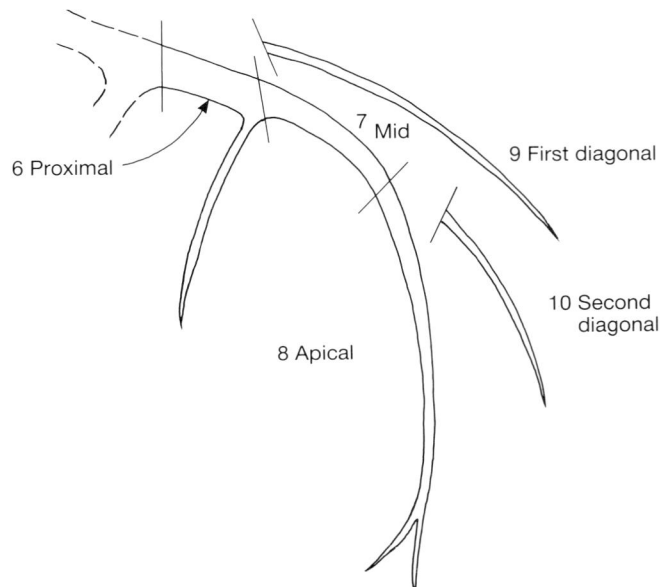

6 Proximal	LAD proximal to and including origin of the first major septal perforator branch.
7 Mid	LAD immediately distal to origin of the first major septal perforator branch and extending to point where LAD forms an angle (RAO view) and often but not always coinciding or close to the origin of second diagonal branch (D_2). If this angle or branch is not identifiable, this segment ends at one-half the distance from the first major septal perforator branch to apex of heart.
8 Apical	Terminal portion of LAD running along interventricular sulcus, beginning with the end of previous segment, and usually extending beyond apex.
9 First diagonal	First diagonal (D_1): The largest, and usually the first, diagonal branch having its origin from proximal segment of LAD. Occasionally, this can be a separate branch off main LCA.
10 Second diagonal	Second diagonal (D_2): The second diagonal branch, which often has its origin at the 'angle' of LAD, descending when visualised in RAO projection.

LEFT CIRCUMFLEX CORONARY ARTERY (CIRC)

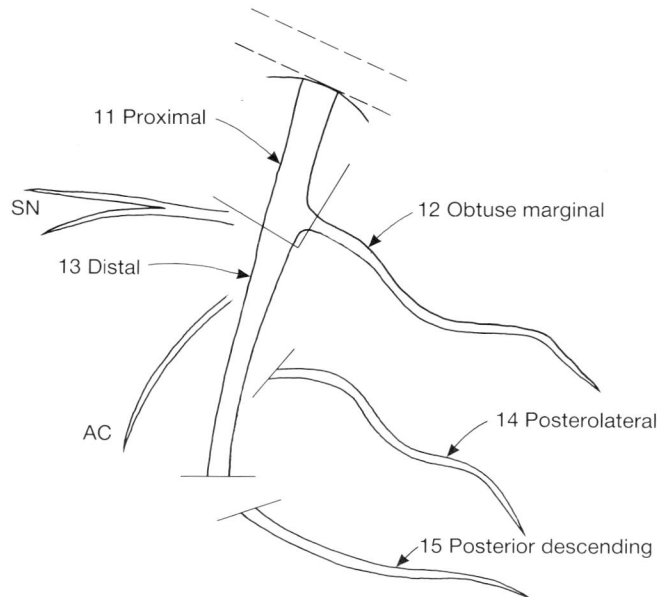

11 Proximal

SN

13 Distal

12 Obtuse marginal

AC

14 Posterolateral

15 Posterior descending

11 Proximal	Main stem of circumflex from its origin off main LCA to and including origin of obtuse marginal branch.
12 Obtuse marginal (OM)	The largest branch of circumflex running in general area of obtuse margin of heart.
13 Distal	The stem of the circumflex distal to origin of obtuse marginal branch and running along or close to posterior left artrioventricular groove. Caliber of this portion may be small.
14 Posterolateral (PL)	Posterolateral branch of circumflex distributing to posterolateral surface of left ventricle; almost always smaller in caliber than obtuse marginal. May be absent or may be a division of obtuse marginal branch.
15 Posterior descending (PD)	Posterior descending, when present as a branch of circumflex. *Note*: Minor or variable branches such as the sinus node (SN) and the atrial circumflex (AC) are indicated in the diagram only for the purpose of general orientation. They may or may not be visualised in the individual patient.

GENERAL READING

1 Abrams HL (ed.) *Coronary arteriography: a practical approach.* Massachusetts, Little, Brown and Co., 1983.
2 King SB, Douglas JS. *Coronary arteriography and angioplasty.* New York, McGraw Hill, 1985.

REFERENCES

1 Vieweg WVR, Alpert JS, Hagen AD. Caliber and distribution of normal coronary arterial anatomy. *Cathet Cardiovasc Diagn* 1976;**2**:269.
2 Vieweg WVR, Smith DC, Hagen AD. A clinically useful coding system for normal coronary artery anatomy. *Cathet Cardiovasc Diagn* 1975;**1**:171.
3 Vieweg WVR, Alpert JS, Hagen AD. Origin of the sinoatrial node and atrioventricular node arteries in right, mixed and left inferior emphasis systems. *Cathet Cardiovasc Diagn* 1975;**1**:361.
4 Sones FM, Shirey EK. Cine coronary arteriography. *Mod Concepts Cardiovasc Dis* 1962;**31**:735.
5 Sheldon WC. Techniques for coronary arteriography. *Cathet Cardiovasc Diagn* 1979;**5**:191.
6 Judkins MP. Selective coronary arteriography: I. A percutaneous transfemoral technique. *Radiology* 1967;**89**:815.
7 Page HL. The Judkins technique. *Cathet Cardiovasc Diagn* 1979;**5**:187.
8 Amplatz K, Formanek G, Stanger P, Wilson W. Mechanics of selective coronary artery catheterization via femoral approach. *Radiology* 1967;**89**:1040.
9 Wells DE *et al.* A simplified method for left heart catheterization including coronary arteriography. *Chest* 1973;**63**:959.
10 Zir LM, Dinsmore RE, Goss C, Harthorne JW. Experience with preformed catheters for coronary angiography by the brachial approach. *Cathet Cardiovasc Diagn* 1975; **1**:303.
11 Schoonmaker FW, King SB. Coronary arteriography by the single catheter percutaneous femoral technique. Experience with 6800 cases. *Circulation* 1974;**50**:735.
12 El Gamal *et al.* Selective coronary arteriography with a preformed single catheter: percutaneous femoral technique. *AJR* 1980;**135**:630.
13 Arani DT. A time-saving technique in angiography of aortocoronary bypass patients. *Cathet Cardiovasc Diagn* 1981;**7**:301.
14 Singh RN. Internal mammary arteriography: a new catheter technique by right brachial approach. *Cathet Cardiovasc Diagn* 1980;**6**:439.
15 Salem BI *et al.* Left main coronary artery ostial stenosis: clinical markers, angiographic recognition and distinction from left main disease. *Cathet Cardiovasc Diagn* 1979;**5**:125.
16 Miller GAH, Honey M, El-Sayed H. Isolated coronary ostial stenosis. *Cathet Cardiovasc Diagn* 1986;**12**:30.
17 Maseri A *et al.* 'Variant' angina: one aspect of a continuous spectrum of vasospastic myocardial ischaemia. *Am J Cardiol* 1978;**42**:1019.
18 Fester A. Ergonovine Maleate — a provocative test. *Cathet Cardiovasc Diagn* 1980;**6**:217.
19 Buxton A *et al.* Refractory ergonovine induced coronary vasospasm: importance of intracoronary nitroglycerin. *Am J Cardiol* 1980;**46**:329.
20 Helfant RH. Coronary arterial spasm and provocative testing in ischemic heart disease. *Am J Cardiol* 1978;**41**:787.
21 Pepine CJ, Feldman RL, Conti CR. Recommendations for use of ergonovine to provoke coronary artery spasm. *Cathet Cardiovasc Diagn* 1980;**6**:423.
22 Thomas AC *et al.* Potential errors in the estimation of coronary arterial stenosis from clinical arteriography with reference to the shape of the coronary arterial lumen. *Br Heart J* 1986;**55**:129.
23 Spears JR, Sandor T, Baim DS, Paulin S. The minimum error in estimating coronary luminal cross-sectional area from cineangiographic diameter measurements. *Cathet Cardiovasc Diagn* 1983;**9**:119.
24 Bjork L, O'Keefe A. Estimation of coronary artery stenosis. Limitation of present methods. *Acta Radiol Diagn* 1976;**17**:777.
25 Austen WG *et al.* A reporting system on patients evaluated for coronary artery disease. *Circulation* 1975;**51**:5.
26 Brandt PWT, Partridge JB, Wattie WJ. Coronary arteriography: method of presentation of the arteriogram report and a scoring system. *Clin Radiol* 1977;**28**:361.
27 Levin DC, Fallon JT. Significance of the angiographic morphology of localised coronary stenoses: histopathologic correlations. *Circulation* 1982;**66**:316.
28 Roberts WC. Major anamalies of coronary arterial origin seen in adulthood. *Am Heart J* 1986;**111**:941.
29 Engel HJ, Torres C, Page HL. Major variations in anatomical origin of the coronary arteries. Angiographic observations in 4,250 patients without associated congenital heart disease. *Cathet Cardiovasc Diagn* 1975;**1**:157.
30 Lipton MJ *et al.* Isolated single coronary artery: diagnosis, classification and clinical significance. *Radiology* 1979;**130**:39.
31 Keeton BR *et al.* Anatomy of coronary arteries in univentricular hearts and its surgical implications. *Am J Cardiol* 1979;**43**:569.

Coronary angioplasty (PTCA)

INTRODUCTION

Angioplasty was introduced by Andreas Gruentzig in 1977 [1]. He modified the technique previously described by Dotter and Judkins for use in the peripheral circulation. He originally imagined that the procedure would have limited application to patients with persistent angina who had a single discrete, concentric stenosis in only one coronary artery. A retrospective analysis of a large number of angiograms at the time suggested that between 2 and 3% of patients undergoing coronary arteriography would be suitable for angioplasty (London Chest Hospital, unpublished data).

Experienced angiographers were surprised to find how difficult angioplasty was. The most unexpected problems were the difficulty in knowing the exact location especially, in three dimensional terms, of the dilatation catheter and guide wire with respect to the target stenosis; and how easy it was to enter small branches that were not necessarily visible angiographically. The problem was increased by the poor visualisation of the coronary tree that was possible when injecting radio-opaque medium through the guiding catheter whose lumen was mostly taken up by the dilatation catheter, and the inability to manoeuvre the dilatation system in the coronary circulation.

In the London Chest Hospital approximately 25% of the patients with coronary artery disease are now treated with angioplasty and in other centres the proportion is much greater. There are a number of reasons for this including increased experience, better technology, and a more aggressive approach.

X-RAY APPARATUS

Guide wires can be very fine, as little as 0.01 inches in diameter, and thus difficult to see with standard image intensification systems which are able to resolve only approximately two pairs of lines per millimetre. The latest systems employ 1249 as opposed to 625 line TV which, when used with a small field size, gives high magnification of the image. This results in a resolution of 3.5 line pairs (lp) per millimetre and greatly increases the ability to see the dilatation system.

Most operators work with what has become known as a road map; that is a still frame of the appropriate coronary arteriogram. Spatial orientation is greatly improved by being able to see two views at right angles to each other simultaneously with biplane fluoroscopy. A number of images can be stored using digital systems for instant recall to match the chosen fluoroscopic views and these stored images can be automatically updated to match the current situation if desired. Such systems are very sophisticated and expensive but it is possible to perform successful angioplasty with much less. However single plane apparatus with good resolution TV, video playback and freeze frame facilities are minimum requirements.

PHYSIOLOGICAL MONITORING

Electrocardiogram

S—T segment shift, usually elevation, is a common occurrence during balloon inflation. Monitoring the changes is, however, important since it may influence the procedure. The duration of each balloon inflation and the total number of inflations may be modified by the changes that are seen. If only a single ECG lead is being monitored it must be chosen to reflect the part of the myocardium supplied by the vessel being treated. Preferably multiple leads should be monitored particularly as a problem such as dissection due to a misdirected guide wire, embolism or thrombosis may occur in an area remote from that supplied by the target vessel. It is possible to monitor the 12 standard leads simultaneously. Small electrodes can be used for the chest leads that do not interfere with visualisation of the dilatation system (see Fig. 14.6).

Blood pressure

Blood pressure is continuously monitored through the guiding catheter but various necessary manoeuvres such as loosening the haemostatic valve to introduce the balloon catheter make this pressure unreliable. Some operators therefore prefer to monitor femoral artery pressure through the side-arm of the femoral introducing sheath in addition. It is possible to measure the transstenotic gradient continuously with some dilatation systems.

It is not necessary to make any other routine physiological measurements although it has been very informative to do so. The pathophysiological changes of transient ischaemia due to balloon inflation will be discussed below.

PATIENT PREPARATION

Premedication

As with every invasive procedure premedication is a matter of personal choice but must be compatible with the possibility of the patient undergoing emergency surgery. Chest pain may occur so its effects should be minimised. Atropine or related substances may be used but if they are sublingual nitrates will not be effective later because of the lack of oral secretions. Hypotension should be avoided because of its deleterious effect on myocardial perfusion. Papaveratum given 2 hours before the procedure has provided good premedication.

Vasodilators

Coronary arterial spasm may occur during angioplasty so that vasodilators are helpful. Hypotension, however, has a deleterious effect on coronary perfusion and enhances the likelihood of thrombosis so that vasodilators should be used sparingly. Many of the patients are already taking long acting vasodilators and a last dose with the premedication is reasonable. Some operators prefer to give continuous

infusions in which case care must be taken to control the infusion rate — especially during transfer of the patient between bed and laboratory — so as to avoid undersirable hypotension.

Antiplatelet agents

The damage to the arterial wall caused by angioplasty produces platelet aggregation with a tendency to thrombosis and platelet adhesion and the local release of substances such as platelet growth factor which are likely to play a part in the restenosis that may occur. Antiplatelet agents such as aspirin and dipyridamole are usually given 24 hours before the procedure to minimise these effects. Concern that aspirin might lead to uncontrollable bleeding if urgent surgery is needed has, fortunately, not been borne out by experience.

TECHNIQUE

General

SEDATION

A low level of anxiety is clearly desirable in the laboratory; there should be dim lighting and a minimum of noise to avoid stimulating the premedicated patient. Additional sedation should be given as indicated. 10 mg of diazepam is often sufficient to enable the patient to sleep for the majority of an average length procedure.

BLOOD PRESSURE CONTROL

The need to avoid hypotension has already been mentioned but this is particularly important in the laboratory. The patient is already sedated and the excessive use of vasodilators readily produces hypotension. It is easy for an operator, especially one not very experienced, to err in the wrong direction and give large doses of vasodilators because of anxiety about the possibility of coronary spasm. Correction of hypotension is difficult in these circumstances as vasoconstrictors have undesirable effects especially on already ischaemic myocardium. It is probably better, in the first instance, to try postural manoeuvres and resort to catecholamines only if these fail.

HEART RATE

The heart rate should be maintained above 70 per minute and this can be achieved with atropine. It is rarely necessary to slow the rate in an adequately sedated patient.

ANTICOAGULATION

The patient should be adequately heparinised throughout the procedure. This can be by continuous infusion or, more usually, by intermittent bolus injections. The dose can be controlled by measuring the activated partial thromboplastin time (APTT). Most laboratories simply give 100 u/kg body weight at the start of the procedure and add 50 u/kg after 1 hour.

Specific technique

ROUTE

The majority of angioplasties are performed from the right femoral artery. This is a convenient situation with the patient being used as a table for the guide wire, balloon catheter and inflation device. It also provides greater protection from radiation since operator and assistants are further from the X-ray source. It is physically easier to introduce further protective shields. Patients may also experience discomfort in the arm and hand during prolonged procedures from the brachial artery.

VENOUS CATHETER

It is desirable to have a venous route for quick administration of drugs, continuous infusions or placement of a pacing catheter if necessary but it is not necessary to have a catheter in place. It is convenient to place a sheath in the vein adjacent to the arterial entry site.

GUIDING CATHETER

The original guiding catheters were designed to overcome difficulties in directing the dilatation system into the appropriate artery and there were, for instance, catheters with different tip orientations for the anterior descending and circumflex branches of the left coronary artery. They were also large, 9F or more, to permit visualisation of the coronary vessels

by dye injection when the dilatation catheter was in place. The tip was not deformable thus increasing the risk of arterial wall damage and they were not very radio-opaque.

General advances in the technique and design improvements have produced guiding catheters with much better characteristics. A large number of different types are available but small size (8F), thin wall, good radio-opacity and a relatively atraumatic tip (e.g. 'soft-tip' Schneider Medintag AG for address see Appendix II) are common to most. A number have radioopaque rings at the tip facilitating its visualisation particularly with respect to movement of the catheter down the coronary artery.

BALLOON/GUIDE WIRE SYSTEM

The original Greuntzig dilatation catheter had a short flexible guide wire attached to its tip. It was not steerable but it had a lumen for pressure measurement or injection of radio-opaque medium. Catheters similar to this are still available although they are more steerable (Hartzler LPS, see Fig. 14.3). The main advances that have occured have been the development of separate steerable guide wires, the production of low profile balloons and the reduction of catheter size allowing good visualisation of the coronary arteries with the dilatation system in situ. There has been some inevitable trade-off and many of the currently used systems do not allow measurement of the transstenotic pressure gradient. There has been much discussion about the value of these gradients. They are undoubtedly affected by two major factors, the presence of the catheter across the stenosis and the unpredictable effect of collateral flow. Reduction of gradient was an important indicator of successful dilatation but improved angiographic visualisation has made it much less so.

Continued development makes it very likely, however, that new systems will become available that have all of the desirable characteristics. The separation of the balloon catheter and guide wire has made it possible to use exchange wires so that catheters with different shape and size balloons can be used without having to recross the lesion with the guide wire.

Two systems have been developed that allow excellent visualisation of the coronary tree without removal of the balloon catheter or the guide wire. The Monorail catheter (see Fig. 14.2) (Schneider

Medintag AG) has a narrow shaft (1 mm diameter) which widens just proximal to the balloon where there is an entry hole for the guide wire which passes through the balloon segment and out of the end-hole in the usual way. The guiding catheter therefore contains only the small guidewire and balloon catheter shaft and contrast medium can be injected at a sufficiently high flow rate for good visualisation. Uniquely the balloon catheter can be threaded over a previously positioned standard length guide wire without having to withdraw it as the balloon is advanced. The manoeuvre can be repeated with different size balloons making it a very versatile system. The snake version has an additional short flexible segment of shaft behind the balloon to help with passage through tortuous arteries. The only disadvantage is that it lacks 'pushability' when attempting to cross difficult stenoses. The second system has similar problems and advantages. It is the Micro Hartzler (ACS) balloon catheter which also has a smaller shaft which contains a fine guide wire that has a larger flexible tip so that the wire cannot be totally withdrawn from the catheter. This system is very manoeuvreable and is especially useful for tortuous vessels and distal lesions. Fig. 14.5c shows how well the coronary arteries can be visualised with this dilatation system in place.

BALLOON PROFILE

The profile of the deflated balloon is usually what determines whether or not a stenosis or occlusion is crossed. Both of the systems described above have low profile balloons, the monorail made of PVC (polyvinylchloride) and the Micro Hartzler of polyethylene. Polyethylene terephthalate (PET) is a material that has characteristics that enable the balloon to be made of a much thinner membrane so that the deflated profile is reduced. It is now being used for some balloons (e.g. USCI Profile Plus, Monorail 'Piccolino'). The lowest profile system of all is a guide wire with an integral PET balloon (USCI Probe). Fig. 14.3 shows a comparison of the deflated profiles of this and the Micro-Hartzler balloons.

Dilatation technique

A great deal of attention has been paid to balloon size, and inflation pressure and duration, with relation to both immediate and long term success.

Early workers suggested that evidence of local dissection was an indicator of adequate dilatation and there was therefore a tendency to use over-sized balloons inflated to high pressures for long periods. This philosophy has now mostly been abandoned and correctly sized balloons are used with the aim of complete dilatation with the minimum of disruption to the artery. The dilatation can often be seen to be angiographically successful either by injection of contrast medium or by seeing the indentation in the inflated balloon caused by the stenosis disappear after a short low pressure inflation with an appropriately sized balloon. There is no evidence that further inflations are helpful. This ability to judge the effectiveness of the inflation with the dilatation system *in situ* is an important consideration when choosing the system. A reasonable policy is therefore to start with an inflation at 3 or 4 atm (303 or 404 kPa) for 20 or 30 seconds, assess the result and then increase both pressure and duration until an adequate result is achieved, no further improvement is seen, a complication occurs or the agreed maximum inflation pressure is reached. A number of operators using systems that allow reliable measurement of pressure gradients use reduction of the gradient to 10 mmHg or less as an indicator of a successful result. The maximum inflation pressure varies considerably from centre to centre. It was previously limited by the balloon materials since balloons ruptured at pressures of approximately 10 atm (1010 kPa). Current balloons resist pressures of 20 atm (2020 kPa) or more.

Most operators set the limit at between 10 and 12 atm (1010 and 1212 kPa). Inflation duration is often limited by the development of pain, S—T segment changes, or more particularly, the appearance of arrhythmias. In the absence of these events the inflation time is theoretically unlimited since the implication is that collateral flow is adequate to prevent ischaemia at rest. Inflation times of between 1 and 2 minutes are common and up to 10 minutes have been used. There is no evidence, however, that such prolonged inflation has any benefit and the prolongation of the procedure is undesirable. An average lesion might be dilated three or four times to a maximum of 6 to 8 atm (606 to 808 kPa) for a maximum of 60 to 90 seconds.

Occluded vessels and severe stenoses

Re-opening occluded vessels requires first penetrating the lesion with a guide wire before the balloon catheter can be advanced and inability to do this is the most frequent cause of failure. Repeated gentle probing of the lesion may achieve success but it is essential to avoid making an artificial track and risk perforation of the vessel. Some operators prefer very fine wires and others use larger stiffer ones. A road map showing the distal vessel filled by dye injected into the contralateral artery is very helpful in this situation. The lesion can sometimes be crossed with the aid of a small (2 mm) low profile balloon with the guide wire just protruding from its endhole. The usual problem is that attempts to advance the dilatation system merely push the guiding catheter out of the coronary orifice. This can be overcome by altering the position and shape of the guiding catheter in the aortic root so that it is splinted against the aortic walls. It can even be cautiously advanced down the coronary artery if it has a soft tip. There is a risk of dislodging a proximal plaque and if this is in the left main vessel the dangers are obvious and the need for caution cannot be over emphasised. A differently shaped guiding catheter may be needed.

Tortuous vessels and distal lesions

The special balloon catheters described above have better tracking characteristics to allow access to distal lesions or those in tortuous vessels. Perseverence is often required to complete the procedure and more than one dilatation system may have to tried.

Complex lesions

Dilatation of lesions involving branches may result in the occlusion of the branch. There are a number of ways of dealing with this problem but they all involve the same principle of having a balloon catheter and/or guide wire in both branches throughout the procedure. It was at first thought that two balloons had to be inflated simultaneously (kissing balloons) to prevent occlusion of one of the involved branches. However it has been demonstrated that a guide wire in the branch at risk is sufficient. If the branch becomes occluded in these circumstances it can almost always be re-opened and successfully dilated.

Dilatation of lesions sited on arterial bends inevitably leads to unnatural straightening of the vessel increasing the risk of damage and dissection. This problem may be overcome with the angulated balloons now becoming available.

PATHOPHYSIOLOGY OF BALLOON INFLATION

Study of the effects of balloon inflation has provided a very good means of elucidating the sequence of events that occur with myocardial ischaemia. It has long been appreciated that cardiac pain is a relatively late and not invariable result of ischaemia. S−T segment change on the electrocardiogram has been looked upon as the gold standard but in a study of 52 patients undergoing angioplasty with continuous 12-lead ECG monitoring [2] it occurred in only 63% of patients whereas left ventricular contraction abnormalities occurred in 98%. A fall in ejection fraction occurred in all but one patient and there was a regional left ventricular wall motion abnormality in the ischaemic segment in the majority. These changes were fully developed by 20 seconds of balloon inflation, often before the ECG changed. Pain was a relatively rare consequence since the ECG changes when they occurred often lead to limitation of the duration of the inflation.

Collateral flow to the ischaemic segment, as judged from the previous coronary arteriogram, does not abolish the contraction abnormalities but does reduce both them and the presence and extent of the ECG changes.

There has been much discussion about the implication of reciprocal ECG changes. One view is that, for instance, S−T depression in the inferior ECG leads in a patient with anterior S−T elevation due to anterior myocardial infarction is due to ischaemia of the inferior wall implying additional right coronary disease. The alternative explanation is that the changes are purely reciprocal and do not indicate more disease. Studies during angioplasty of the anterior descending coronary artery in patients known not to have additional coronary disease have shown that ECG changes do occur in the inferior leads and that they are dependant on the degree of the anterior S−T elevation that occurs and are therefore truly reciprocal. This does not mean that these changes are always reciprocal but it has provided good evidence that they may be and has helped to resolve the issue.

COMPLICATIONS

Angioplasty carries both the risk of complications due to any cardiac catheterisation and, in addition, special risks related to the procedure itself. The major complications are due to the effects of myocardial ischaemia; either transient during balloon inflation, or more long lasting because of occlusion of the vessel.

Arrhythmias

Minor rhythm problems are common. Bradycardia can almost invariably be controlled with atropine but if not temporary pacing can be used. This can be rapidly instituted using the venous sheath inserted at the beginning of the procedure. Ectopic beats may occur during balloon inflation or if the guide wire is occluding a small branch. The latter should be promptly recognised and corrected by repositioning the wire.

Potentially serious ventricular tachyarrhythmias can usually be prevented by anticipation of the possibility of their occurence and taking prompt avoiding action. They are therefore rare but if they occur they have to dealt with in the usual way. The procedure does not necessarily have to be abandoned because of them but it may have to be because of their cause.

The incidence of other arrhythmias is similar to that occurring during other forms of catheterisation. They are dealt with in the standard way.

Plaque disruption

Pathological examination has revealed plaque rupture and disruption caused by angioplasty and it seems likely that this is a frequent, if not invariable, consequence of the procedure.

1 *Spasm.* Vasoactive substances are released from both the arterial wall and from platelets that adhere to the damaged intima. This may produce local spasm which may be very intense and not responsive to vasodilators. It can sometimes be relieved by repeat dilatation.

2 *Dissection.* The plaque disruption may produce dissection. If this is localised it may not predjudice the immediate result but may be associated with a higher early restenosis rate. Longer spiral dissections almost invariably produce occlusion of the vessel.

3 *Thrombosis.* It has now been well demonstrated, with both angiography and angioscopy that thrombus often complicates the plaque ulceration that is frequently present in patients with unstable angina and cardiac pain at rest. The low flow conditions that inevitably accompany balloon inflation make the increase of pre-existing thrombus likely. Even in patients with stable angina and a low incidence of complicating thrombus the plaque disruption that angioplasty may cause is also likely to initiate thrombus formation. Fig. 14.5a shows a filling defect in the posterolateral circumflex branch of the left coronary artery of a patient with unstable angina.

There is presently much discussion as to whether thrombolytic agents should be used routinely in at least the most susceptible group of patients with pre-existing thrombus. There is, however, a relatively high risk of haemorrhage with currently available agents which would seriously predjudice the outcome of surgery if it was needed and for this reason they are not used in most centres.

Adequate levels of heparin are essential but despite this partial or totally occlusive thrombosis may occur. It can sometimes be dispersed by repeating the dilatation and contrary to what might be expected distal occlusion by dislodged thrombus does not appear to be an important problem.

4 *Perforation.* Perforation of a coronary artery with a guide wire rarely occurs. If it does it usually leads to tamponade and requires urgent surgery — with or without pericardial aspiration.

EMERGENCY SURGERY

The aim of emergency surgery is almost always to salvage myocardium which has been put at risk by occlusion of a coronary artery. The time available for this cannot be determined accurately but depends mostly on the degree of collateral flow to the myocardium at risk. The perfusion pressure in the distal arterial segment with the balloon inflated gives some indication of this but it is not always possible to measure this pressure. Angiographic demonstration of collateral flow is not a very reliable indicator. The myocardium will survive approximately 45 to 60 minutes without collaterals so that intervention has to be prompt in the worst case situation. There is thus a dilemma for the operator between attempting to re-open the occluded vessel and not delaying surgical revascularisation. The decision is often a pragmatic one depending on the availability of the operating theatre and surgical team. Prolonged efforts in the catheter laboratory to restore the blood supply should however be avoided.

Perfusion catheters

Perfusion can be maintained using a 'bale-out' catheter. This is a specially designed catheter that has a number of side-holes that are positioned in the aorta when the tip is in the coronary artery. If the problem is one of recurrent occlusion it can be introduced into the vessel beyond the occlusion over the guide wire which can then be withdrawn allowing perfusion of the distal coronary bed via the side-holes in the aorta.

POST-PTCA CARE

Drugs

The use of medication after the procedure is governed by the same principles that apply to pretreatment and during the procedure itself.

ANALGESICS

Pain after angioplasty is most likely due to a complication occurring and every effort should be made to confirm this even by repeat catheterisation if there is doubt. Having said that, cardiac pain may occur without an obvious complication and it can then be treated conventionally. The effect of balloon inflation on the ECG will have been observed during the procedure and this will provide a useful guide as to whether the vessel is occluded. It cannot however be taken as absolute and if the other evidence strongly suggests occlusion angiography should be repeated.

VASODILATORS

At least some coronary spasm is quite likely to occur after the procedure and most centres use vasodilators for at least the first 24 hours after the procedure. As mentioned previously hypotension should be avoided. It is convenient to give a nitrate by continuous intraveneous infusion titrating the dose to avoid both hypotension and severe headache. Some headache is almost invariable. Calcium antagonists are used in many centres particularly for their vasodilator effect.

ANTICOAGULANTS

Heparin is usually continued for the first 24 hours whilst the femoral sheaths are in place. It is important to wait 4 hours after stopping the heparin before removing the sheaths to avoid excessive bleeding.

Warfarin is not at present routinely used in most centres but there are a number of trials in progress to evaluate whether or not long term anticoagulation has any beneficial effects.

ANTIPLATELET DRUGS

Most patients are asked to take aspirin or dipyridamole or both. Some centres continue medication long term and others for the first 3 to 6 months. None of these regimes has been demonstrated to be better than any other and once again trials are in progress to test various of them.

Investigations

Cardiac enzymes and 12-lead ECG are usually checked on the day of the angioplasty and 24 hours later although further intervention is only indicated on clinical grounds. No other routine investigations are needed. Some centres perform an early exercise test before the patient leaves hospital.

Results

PRIMARY SUCCESS

Definition

Comparison of results obtained by different centres or among different groups of patients is made difficult by the use of different definitions of success. Primary success was defined conservatively by Greuntzig as a reduction of 20 percentage points in lumen diameter stenosis so that a 95% stenosis reduced to 75% was considered successful dilatation. In some series 75% stenosis is the lowest level thought to be significant since this is the level at which resting coronary flow is reduced and is well above the degree of stenosis that reduces coronary flow reserve. It is certainly, therefore, haemodynamically and clinically important. Thus it is not very logical to consider a residual stenosis of the order of 70% or more a successful dilatation. Stenosis reduction to less than 50% is now much more commonly used as an index of success.

In practice the actual average reduction achieved in reported series has usually been much greater than 20% so that differences in the definition of success have probably been less important than might have been the case.

Learning curve

As with any procedure there is a learning period during which experience is gained and results improve. This has been particularly so with angioplasty; perhaps related to the unexpected difficulties experienced angiographers had in learning the technique. In 1977, when angioplasty was just beginning, a registry was set up by the National Heart Lung and Blood Institute (NHLBI) in the US to which 105 centres contributed information. Primary success was defined as by Greuntzig, a reduction of 20% in diameter stenosis. The success rate increased from 54% in 1979 to 66% in 1981. Investigators who had performed less than 50 cases had 55% success rate compared with 77% for those who had performed 150 procedures [3].

Using the same criterion of success Greuntzig's group evaluated both the learning curve and the change in success over the 5 years from 1980 to 1984 related to the improvements in dilatation systems — particularly the introduction of steerable guide wires in patients undergoing single vessel angioplasty [4].

The introduction of steerable catheter systems lead to significant improvements in success rates in the right coronary artery from 78 to 88% and the introduction of low-profile balloons lead to increasing success in the anterior descending from 90 to 94%. At the end of the period there was no difference in the ability to reach and cross lesions in the three coronary arteries. Finally the proportion of patients with anterior descending angioplasty decreased and those with circumflex angioplasty increased.

Similar results can be achieved in patients with multivessel disease. In one report of 428 patients who underwent multilesion angioplasty with an average of 2.4 attempts per patient the angiographic success rate, using the Greuntzig definition, was

94% [5]. The average reduction in stenosis was from 80 to 17% so that this report represents truly effective multilesion angioplasty.

Although it is difficult to be certain, from published reports, how various centres compare with each other because of great differences in patient selection and grouping, complication rates are in general higher in patients with multivessel disease than in those with single vessel disease when these two groups are compared in a single centre [6, 7].

Unstable angina was initially considered to be a contraindication to angioplasty because of the possible role of coronary vasospasm in its causation. It has however now been demonstrated that primary success rates are similar to those achieved in patients with stable angina [8] although the complication rate might be a little higher.

Urgent surgery

The decision about the need for urgent bypass surgery is a difficult one the operator having to decide between attempting to re-open the occluded vessel and transferring the patient rapidly to the operating theatre. Some centres prefer to allow the patient to have a limited myocardial infarction if the territory supplied by the occluded vessel is not large, rather than subject him to the additional risk of bypass surgery. The frequency of urgent surgery in the centres mentioned ranges between 1.4 and 8.4%. In the author's institution the overall rate for the last 165 patients (last data review) was 2% for patients with single vessel disease and 2.2% for those with multivessel disease. It was 4.3% for patients with unstable angina and 2.1% for those with stable symptoms.

The ability to intervene quickly is considerably reduced by previous surgery so that the risks of myocardial infarction and its sequelae are greater in patients who have had previous cardiac surgery.

Myocardial infarction

The rates for myocardial infarction range from 0.5 to 6.5% and in the author's centre they were 1% for single vessel disease and 5.5% for multivessel disease at the last review.

Mortality

Comparable overall mortality figures range between

1 and 2.8%. In the author's institution the overall rate has been 1.6%; 0.6% for patients with single vessel disease and 4.4% for those with multivessel disease. There have been no deaths in the last 165 cases.

FOLLOW-UP

Clinical results

In a recently published series of 1352 consecutive patients 77.9% of the 1163 (86%) in whom the angioplasty had been successful remained free of symptoms and cardiac events for 5 years [9]. When symptoms recurred they did so in the first 3 to 6 months — a finding reported by most other groups. 5% of the patients required aortocoronary bypass surgery and 8% required repeat angioplasty. These patients were similar to those treated in most centres, the majority having stable angina but about a quarter having unstable angina and 5% each with myocardial infarction after thrombolytic therapy and post by-pass surgery. 75% of the patients had single vessel disease.

The long-term results in patients all of whom had multivessel disease are less good. In the study by Dorros *et al.* [5] only 68% of patients were free of angina after an average of 28 months follow-up. 10% of the patients had undergone bypass surgery and 24% repeat angioplasty.

Much has been said about treatment of the culprit lesion in patients with multivessel disease with the aim both of relieving the symptoms and converting a patient with triple vessel disease to one with double vessel disease; implying that the prognosis will thus be improved. The clinical results of this approach, in patients with unstable angina at least, appear to be satisfactory although only small numbers of patients have been studied [8, 10]. It is reasonable to be conservative in this group because of the generally higher complication rate of any intervention. There is no reason to believe, however, that incomplete revascularisation will be any more effective with angioplasty than it was with bypass surgery [11] and this has been shown to be the case. In a group of 229 patients 69% of those who underwent an incomplete angioplasty later required aortocoronary bypass compared with 29% of those who had complete revascularisation [12].

There is, as yet, very little information on the effect of angioplasty on long term survival. The good 5 year outcome referred to above was for patients most of whom had single vessel disease who are known to have a good outcome with or without intervention.

RESTENOSIS

Restenosis seems mostly to occur in the first 3 to 6 months after angioplasty and occurs in about 25 to 30% of patients. In most reported series the angiographic data has been obtained from patients biased towards those with recurrent symptoms because of the natural reluctance to perform angiography on symptom free postangioplasty patients. The large recently published series referred to above [9] has provided particularly useful information on this point. Angiographic data was available from 63% of the patients whose angioplasty had been successful initially. Restenosis was defined as loss of 50% of the initial gain. Only 2% of the symptom-free patients had restenosis compared with 75% of the patients with recurrent angina. The restenosis rate in the native coronary vessels is highest in the proximal anterior descending but it is still higher in dilated bypass grafts.

Restenosis therefore remains one of the most important unsolved problems of angioplasty and is the subject of much research mostly centred on the prevention of the haematological sequelae of plaque disruption. There is some hope that using bio-engineering techniques substances will be developed that will render the dilated segment non-thrombogenic.

PATIENT SELECTION

It follows from what has already been said that angioplasty has so far been shown to be an effective means of relieving symptoms in the patients who have undergone the procedure. The majority of these have had single vessel disease and even in the centres where patients with multivessel disease have been treated they have been carefully selected from a larger group of patients many of whom have been treated surgically.

The patients who are rejected usually have unsuitable coronary lesions. Unsuitability varies from centre to centre and indeed from operator to operator. It is universally agreed that unprotected left main stem stenosis (without a functioning left coronary bypass graft) and very diffuse disease are absolute contraindications to the angioplasty. Calcification of the vessel is not but the likelihood of successful dilatation is much reduced if the lesion is calcified. The ability to tackle complex lesions is very dependant on the operators experience. There is some preliminary data to suggest that the results of dilatation are better and the complication rates lower for smooth lesions when compared to irregular ones. Eccentricity alone does not seem to affect the outcome.

Inevitably there is discussion as to whether or not minor stenosis (less than 50%) should be treated — as there was with bypass surgery. At the present time angioplasty is used to relieve symptoms which it is agreed are not caused by minor lesions and, since the risk is probably similar for all degrees of stenosis, treatment of minor lesions is not recommended. There is some evidence to suggest that it is in fact harmful [13].

The complication rates, especially in patients with single vessel disease, are acceptably low and some centres have achieved similarly low rates in patients with multivessel disease.

Data on the effect of the procedure on survival are not yet available although it is hoped that the various trials currently in progress will provide this information so that the place of angioplasty can be more clearly defined, especially for patients with multivessel disease.

Single vessel disease

Angioplasty is probably the treatment of choice for patients with single vessel disease whose symptoms are not satisfactorily controlled by medical means. Since the risks of the procedure are so low in this group it should not be reserved for patients with intractable symptoms but can be used fairly freely. There are a number of centres that now advise angioplasty in patients with single vessel disease on angiographic grounds alone despite the absence of symptoms.

Multivessel disease

Patients with left main stem stenosis or proximal triple vessel disease (especially those with some left ventricular damage in whom there is good evidence that prognosis is improved by bypass surgery) should be treated surgically unless it is contraindicated. The remainder of patients should be considered for angioplasty although many of them may eventually prove to be unsuitable. The likelihood that all of the lesions can be satisfactorily dilated should be the most important factor in the decision. It is not necessary to dilate all stenoses at one time. In the author's centre the femoral sheaths are frequently left in place and the procedure is completed the day after the first dilatations. This has the considerable advantage of demonstrating that the initially dilated lesions are stable and the risk of a simultaneous complication involving more than one vessel is very unlikely.

Myocardium at risk

Another important factor is the amount of viable, myocardium that would be at risk if the vessel to be dilated were to become occluded. For example an anterior descending artery with a major stenosis often provides the blood supply to the inferior left ventricular wall retrogradely by collateral vessels because of a major stenosis or occlusion of the right coronary artery. In these circumstances it would be safe to first re-open the right coronary and only then attempt dilatation of the anterior descending stenosis. This consideration has even greater importance if there is already a degree of left ventricular damage.

Postoperative patients

These patients suffer from two disadvantages. Firstly, because of the effects of the previous surgery emergency surgical revascularisation, should it become necessary, is less likely to be completed in time to prevent myocardial infarction. Secondly, the chance of long term success of graft dilatation has been shown to be lower. Dilatation of lesions in native vessels has the same chance of success as in nonsurgical patients. Angioplasty may, however, be the only option for such patients and they represent an increasing proportion of the patients treated.

FUTURE DEVELOPMENTS

A great deal of research is currently in progress into interventional techniques to either compliment or replace angioplasty.

Lasers

Laser recanalisation of peripheral arteries is now possible. Laser devices delivering heat energy ('hot tip') have been used in the coronary circulation with less success [14]. The problems are related to the size and relative rigidity of the delivery systems and the lack of control over the heat energy. The most promising type at present is the excimer pulsed laser but this is not yet ready for use *in vivo*.

Stents

Stents work on the principal of tunnel supports with the aim of maintaining the internal lumen of the artery after balloon dilatation. A stent in the form of a stainless steel mesh has been placed in the coronary circulation in more than 100 patients [15]. It can be placed across branches without prejudicing flow in them although it does preclude later angioplasty of those branches. Subsequent thrombosis is the main early problem although it is hoped that it will be possible to bind an anticoagulant, like heparin, to the surface of the stent to prevent it.

Atherectomy

Like laser devices the atherectomy catheter [16] and the rotational atherectomy device [17] have been used successfully in peripheral arteries and the atherectomy catheter in a number of patients in the coronary circulation. These are similar devices, the pulveriser employs a high speed drill and the atherectomy catheter a tubular cutting mechanism. They both suffer from similar problems to the laser catheters in that they are relatively large and inflexible. Development is taking place very quickly and it seems likely that in the future a number of different devices will be used in sequence; perhaps guided by angioscopy.

EQUIPMENT

Fig. 14.1 (a) 8F 'soft-tip' guiding catheter (A) is inserted through a 9F valved sheath (B). (Longer, 24 cm, sheaths can be used to protect the iliac artery — especially if this vessel is diseased or tortuous.) The catheter is lead to the ascending aorta by an 0.035 or 0.038 guide wire and the coronary artery cannulated in the usual way. Coronary arteriograms are performed, and stored for subsequent replay, to provide a road map during angioplasty. The side-arm of the Y-connector (C) allows the injection of non-ionic contrast medium through the guiding catheter. The other arm of the Y-connector is equipped with a Tuohy–Borst valve (closed during the injection of contrast medium) through which the angioplasty catheter will be inserted. Opening the Tuohy–Borst valve allows the guiding catheter and Y-connector to be purged of air.

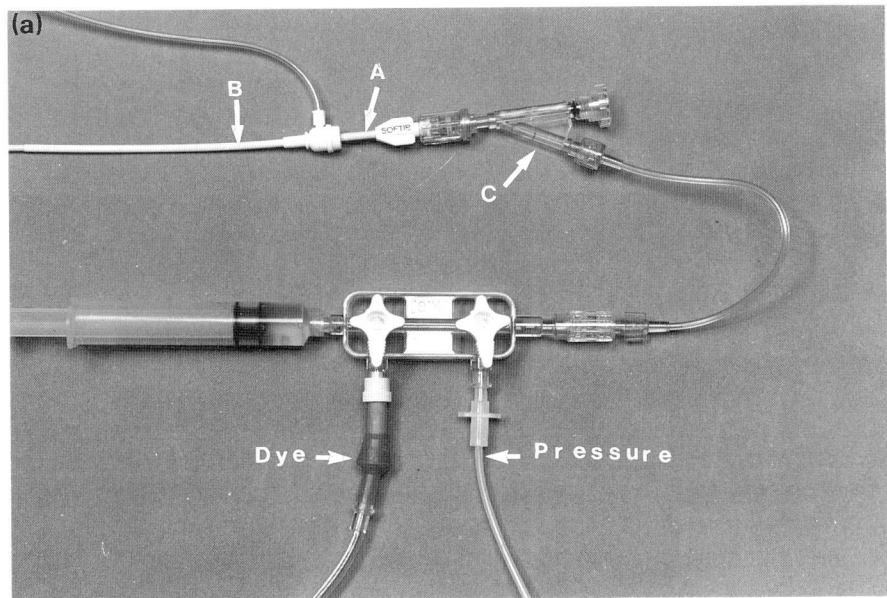

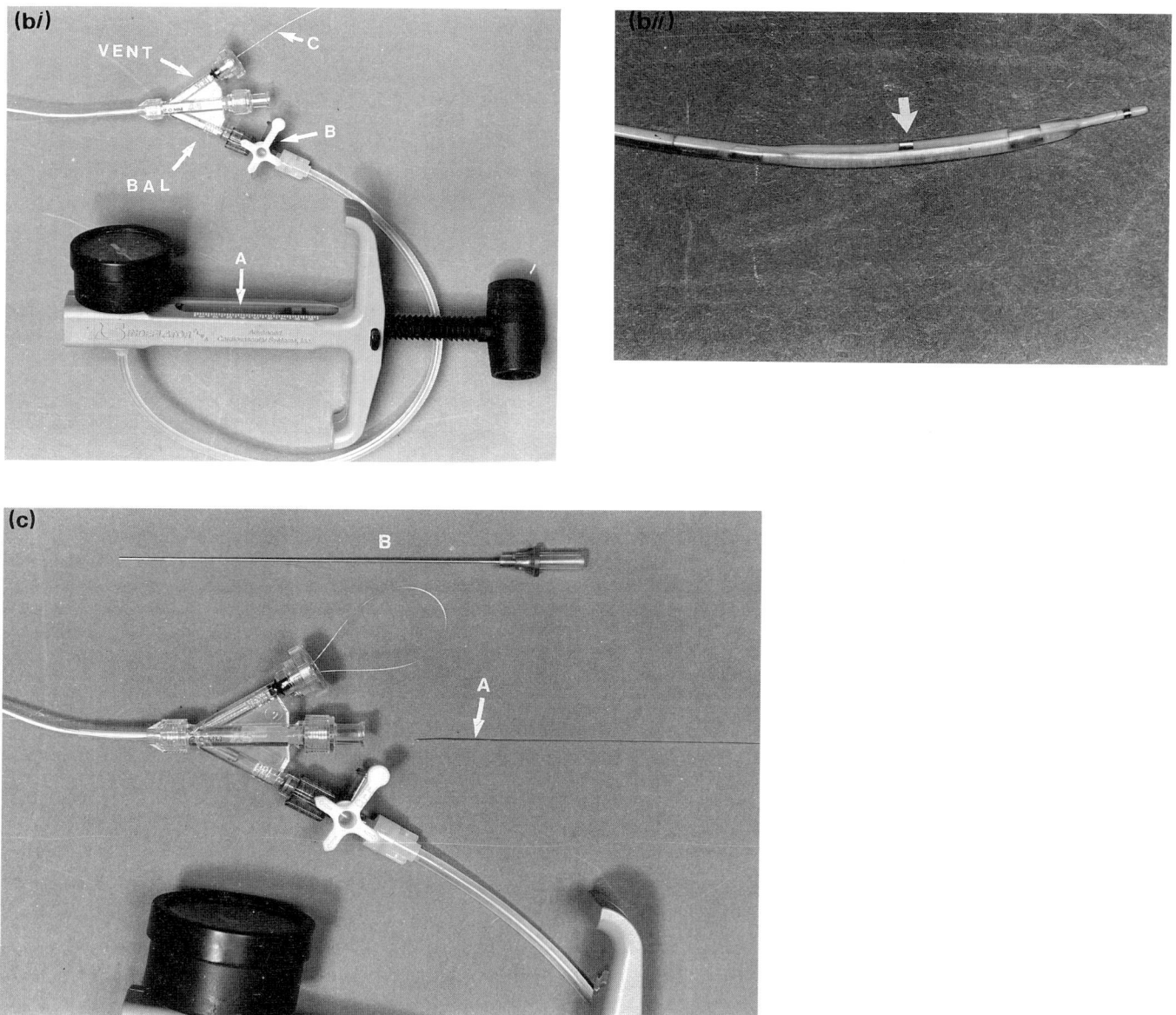

Fig. 14.1 (b) Preparation of the angioplasty catheter. The 'indeflator' (A) is filled with dilute contrast medium and any air expelled through the side-arm of a three-way tap (B). After removing a small, protective sleeve the balloon is briefly inflated using the indeflator attached to the appropriate arm (BAL) of the three-way manifold. The Tuohy–Borst valve on the other side-arm (VENT) is loosened allowing the venting tube (C) to be advanced to within 1 mm of the distal end of the balloon. The balloon is then inflated at 101–202 kPa (1–2 atm), until all air has been expelled and contrast medium emerges from the proximal end of the fine venting tube. Note that a gold marker (arrow) is positioned at the centre of the balloon. The venting tube is then withdrawn some 10 cm and closed by inserting its proximal end back through the Tuohy–Borst valve and tightening the valve (see Fig. 14.2c). Negative pressure is applied to collapse the balloon. The protective sleeve can be passed over the balloon to ensure complete furling and the lowest possible profile. The sleeve is then discarded. (c) The tip of the fine guide wire (0.014″, hi-torque, floppy tip) may be curved by hand before inserting the wire (A) through the middle arm of the manifold. A special introducing needle (B) is available to aid insertion of the wire.

Fig. 14.1 (d) After purging the manifold the angioplasty catheter and guide wire can now be inserted through the Tuohy–Borst valve of the guiding catheter and advanced, under fluoroscopic control, to within 1 cm of the tip of the guiding catheter. The torqueing device (A) is threaded over the end of the guide wire preparatory to advancing the guide wire and steering the wire past the target lesion. When the guide wire is in place (advanced as far as possible down the distal vessel) and its position checked by fluoroscopy in at least two projections the angioplasty catheter is advanced (with countertraction on the guide wire) until the central gold marker is centred at the lesion. Difficulty in crossing the lesion may require additional back-up support by the guiding catheter — see Fig. 14.7. The balloon is then inflated, using the indeflator. Screwing the handle of the indeflator in a clockwise direction allows effortless inflation to the desired pressure; counter-clockwise rotation, or traction on the handle after releasing the catch, will cause the balloon to deflate.

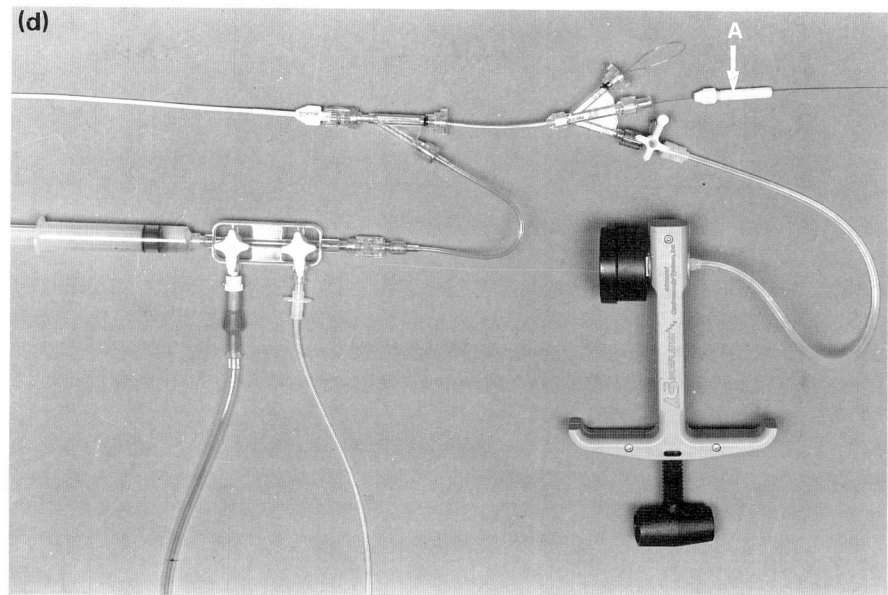

Notes:

1 Contrast medium can be injected through the angioplasty catheter (using the central arm of the three-way manifold) or, more usefully, through the guiding catheter. The Tuohy–Borst valve of the guiding catheter should be tightened during the injection of contrast medium to prevent its escape and thus improve opacification. The Tuohy–Borst valve must be loosened, slightly, during manipulation of the angioplasty catheter and during balloon inflation.

2 In some ACS catheters the venting tube is replaced by an micropore at the end of the balloon which allows the balloon to be purged since the micropore is permeable to air but not to contrast medium. Other manufacturers employ other venting systems.

Fig. 14.2 (a) Schneider Shiley 'monorail' system. In this system the guide wire passes through the balloon but emerges through the side of the catheter 18 cm proximal to the tip. This has several important consequences. It is possible to change the angioplasty catheter (e.g. to one with a larger or smaller balloon diameter) while still using the standard length (175 cm) guide wire and without the need to change to a long (300 cm) exchange wire or to add an extra length of wire. The Y-connector and Tuohy–Borst valve will accept several wires as well as the catheter and double-wire techniques are readily accomplished with this system. Since the catheter shaft is only 1 mm in diameter there is plenty of space within the guiding catheter and excellent coronary angiograms can be obtained with the angioplasty catheter in place thus facilitating correct placing of the balloon. The angioplasty catheter need not be prepared until the wire has been positioned; thus saving material if it is impossible to cross the lesion. The technique is otherwise similar on that described for the ACS system above. There is, however, no venting tube and air has to be removed from the balloon by repeated inflation and deflation with dilute contrast medium.

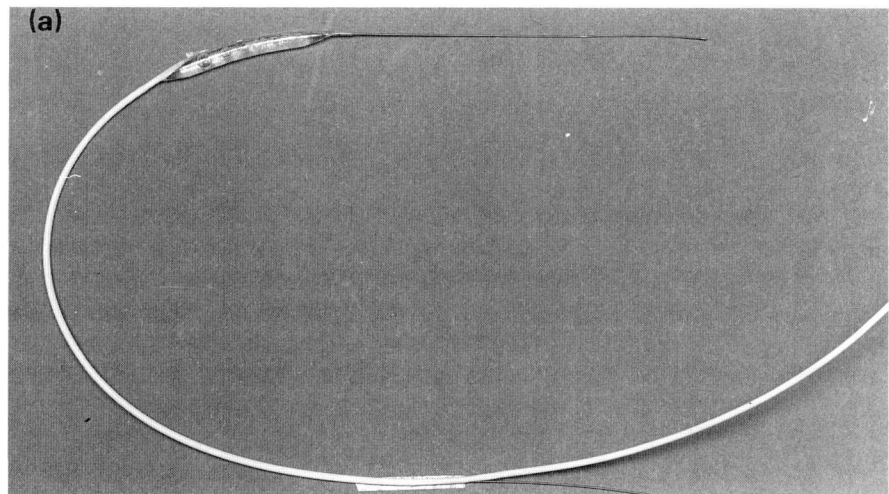

(b)

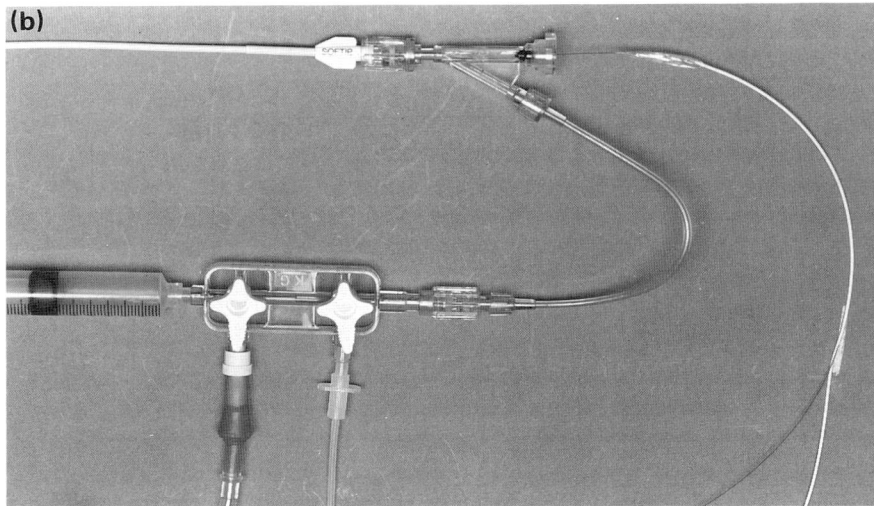

Fig. 14.2 (b) With the wire in place the catheter is threaded over the distal end of the wire and through the (loosened) Tuohy—Borst valve of the Y-connector. The catheter is then advanced, with countertraction on the wire, until the balloon is centred at the target lesion. At the end of the procedure the balloon can be withdrawn into the 'balloon garage' of the Y-connector and the result checked by arteriograms performed with the guide wire still in place. If the result is satisfactory all catheters are removed but the introducing sheath is sutured in place and left for several hours until the postangioplasty period has been seen to be free of complications. Heparinisation may then cease and the sheath can be removed 2 hours later.

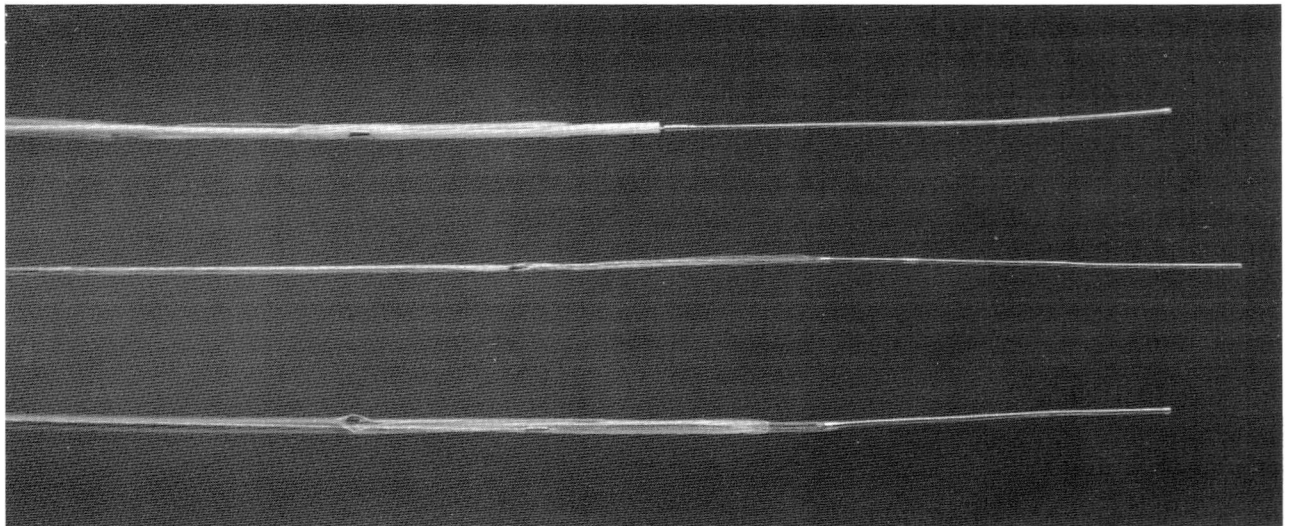

Fig. 14.3 The balloon tips of three low profile balloon catheters are shown. They are (a) ACS Micro Hartzler, (b) USCI probe and (c) ACS Hartzler LPS. The USCI probe has the lowest profile.

Fig. 14.4 (opposite) Angioplasty using the 'monorail' system. (a) Original lesion — severe stenosis in the middle third of the right coronary artery (arrow). (b) Guide wire (hi-torque, floppy tip) in place — note that the tip of the wire (closed arrow) has been placed as far as possible in the distal branches of the right coronary artery. The deflated balloon (3.5 mm 'Piccolino monorail') has been threaded over the guide wire and the central gold marker (open arrow) centred at the target stenosis. (c) The balloon has been inflated to 202 kPa (2 atm) and is indented by the target stenosis (arrow). (d) Further inflation to 808 kPa (8 atm) has resulted in the disappearance of the indentation indicating that the stenosis has been dilated. (e) The balloon has been withdrawn into the guiding catheter but the wire (not well seen) is still in place. Note that good opacification can be obtained, with this system, by injection through the guiding catheter despite the presence of the angioplasty catheter within it. If necessary the angioplasty catheter can be re-advanced, or exchanged for a different one, over a standard length guide wire without the need to recross the lesion or substituting an exchange guide wire. (f) Final result.

TECHNIQUES AND RESULTS

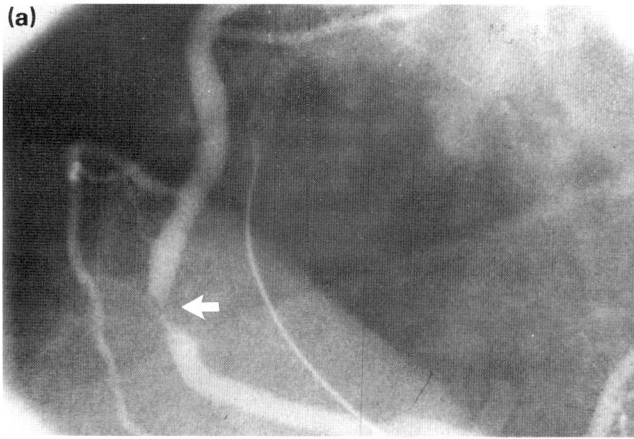

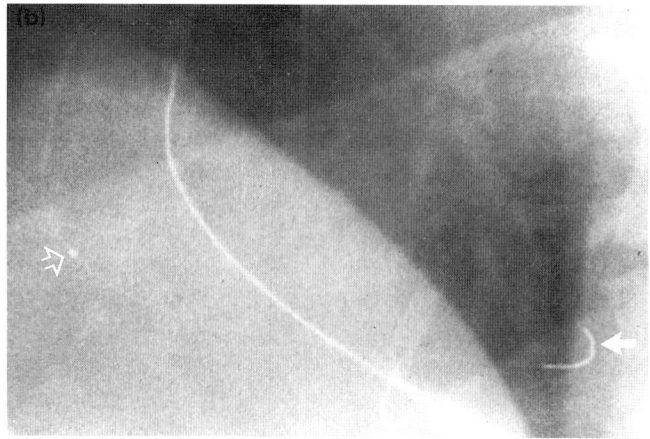

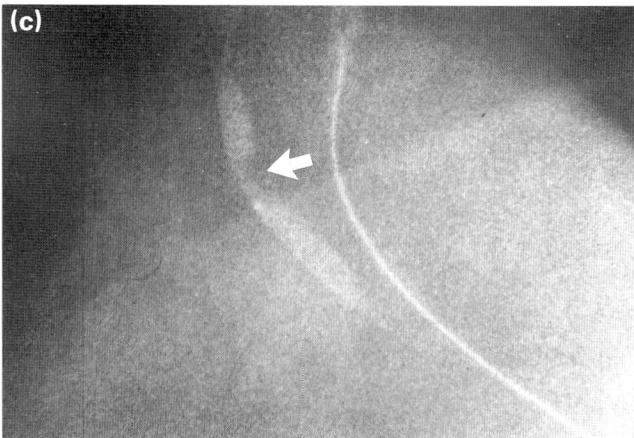

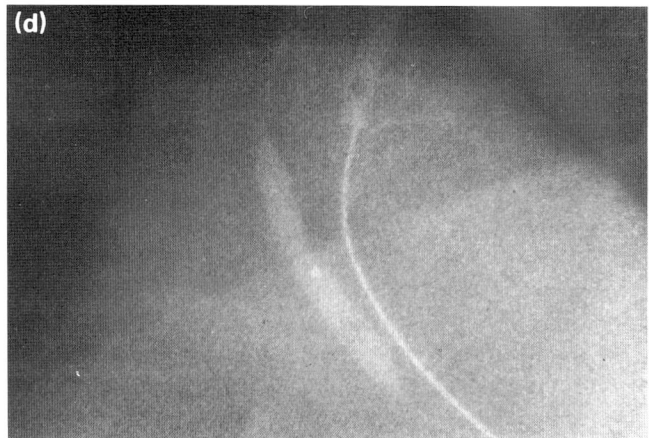

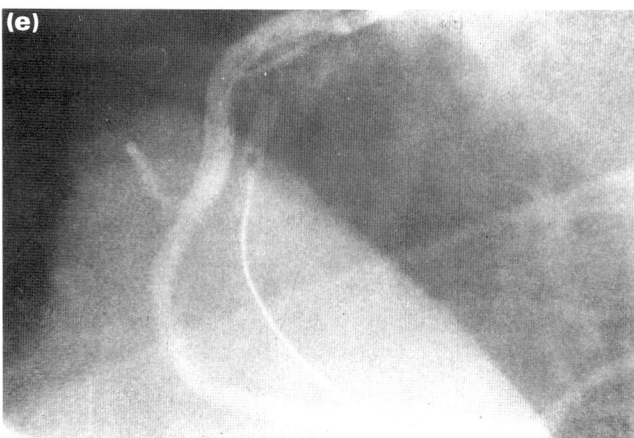

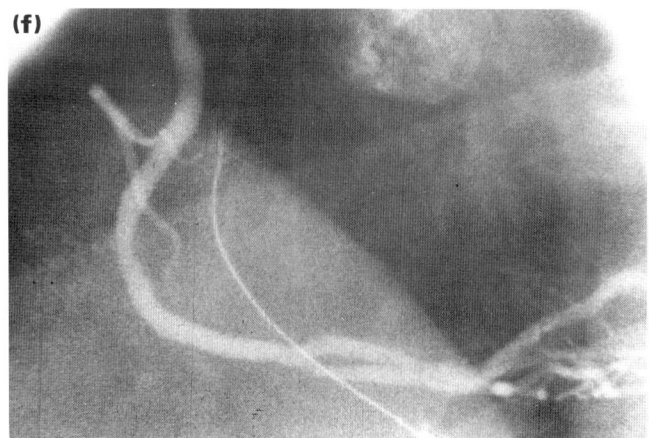

(a)

(b)

(c)

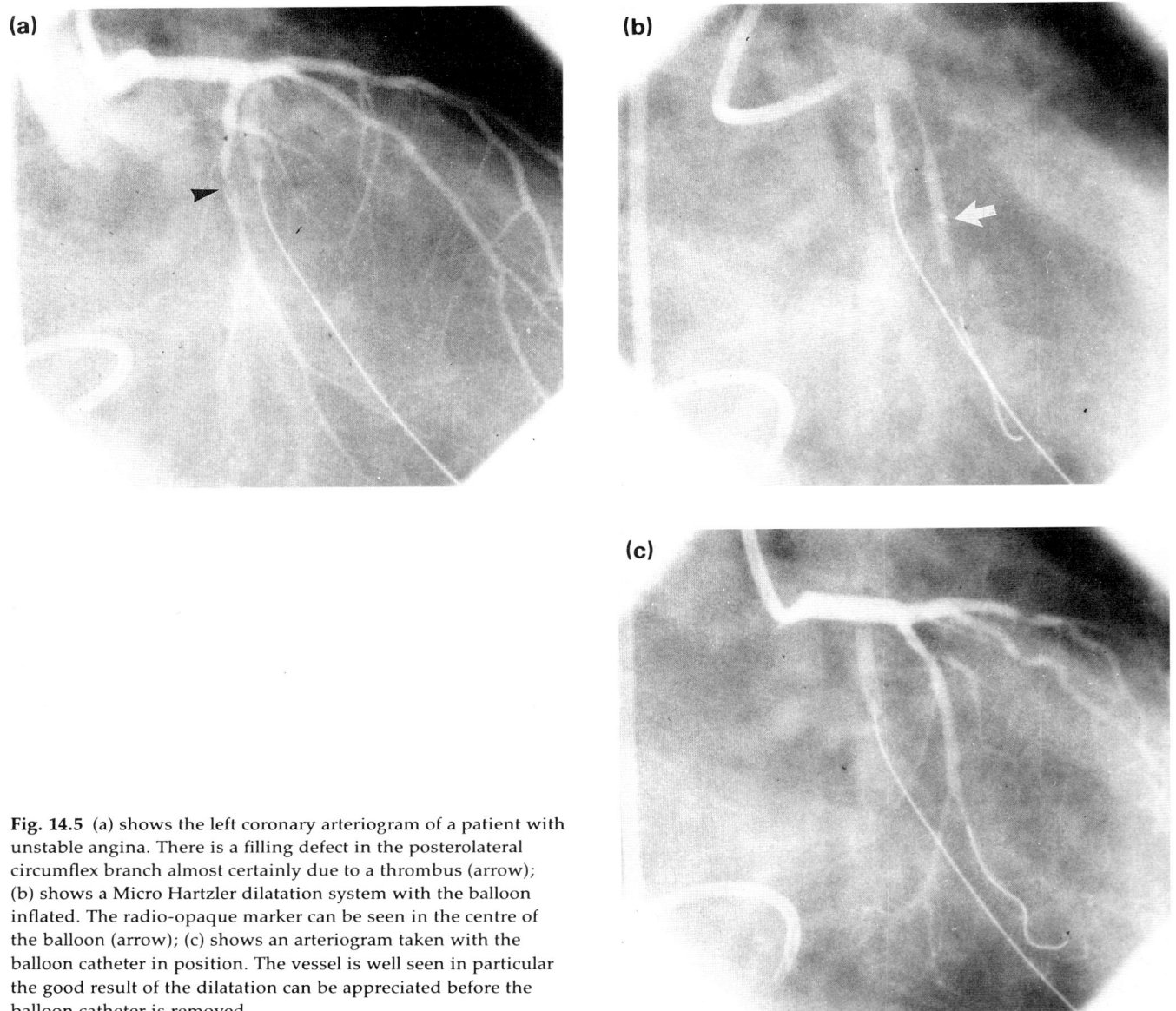

Fig. 14.5 (a) shows the left coronary arteriogram of a patient with unstable angina. There is a filling defect in the posterolateral circumflex branch almost certainly due to a thrombus (arrow); (b) shows a Micro Hartzler dilatation system with the balloon inflated. The radio-opaque marker can be seen in the centre of the balloon (arrow); (c) shows an arteriogram taken with the balloon catheter in position. The vessel is well seen in particular the good result of the dilatation can be appreciated before the balloon catheter is removed.

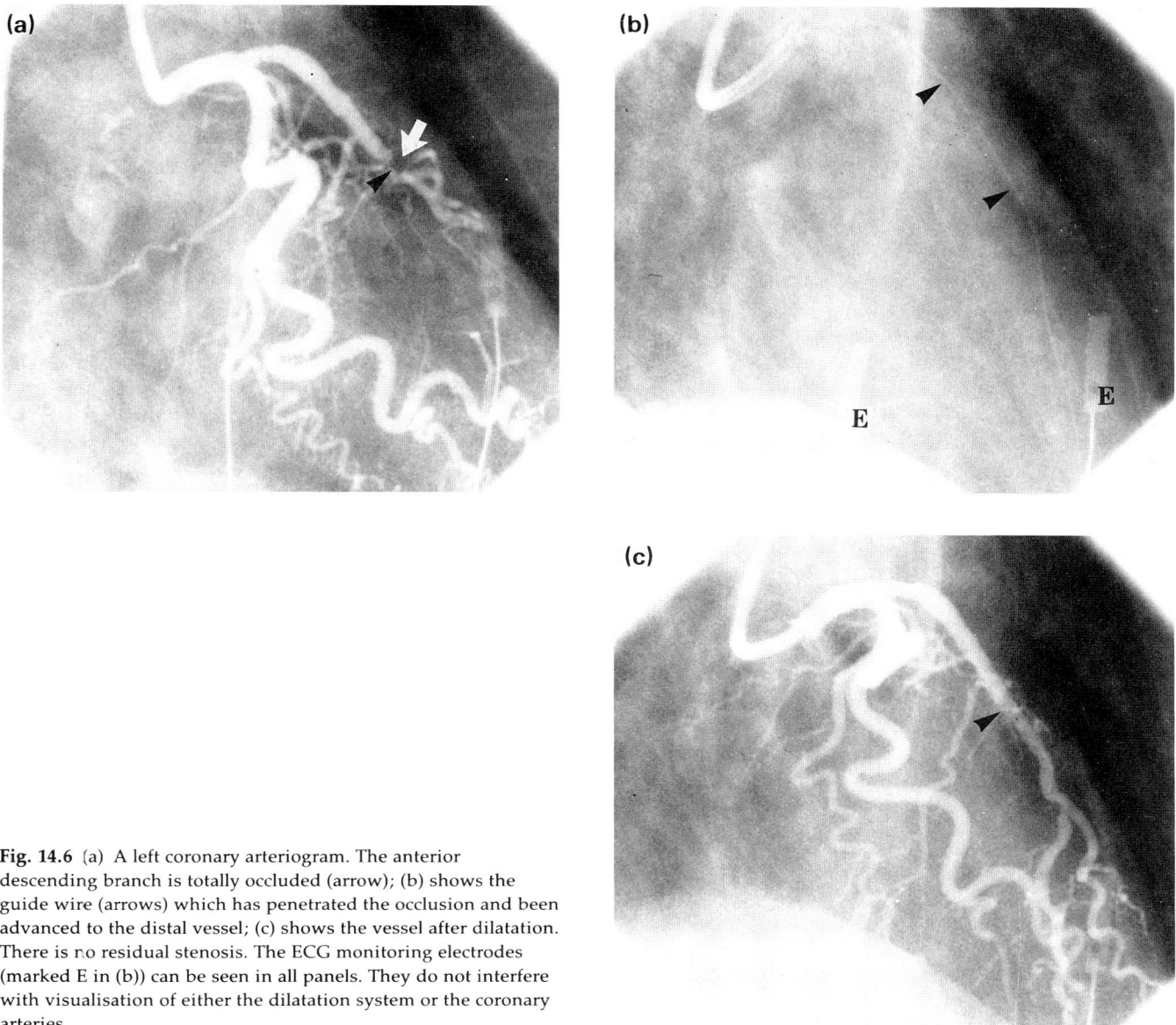

Fig. 14.6 (a) A left coronary arteriogram. The anterior descending branch is totally occluded (arrow); (b) shows the guide wire (arrows) which has penetrated the occlusion and been advanced to the distal vessel; (c) shows the vessel after dilatation. There is no residual stenosis. The ECG monitoring electrodes (marked E in (b)) can be seen in all panels. They do not interfere with visualisation of either the dilatation system or the coronary arteries.

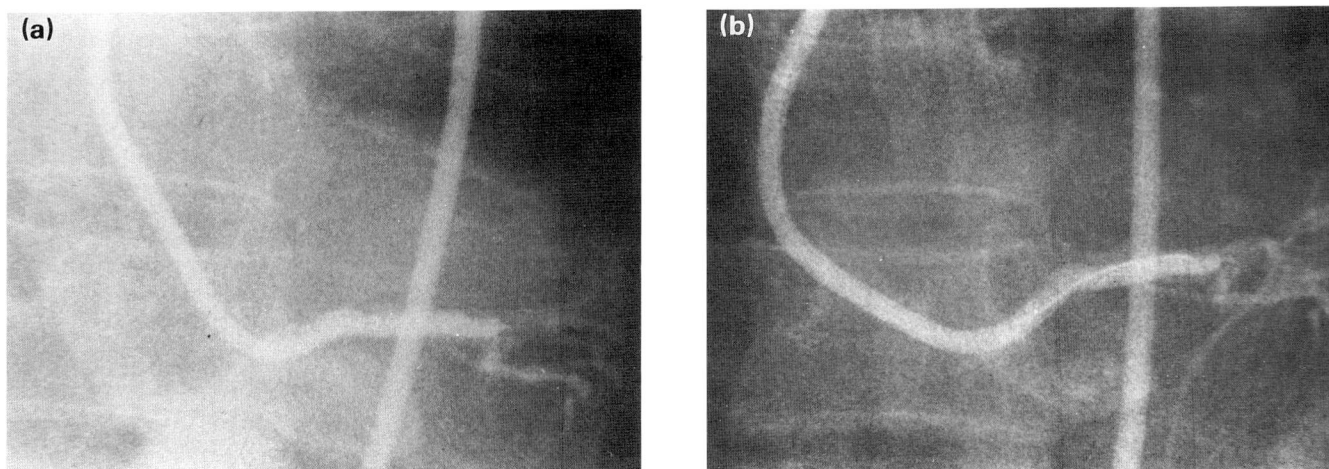

Fig. 14.7 'Butressing' the guiding catheter against the aortic wall. (a) Occluded anterior descending. The guide wire would not traverse the lesion and attempts to advance the wire caused the guiding catheter to become disengaged from the left coronary ostium. (b) The guiding catheter has been advanced so that it is pressing against the opposite wall of the aorta and its tip is deeply engaged in the coronary ostium thus providing additional support during attempts to advance the guide wire or balloon catheter through the lesion.

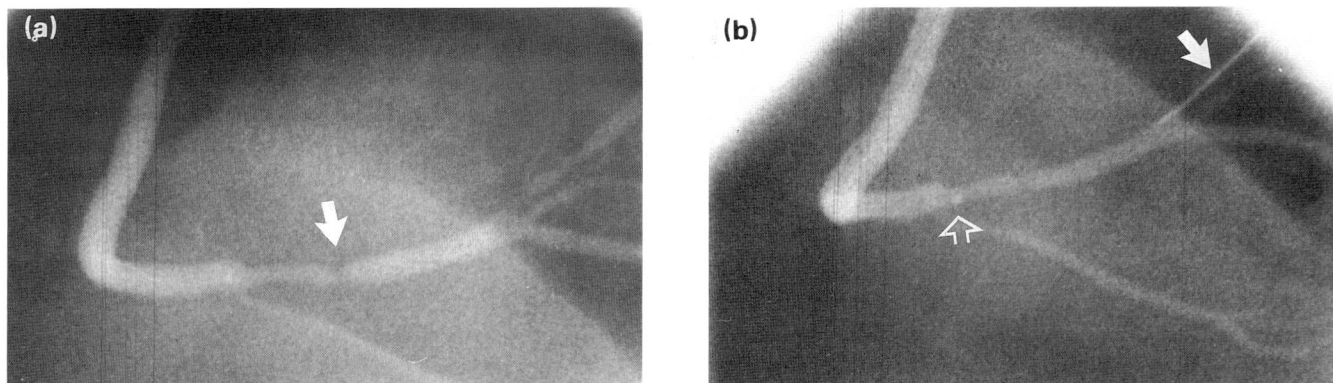

Fig. 14.8 Angioplasty via a vein graft. (a) The native right coronary artery is occluded proximally; contrast medium has been injected into a saphenous vein bypass graft demonstrating a stenosis of the native vessel just distal to the point of graft insertion (arrow). (b) Guide wire in place in the distal vessel (solid arrow). A monorail angioplasty catheter has been threaded over the wire and contrast medium injected through the guiding catheter. Despite the presence of the catheter good opacification has been obtained showing that the central gold marker of the balloon (open arrow) is just proximal to the stenosis.

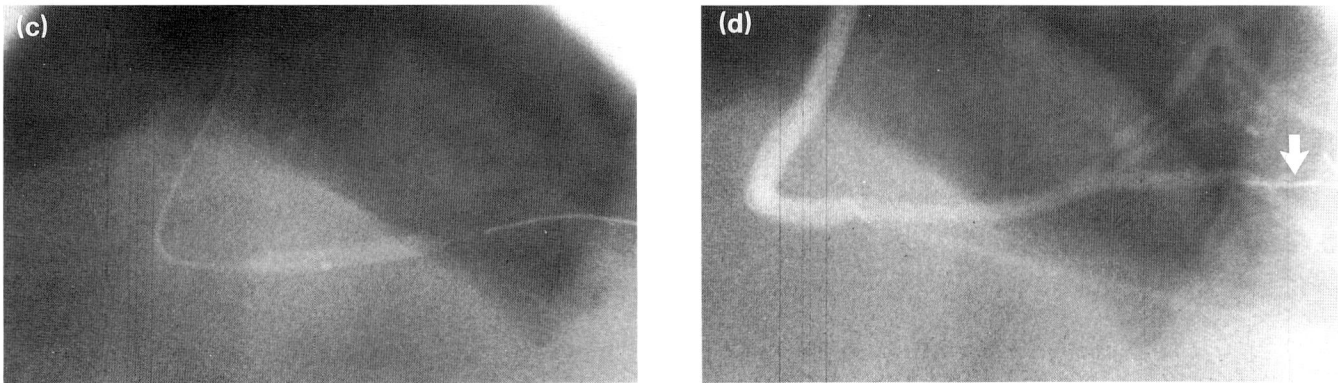

Fig. 14.8 *cont.* (c) The balloon has been advanced, slightly, and inflated with the dilute contrast medium. (d) Final result showing diagnostic opacification obtained despite the continued presence of the guide wire (arrow) and of the angioplasty catheter within the guiding catheter.

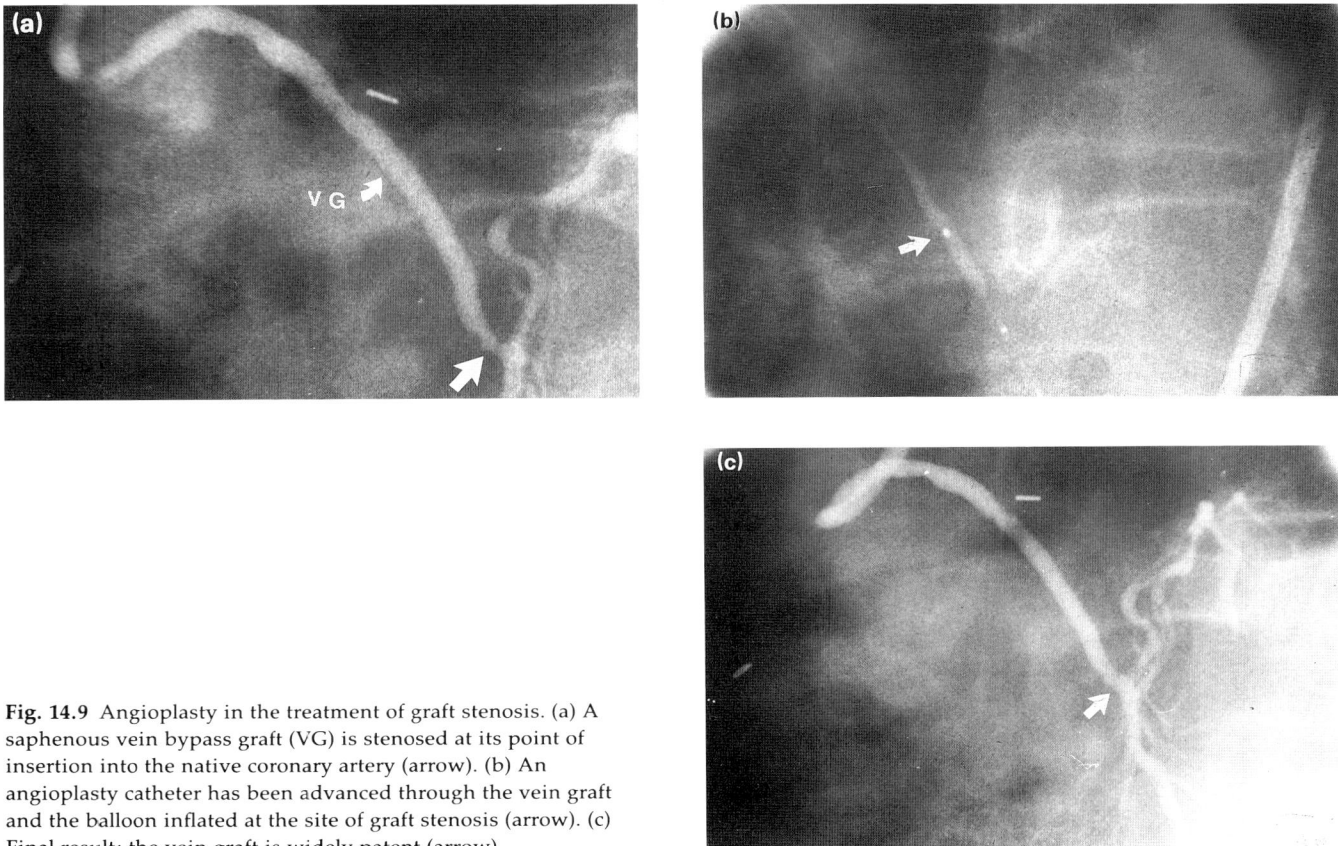

Fig. 14.9 Angioplasty in the treatment of graft stenosis. (a) A saphenous vein bypass graft (VG) is stenosed at its point of insertion into the native coronary artery (arrow). (b) An angioplasty catheter has been advanced through the vein graft and the balloon inflated at the site of graft stenosis (arrow). (c) Final result; the vein graft is widely patent (arrow).

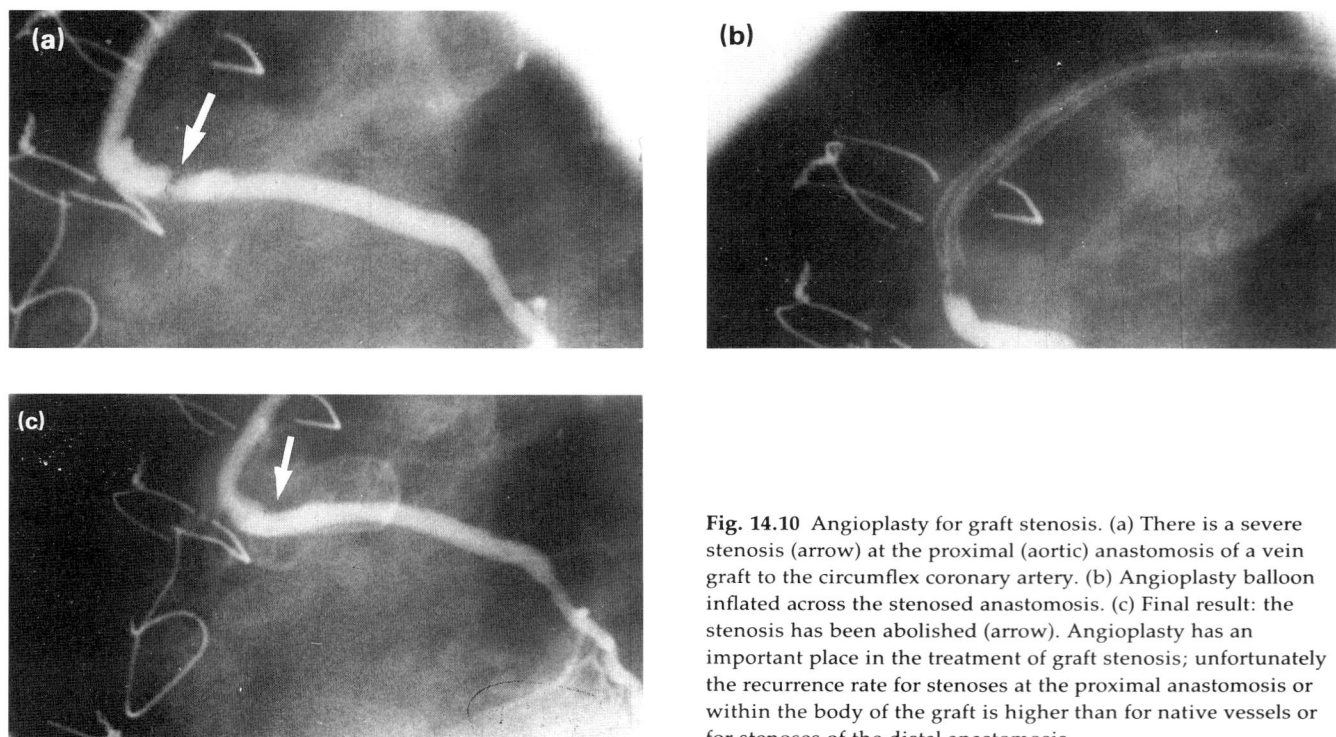

Fig. 14.10 Angioplasty for graft stenosis. (a) There is a severe stenosis (arrow) at the proximal (aortic) anastomosis of a vein graft to the circumflex coronary artery. (b) Angioplasty balloon inflated across the stenosed anastomosis. (c) Final result: the stenosis has been abolished (arrow). Angioplasty has an important place in the treatment of graft stenosis; unfortunately the recurrence rate for stenoses at the proximal anastomosis or within the body of the graft is higher than for native vessels or for stenoses of the distal anastomosis.

GENERAL READING

1 Meier B. *Coronary angioplasty*. Grune & Stratton. 1987.
2 King SB, Douglas JS. *Coronary arteriography and angioplasty*. McGraw-Hill Book Co. 1985.

REFERENCES

1 Greuntzig A. Transluminal dilatation of coronary artery stenosis. *Lancet* 1978;**1**:263.
2 Norell M *et al*. Assessment of left ventricular performance during percutaneous transluminal angioplasty: a study by intravenous digital subtraction ventriculography. *Br Heart J* 1988;**59**:419.
3 Kelsey SF *et al*. Effect of investigator experience on percutaneous transluminal coronary angioplasty. *Am J Cardiol* 1984;**53**:56C.
4 Anderson HV *et al*. Primary angiographic success rates of percutaneous transluminal coronary angioplasty. *Am J Cardiol* 1985;**56**:712.
5 Dorros G, Lewin RF, Janke L. Multiple lesion transluminal coronary angioplasty in single and multivessel coronary artery disease: acute outcome and long-term effect. *J Am Coll Cardiol* 1987;**10**:1007.
6 Sowton E *et al*. Early results after percutaneous transluminal coronary angioplasty in 400 patients. *Br Heart J* 1986;**56**:115.
7 Mid America Heart Institute of St Luke's Hospital. Complex angioplasty course September 1986 (personal communication).
8 De Feyter PJ *et al*. Emergency coronary angioplasty in refractory unstable angina. *N Engl J Med* 1985;**313**:342.
9 Ernst SMPG *et al*. Long term angiographic follow up, cardiac events, and survival in patients undergoing percutaneous transluminal coronary angioplasty. *Br Heart J* 1987;**57**:220.
10 Wohlgelertner D, Cleman N, Highman HA, Zaret BL. Percutaneous transluminal coronary angioplasty of the "culprit" lesion for management of unstable angina pectoris in patients with multivessel coronary artery disease. *Am J Cardiol* 1986;**58**:460.
11 Jones EL *et al*. Importance of complete revascularisation in performance of the coronary bypass operation. *Am J Cardiol* 1983;**51**:7.
12 Mabin TA *et al*. Follow-up clinical results in patients

undergoing percutaneous transluminal coronary angioplasty. *Circulation* 1985;**71**:754.

13 Ischinger T *et al.* Should coronary arteries with less
than 60% diameter stenosis be treated by angioplasty?
Circulation 1983;**68**:148.
14 Cumberland DC *et al.* Percutaneous laser-assisted
coronary angioplasty. *Lancet* 1986;**ii**:214.
15 Sigwart U *et al.* Intravascular stents to prevent occlusion
and restenosis after transluminal angioplasty. *New Engl
J Med* 1987;**316**:701.
16 Simpson JB *et al.* Transluminal atherectomy: initial
clinical results in 27 patients. *Circulation* 1986; suppl
2:**203**.
17 Zacca N *et al.* First in-vivo human experience with
a recently developed rotational atherectomy device.
Circulation 1987;**76**:(suppl IV)46.

Valvar heart disease

Cardiac catheterisation in valvar heart disease is concerned with identifying which valves are abnormal, with estimating the severity of regurgitation or stenosis and with assessing the consequences of valvar heart disease — primarily the effect on ventricular function and on the pulmonary vasculature. Finally it is sometimes possible to determine the aetiology of a lesion; as when mitral regurgitation is due to cusp prolapse. Abnormalities of cardiac valves become clinically important when they cause stenosis or regurgitation (or both). Before describing the investigation of individual valves it is appropriate to discuss the investigation of valve stenosis and regurgitation in general.

STENOSIS

Valve stenosis is revealed by a *gradient* across it. The gradient will only be present when there is flow across the valve; during ventricular systole at the aortic and pulmonary valves and during diastole at the tricuspid and mitral valves. The magnitude of the gradient is dependent on (1) the flow across the valve (the cardiac output plus any regurgitant flow or left-to-right shunt), (2) the time available for flow to take place (the 'systolic ejection period' for the pulmonary and aortic valves and the 'diastolic filling period' for the tricuspid and mitral valves), and (3) the area of the valve opening. This relationship between cardiac output, systolic ejection period or diastolic filling period and gradient forms the basis of the 'Gorlin formula' for the calculation of valve area [1]. The Gorlin formula as applied to the mitral valve is:

$$MVA = \frac{MVF}{38 \times \sqrt{Gradient}}$$

where MVA = cross sectional area in cm^2 of the

orifice, and MVF = mitral valve flow in cc/second. Mitral valve flow is given by

$$CO \ / \ (HR) \times (Dfp)$$

where CO = cardiac output (ml/min), and HR = heart rate (beats/min), and Dfp = diastolic filling period (second/beat).

For the aortic valve the formula is:

$$AVA = \frac{AVF}{44.5 \times \sqrt{Gradient}}$$

and AVF is given by:

$$CO \ / \ (Sep) \times (HR)$$

and Sep = systolic ejection period (second/beat).

As originally described the Gorlin formula was derived from data obtained at right heart catheterisation only. Thus the diastolic filling period (Dfp) for the mitral valve was derived from analysis of the brachial arterial pulse (from the beginning of the dicrotic notch to the beginning of the next upstroke and thus including isometric contraction and relaxation periods). Similarly left ventricular diastolic pressure was not known and was assumed to be a mean of 5 mmHg. With the advent of left heart catheterisation as part of the routine investigation of mitral and aortic valve disease it became possible to measure the diastolic filling period with greater accuracy as being from the moment when the two pressure traces crossed (left atrium or wedge and left ventricle) to the moment when they again equalised. In recognition of this Cohen and Gorlin [2] recalculated the empirical constant as it applied to direct measurements of the diastolic filling period and gradient and proposed the new constant of 38 (the original constant being 44.5).

Although the Gorlin formula is the best available method of determining the severity of valve stenosis in the catheterisation laboratory the calculations involved are tedious. Fortunately a simplified version of the formula is available which has been shown to give values for valve area which correlate well with areas calculated by the original formula. The derivation of this simplified formula is as follows. The Gorlin formula for the mitral valve can be written as:

$$MVA = (CO / \sqrt{VG}) \times 1000 / Dfp \times 38)$$

and for the aortic valve as:

$$AVA = (CO / \sqrt{VG}) \times (1000 / Sep \times 44.5)$$

where MVA = mitral valve area (cm^2), AVA = aortic valve area (cm^2), CO = cardiac output (l/min), VG = valve gradient (mmHg), Dfp = diastolic filling period (second/min), and Sep = systolic ejection period (second/min).

Thus, if the values of Dfp $\times$ 38 and Sep $\times$ 44.5 are close to 1000 the Gorlin formula could be rewritten in a much simpler form as:

$$VA = CO / \sqrt{VG}$$

That these values are close to 1000 over a wide range of valve areas has been shown by Hakki *et al.* [3] who proposed the above simplified formula.

Calculation of valve area by the Gorlin formula or by the simplified formula proposed by Hakki *et al.* involves planimetry in order to obtain the mean gradient; a tedious procedure which contributes to the general reluctance to employ the Gorlin formula routinely. The final step in the development of a

simple and reliable method of calculating valve areas is to substitute the 'three-point method' for determining the mean transvalvar gradient. This involves a simple calculation of the average gradient at three equidistant points which divide the systolic ejection period or diastolic filling period into four equal intervals (Fig 15.1). Nigri *et al.* [4] have shown that both aortic and mitral valve areas can be calculated using the simplified Gorlin formula (VA = CO / $\sqrt{VG}$) and the three-point method of finding the mean gradient with results that agree remarkably closely with those obtained by the traditional Gorlin method. Moreover, for the aortic valve, either the mean gradient or the peak systolic gradient may be used with essentially the same results. These findings make it possible to construct a single table (Table 15.1) from which valve areas for both (a) the aortic, and (b) the mitral valve can be read provided the cardiac output and the mean gradient (or peak aortic valve gradient) are known.

The substitution of a simplified formula and of the three-point method for the original time consuming calculations and planimetry has not removed all of the problems involved in calculating valve areas. In the first place calculations of cardiac output based on an assumed value for oxygen consumption

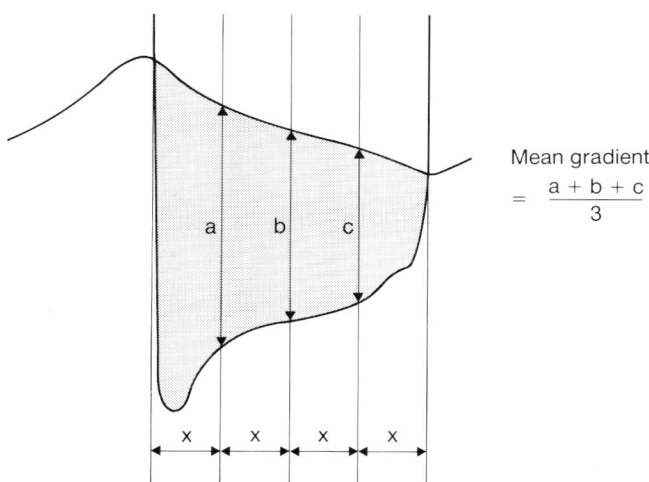

Fig. 15.1 Calculation of mitral valve gradient by the 'three-point method?

Table 15.1a Aortic valve area derived from cardiac output and gradient. Valve area (cm^2) calculated as CO (l/min)/gradient.

Gradient	Cardiac output l/min									
	1.0	1.5	2.0	2.5	3.0	3.5	4.0	4.5	5.0	
2	0.71	1.06	1.41	1.77	2.12	2.47	2.83	3.18	3.54	
4	0.50	0.75	1.00	1.25	1.50	1.75	2.00	2.25	2.50	Normal
6	0.41	0.61	0.82	1.02	1.22	1.43	1.63	1.84	2.04	
8	0.35	0.53	0.71	0.88	1.06	1.24	1.41	1.59	1.76	
10	0.31	0.47	0.63	0.79	0.95	1.10	1.26	1.42	1.58	
12	0.29	0.43	0.58	0.72	0.87	1.01	1.15	1.29	1.44	
14	0.27	0.40	0.53	0.67	0.80	0.94	1.07	1.20	1.34	Mild AS
16	0.25	0.37	0.50	0.63	0.75	0.88	1.00	1.13	1.25	
18	0.24	0.35	0.47	0.59	0.71	0.82	0.94	1.06	1.18	
20	0.22	0.34	0.45	0.56	0.67	0.78	0.89	1.00	1.12	
30	0.18	0.27	0.37	0.46	0.55	0.64	0.73	0.82	0.91	Moderate AS
40	0.16	0.24	0.32	0.39	0.47	0.55	0.63	0.71	0.79	
50	0.14	0.21	0.28	0.35	0.42	0.49	0.57	0.64	0.71	
60	0.13	0.19	0.26	0.32	0.39	0.45	0.52	0.58	0.65	
70	0.12	0.18	0.24	0.29	0.36	0.42	0.48	0.54	0.59	Severe AS
80	0.11	0.17	0.22	0.28	0.34	0.39	0.45	0.50	0.56	
90	0.11	0.16	0.21	0.26	0.32	0.37	0.42	0.47	0.52	
100	0.10	0.15	0.20	0.25	0.30	0.35	0.40	0.45	0.50	

Table 15.1b Mitral valve area derived from cardiac output and gradient. Valve area (cm^2) calculated as CO (l/min)/gradient.

Gradient	Cardiac output l/min								
	1.0	1.5	2.0	2.5	3.0	3.5	4.0	4.5	5.0
2	0.71	1.06	1.41	1.77	2.12	2.47	2.83	3.18	3.54
4	0.50	0.75	1.00	1.25	1.50	1.75	2.00	2.25	2.50
6	0.41	0.61	0.82	1.02	1.22	1.43	1.63	1.84	2.04
8	0.35	0.53	0.71	0.88	1.06	1.24	1.41	1.59	1.76
10	0.31	0.47	0.63	0.79	0.95	1.10	1.26	1.42	1.58
12	0.29	0.43	0.58	0.72	0.87	1.01	1.15	1.29	1.44
14	0.27	0.40	0.53	0.67	0.80	0.94	1.07	1.20	1.34
16	0.25	0.37	0.50	0.63	0.75	0.88	1.00	1.13	1.25
18	0.24	0.35	0.47	0.59	0.71	0.82	0.94	1.06	1.18
20	0.22	0.34	0.45	0.56	0.67	0.78	0.89	1.00	1.12

Mild MS

Moderate MS

Critical MS   Severe MS

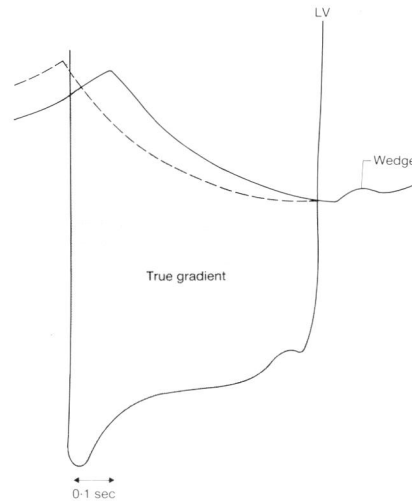

Fig. 15.2 Wedge/LV diastolic gradient. The delayed record of wedge pressure is redrawn so that the peak of the v wave coincides with isometric relaxation — usually a leftward shift of 0.1 seconds.

can introduce significant errors. For example if the calculated cardiac output was 3.0 l/min a mitral valve gradient of 9 mmHg would lead to a calculated valve area of 1.0 cm whereas if the true output was only 2.5 l/min the same gradient would result from a valve area of only 0.83 cm^2. The first value represents moderate stenosis but the second, true, value represents severe mitral stenosis.

Secondly atrial fibrillation, with varying cycle lengths, results in gradients that differ from beat to beat; the gradient must be averaged over several cycles and the average value used in the calculations.

Thirdly the use of the wedge pressure instead of the left atrial pressure can lead to serious errors. While the wedge pressure reflects, with accuracy, the mean left atrial pressure the wave form tends to be damped and the resulting delay in the Y descent can lead to an overestimate of the mitral valve gradient. The beginning of the Y descent should coincide with the downstroke of the left ventricular pressure but, in the wedge pressure tracing, it is often delayed by about 0.1 second. This should be corrected for by redrawing the wedge pressure tracing in the superimposed wedge and left ventricular pressure record (Fig. 15.2). The delayed course of the Y descent in the wedge pressure may be especially marked in patients with prosthetic mitral valves. In such patients an average under estimate of valve area of 0.3 cm^2 has been reported to result from use of the wedge instead of the direct left atrial pressure [5]. In such patients it may be wise, when assessing wedge/left ventricular gradients, to add 0.3 cm^2 to the calculated valve area in order to avoid an overestimate

of obstruction at a mitral prosthesis leading to unecessary reoperation.

Finally calculations of valve area are invalidated by the presence of significant regurgitation. Under these circumstances the flow across the valve cannot be calculated as it is made up of the forward flow (cardiac output) which *can* be calculated *plus* the regurgant flow which *cannot* be measured with any accuracy.

REGURGITATION

The assessment of regurgitation may be based on (1) subjective evaluation of the cine angiogram, (2) indicator dilution techniques, or (3) measurements of left ventricular volumes. In addition the haemodynamic consequences of regurgitation — the height of the left atrial pressure and its waveform, the severity of pulmonary hypertension or the height of the left ventricular end-diastolic pressure, for example — provide clues to its severity.

Cine-angiographic estimates of regurgitation depend on injecting radio-opaque contrast medium beyond the suspect valve and noting the speed and density of opacification of the proximal chamber.

The estimate is usually subjective — by eye — though video-densitometry can be used to give the estimate an appearance of objectivity. A number of problems beset this method. Thus the density of opacification of the proximal chamber will, for a given regurgitant volume, be inversely proportional to the size of the chamber. A large left atrium, as is found in long standing mitral valve disease, will be less densely opacified than the small left atrium of recent onset mitral regurgitation.

Spurious regurgitation may result from ventricular ectopic beats during the injection of contrast medium. The position of the catheter in relation to the suspect valve is important; too near the valve and it may interfere with valve function, too far away and regurgitation may be underestimated. A catheter which is traversing a valve can certainly cause spurious regurgitation by interfering with valve closure. In practice the great advantage of 'eye-ball' evaluation is that an experienced operator will take all these factors into account when assessing the severity of regurgitation. He will also bear in mind the relation between ventricular end-diastolic volume and the volume load. Severe aortic or mitral regurgitation *must* result in an increase in ventricular volume which is proportional to the severity of regurgitation thus providing another aid to assessment of severity.

Indicator dilution techniques for assessing regurgitation are of two types. The simplest depends on the effect of regurgitation in reducing the peak concentration and prolonging the disappearance phase of indicator dilution curves obtained from a peripheral artery. More sophisticated is the 'double indicator dilution technique' in which indicator injected downstream of the suspect valve is sampled simultaneously in the upstream chamber and in a peripheral artery. The relationship between the two curves is used to provide a 'regurgitant index' (see Chapter 10). A simplification of this technique is to perform the two curves in sequence. Problems with indicator dilution techniques are to do with non-uniform mixing of indicator and non-representative sampling. The techniques also add complexity to the study; the double sampling technique for assessing mitral regurgitation, for example, requires transseptal catheterisation for upstream sampling.

Measurements of left ventricular volume derived from the left ventricular angiogram can provide a third method of quantifying regurgitation. The theory is simple; total left ventricular stroke volume is ob-

tained by subtracting end-systolic (LVESV) from end-diastolic (LVEDV) left ventricular volume. Forward stroke volume is obtained by dividing the cardiac output (CO) by the heart rate. When there is no regurgitation the two values should be the same; when there is regurgitation the total stroke volume of the ventricle will exceed the forward stroke volume by an amount equal to the regurgitant volume. This can be expressed as the 'regurgitant fraction' (RF):

$$RF = \frac{\text{Total LV stroke volume} - \text{Forward stroke volume}}{\text{Total LV stroke volume}} \times 100$$

Total LV stroke volume is given by LVEDV − LVESV, and forward stroke volume by CO/heart rate.

Although providing a reasonably accurate measure of regurgitation the method is tedious requiring, as it does, the measurement of ventricular volumes from cine angiograms (Chapter 8). Errors in measurement of ventricular volumes result in some 'misestimate' of regurgitation so that regurgitant volume is seldom zero when the technique is 'calibrated' in patients without regurgitation.

Cardiology and medicine are not exact sciences and it is not surprising that no precise measure of regurgitation exists nor that those indices that are used sometimes give misleading information. The severity of valve disease is assessed not only by catheterisation but also on the basis of the symptoms, physical signs and results of non-invasive investigations — echocardiography in particular. This being so it is probably best to use the simplest invasive method available — subjective analysis of the cine angiogram — while accepting that the findings can be misleading; as they can with any of the alternative techniques.

THE MITRAL VALVE

Mitral stenosis

With very rare exceptions mitral stenosis is rheumatic in origin. Exceptions include rheumatoid arthritis and congenital mitral stenosis. A number of different forms of congenital left ventricular inflow obstruction have been described; not all are due to valve anomalies since congenital left ventricular inflow obstruction can be due to a supravalve stenosing ring of the left atrium or to cortriatriatum.

The objectives of catheterisation in cases of mitral

stenosis have changed over the past 20 years. At the time when mitral valvotomy was the only operation available it was important to assess the presence and severity of coexisting mitral regurgitation as there was no effective surgical treatment for a significantly regurgitant valve. With the development of mitral prostheses in the mid-1960s this became less important as open operations could be performed (using cardiopulmonary bypass) and the valve replaced if necessary. The emphasis changed towards confirmation of the diagnosis and assessment of severity. Today the diagnosis is seldom in doubt; it can be confirmed, and the severity assessed, by echocardiography as well as by symptoms. There remain, however, some patients in whom the severity of stenosis is in doubt and catheterisation is required for full assessment. Additionally catheterisation may be needed to detect and assess the severity of other valve lesions (aortic and tricuspid) or to study the coronary circulation. The question posed is not so much 'Is mitral valve surgery indicated?' as 'Is surgery required for other valve or coronary artery lesions as well?'

The assessment of mitral regurgitation and of other valve lesions will be discussed in the appropriate sections; here we are concerned with the assessment of the severity of mitral stenosis and of the haemodynamic consequences. The severity of stenosis is assessed using measurements which are related to estimates of *orifice size or area*. The consequences of mitral stenosis are (1) to modify the height and waveform of the left atrial pressure, (2) to lead to a pressure gradient across the mitral valve, and (3) to raise pulmonary artery pressure both 'passively' as the consequence of a raised downstream (left atrial) pressure and as a result of a secondary increase in pulmonary arteriolar resistance. Pulmonary hypertension resulting from left ventricular inflow obstruction itself has secondary effects such as dilatation of the right ventricle and consequent tricuspid incompetence. Finally there are downstream consequences of obstruction to left ventricular inflow; a reduced cardiac output and stroke volume and altered ventricular performance.

LEFT ATRIAL PRESSURE AND WAVEFORM

In moderate degrees of mitral stenosis the mean left atrial pressure will be found to be around 15 to 20 mmHg (normal 10 to 12 mmHg). When mitral

stenosis is severe the mean pressure may be as high as 30 to 40 mmHg — levels at which pulmonary oedema can occur. Delayed left atrial emptying results in prolongation of the y descent, and atrial fibrillation, if present, results in loss of the a wave. Prolongation of the y descent has been used as an index of the severity of mitral stenosis and a guide to the degree of coexisting regurgitation. In mitral regurgitation the tendency is for the v wave to be accentuated followed by a rapid y descent; the converse is true when mitral stenosis is the dominant lesion. Thus the more severe the stenosis and the less the regurgitation the slower the y descent in relation to the height of the v wave. The ratio between the two, the Ry/v ratio, is calculated as follows:

$$\text{Ry (the rate of descent in mmHg/second)} = \frac{P_1 - P_2}{T_2 - T_1}$$

where $P_1 - P_2$ is the difference in pressure between the peak of the v wave and its trough at the end of the y descent and $T_2 - T_1$ is the time in seconds between these two points. Ry is divided by V, the height of the v wave in mmHg to provide the ratio [6]. A ratio between 0.6 and 1.0 is found in pure mitral stenosis while in pure mitral regurgitation ratios between 2.0 and 6.0 are found (Fig. 15.3).

Morrow *et al.* [7] used the relationship between the rate of the y descent (Ry) and the mean left atrial pressure (LAMP) to derive an index, Ry/LAMP, for which values less than 4 were found in patients needing mitral valvotomy while values larger than this suggested dominant mitral regurgitation.

For reasons discussed above we are not much concerned, today, with evaluating relative degrees

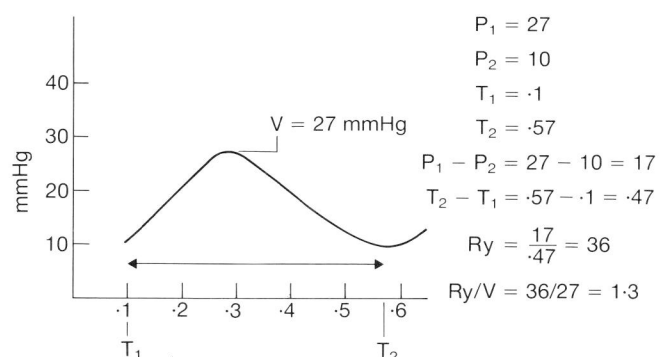

Fig. 15.3 Calculation of the Ry/V ratio.

of stenosis and regurgitation; in any case there are more direct ways of evaluating the degree of stenosis while regurgitation is estimated from left ventricular angiocardiograms.

GRADIENT

The most direct way of assessing the severity of mitral stenosis is to measure the transvalvar *gradient*. This measurement was combined with a measure of the rate of the y descent by Libanoff and Rodbard [8, 9] to provide yet another index of severity: the 'atrioventricular pressure half-time'. The time at which the pressure gradient between the left atrium and ventricle reaches half its value at the beginning of ventricular filling is measured from the beginning of ventricular filling; values of 100 msec were found in patients with mild mitral stenosis and of 200 msec in those with moderate stenosis. In patients with severe mitral stenosis values of 300 msec or more were found.

It remained for Gorlin and Gorlin to apply hydraulic principles to provide a measure of *valve area*. The calculation of valve area by the Gorlin formula and its derivatives has been discussed in the introductory section to this chapter since the principle can be applied to the calculation of all valve areas, not just the area of the mitral valve. In its original form [1] the Gorlin formula for the calculation of mitral valve area is:

$$MVA = \frac{MVF}{31 \times \sqrt{PC - 5}}$$

where MVA = area of the mitral valve in cm^2, MVF = mitral valve flow in cc/(diastolic) second, PC = pulmonary capillary (wedge) mean pressure, mmHg, 5 = assumed left ventricular diastolic pressure, mmHg and 31 = empirical constant.

MVF is obtained by dividing the cardiac output, in cc/min, by the product of the heart rate and the diastolic filling period in second/beat;

$$MVF = \frac{CO}{(HR) \times (Dfp)}$$

As discussed in the introduction to this section the diastolic filling period was calculated from the beginning of the dicrotic notch of the brachial arterial tracing to the beginning of the upstroke of the next pressure pulse. As modified by Cohen and Gorlin [2] for direct measurements of gradient and Dfp the

formula becomes:

$$MVA = \frac{MVF}{37.9 \times \sqrt{Gradient}}$$

The simplified formula as proposed by Hakki *et al.* [3] is:

$$MVA = \frac{CO \ (l/min)}{\sqrt{Valve \ gradient}}$$

Angel *et al.* [10] investigated the accuracy of this simplified formula and found significant errors in relation to differing heart rates. For patients with mitral stenosis they proposed correcting Hakki's formula by dividing by 1.35 if the heart rate was less than 75 beats/minute.

The area of the normal mitral valve is between 4 and 6 cm^2 but there is no significant obstruction until stenosis has narrowed the orifice to less than 2.5 cm^2. The following are a rough guide to the severity of stenosis in relation to valve area (see Table 15.1):
1 2.0 to 2.5 cm^2 = mild stenosis (Class I). No limitations, only breathless on severe exertion.
2 1.0 to 2.0 cm^2 = moderate stenosis (Class II). Slight limitation of physical activity, breathless on ordinary exertion.
3 0.75 to 1.0 cm^2 = severe stenosis (Class III). Marked limitation of physical activity, breathless on mild exertion.
4 0.5 to 0.75 cm^2 = critical stenosis (Class IV) Unable to carry on any physical activity, breathless at rest.

PULMONARY ARTERY PRESSURE

The normal mitral valve is able to transmit a considerable increase in flow, during exercise for example, without an increase in left atrial pressure. When mitral stenosis is mild the left atrial pressure may be normal at rest but the increased flow during exercise can only be accomodated by a rise in left atrial pressure and the appearance of a mitral valve gradient. The tachycardia of exercise shortens diastole more than systole; as a result the increased flow has to be accomodated during a shortened diastolic filling period thus further increasing the mitral valve gradient and the height of the left atrial pressure. Finally, with increasing severity of stenosis, the left atrial pressure is elevated at rest.

The inevitable result of a raised left atrial pressure is that the pulmonary arterial pressure must rise to maintain forward flow. If this were the only consequence of mitral stenosis the height of the pulmonary arterial pressure would be a measure of the severity of mitral stenosis. While there is some relationship between the degree of pulmonary hypertension and the severity of stenosis the relationship is not a simple one. This is because, as mitral stenosis becomes more severe and left atrial pressure rises, two 'compensatory mechanisms' come into play: a rise in pulmonary arteriolar resistance and a fall in cardiac output. These changes can be regarded as compensatory or 'protective' since they protect against the occurrence of pulmonary oedema. When the mitral valve area is around $1\,cm^2$ mitral flow cannot increase and exercise would result in an increase in left atrial pressure to levels at which pulmonary oedema would result. If, however, there is an increased resistance to pulmonary flow at arteriolar level this tends to prevent a marked increase in right ventricular output causing an increase in pulmonary venous return and a consequent rise in left atrial pressure. In practice levels of pulmonary arteriolar resistance tend to rise sharply when the mitral valve area is reduced to $1\,cm^2$ and resting cardiac output is low ($<2.5\,l/min/m^2$). However the relationship between valve area, pulmonary arteriolar resistance and cardiac output varies from patient to patient; in some patients the pulmonary arteriolar resistance remains relatively low and such patients may be particularly liable to develop pulmonary oedema [11]. For our purposes what is important to remember is that the degree of pulmonary hypertension present is only a rough guide to the severity of mitral stenosis; in theory it is possible for a patient to have severe mitral stenosis and a normal pulmonary artery pressure provided the arteriolar resistance and the cardiac output are both low enough.

The increased pulmonary arteriolar resistance associated with downstream obstruction tends to regress when obstruction is relieved (e.g. by mitral valvotomy/replacement) and therefore has a less sinister significance than a rise in resistance occurring in response to a high flow/high pressure situation in congenital heart disease.

LEFT VENTRICULAR FUNCTION

It has been known for many years that left ventricular systolic function may be abnormal in patients with mitral stenosis [12]. In some this may be due to rheumatic carditis [13] but this is not necessarily the case and Cotter et al. [14] have shown that the abnormalities can regress after surgery and do not necessarily, therefore, imply irreversible left ventricular damage. Heller and Carleton [15] found ejection fractions which averaged 55.7% in patients with mitral stenosis as against 76.7% in normal subjects. They also described 'distortion, immobility and rigidity' of the posterobasal segment of the left ventricle associated with mitral stenosis. The message is that while left ventricular systolic function (ejection fraction) may be reduced in mitral stenosis it is wrong, as a result, to make a diagnosis of 'cardiomyopathy' in addition to the diagnosis of mitral stenosis.

Mitral regurgitation

In contrast to mitral stenosis there are many causes of mitral regurgitation other than rheumatic fever and catheterisation and angiography can often determine the likely cause. These causes include mitral valve prolapse, floppy mitral valve, ruptured chordae tendinea, ruptured papillary muscle or papillary muscle dysfunction, dilated mitral annulus secondary to left ventricular enlargement and dysfunction, infective endocarditis, systemic lupus, annular calcification and congenital causes. To these we must add regurgitation due to malfunction of a prosthetic valve or paraprosthetic leak.

Mitral prolapse (Fig. 15.4) is common but in a small minority of patients progressive mitral regurgitation can develop. The leaflet, usually the posterior leaflet, is seen to balloon backwards into the left atrium during late systole. When regurgitation occurs this is also, initially, late systolic in timing and an eccentric jet is often seen with contrast medium swirling round the left atrium. Ruptured chordae and papillary muscle dysfunction can produce a distinctive syndrome of *acute mitral regurgitation* but can also result in chronic regurgitation. Papillary muscle rupture following myocardial infarction causes acute mitral regurgitation and has to be distinguished from postinfarction ventricular septal defect (ruptured interventricular septum). Mitral regurgitation secondary to left ventricular enlargement and dysfunction is commonly observed but is seldom severe; when ventricular dysfunction is due to chronic ischaemic heart disease then papillary

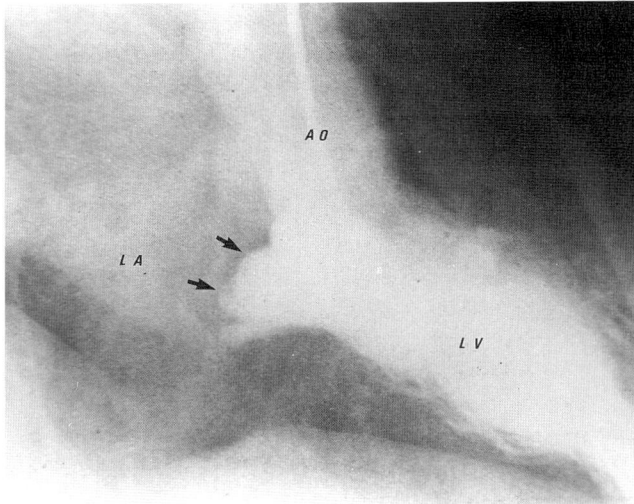

Fig. 15.4 Mitral valve prolapse. The prolapsing posterior cusp of the mitral valve (arrows) is seen. There is some associated mitral regurgitation as evidenced by opacification of the left atrium (LA).

muscle dysfunction may play a part in causing mitral regurgitation. Infective endocarditis can affect a previously normal valve but more usually affects a rheumatic or prolapsing valve with rapid worsening of regurgitation as a result. Annular calcification

(Fig. 15.5) has to be distinguished from calcification of the valve leaflets, such as occurs in rheumatic valves. Annular calcification is not uncommon in the aged, particularly in women. It is usually benign but can result in mitral regurgitation and, rarely, mitral stenosis.

Congenital causes of mitral regurgitation include atrioventricular defects (atrioventricular canal) and regurgitation at a morphologic, left sided, tricuspid valve in conditions with atrioventricular discordance. In adults the development of mitral regurgitation may be the first clue to the presence of atrioventricular and ventriculo-arterial discordance (corrected transposition).

The detection and assessment of mitral regurgitation in the catheterisation laboratory depends on left ventricular cine-angiography. Assuming that the catheter is correctly positioned away from the mitral valve contrast medium appearing in the left atrium indicates the presence of mitral regurgitation. (Fig. 15.6). A right oblique projection is selected so as to profile the mitral valve and separate the left atrium from the left ventricle. Spurious regurgitation can result when the pressure injection leads to multiple ventricular ectopic beats. Estimates of the severity of regurgitation should be interpreted with caution under these circumstances. If there is adequate contrast medium remaining in the ventricle when the run of ectopics is over it may be possible to see that there is no (true) regurgitation during sinus rhythm. Spurious regurgitation may also occur towards the

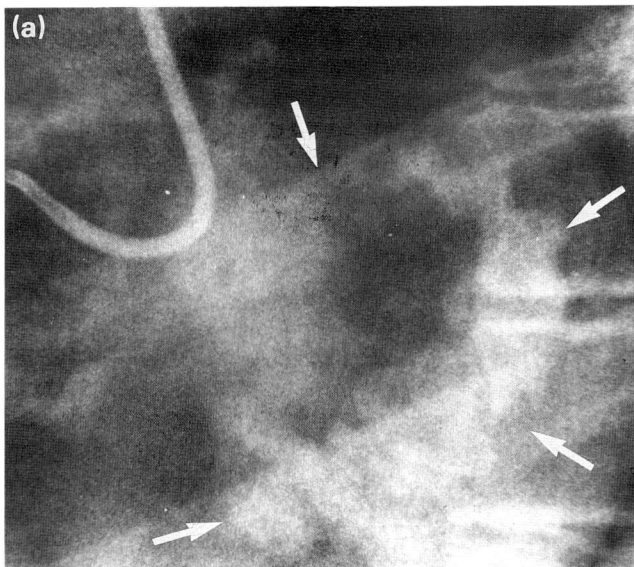
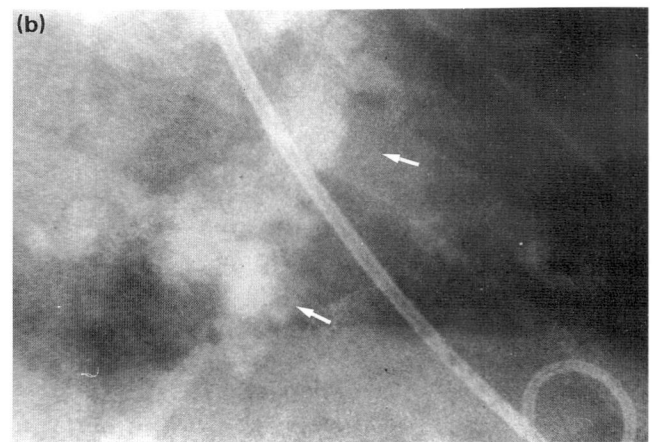

Fig. 15.5 (a) Calcification of the mitral valve annulus (annular calcification). Such annular calcification occurs in elderly patients. The ring-shaped calcification (arrows) is well seen in this left oblique view. In the right oblique view (b) heavy calcification (arrows) is obvious but the annulus is seen on edge and the ring-shape is obscured.

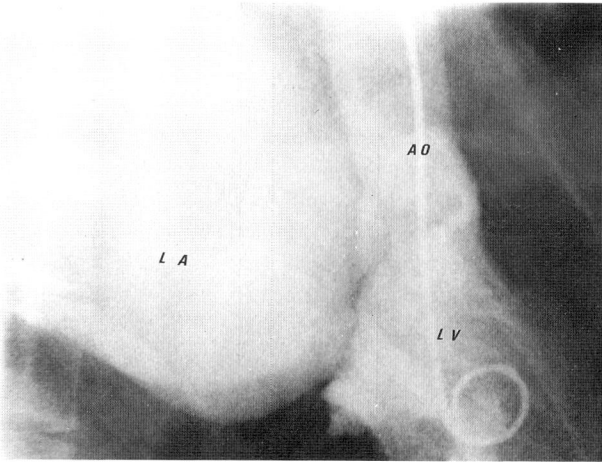

Fig. 15.6 Rheumatic mitral valve disease. Injection of contrast medium into the left ventricle (LV) has resulted in dense opacification of a grossly enlarged left atrium (LA) indicating severe mitral regurgitation.

end of prolonged diastasis such as may follow a rapid series of ectopics. Such spurious regurgitation is easily recognised; contrast medium appears to float lazily backwards into the left atrium. True regurgitation results in a forceful jet of contrast medium passing backwards into the left atrium during ventricular systole. The severity of regurgitation is estimated from the rapidity of left atrial opacification, the density of opacification (allowing for left atrial size) and the width of the regurgitant jet. A subjective grading of mitral regurgitation that is widely accepted is:

Grade 1: visible jet during systole with only minimal left atrial opacification which clears rapidly.

Grade 2: as above but moderate left atrial opacification.

Grade 3: broad regurgitant jet with dense left atrial opacification which clears slowly.

Grade 4: as above but left atrium more densely opacified than the left ventricle and contrast remains in the left atrium throughout filming.

It must be remembered that, as long as myocardial function is unimpaired (normal ejection fraction), there is a linear relation between the volume load on a ventricle and its end-diastolic volume; thus any significant degree of mitral regurgitation must result in an increased left ventricular end-diastolic volume. This feature can be used as an 'eye-ball' check of the severity of regurgitation.

A more precise use of ventricular volume measurements for quantitating regurgitation depends on calculating the regurgitant fraction from the difference between the angiographically derived left ventricular stroke volume and the forward stroke volume [16, 17].

The accuracy of the various methods of estimating mitral regurgitation has been studied by Lopez *et al.* [18].

The forceful arrival of blood in the left atrium during ventricular systole raises the left atrial pressure and alters the left atrial pressure wave form. Characteristically the left atrial pressure exhibits a dominant v wave with a rapid y descent and the Ry/v ratio can calculated as described in the preceding section on mitral stenosis.

Accentuation of the v wave is most marked (giant v waves) when mitral regurgitation is of recent onset (acute mitral regurgitation) and the left atrium is still small and relatively non-compliant. Such left atrial pressure tracings are associated with non-rheumatic mitral regurgitation from, for example, ruptured chordae or ruptured papillary muscle. On occasion the v wave in such patients may be higher than the pulmonary artery systolic pressure (though the *mean* left atrial pressure must be less than the mean pulmonary artery pressure) and the v wave is seen as a separate spike immediately following the initial pulmonary artery systolic pressure wave. The concept that tall v waves are associated with acute, non-rheumatic, mitral regurgitation has recently been questioned [19] but the observation is so commonplace that it must still be regarded as a pointer towards the aetiology of regurgitation though not an invariable finding and to be assessed in conjunction with all other relevant clinical and investigatory findings.

In acute or recent onset mitral regurgitation left ventriculography results in dense left atrial opacification as the left atrium is not greatly enlarged. Contrast medium will be seen to fill the pulmonary veins.

Acute mitral regurgitation as a complication of myocardial infarction (usually inferior infarction with rupture of a head of the posteromedial papillary muscle) is a life-threatening event. The differential diagnosis is from ruptured ventricular septum. Ruptured ventricular septum is most easily proved by bedside catheterisation using a balloon-tipped, flow-guided, catheter. A series of samples will demonstrate a marked increase in oxygen saturation at ventricular and pulmonary artery level. Mixed venous saturation is likely to be very low, reflecting the low cardiac output. In acute mitral regurgitation there will be no such step-up and giant v waves may be seen if the catheter is allowed to advance to the wedge position. It must be remembered that the detection of a shunt at ventricular level (VSD) does not exclude acute mitral regurgitation since the two conditions can coexist. Despite the large shunt detected in ruptured ventricular septum right ventricular systolic pressure, though high, is seldom as high as the systemic pressure. The septal defect lies in the muscular portion of the septum and, as a rule, towards the apex inferiorly. Formal catheterisation with left ventriculography and coronary arteriography is often advised in these conditions. This, in my view, is unwise and should be avoided if at all possible in these very sick, high risk, patients. It is unlikely that coronary artery grafting will make any difference to the outlook in patients whose infarct typically occurred several days previously. Certainly coronary arteriography and a prolonged operation will add significantly to the, already high, risk. Urgent mitral valve replacement/repair and/or closure of the septal defect is needed to save the patient's life. Ideally operation should be postponed until scar tissue has replaced necrotic myocardium — but this is often impossible.

THE AORTIC VALVE

Aortic stenosis

The causes of left ventricular outflow obstruction include:
1 *Acquired*:
  Rheumatic valvular aortic stenosis.
  Fibrosis/calcification of a congenitally abnormal valve (e.g. bicuspid).
  Fibrosis/calcification of a normal (tricuspid) valve.
2 *Congenital*:
  Valvar aortic stenosis.
  Discrete subvalvar fibromuscular membrane.
  'Tunnel' subaortic stenosis.
  Hypertrophic cardiomyopathy (see Chapter 16).
  Supravalve aortic stenosis.
  Rheumatic aortic stenosis may be an isolated lesion or there may be associated aortic regurgitation

or other rheumatic valve disease (e.g. mitral stenosis). Many case of isolated aortic valve disease (stenosis or regurgitation) presenting in adult life are due to degenerative changes or calcification in a congenitally bicuspid valve. Fibrosis and calcification can also occur in a previously normal valve; such valves may be stenotic but this is not always the case and many have no valve gradient (aortic sclerosis).

Congenital valvar aortic stenosis is due to a unicuspid valve (in the neonate) or to cusp fusion of a bicuspid valve (Figs 15.10 and 15.8). The stenosis may be severe and patients with critical aortic valve stenosis can present in the neonatal period. Bicuspid aortic valve may be the commonest congenital cardiac defect but patients do not present until (and if) calcification and stenosis or regurgitation have developed in adult life at which time it may be impossible to determine that the valve was originally a congenitally malformed one (Fig. 15.9).

Congenital subaortic stenosis is of two types. In the first type there is a discrete fibrous 'diaphragm' which may be immediately below the valve or a centimetre or so beneath it (Fig. 15.14). Some, mild, aortic regurgitation is common and, as a result, the subvalvar chamber may be outlined by aortography. The valve cusps themselves may be somewhat thickened — perhaps from a jet lesion — and this is the only form of subaortic stenosis in which there may be some poststenotic dilatation of the aorta. The diagnosis is made from the pressure records and by left ventriculography. A 'pull-back' pressure

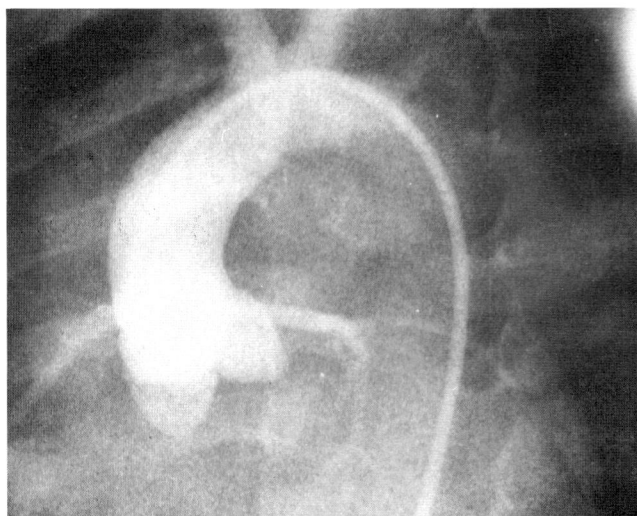

Fig. 15.7 Normal, three-cusp aortic valve.

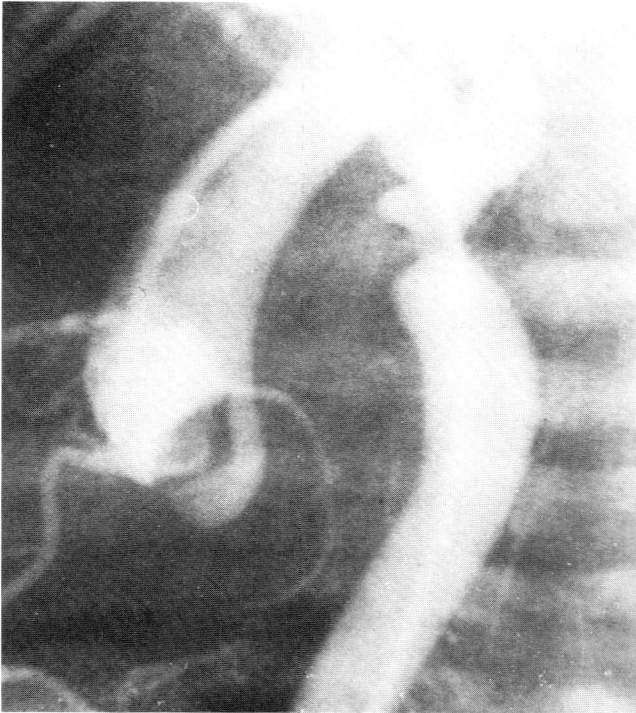

Fig. 15.8 Congenitally stenotic, bicuspid, aortic valve. Coarctation is also present.

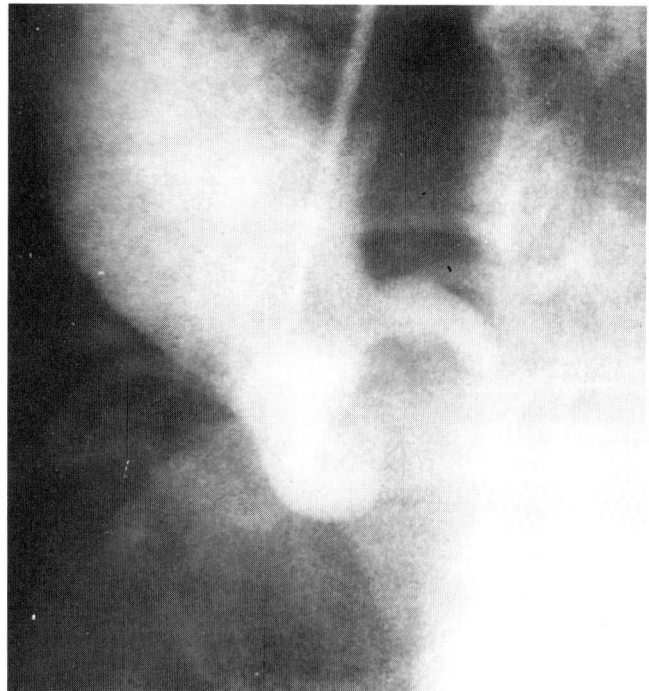

Fig. 15.9 Aortic valve stenosis in an adult. The valve is thickened and irregular and does not open fully. There is some poststenotic dilatation and there is aortic regurgitation since the left ventricle has opacified following the injection of contrast medium into the aorta.

record may demonstrate, in sequence, (1) a high pressure ventricular pressure tracing, (2) a lower, but still ventricular, pressure, and (3) an aortic tracing with a systolic pressure the same as, or little lower than, the systolic pressure in the subaortic chamber. Often, however, the subvalve membrane is so close to the valve that it is impossible to record a separate pressure from the subvalve chamber. These records should be obtained with a single end-hole catheter; catheters with multiple side-holes can produce 'artefactual subaortic stenosis' as some side-holes are in the ventricle while others are in the aorta. Ventriculography should be performed in the left oblique projection *with cranial tilt* so as to display the outflow tract without foreshortening. Even with this precaution it is easy to miss the diagnosis; biplane filming is desirable as the diaphragm is close to the valve and may not be visible in all projections. Some cases develop severe hypertrophy of left ventricular myocardium which is indistinguishable from hypertrophic cardiomyopathy. It is uncertain if this is merely secondary to the increased afterload or an association between two, congenitally determined,

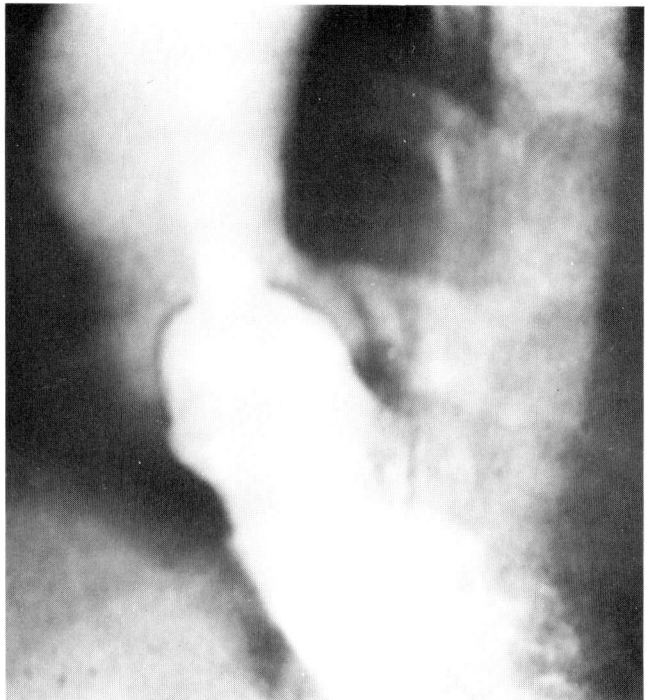

Fig. 15.10 Congenital aortic valve stenosis. The valve is thin but does not open fully; there is 'doming' in systole and a central jet of contrast medium together with some poststenotic dilatation. Compare with Fig. 15.9.

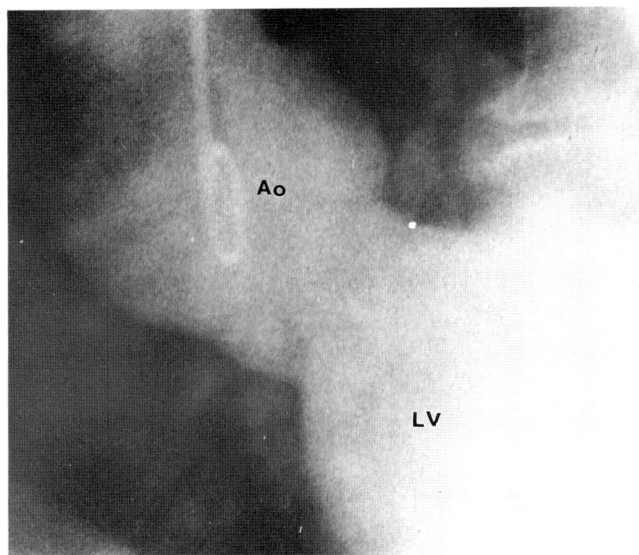

Fig. 15.11 Severe aortic valve regurgitation. An injection of contrast medium into the ascending aorta (Ao) has resulted in rapid and dense opacification of the left ventricle (LV) which clears slowly.

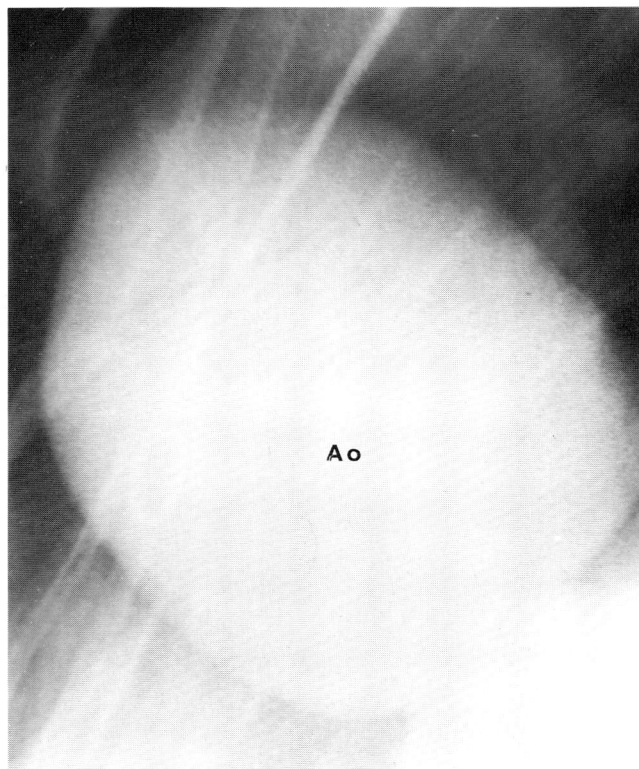

Fig. 15.12 Annulo-aortic ectasia; the dilated aortic root (Ao) fills most of the frame, the aortic valve is just visible at the bottom right corner of the figure and there is aortic regurgitation.

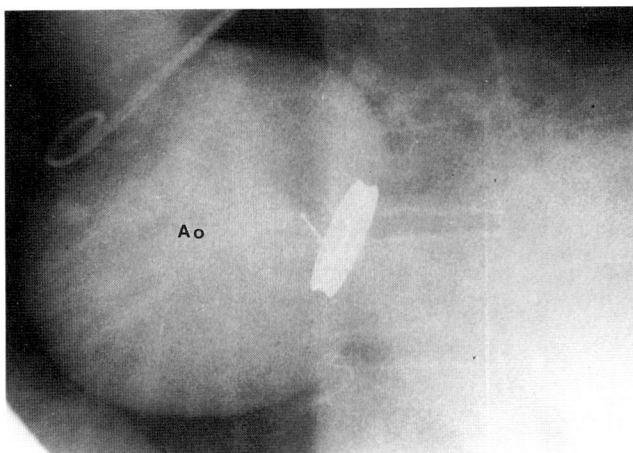

Fig. 15.13 Annulo-aortic ectasia has lead to aortic regurgitation and a prosthetic (Bjork−Shiley) valve has been inserted.

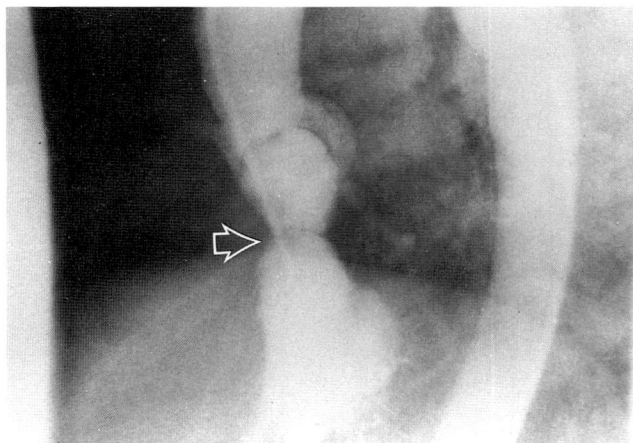

Fig. 15.14 Subaortic stenosis due to a discrete, fibromuscular, diaphragm below the aortic valve (arrow). Cranial angulation is needed to display this lesion which is obscured by foreshortening of the ventricle in standard oblique or lateral projections.

anomalies. Discrete, subaortic, stenosis may be associated with other, usually left-sided, congenital cardiac defects. In particular it forms part of Shone syndrome [20] of coarctation, supra- and subvalve aortic stenosis, parachute mitral valve and supravalve stenosing ring of the left atrium.

The second form of congenital, subaortic, stenosis — tunnel stenosis — takes the form of a diffuse narrowing of the outflow tract (Fig. 15.16). Both tunnel subaortic stenosis and the discrete variety

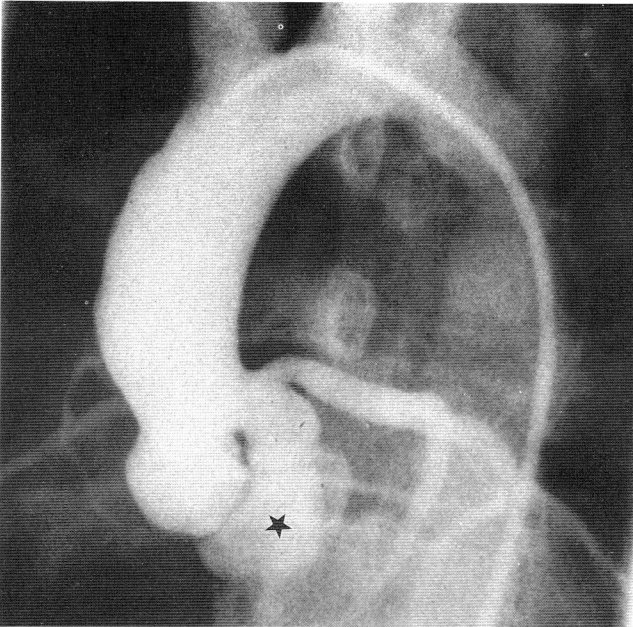

Fig. 15.15 In the same patient as Fig. 15.14, an aortogram appears to show aortic cusp prolapse. In fact the aortic valve, though malformed, is in the normal position but aortic regurgitation has outlined a subaortic chamber (asterisk) bounded below by the upper surface of the subaortic diaphragm. Mild aortic regurgitation and cusp deformity are common in this condition and left ventricular hypertrophy may mimic hypertrophic cardiomyopathy.

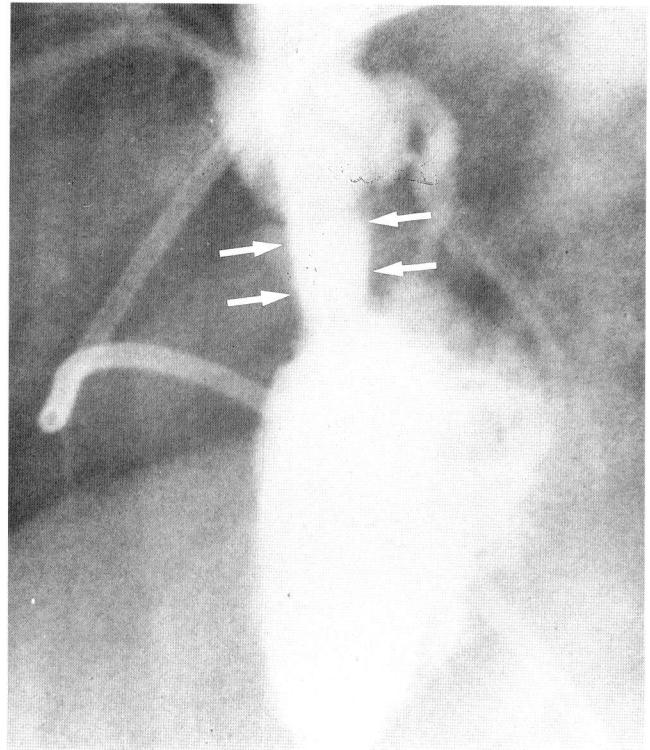

Fig. 15.16 Another form of subaortic stenosis due to a tunnel-like narrowing of the left ventricular outflow tract (arrows). There are many other causes of subaortic obstruction associated with other, often complex, congenital cardiac malformations. Hypertrophic cardiomyopathy may result in subaortic obstruction and is illustrated elsewhere.

occur in Shone syndrome. In some patients tunnel stenosis merges into a hypoplasia of the whole of the outflow with a hypoplastic valve annulus and hypoplastic ascending aorta. Surgical reconstruction may involve valve replacement. The diagnosis is again made on the angiographic appearances.

Supravalve aortic stenosis is of three types; hour-glass constriction, diffuse narrowing and a membrane or crescentic shelf [21]. Of these an hour-glass narrowing is most frequently seen while the membranous, or shelf, lesion is rare. In the hour-glass form there is a localised constriction at the level of the upper border of the sinuses of Valsalva. Supravalve aortic stenosis occurs in the Williams syndrome [22] — infantile hypercalcaemia, elfin facies, mild mental retardation, supravalve aortic stenosis and peripheral pulmonary artery stenosis or diffuse pulmonary arterial hypolasia. If suspected the investigation should include pulmonary arteriography or a right ventricular angiocardiogram in the four-chamber projection. The coronary arteries are

often large and tortuous in supravalve aortic stenosis but ostial stenosis has been described as resulting from fusion of the valve leaflet with the ridge at the upper edge of an aortic sinus thus excluding the coronary ostium.

LABORATORY INVESTIGATION

Cardiac catheterisation in cases of aortic stenosis is undertaken (1) to confirm the diagnosis, (2) to assess severity, (3) to detect and assess other, coexisting valve disease, (4) to demonstrate the morphology and the aortic root, (5) to assess left ventricular function, and (6) to perform coronary arteriography. There may also be a place for balloon valvuloplasty in selected cases (Chapter 5).

Abnormalities of pressure records are described in Chapter 6. The important abnormalities seen in valvar aortic stenosis are (1) a slow upstroke arterial pulse — often with vibrations due to turbulence, and (2) a gradient between the left ventricular and aortic pressures. In most cases measurement of the gradient provides an adequate estimate of severity. A gradient of more than 50 mmHg, indicates severe aortic stenosis requiring surgical correction. Ideally aortic valve area should be measured since a high output state could result in a significant gradient despite only moderate valve narrowing. More importantly a small or trivial gradient is sometimes found in patients with severe aortic stenosis and a very low cardiac output. Such patients have severely impaired left ventricular function and are examples of end-stage aortic stenosis. Despite the increased risk these patients require urgent surgical treatment (or balloon valvuloplasty) since the prognosis is otherwise hopeless.

The normal aortic valve area is about 3 cm^2, and a gradient will be detected when the valve is narrowed to less than 2 cm^2. Valve areas of 0.75–1.0 cm^2 represent moderately severe aortic stenosis requiring surgical treatment while a valve area of less than 0.75 cm^2 represents severe or critical aortic stenosis (see Table 15.1).

Left ventriculography allows assessment of left ventricular function and, if performed in the right oblique projection, allows detection and assessment of any coexisting mitral regurgitation. Aortography should be performed in the left oblique projection, with or without cranial tilt, and will demonstrate any aortic regurgitation as well as the aortic root anatomy. Valve movement will be seen to be restricted and a negative jet is likely to be seen as unopacified blood is forcefully ejected into the dilated aortic root. Valve calcification is best seen during fluoroscopy and may extend into the upper part of the ventricular septum.

It can be argued that little of this investigation is really necessary in the adult patient with aortic stenosis. Once the presence of severe aortic stenosis has been established from the pressure gradient then surgical treatment is required. Poor left ventricular function may increase the operative risk but is seldom a contraindication to valve replacement since it will not improve without relief of obstruction. Remaining indications for cardiac catheterisation are the assessment of other valve lesions — if these are in doubt — and the need for coronary arteriography. The indication for coronary arteriography in aortic stenosis is a subject of debate [23, 24]. Angina is a symptom in some two-thirds of patients with aortic stenosis but only about half of these patients have significant, atherosclerotic, coronary artery disease. Angina may be abolished by aortic valve surgery without the need for coronary bypass grafting and it is not yet known if combining coronary artery surgery with aortic valve surgery improves the long-term prognosis. None the less it seems entirely reasonable to perform coronary arteriography in patients with aortic stenosis and angina; the risk involved is very small and the added information may allow more rational treatment. Coronary arteriography in these patients can be technically difficult; large curve catheters may be needed (e.g. Judkins no. IV, 6 cm curve or Castillo no. III) because of aortic root dilatation and the forceful systolic jet may interfere with catheter manipulation. Cannulation of the right coronary ostium can be particularly difficult.

Catheterisation, in patients with valvar aortic stenosis, is best performed from a (right) brachial arteriotomy with retrograde entry to the left ventricle across the aortic valve. Catheterisation from the leg is perfectly possible but allows rather less control of the catheter in the ascending aorta. Hints on crossing a stenotic aortic valve are given in Chapter 4. If the aortic valve cannot be crossed retrogradely the remaining alternatives are the transseptal approach and percutaneous, transapical, left ventricular puncture using a 10 cm long 21 gauge needle. Transseptal puncture carries a significant risk; unless the operator is very experienced in the technique the aortic valve gradient is best obtained by left ventricular puncture. Both techniques are described in Chapter 3. Transapical needle puncture does not allow left ventriculography. If a left ventriculogram is needed for assessment of left ventricular function a pulmonary arteriogram with follow-through will suffice. If a left ventriculogram is needed to detect and assess mitral regurgitation and both antegrade (transseptal) and retrograde left ventricular access is impossible an angiographic catheter can be introduced, transapically, by a modification of the transapical technique [25], see Chapter 3.

Aortic regurgitation

Aortic regurgitation may be due to conditions which affect the valve itself, as in rheumatic aortic valve disease, or may be secondary to abnormalities of the

ascending aorta, as in Marfan disease or aortic dissection. Thus a classification of the causes of aortic regurgitation would include:
1 Abnormalities of the aortic valve:
Congenital: congenitally malformed valve — bicuspid, unicuspid, etc; and aortic valve prolapse in supracristal VSD.
Acquired: Rheumatic fever, infective endocarditis, rheumatoid arthritis, and ankylosing spondylitis.
2 Abnormalities of the aortic root and ascending aorta:
Congenital: Marfan disease, Ehlers−Danlos, pseudoxanthoma elasticum, and sinus of Valsalva aneurysm with distortion of aortic valve.
Acquired: aortic dissection, syphilis, ankylosing spondylitis, and Bechet syndrome.

LABORATORY INVESTIGATION

Cardiac catheterisation in aortic regurgitation is indicated for much the same reasons as in aortic stenosis. Aortography will outline the anatomy of the aortic root and also allow subjective assessment of the severity of regurgitation. Left ventriculography will provide information about left ventricular function and detect the presence of associated mitral regurgitation. Simultaneous right heart catheterisation provides a measure of the wedge/LV gradient to assess coexisting mitral stenosis and coronary arteriography allows detection of coexisting atherosclerotic coronary artery disease.

Aortography and the angiographic appearances of aortic disease are described in Chapter 20.

A subjective assessment of the severity of regurgitation can be based on the aortographic appearances:
Grade 1 (mild): opacification of left ventricular outflow (only) during early diastole which clears completely during systole.
Grade 2 (moderate): opacification of whole of left ventricular cavity which increases in density during several cycles.
Grade 3 (severe): as above but ventricular opacification is complete within one diastole and contrast remains in the ventricle for 10 seconds or more.

In chronic aortic regurgitation left ventriculography will always demonstrate an increase in end-diastolic and end-systolic volumes consistent with the increased volume load but the ejection fraction only becomes reduced in the later stages of the disease as left ventricular dysfunction supervenes.

The haemodynamic findings depend on whether regurgitation is acute (e.g. following infective endocarditis) or chronic and whether or not left ventricular function has become impaired as a result of long standing aortic regurgitation. The characteristic findings in chronic aortic regurgitation include:
1 A wide pulse pressure due to an increased systolic and low diastolic pressure.
2 Left ventricular end-diastolic pressure is initially normal but becomes raised as left ventricular function becomes impaired.
3 Similarly the ejection fraction, initially normal, becomes reduced as left ventricular function becomes impaired. At this stage:
4 Left atrial pressure rises and there is a comensurate rise in pulmonary arterial pressure; eventually right heart 'failure' supervenes and cardiac output falls while right ventricular filling pressure and right atrial pressure rise. In acute aortic regurgitation the most striking abnormality is a very high left ventricular end-diastolic pressure which may equalise with aortic diastolic pressure as early as mid-diastole [26]. The steeply rising left ventricular diastolic pressure exceeds left atrial pressure resulting in premature closure of the mitral valve. The findings in acute aortic regurgitation can be explained on the basis that the ventricle has not had time to enlarge in response to a volume load and is therefore noncompliant. Thus the aortic diastolic pressure is maintained by the high ventricular diastolic pressure and the pulse pressure is not especially wide. This is the most noticeable difference from chronic aortic regurgitation. However end-stage chronic aortic regurgitation with impaired ventricular function and a high ventricular end-diastolic pressure can produce similar haemodynamic findings with the exception that ventricular volumes are considerably increased in this state and are not so increased in acute aortic regurgitation.

TRICUSPID VALVE DISEASE

Tricuspid regurgitation is much more common than tricuspid stenosis and functional tricuspid regurgitation, secondary to right ventricular hypertension, much more common than organic tricuspid valve disease.
1 Tricuspid regurgitation:
a Secondary to RV hypertension, e.g. rheumatic

mitral valve disease, pulmonary vascular disease (Eisenmenger, primary PHT, cor pulmonale), pulmonary stenosis.

b Primary tricuspid valve disease: *congenital*, e.g. Ebstein's malformation of the tricuspid valve, congenitally absent valve, transient myocardial ischaemia of the newborn and Marfan syndrome. *Acquired*, e.g. rheumatic, carcinoid heart disease, endomyocardial fibrosis, right ventricular infarction and Staphylococcal endocarditis.

2 Tricuspid stenosis:
   Rheumatic involvement, ?carcinoid.

Tricuspid regurgitation

Of the causes listed above rheumatic involvement of the tricuspid valve occurs in some 5% of patients with rheumatic valvular disease; tricuspid regurgitation is more commonly functional as a result of pulmonary hypertension due to rheumatic mitral valve disease. Carcinoid heart disease occurs in about half of the patients with liver metastases from carcinoid ileal tumours. The plaque lesions result, most commonly, in pulmonary valve stenosis and tricuspid regurgitation [27]. Staphylococcal endocarditis of the tricuspid valve occurs in drug addicts who introduce infection intravenously. With the exception of Ebstein's malformation congenital tricuspid regurgitation is a very rare lesion. Congenital absence, or dysplasia, of the tricuspid valve occurs as an isolated lesion and in association with a few cases of pulmonary atresia with intact ventricular septum; such patients have gross enlargement of the right atrium and cavity of the right ventricle.

LABORATORY DIAGNOSIS

Pressure recordings

In the rare cases of isolated, primary, tricuspid disease the right ventricular pressure is normal or low. In patients with functional tricuspid regurgitation right ventricular pressure will be very high. In those with rheumatic tricuspid valve disease who have other rheumatic valvular involvement right ventricular pressure will also be raised as a result of mitral and/or aortic valve involvement.

Right atrial and right ventricular end-diastolic pressure is raised and, typically, the normal x descent is replaced by a regurgitant v or c—v wave. This wave is plateau shaped or upwardly convex until terminated by the y descent following isovolumic relaxation of the ventricle. In severe tricuspid regurgitation the right atrial pressure resembles, increasingly, the right ventricular pressure (ventricularisation). These findings, though characteristic of tricuspid regurgitation, can be mimicked by atrial fibrillation in the presence of pulmonary hypertension. An important finding is that, in contrast to the normal inspiratory fall in pressure, right atrial pressure either rises, or is unchanged, during deep inspiration [28].

Angiography

Tricuspid regurgitation is difficult to assess angiographically; the presence of a catheter across the valve may itself induce 'spurious' regurgitation while gross right atrial and right ventricular enlargement dilutes the contrast medium so that angiography is often of poor quality. Gross enlargement of the right atrium and the forceful regurgitant jet also make entry to the right ventricle technically difficult — especially if the approach is from the leg. Lingamneni *et al.* [29] have employed a specially modified NIH angiographic catheter and low flow rates (40—45 ml at 10—12 ml/second) with apparently reliable results. The severity of regurgitation is estimated, subjectively, on a four point scale:

1 Minimal regurgitant jet in systole, which clears rapidly.

2 Regurgitant jet with persistent partial opacification of the right atrium.

3 Dense opacification of the entire right atrium.

4 Dense opacification of the entire right atrium and both vena cavae.

Indicator dilution techniques can be used to assess tricuspid regurgitation

If indicator is injected upstream and sampled at a downstream site the characteristic distortion of regurgitation is seen. The peak concentration is delayed and reduced in magnitude and the disappearance phase is prolonged. Alternatively a double-sampling technique can be used; indicator is injected into the right ventricle and sampled from the right atrium. The immediate appearance of dye in the right atrium signals the presence of tricuspid regurgitation and the magnitude of the deflection gives some indication of severity. The usual problems associated with indicator dilution beset this method; in particular non-representative sampling and incomplete mixing of dye. The angiographic technique has the advantage that the 'sample' is taken from the whole of the right atrium — the sampling technique being 'eyeball' assessment of the angiographic appearances. Allowance can be made for the diluting effect of a large right atrium. Two-dimensional echocardiography is perhaps the best technique for assessing tricuspid regurgitation since there is no catheter across the valve to cause spurious regurgitation and the distribution of the indicator (micro-bubbles) throughout the right atrium and cavae is readily assessed by eye.

Tricuspid stenosis

The key to the laboratory diagnosis of tricuspid stenosis is, as always, the presence of a transvalvar gradient. However gradients of as little as 2 mmHg across the tricuspid valve can be associated with significant stenosis. It follows that, if tricuspid stenosis is suspected, a double catheter or double-lumen catheter technique must be used. It is not sufficient to record a gradient on pull-back. One catheter (or one port of a double-lumen catheter) is placed in the right atrium and the other in the right ventricle. The pressure transducers must be equisensitive and great care must be taken to ensure that both are zeroed to the same level and that both are producing undamped records. The lumens of a double-lumen catheter are small and any blood clot or air bubbles present will result in a damped recording. The simplest way of checking that the record is satisfactory is to record, initially, with both ports in the right atrium — identical, and superimposed, records should be displayed. Mean diastolic gradients of 2 mmHg or more are significant and gradients of 5 mmHg and a calculated valve area of $0.8-1.5\,\text{cm}^2$ are enough to cause symptoms.

Other haemodynamic findings in tricuspid stenosis are (1) a large or 'giant' a wave, (2) raised right atrial pressure and valve gradient which increase on deep inspiration, and (3) slow y descent. Most cases of rheumatic tricuspid valve disease have a valve which is both stenosed and regurgitant.

PULMONARY VALVE DISEASE

Almost all cases of pulmonary valve disease are of congenital origin, indeed valvar pulmonary stenosis is one of the commonest congenital cardiac defects. As the prognosis is good pulmonary valve stenosis forms a significant proportion of the cases of congenital heart disease surviving into adult life. Acquired pulmonary valve disease, other than that resulting from cardiac surgery, is rare. Carcinoid heart disease may cause pulmonary stenosis and regurgitation and rheumatic heart disease very occasionally affects the pulmonary valve. Finally pulmonary regurgitation can occur in syphilis and in drug users as a result of infection introduced by intravenous injections. Extrinsic compression by tumours can result in right ventricular outflow obstruction.

Pulmonary stenosis

Congenital, valvar, pulmonary stenosis is of two types. The majority of patients have thin, mobile, valve cusps which 'dome' in systole (Fig. 15.17). A minority of patients have thickened, dysplastic

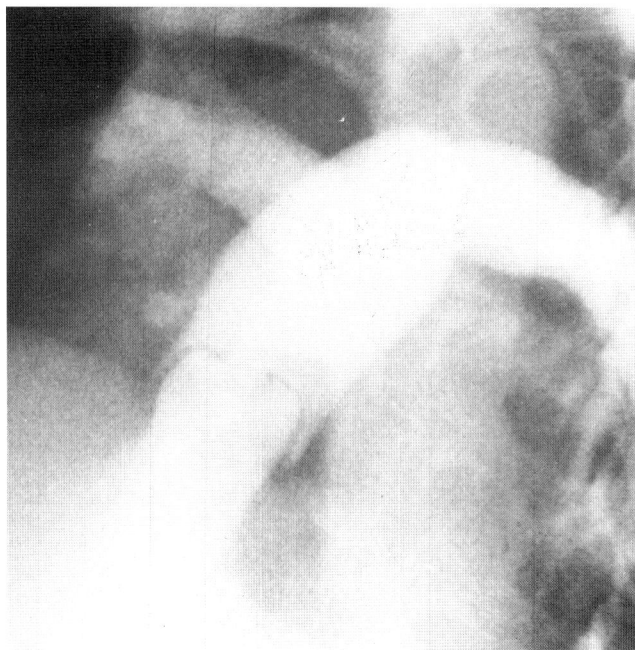

Fig. 15.17 'Typical' pulmonary valve stenosis. The pulmonary valve is thin and 'domes' in systole. Such valves are ideally treated by balloon valvuloplasty.

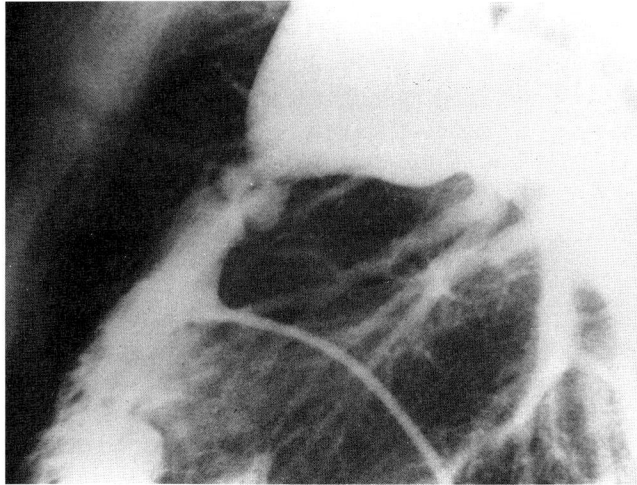

Fig. 15.18 Pulmonary stenosis with a dysplastic valve and narrow valve ring. There is marked poststenotic dilatation of the pulmonary artery. Such valves are unlikely to respond to balloon valvuloplasty.

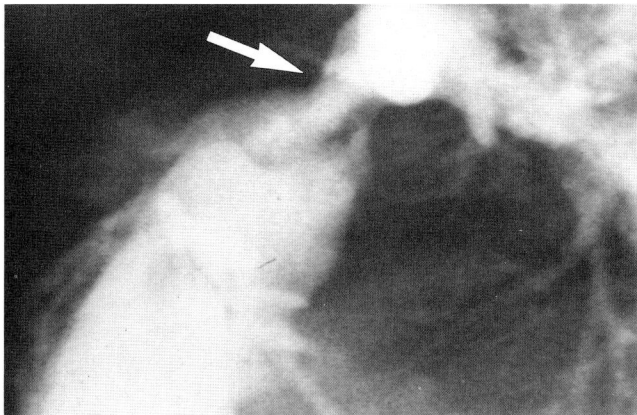

Fig. 15.19 Supravalve pulmonary stenosis (arrow). Supravalve aortic stenosis was also present in this patient.

valves; (Fig. 15.18) classically this type of pulmonary valve is found in patients with Noonan syndrome. Critical pulmonary valve stenosis presents in the neonatal period and closely resembles the condition of pulmonary atresia with intact ventricular septum.

Infundibular stenosis may develop as the right ventricle hypertrophies; isolated infundibular stenosis is uncommon, there is usually an associated ventricular septal defect though it may be small or there may be evidence that one has been present but has closed.

The diagnosis of pulmonary stenosis is made, in the catheterisation laboratory, on the basis of the pressure recordings and right ventricular angiography.

PRESSURE RECORDS

In anything more than mild pulmonary stenosis the right atrial pressure record is likely to exhibit a large a wave but the mean right atrial pressure will only be raised in severe pulmonary valve stenosis. Right ventricular pressure is raised and there is an abrupt fall in pressure as the catheter enters the pulmonary artery. The severity of pulmonary stenosis is classified according to the right ventricular systolic pressure (see Table 15.2).

Table 15.2 The severity of pulmonary stenosis.

Severity	RV systolic pressure	Valve area (cm²)
Mild	<50 mmHg	>1.0
Moderate	50–100 mmHg	0.5–1.0
Severe	>100 mmHg	<0.5

ANGIOGRAPHY

The pulmonary valve is best visualised by right ventricular angiography in the lateral projection. In classical pulmonary valve stenosis angiography demonstrates thin valve leaflets which do not open widely but dome upwards in systole. There is a central jet of contrast into the dilated pulmonary trunk (poststenotic dilatation). In the less common form of valvar stenosis due to a dysplastic valve the leaflets are thickened and do not dome in the same manner. When stenosis is moderate or severe there may be secondary infundibular hypertrophy causing subvalve obstruction. This infundibular hypertrophy is best visualised in the right oblique projection suggesting that, if biplane angiography is available, a combination of left lateral and right oblique projections are the ideal. If the valve is not obviously abnormal but there is obvious infundibular narrowing the probability is that the correct diagnosis is of primary infundibular stenosis. If the angiographic appearances suggest infundibular stenosis a second, left ventricular, angiogram should be performed using a long axis projection so as to profile the ventricular septum and demonstrate a VSD or aneurysm of the membranous septum.

Pulmonary regurgitation

The laboratory diagnosis of pulmonary regurgitation depends on (1) the demonstration of an abnormally low pulmonary diastolic pressure or, more commonly, ventricularisation of the pulmonary pressure, and (2) the angiographic demonstration of abnormal anatomy. Pulmonary arteriography *has* to employ a catheter which crosses the valve; as a result it is not easy to determine the significance of angiographic regurgitation — unlike the situation in aortic regurgitation when the catheter is clear of the valve. The purpose of angiography is, therefore, to elucidate the *cause* of pulmonary regurgitation. The commonest cause is surgical — following reconstruction of the right ventricular outflow tract. Angiography may reveal aneurysm formation at the site of outflow reconstruction (Fig. 17.75) or calcification of a tissue valve or of a conduit made of biological material. Pulmonary artery banding (Fig. 19.16) results in functional pulmonary regurgitation and the pressure in the pulmonary trunk proximal to the band is often indistinguishable from the right ventricular pressure tracing.

Some degree of pulmonary regurgitation is common following right ventricular outflow surgery but is seldom of importance; more important is the assessment of right ventricular function and right ventricular angiography will be needed to assess this.

Functional pulmonary regurgitation occurs in conditions resulting in severe pulmonary hypertension; it is seldom of importance and again catheterisation is more likely to be undertaken to discover the cause of the pulmonary hypertension than to assess the degree of regurgitation.

One congenital anomaly deserves mention; the syndrome of congenital absence of the pulmonary valve (Figs 19.16 and 19.17). The findings are diagnostic. There is some degree of right ventricular outflow obstruction with right ventricular pressure at systemic level and a low pulmonary artery pressure. There is a ventricular septal defect with, usually,

some left-to-right shunting and there is enormous dilatation of the right and left pulmonary arteries with an abrupt diminution in calibre at their first-order branches. The dilated left pulmonary artery may compress the upper surface of the left atrium and can cause bronchial compression with resulting pulmonary disease.

ARTIFICIAL VALVES

Since the introduction of the original Starr—Edwards caged ball valve in 1960 a bewildering variety of artificial valves have been developed. They can be divided into (1) mechanical valves, and (2) tissue valves. Of the mechanical valves that are currently available there are three basic designs; the caged ball valve in which blood has to flow around the ball, the low profile caged disc valve in which the ball is replaced by a flattened disc but flow is still around the disc and the various tilting disc valves which allow central flow. It is possible to determine the make and model of these valves from their X-ray appearance [30—33]. Currently available artificial valves are:

1 *Mechanical valves*:
a Caged ball: Starr—Edwards silastic ball, model 1200, 1260 aortic prostheses or 6120 mitral prosthesis (Fig 15.20), and Smeloff—Cutter.
b Low-profile caged disc: Beall—Surgitool.

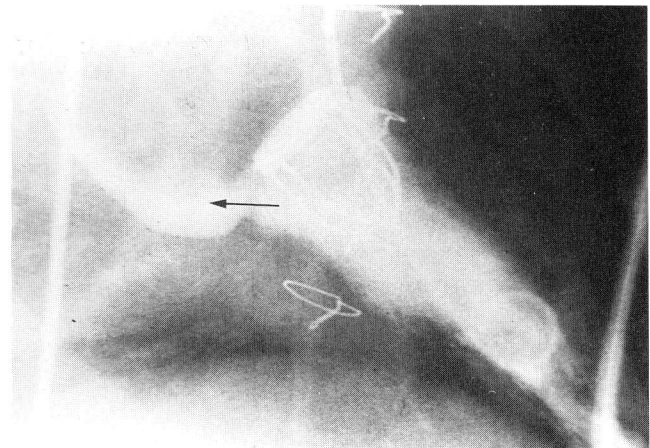

Fig. 15.20 Paraprosthetic mitral regurgitation. A ball valve prosthesis (Starr—Edwards) is in place but has become detached inferiorly (arrow) allowing regurgitation of contrast medium to the left atrium.

c Central flow, tilting disc: Lillehei—Kaster, Bjork—Shiley (standard and convexo-concave) (Fig. 15.21), Medtronic—Hall, St Jude Medical (twin leaflet), and omniscience.

2 *Tissue valves*:

a Frame-mounted, glutaraldehyde-treated porcine aortic valves (xenograft) e.g. Carpentier—Edwards 2625 (aortic prosthesis) and 6625 (mitral prosthesis) (Fig. 15.22) Wessex porcine bioprosthesis, Hancock porcine bioprosthesis (Fig. 15.23).

b Frame-mounted bovine or porcine pericardial bioprosthesis e.g. Ionescu—Shiley.

c Human (homograft) valves.

All prosthetic valves are stenotic in the sense that they pose more potential obstruction to flow than do native valves. Whether or not the obstruction is significant depends on the effective orifice area (prosthetic valves are made in a range of sizes and the smaller sizes may be stenotic), the cardiac output and the heart rate; in other words the same variables that are needed to calculate valve area by the Gorlin formula [1]. It is important to recognise that the effective valve area, as calculated in postoperative patients, is always less than the valve area obtained from *in vitro* measurements of the prosthesis or from pulse-duplicator testing [34]. This has great practical importance; the catheterising physician must be

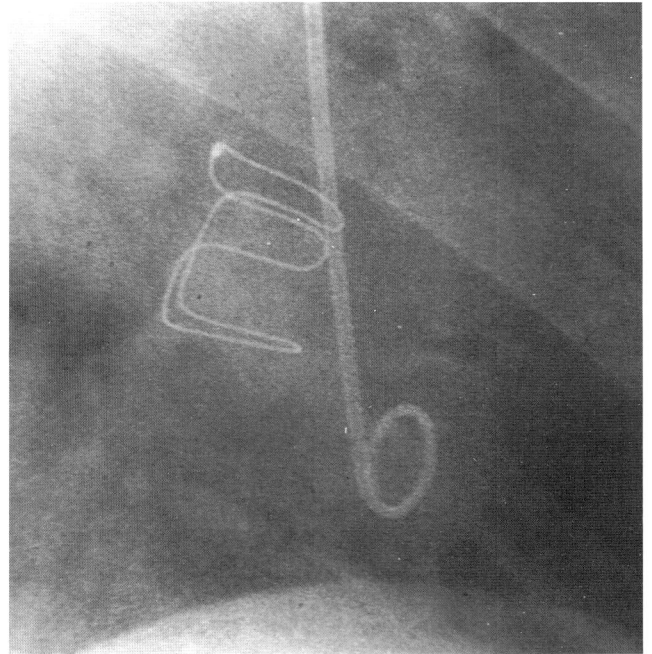

Fig. 15.22 The appearances of a frame-mounted mitral xenograft (Carpentier—Edwards); only the radio-opaque wire stent is seen.

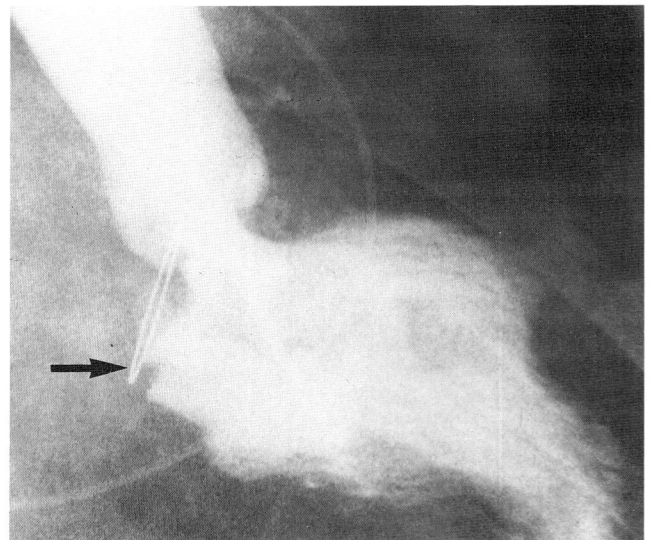

Fig. 15.23 Hancock xenograft in the mitral position. Only the base ring (arrow) is seen, the stent is radiolucent.

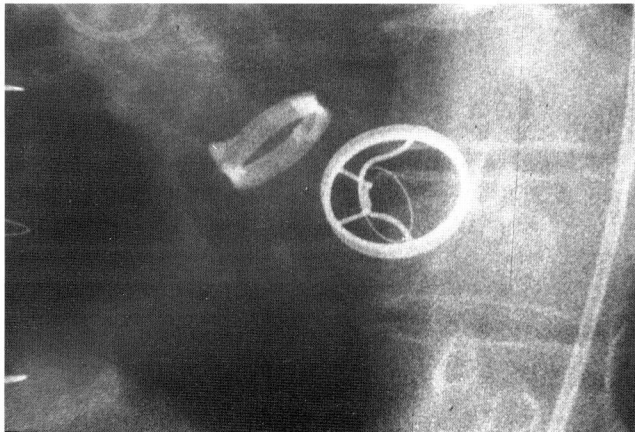

Fig. 15.21 Omniscience prosthetic valve in the aortic position and a Bjork—Shiley prosthesis in the mitral position. For a complete description of the radiographic identification of prosthetic valves see: Mehlman DJ, Resnekov L. A guide to the radiographic identification of prosthetic heart valves. *Circulation* 1978;**57**:613; *and* Mehlman DJ. A guide to the radiographic identification of prosthetic heart valves; an addendum. *Circulation* 1984;**69**:102.

aware that significant gradients can exist across normally functioning prosthetic valves. There is seldom a problem in assessing the severity of stenosis of native valves; gradients are not normally found and

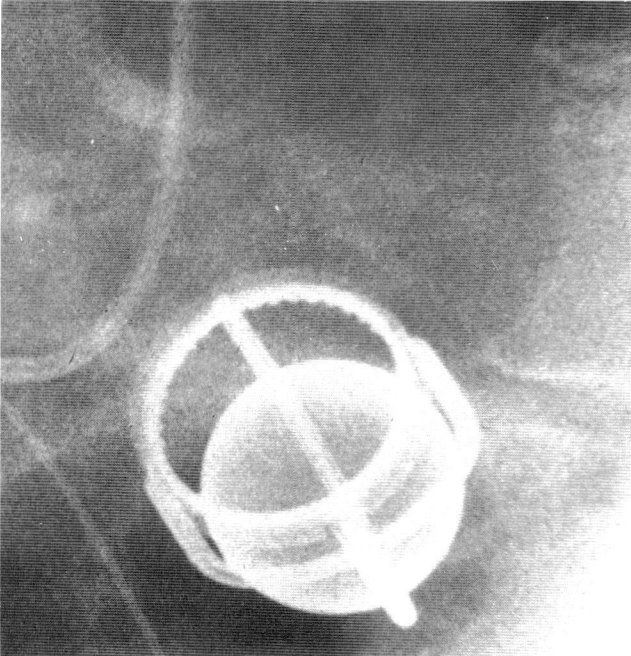

Fig. 15.24 Composite-seat Starr—Edwards caged ball valve in the mitral position.

there are many other clues to the severity of valve disease, these include the patient's symptoms, the physical signs and the echocardiographic findings. Indeed it has been suggested that catheterisation is seldom needed for preoperative assessment in patients with, for example, mitral valve disease [35]. But in patients who have undergone cardiac surgery symptoms *may* be due to prosthetic malfunction but they may also be due to residual pulmonary vascular disease, to left ventricular dysfunction, to haemolysis and anaemia and to the stenotic nature of all prosthetic valves. When true prosthetic valve stenosis occurs it may be due to thrombus formation or tissue overgrowth in the case of mechanical valves or to increasing immobility or calcification of the leaflets of tissue valves. A measured gradient may be due to one of these complications but may be due to the inherent characteristics of the prosthesis. To advise a hazardous reoperation in the second situation is a mistake that should be avoided. Thus we need to know the maximum permitted gradient for each type and size of prosthetic valve. Many studies have attempted to define the gradients and calculated valve areas that are to be expected with the various models and sizes of prosthetic valves

[34, 37—40]. The reported results are difficult to summarise but some guidelines can be defined:

1 Ball valves (e.g. Starr—Edwards) are more stenotic than disc valves.

2 Caged disc valves (e.g. 'low-profile' valves such as the Beall valve) are more stenotic than tilting-disc valves.

3 Cloth-covered ball valves (e.g. Starr—Edwards models 2300—2400), which may still be in place in a few patients, are more stenotic than bare-strut valves [36] — and have been discontinued for this reason.

4 Tilting-disc valves (e.g. Bjork—Shiley) are among the least stenotic valves though tissue valves (e.g. porcine xenograft) and the latest mechanical valves (e.g. St. Jude Medical prosthesis) have the smallest gradients of all.

5 Calcification of tissue valves, leading to stenosis, occurs more frequently and more rapidly in children than in adults.

6 The smaller sizes of prosthesis have the largest gradients. For aortic prostheses annulus diameters of 25 mm or less can be considered small. In the new designation of Starr—Edwards aortic valves the annulus diameter is given as part of the valve number (e.g. model 1200 16A and 18A and model 1260 21A—24A refer to annulus diameters between 16 and 24 mm. These are equivalent to 6A—10A in the old designation). Mitral annulus diameters less than 28 mm may be considered small (e.g. Starr—Edwards model 6120 from 20M—28M which are equivalent to 00M—2M in the old designation).

Table 15.3 overleaf lists some reported, postoperative, resting gradients for four representative types of prosthetic valves in the aortic and mitral position. The figures are for the smaller sizes of prosthesis since it is in these that the largest gradients are found.

The investigation of prosthetic valve malfunction

Prosthetic valve malfunction can usually be diagnosed clinically and by echocardiography. In cases where there is doubt catheterisation should provide the answer. Cine-fluoroscopy, performed before any catheters are inserted, may be helpful. Dehiscence may result in excessive movement of the sewing ring though lack of abnormal movement does not exclude dehiscence. The angular movement of the sewing ring between systole and diastole should not

Table 15.3 Aortic prostheses.

Valve	Annulus (mm)	Average gradient (mmHg) peak/range or SD	Average valve area (cm^2) range or SD
Starr–	21 (8A)	29 (13–54)	0.9 (0.7–1.4)
Edwards	23 (9A)	18 (1–32)	1.1 (0.8–1.5)
[34]	25 (10A)	13 (6–26)	1.3 (0.9–1.7)
Bjork–	21	22 (NA)	1.3 (+0.25)
Shiley	23	13.8 (NA)	1.7 (+0.49)
[37]	25	9.3 (NA)	2.2 (+0.5)
Porcine	21	13 (5–28)	1.2 (0.52–1.56)
Xenograft	23		
[38]	25	10.5 (3–20)	1.37 (1.0–1.79)
St Jude	21	6 (+0.6)	(NA)
Medical	23	2 (+2.0)	(NA)
[39]	25	2.4 (+1.0)	(NA)
Mitral prostheses			
Starr–	23 (OM)	(NA)	(NA)
Edwards	25 (1M)	10	1.4
[34]	27.5 (2M)	8 (4–13)	1.4 (0.8–1.8)
Bjork– Shiley [40]	?	4	(NA)
Porcine Xenograft [38]	27	7	1.7 (1.4–1.8)
St Jude Medical [39]	23	4 (end-diastolic)	(NA)
	27	2 (+2, end-diastolic)	

normally exceed 10° [41]. Prosthetic obstruction resulting in diminished movement of the poppet or, more usually, the disc, may be obvious though the findings need to be interpreted with caution since haemodynamic abnormalities (low output, atrial fibrillation, aortic regurgitation preventing full opening of a mitral tilting disc prosthesis) might also cause reduced movement. It may not always be possible to visualise the disc or poppet; a radio-opaque ring was not inserted into the (radiolucent) Pyrolyte disc of the Bjork–Shiley valve until 1975. Normally the disc of this valve should open to about 60° and impaired opening of the disc of a mitral Bjork–Shiley prosthesis due to thrombotic occlusion can be recognised fluoroscopically [42]. Similarly it may be possible to detect failure of a poppet to seat properly due to thrombotic occlusion [42]. Component failures, such as ball variance, uneven wear of a disc or fracture of a strut are now very rare. Failure of a mechanical valve is likely to be due to paraprosthetic

leak or to obstruction by thrombus formation or ingrowth of tissue. Tissue valve failure may be due to calcification, visible fluoroscopically, or fibrosis. Stiffening or retraction of the leaflets results in stenosis or regurgitation (or both). Infection may result in dehiscence and a paraprosthetic leak — as in mechanical prostheses.

Again, therefore, we are concerned with the detection and assessment of stenosis and of regurgitation. The importance of distinguishing between a gradient which is pathological and one which is no more than can be expected for the size and type of prosthesis has been discussed above. The gradient across a mitral prosthesis is measured in just the same way as is the gradient across a native mitral valve — retrograde catheterisation of the left ventricle with simultaneous recording of the indirect left atrial (wedge) pressure. However particular care is needed to ensure that the wedge pressure is a valid record; the tracing should be phasic, that is it should exhibit a and v waves (or v waves alone if there is atrial fibrillation). If there is doubt and if other, non-invasive, studies are not diagnostic then transseptal catheterisation is called for.

Paraprosthetic regurgitation at a mitral prosthesis is readily demonstrable by left ventriculography — provided entry to the ventricle is not barred by a second (aortic) prosthesis. If an aortic prosthesis is in place there are a number of alternatives:

1 Transseptal catheterisation will permit measurement of the gradient across an aortic prosthesis and allow left ventriculography. But the technique is not without risk and is excluded if there is a mitral prosthesis.

2 Percutaneous, transapical, needle puncture of the left ventricle is a simple technique and allows measurement of both aortic and mitral valve gradients. Left ventriculography is not possible but a follow-through pulmonary arteriogram will provide left ventricular opacification for assessment of ventricular function (ejection fraction) if this is all that required.

3 The aortic prosthesis may be crossed retrogradely, or

4 Transapical left ventriculography is possible by a modification of the needle puncture technique [25]. Many investigators choose to cross an aortic ball valve in order to obtain left ventricular pressure and a left ventriculogram. If this is done it is important to use the smallest diameter catheter that will provide the information required. A Shirey catheter with its fine (5F) tip and multiple side-holes is ideal. However there is no doubt that the inevitable interference with poppet movement causes a profound haemodynamic disturbance. Acute aortic regurgitation and, often, a significant degree of aortic obstruction are inevitable consequences. Apart from the unreliability of results obtained in such unphysiological circumstances there is also the danger of precipitating acute pulmonary oedema; wedge pressures rise rapidly to 40 mmHg both in our experience and in that of others [43].

Tilting disc (e.g. Bjork—Shiley) aortic prostheses have been crossed in retrograde fashion with apparent safety [44] but this technique has a significant risk; if the catheter should pass through the small strut the disc will be fixed in a wide-open position with resulting acute aortic regurgitation [45].

It is not our practice to attempt to cross tilting disc aortic prosthesis. Instead, if left ventriculography is

mandatory, (for example to assess paraprosthetic mitral regurgitation in a patient with an aortic prosthesis) we employ the transapical technique of left ventriculography. This technique is described in Chapter 3. Since reporting our early results [25] we have continued to employ this technique, on the infrequent occasions that it is indicated, without significant problems.

Retrograde, or antegrade, passage of a catheter across a tissue valve poses no problems other than those commonly encountered when attempting to cross stenotic or regurgitant native valves. A flow-guided, balloon-tipped, catheter will usually overcome any difficulties that are encountered in attempting antegrade crossing of a tissue valve.

GENERAL READING

Dalen JE, Alpert JS (eds.) *Valvular heart disease.* 2nd edn. Toronto, Little, Brown and Co., 1987.

REFERENCES

1 Gorlin R, Gorlin SG. Hydraulic formulae for calculation of area of stenotic mitral valve, other cardiac valves and central circulatory shunts. *Am Heart J* 1951;**41**:1.

2 Cohen MV, Gorlin R. Modified orifice equation for the calculation of mitral valve area. *Am Heart J* 1972;**84**:839.

3 Hakki AH *et al.* A simplified valve formula for the calculation of stenotic cardiac valve areas. *Circulation* 1981;**63**:1050.

4 Nigri A *et al.* Nomogram for calculation of stenotic cardiac valve areas from cardiac output and mean transvalvular gradient. *Cathet Cardiovasc Diagn* 1984;**10**:613.

5 Hosenpud JD, McAnulty JH, Morton MJ. Overestimation of mitral valve gradients by phasic pulmonary capillary wedge pressure. *Cathet Cardiovasc Diagn* 1983;**9**:283.

6 Owen SG, Wood P. A new method of determining the degree or absence of mitral obstruction: an analysis of the diastolic part of indirect left atrial pressure tracings. *Br Heart J* 1955;**17**:41.

7 Morrow AG *et al.* Left atrial pressure pulse in mitral valve disease. A correlation of pressures obtained by transbronchial puncture with the valvular lesion. *Circulation* 1957;**16**:399.

8 Libanoff AJ, Rodbard S. Evaluation of the severity of mitral stenosis and regurgitation. *Circulation* 1966;**33**:218.

9 Libanoff AJ, Rodbard S. Atrioventricular pressure half-time. Measure of mitral valve orifice area. *Circulation* 1968;**38**:144.

10 Angel J *et al.* Haemodynamic evaluation of stenotic cardiac valves: II, modification of the simplified formula for mitral and aortic valve area calculation. *Cathet Cardiovasc Diagn* 1985;**11**:127.

11 Lewis BM *et al.* Clinical and physiological correlations in patients with mitral stenosis. *Am Heart J* 1952;**43**:2.

12 Flemming HA, Wood P. The myocardial factor in mitral valve disease. *Br Heart J* 1959;**21**:117.

13 Ibrahim MO. Left ventricular function in rheumatic mitral stenosis. Clinical echocardiographic study. *Br Heart J* 1979;**42**:514.

14 Cotter L, Dawkins K, Gibson D. Incidence and mechanism of left ventricular disease in mitral stenosis. *Br Heart J* 1983;**49**:302P.

15 Heller SJ, Carleton RA. Abnormal left ventricular contraction in patients with mitral stenosis. *Circulation* 1970;**42**:1099.

16 Sandler H, Dodge HT, Hay RE, Rackley CE. Quantitation of valvular insufficiency in man by angiography. *Am Heart J* 1963;**65**:501.

17 Miller GAH, Kirklin JW, Swan HJC. Myocardial function and left ventricular volumes in acquired valvular insufficiency. *Circulation* 1965;**31**:374.

18 Lopez JF, Hanson S, Orchard RC, Tan L. Quantification of mitral valvular incompetence. *Cathet Cardiovasc Diagn* 1985;**11**:139.

19 Pizzarello RA *et al.* Left atrial size, pressure and V wave height in patients with isolated, severe, pure mitral regurgitation. *Cathet Cardiovasc Diagn* 1984;**10**:445.

20 Shone JD *et al.* The developmental complex of 'parachute mitral valve'. Supravalvar ring of the left atrium, sub-aortic stenosis and coarctation of the aorta. *Am J Cardiol* 1963;**11**:714.

21 Peterson TA, Todd DB, Edwards JE. Supravalvar aortic stenosis. *J Thoracic Cardiovasc Surg* 1965;**50**:734.

22 Williams JCP, Barratt-Boyes BG, Lowe JB. Supravalvar aortic stenosis. *Circulation* 1961;**24**:1311.

23 Bonow RO *et al.* Aortic valve replacement without myocardial revascularisation in patients with combined aortic valvular and coronary artery disease. *Circulation* 1981;**63**:243.

24 Kirklin JW, Kouchoukos NT. Editorial: Aortic valve replacement without myocardial revascularisation. *Circulation* 1981;**63**:252.

25 Wong CM, Wong PHC, Miller GAH. Percutaneous left ventricular angiography. *Cathet Cardiovasc Diagn* 1981;**7**:425.

27 Morganroth J *et al.* Acute, severe aortic regurgitation. *Ann Int Med* 1977;**87**:223.

28 Roberts WC, Sjoerdsma A. The cardiac disease associated with the carcinoid syndrome (carcinoid heart disease). *Am J Med* 1969;**36**:5.

29 Lingamneni R *et al.* Tricuspid regurgitation: clinical and angiographic assessment. *Cathet Cardiovasc Diagn* 1979;**5**:7.

30 Bonchek LI *et al.* Roentgenographic identification of Starr–Edwards prostheses. *Circulation* 1973;**47**:154.

31 Silver MD, Datta BN, Bowes VF. A key to identify heart valve prostheses. *Arch Pathol* 1975;**99**:132.

32 Mehlman DJ, Resnekov L. A guide to the radiographic identification of prosthetic heart valves. *Circulation* 1978;**57**:613.

33 Mehlman DJ. A guide to the radiographic identification of prosthetic heart valves: an addendum. *Circulation* 1984;**69**:102.

34 Pyle RB *et al.* Hemodynamic evaluation of Lillehei–Kaster and Starr–Edwards prostheses. *Ann Thoracic Surg* 1978;**26**:336.

35 St John Sutton MG *et al.* Valve replacement without preoperative cardiac catheterisation. *New Engl J Med* 1981;**306**:1233.

36 Reis RL *et al.* Clinical and hemodynamic assessments of fabric-covered Starr–Edwards prosthetic valves. *J Thoracic Cardiovasc Surg* 1970;**59**:84.

37 Bjork VO, Holmgren A, Olin C, Ovenfors CO. Clinical and haemodynamic results of aortic valve replacement with the Bjork–Shiley tilting disc valve prosthesis. *Scand J Thoracic Cardiovasc Surg* 1971;**5**:177.

38 Chaitman BR *et al.* Hemodynamic evaluation of the Carpentier–Edwards porcine xenograft. *Circulation* 1979;**60**:1170.

39 Nicoloff DM *et al.* Clinical and hemodynamic results with the St. Jude Medical cardiac valve prosthesis. *J Thoracic Cardiovasc Surg* 1981;**82**:674.

40 Rostad H, Fjeld NB, Hall KV. Experiences with various types of mitral valve prostheses. *Scand J Thoracic Cardiovasc Surg* 1976;**10**:113.

41 Giminez JL, Soulen RL, Davilla JC. Prosthetic valve detachment: its roentgenographic recognition. *Am J Roentgenol Radium Ther Nucl Med* 1968;**103**:595.

42 Sands MJ *et al.* Diagnostic value of cinefluoroscopy in the evaluation of prosthetic heart valve dysfunction. *Am Heart J* 1982;**104**:622.

43 Shabetai R, Krotkiewski A, Reeves JT. A pitfall in the postoperative evaluation of aortic Starr–Edwards valves. *J Thoracic Cardiovasc Surg* 1967;**53**:288.

44 Maranhao V *et al.* Experience with retrograde left heart catheterisation through the Bjork–Shiley aortic valve prosthesis: a preliminary report. *Chest* 1975;**67**:348.

45 Falicov RV. Retrograde crossing of aortic Bjork–Shiley prosthesis. *Am J Cardiol* 1979;**43**:1062.

CHAPTER 16

Myocardial and pericardial disease

CLASSIFICATION

By some the term 'cardiomyopathy' has been reserved for primary disease of the myocardium (excluding disease secondary to causes such as chronic overload). By others it has been used to describe both primary and secondary disease. It has been reserved for conditions without known cause (ideopathic) and applied to those whose cause is known. In the catheterisation laboratory we detect abnormal myocardial function and observe different haemodynamic and angiographic profiles which allow us to classify the type of cardiomyopathy present and which provide clues to the probable aetiology in many instances. In this chapter, therefore, 'cardiomyopathy' will be used to describe all forms of impaired myocardial function; primary and secondary and of known and unknown aetiology.

A classification of myocardial (and pericardial) disease which emphasises their haemodynamic and angiographic differentiation is described in Table 16.1.

DILATED CARDIOMYOPATHY

In the normal heart there is a linear relationship between the volume load on a ventricle and its end-diastolic volume. The end-diastolic volume of an infant's heart is less than an adult's and the end-diastolic volume is even greater when there is a volume load due to valve regurgitation or a left-to-right shunt. Nonetheless the linear relationship is preserved so that the *ejection fraction*:

$$(LVEDV - LVESV) / LVEDV = \text{(approximately)}\ 0.70\ \text{or}\ 70\%$$

where LVEDV and LVESV are left ventricular end-diastolic and end-systolic volumes respectively and

LVEDV − LVESV is the total left ventricular stroke volume (LVSV) (see Chapter 8). When myocardial *systolic* function is impaired the slope of the line relating end-diastolic volume load is depressed downward so that there is an 'inappropriate' increase in end-diastolic volume (chamber size) for the volume load. This is the hall-mark of a dilated cardiomyopathy. Angiographically the ventricle (usually the left) is enlarged with increased end-diastolic and end-systolic volumes. It contracts poorly; if ejection fraction is measured it is found to be reduced below the normal of 0.7 ± 0.8. The ventricle tends to be unusually spherical in shape so that the usual 2:1 relation between the lengths of the long and minor axes approaches 1:1 [1]. Asynergy — impaired contraction of some segments with preserved function of others — points towards an ischaemic aetiology

Table 16.1 Classification of myocardial (and pericardial) disease.

Dilated cardiomyopathy
Cavity size increased, ejection fraction reduced, (predominantly impaired *systolic* function)

Hypertrophic cardiomyopathy
Cavity size (initially) normal, ejection fraction normal, (predominantly impaired *diastolic* function), gross myocardial hypertrophy

Restrictive cardiomyopathy and pericardial disease
As hypertrophic cardiomyopathy but without gross myocardial hypertrophy:
  Right and left atrial pressures dissimilar: restrictive cardiomyopathy
  Right and left atrial pressures differ by <5 mmHg: pericardial constriction, tamponade

Obliterative cardiomyopathy
Cavity size reduced

Endocardial fibroelastosis
Cavity size increased, systolic and diastolic function impaired

(coronary artery disease) but can be observed in other forms of dilated cardiomyopathy. Coronary arteriography is an integral part of the angiographic investigation of patients with a dilated cardiomyopathy in order to exclude coronary artery disease (ischaemic cardiomyopathy). This investigation must be performed cautiously, or omitted altogether if myocardial function is severely depressed as further myocardial depression due to the contrast medium could precipitate pulmonary oedema. A non-ionic contrast medium can be used and the number of injections reduced to a minimum.

Pressure records from the left ventricle show a slow rise and fall giving a triangular shape instead of the normal 'square wave' appearance of the left ventricular systolic pressure. This may sometimes be appreciated by the naked eye and can be displayed as reduced positive and negative dp/dt (Chapter 8). Arterial pressure will be normal or low and cardiac output normal or reduced depending on the severity of the disease.

Although primarily an abnormality of systolic function the dilated ventricle also exhibits impaired filling so that it is 'stiffer' than normal. As a result both early and late diastolic pressure may be raised with commensurate rise in left atrial (or wedge) pressure. There is often some increase in pulmonary (and systemic) arteriolar resistance and, with gross ventricular dilatation, there may be 'functional' mitral regurgitation. All these effects can lead to a moderate increase in pulmonary arterial pressure; usually to no more than 50 mmHg.

As with any disease process there is a spectrum of severity, in milder forms diastolic pressures may be normal at rest but will rise with exercise. The disease most obviously affects the left ventricle so that it is the left-sided filling pressures that are found to be high — not the right.

Causes of dilated cardiomyopathy

Dilated cardiomyopathy can be the end result of many disease processes. These include end-stage aortic or mitral valve disease and end-stage congenital heart disease. Restrictive and hypertrophic cardiomyopathy can eventually produce chamber dilatation with a reduced ejection fraction. Among the more common and more important causes of dilated cardiomyopathy are:

1 Coronary artery disease (ischaemic cardiomyopathy).
2 Ideopathic [2].
3 Alcoholic cardiomyopathy [3].
4 Postinfective (?viral myocarditis).
5 Toxic — adriamycin (doxorubicin) and cyclophosphamide therapy [4, 5], cobalt [6].
6 Peripartum cardiomyopathy [7].
7 End-stage volume or pressure overload.

Notes

1 *Ischaemic cardiomyopathy*. Diagnosed by positive coronary arteriogram and usually uneven involvement of segments. Diabetic patients are prone to diffuse atherosclerosis of major coronary arteries with resulting ischaemic cardiomyopathy. In young insulin-dependent diabetics there may be microvascular disease of the coronary circulation leading to myocardial dysfunction without angiographically detectable disease of the major coronary arteries.
2 *Alcoholic cardiomyopathy* is associated with excessive consumption but many cases may, in reality, be examples of ideopathic cardiomyopathy.
3 *Peripartum cardiomyopathy* occurs in the last trimester and the puerperium. Associated risk factors are: age above 30, twin pregnancy and previous hypertension.
4 *Myocarditis* can complicate many infections — notably Coxsackie B virus — chronic dilated cardiomyopathy is presumed to be the end result of such infections when antibody titres are found to be raised.
5 *Generalised myocardial dysfunction with chamber dilatation* can be the end result of chronic pressure or volume overload; hypertensive cardiac failure can be included here.
6 *Cancer therapy with adriamycin* can lead to lethal cardiac dysfunction — usually only when the cumulative dose was in excess of 450 mg/m^2. Previous deep X-ray or cyclophosphamide therapy may enhance susceptibility to adriamycin and cyclophosphamide can itself cause an acute dilated cardiomyopathy.

HYPERTROPHIC CARDIOMYOPATHY

In the past this condition has been known as hypertrophic *obstructive* cardiomyopathy (HOCM) and ideopathic hypertrophic subaortic *stenosis* (IHSS).

Both names refer to the possible detection of an intracavity gradient produced by systolic anterior motion (SAM) of the mitral valve causing it to impinge against the hypertrophied septum. However many patients with this condition never exhibit intracavity obstruction and, in those that do, the gradient is labile, being accentuated by an increased inotropic state and reduced or abolished by β-blockade. It is now recognised that the primary functional abnormality is not systolic but diastolic — impaired ventricular filling due to pathological muscular hypertrophy.

The hall-mark of hypertrophic cardiomyopathy is gross increase in the thickness of ventricular myocardium. The condition tends to occur in families (autosomal dominant) but many sporadic cases occur. It has been recognised in neonates and infants. Hypertrophic cardiomyopathy, indistinguishable in every way from the ideopathic form, can occur in association with fixed outflow obstruction — especially when due to discrete fibromuscular sub-aortic stenosis. This may represent an abnormal response to the stimulus to hypertrophy. Hypertrophic cardiomyopathy may, less commonly, affect the right ventricle and pressure gradients due to the septum bulging into the right ventricular outflow tract have been described.

Angiography reveals the myocardial hypertrophy; this is often assymetrical with increased septal thickness (assymetrical septal hypertrophy, ASH) giving a characteristic bent banana appearance (Fig. 16.1) to the cavity of the left ventricle. Thickened papillary muscles may form filling defects (Fig. 16.2). Many cases, however, have concentric hypertrophy without the bulging septum and without intracavity gradients. Contraction is vigorous with almost complete emptying and, often, systolic apical cavity obliteration (Fig. 16.3). The coronary arteries are normal or large though coexisting atherosclerotic coronary disease can occur. There may be muscular systolic compression of the anterior descending coronary artery or its branches.

The haemodynamic abnormalities associated with hypertrophic cardiomyopathy are (1) those due to impaired filling, and (2) those associated with mid-systolic outflow obstruction — when present.

Impaired filling due to a thick, abnormally stiff, left ventricle results in loss of the normal early diastolic dip and elevation of the end-diastolic pressure. Filling is slow and may be associated with an

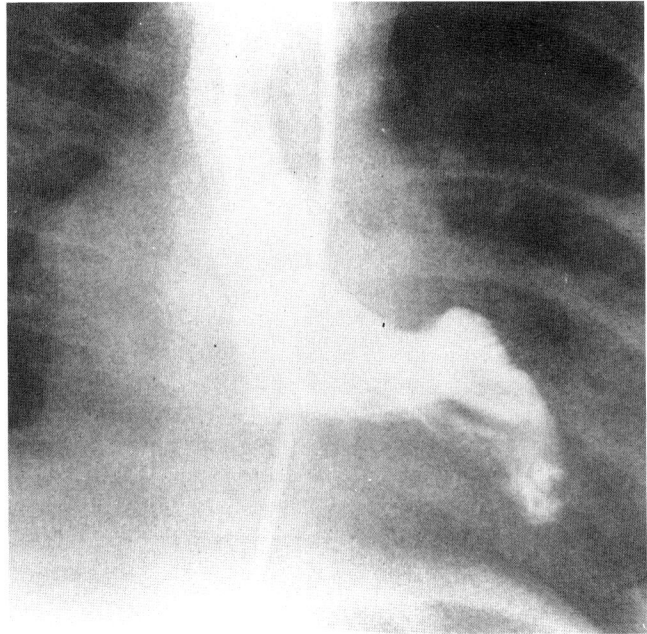

Fig. 16.1 Hypertrophic cardiomyopathy in an infant. The hypertrophied septum bulges into the cavity of the left ventricle giving the appearances of a 'bent banana' or 'dog leg' seen here.

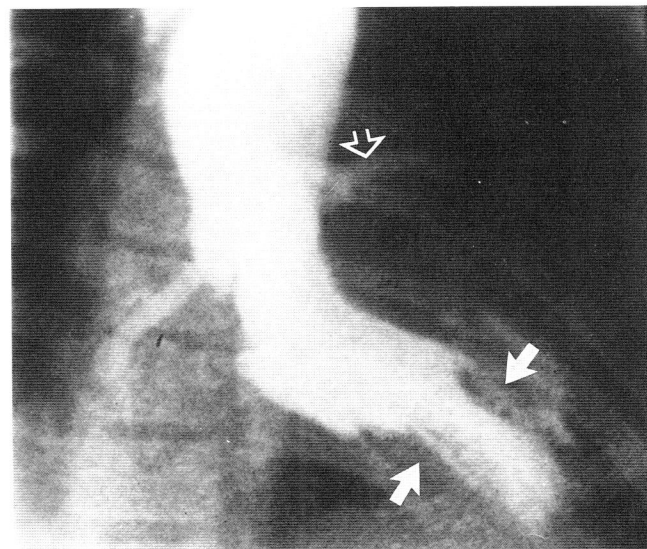

Fig. 16.2 Hypertrophic cardiomyopathy. Hypertrophied papillary muscles causing filling defects (arrows). The increased thickness of the ventricular wall can be judged from the distance between the opacified cavity and the left coronary artery (open arrow).

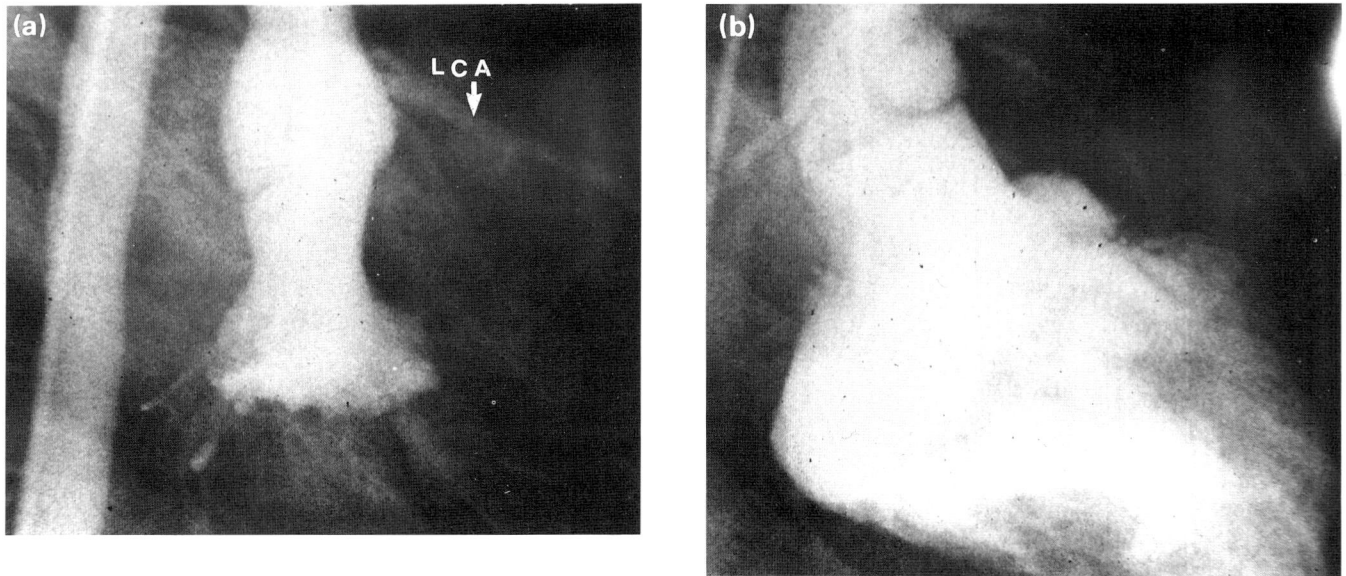

Fig. 16.3 There may be apical cavity obliteration in hypertrophic cardiomyopathy. In (a) the left ventricular cavity is almost obliterated, during systole, in a patient with hypertrophic cardiomyopathy. During diastole, (b), the ventricular cavity is seen to be of almost normal size. The gross increase in wall thickness can be judged by the distance between the left coronary artery (LCA, arrow, Fig. 16.3a) and the left ventricular cavity.

abnormal pressure trace in which the normal early diastolic dip is replaced by a continuing decline of pressure after mitral valve opening until atrial contraction produces a rise in pressure (a wave). The raised left ventricular diastolic pressure, together with moderate mitral regurgitation which is often present, results in an elevated left atrial pressure, a large left atrium and the possibility of moderate pulmonary hypertension.

In those cases in whom mid-systolic gradients occur or can be precipitated the haemodynamic abnormalities observed are:
1 Spike-and-dome arterial waveform.
2 Loss of post extrasystolic potentiation.
3 Intracavity gradient.
In hypertrophic cardiomyopathy early ejection is rapid giving a sharp upstroke to the first part of the arterial pulse. If obstruction develops in mid-systole the sharp upstroke is halted and followed by dip and then a more rounded ejection phase — the spike-and-dome pattern [8]. If intraventricular pressure is being recorded the point at which the spike is halted is marked by a similar halt on the upstroke of the ventricular pressure [8]. It is at this point that intracavity gradients can be recorded.

Post extrasystolic accentuation of the arterial pulse

is a *normal* phenomenon. Following an early, extrasystolic, beat diastole is prolonged resulting in increased filling and a more powerful post extrasystolic beat with a higher pulse pressure. In hypertrophic *obstructive* cardiomyopathy this powerful beat accentuates the intracavity gradient and the post extrasystolic beat has a *lower* pulse pressure than normal and may exhibit a spike-and-dome configuration. This reversal of the normal post extrasystolic accentuation is very characteristic of hypertrophic cardiomyopathy *with obstruction*.

Intracavity gradients have received much attention in the past but are of doubtful importance [9]. They can be provoked or accentuated by any intervention which (1) increases 'contractility', (2) decreases afterload, or (3) decreases preload. Such manoeuvres include:
1 The Valsalva manoeuvre.
2 Exercise.
3 Isoprenaline injection.
4 Amylnitrite inhalation.
5 Extrasystoles — see above.
False gradients may easily be recorded due to trapping of an end-hole catheter within the hypertrophied trabeculae.

Associated conditions

A number of disease states may produce patho- logical hypertrophy indistinguishable from ideo- pathic hypertrophic cardiomyopathy. They include phaeochromacytoma, neurofibromatosis, lentigi- nosis, acromegaly, Turner and Noonan syndromes, infants of diabetic mothers and Friedreich's ataxia.

RESTRICTIVE CARDIOMYOPATHY

The combination of a raised ventricular diastolic pressure with normal chamber size, no gross hyper- trophy and apparently normal systolic function suggests pericardial constriction or a restrictive car- diomyopathy. Distinction between the two con- ditions is not always possible. In pericardial constriction (constrictive pericarditis) the right atrial pressure is raised to 12 mmHg or more and may occasionally be as high as 20 mmHg. The atrial pressure trace is marked by prominent x and y descents giving a characteristic M- or W-shaped waveform. Usually the x and y descents are equal in magnitude or the x descent is dominant (Fig. 16.4). Occasionally it is the x descent which is the most marked. In constriction the rigid pericardium limits ventricular filling; following ejection the volume of the heart is less than that of the pericar- dium and filling is rapid in early diastole until halted abruptly by the constricting pericardium. This results in the so called 'square-root' sign; a ventricular pressure which exhibits a sharp early diastolic dip which is terminated by a plateau for the rest of diastole. This rapid early filling explains the sharp y descent. In restrictive cardiomyopathy ventricular filling is slow; none the less the ventricular and atrial pressure traces are identical to those seen in pericardial constriction; there are prominent x and y descents and a dip-and-plateau ventricular pressure trace. *The most useful point of differentiation is that in pericardial constriction right and left ventricular filling is impaired to an equal extent and as a result right and left atrial and right and left ventricular diastolic pressures seldom differ by more than 5 mmHg (Fig. 16.5). In restrictive cardiomyopathy the left ventricle is more often affected than the right and left atrial and left ventricular end-diastolic pressures are significantly higher than on the right.* Catheterisation in patients with suspected constriction/restriction demands

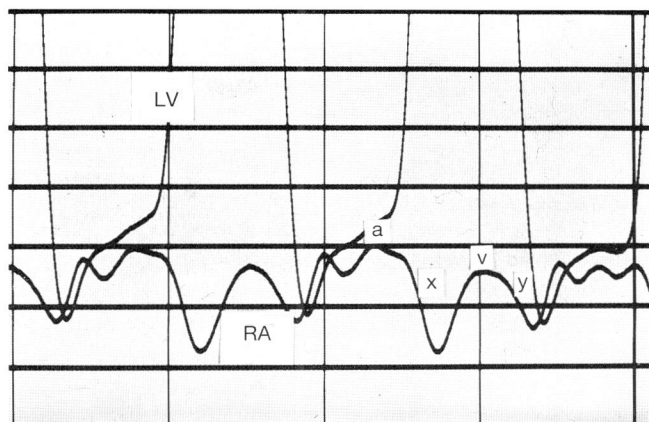

Fig. 16.4 Constrictive pericarditis. Superimposed right atrial (RA) and left ventricular (LV) pressure tracings. Both x and y descents are prominent in the right atrial pressure tracing but the x descent is dominant. There is near equality of the right atrial and left ventricular diastolic pressures (and left and right atrial pressures) suggesting the diagnosis of constriction rather than a restrictive or congestive cardiomyopathy in which left ventricular (and left atrial) diastolic pressures are usually significantly higher than right sided diastolic pressures.

simultaneous recording of right and left ventricular diastolic pressures having ensured equal calibration and baseline settings for the two manometers. *The effect of exercise in restrictive cardiomyopathy is to further increase the difference between left and right ventricular diastolic pressures. A further point of differentiation is that pulmonary hypertension is usually more severe in restrictive cardiomyopathy than in constric- tion; a systolic pressure above 50 mmHg is unusual in constriction and common in restrictive cardiomyopathy.* As a result the right ventricular end-diastolic pressure in constriction is typically one-third or more the height of peak right ventricular pressure — not so in restrictive cardiomyopathy.

Athough these points of difference are helpful there are exceptions. A form of constriction has been described in which left atrial emptying is selectively impaired with haemodynamics resembling mitral stenosis. Another form of pericardial constriction has been labelled 'occult' and may simply represent early constriction. In this condition resting haemo- dynamics are normal and the characteristic abnor- malities of constriction only become apparent after giving a volume load [10].

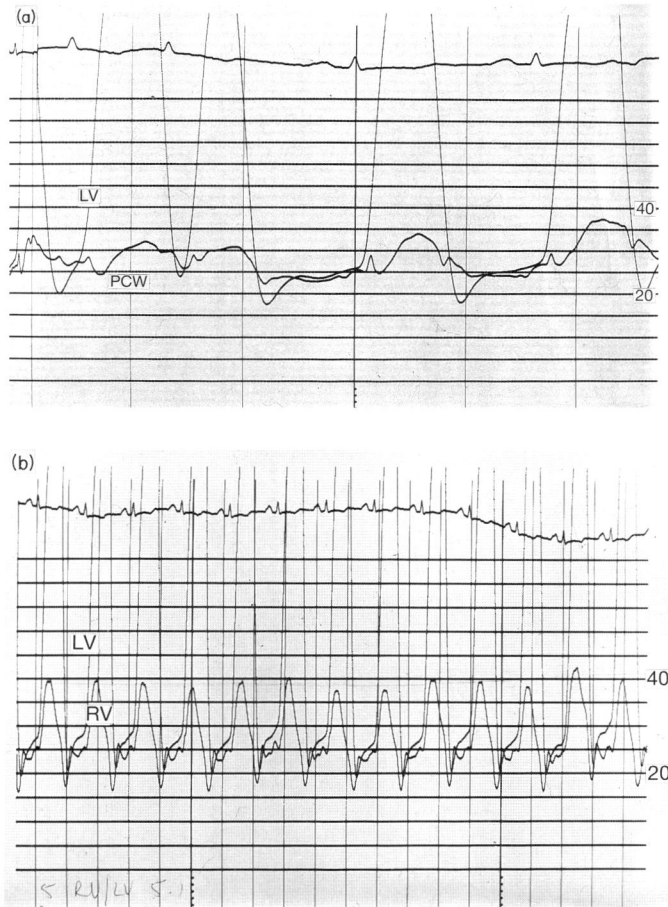

Fig. 16.5 Constrictive pericarditis. Superimposed left ventricular (LV) and pulmonary capillary wedge (PCW) pressures (a) and left (LV) and right (RV) pressures (b) showing near equality (25 mmHg) of diastolic pressures in both sides of the heart.

Causes of restrictive cardiomyopathy

Diseases that may be accompanied by a restrictive pattern of myocardial involvement include:
1 Amyloid heart disease [11, 12].
2 Haemochromatosis and haemosiderosis [13].
3 Sarcoid [14, 15].
4 Eosinophilic heart disease [16].
5 Glycogen storage diseases. Fabry's disease [17–19].
   Cardiac involvement is the commonest cause of

death in patients with primary amyloid (e.g. myeloma) but involvement is rare in amyloid secondary to chronic infection (secondary amyloid). Cardiac involvement occurs infrequently in the rare condition of familial amyloid.

Although included among the restrictive cardiomayopathies amyloid heart disease frequently presents with impaired *systolic* function and chamber enlargement. When the restrictive form is found right sided abnormalities predominate with raised venous pressure and a square root type of right ventricular diastolic pressure.

Haemochromatosis, haemosiderosis and sarcoid can also present both as dilated and restrictive cardiomyopathies. Eosinophillic heart disease is discussed under 'obliterative cardiomyopathy' below. Endomyocardial biopsy (see below) is probably of most value in amyloid and other infiltrative causes of restrictive cardiomyopathy though patchy involvement (e.g. in sarcoid) may result in a false negative biopsy if the specimens have been taken from uninvolved areas.

CONSTRICTIVE PERICARDITIS

The haemodynamics of pericardial constriction have been described in the section on restrictive cardiomyopathy; however there are a few further features of constriction which can be helpful in making the diagnosis. Pericardial calcification (Figs 16.6 and 16.7) suggests the diagnosis but is present in less than half of cases. Calcification may be visible during fluoroscopy but not on the plain chest X-ray. A right atrial (or superior caval) angiogram may show a thickened right atrial wall and distended superior vena cava. A left ventricular angiogram may also show a thickened left ventricle but hypertrophy is present in restrictive cardiomyopathy and indistinguishable from pericardial thickening unless a coronary arteriogram has been performed with oblique views demonstrating the epicardial coronary arteries lying *within* the thickened pericardium. Both restrictive cardiomyopathy and pericardial constriction may, at end-stage, exhibit left ventricular cavity enlargement at ventriculography with impaired systolic function — low ejection fraction — as, rarely, may end-stage hypertrophic cardiomyopathy.

Causes of pericardial constriction

1 Infection (bacterial, viral, fungal and parasitic as well as tuberculous).
2 Chronic renal failure.
3 Connective tissue disease — rheumatoid, periarteritis nodosa, systemic lupus.
4 Previous trauma — including cardiac surgery.
5 Previous myocardial infarction.
6 Previous deep X-ray therapy.
7 Methysergide treatment [20]
8 Involvement by neoplastic disease — usually secondary deposits e.g. lung and breast cancer, leukaemia, lymphoma.

CARDIAC TAMPONADE

Tamponade occurs when, as the result of accumulation of fluid within the pericardial space, the intrapericardial pressure equals the right atrial and right ventricular diastolic pressures. The amount of fluid accumulation that will cause tamponade depends on the rapidity with which it has accumulated; an acute increase of some 2–300 ml above the normal 30–50 ml of pericardial fluid will cause tamponade. In the chronic situation 2–3 1 may accumulate before

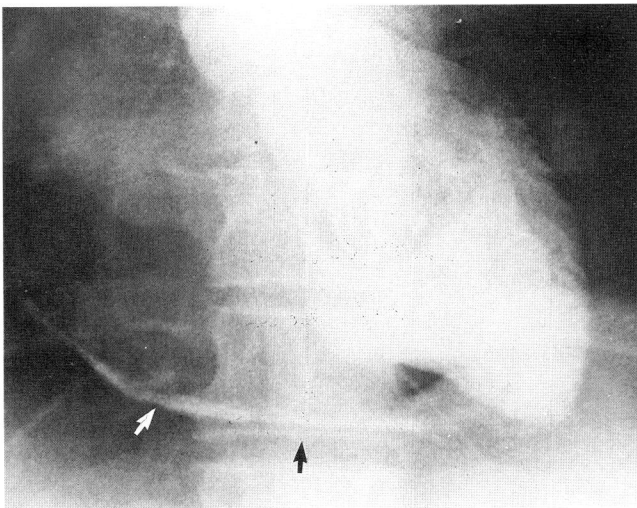

Fig. 16.7 Constrictive pericarditis. Another example with heavy pericardial calcification (arrows).

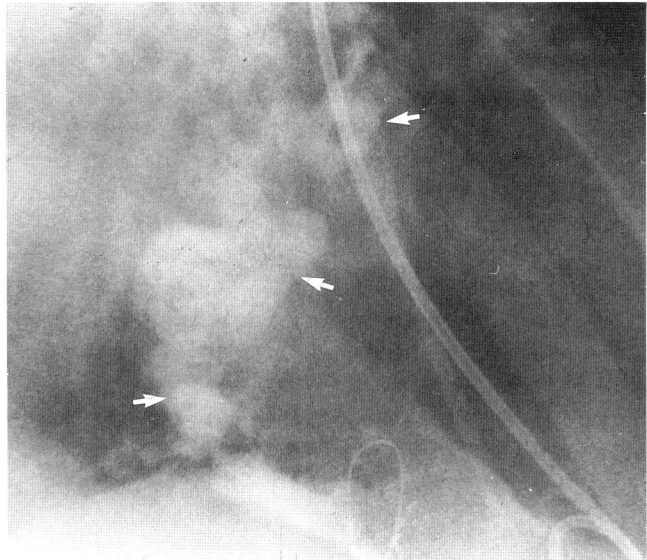

Fig. 16.6 Constrictive pericarditis. There is linear calcification (arrows) due to pericardial calcification. While such appearances are diagnostic pericardial calcification is present in less than 50% of cases.

distress is apparent. The haemodynamic findings in tamponade resemble those of pericardial constriction in that there is equalisation of right and left atrial pressures and of right and left ventricular diastolic pressures but differ in several ways [21];
1 In tamponade there is a prominent x descent but the y descent is small or absent. Both x and y are prominent in constriction.
2 In tamponade the dip-and-plateau pattern of right ventricular diastolic pressure (square root sign) is absent. It is characteristic of constriction (and restrictive cardiomyopathy).

The above two differences are explained as being due to compression of the heart in tamponade throughout the cardiac cycle so that only during systole is there a brief reduction in intrapericardial volume allowing brief inflow — the x descent. During diastole the heart is compressed and the normal rapid inflow of blood in early diastole does not occur, hence no y descent or early diastolic 'dip'.
3 Pulsus paradoxus is a feature of tamponade but is absent or less marked in constriction. Paradox is not truly 'paradoxical' since a fall in arterial pressure during inspiration occurs in the normal heart. Paradox refers to an exaggeration of the normal fall in pressure (seldom more than 10 mmHg) to 15 mmHg

or more. Part of the explanation for paradox is that it is due to increased venous inflow dilating the right ventricle at the expense of the left ventricle whose output briefly falls. This phenomenon is most marked when, as in tamponade, the pericardial space cannot stretch to accomodate the increased right heart filling.

4 In tamponade right atrial pressure falls during inspiration; it may actually rise at this time in constriction (Kussmaul's sign).

Pericardial aspiration

The diagnosis of cardiac tamponade is usually made clinically and the pericardial effusion best demonstrated by echocardiography. However pericardial aspiration is best performed in the catheterisation laboratory with full haemodynamic and fluoroscopic monitoring. Under these circumstances right heart catheterisation will demonstrate the above haemodynamic abnormalities. It may be observed that the tip of the catheter against the right border of the atrium is still 1 cm or so from the right heart border due to the presence of the effusion. An angiogram performed with injection into the superior vena cava will demonstrate the same feature and will serve to exclude superior caval compression (e.g. due to neoplasm) as a cause of the elevated venous pressure — a diagnosis sometimes confused with tamponade. If pericardial aspiration is performed it provides an opportunity to measure pericardial pressure and at the same time right heart catheterisation can be used to monitor the effect of removing the effusion. To begin with pericardial pressure will be identical to right atrial pressure throughout the cardiac cycle; as aspiration proceeds pericardial pressure falls below right atrial pressure and a y descent may appear in the right atrial trace. In patients with both an effusion and constriction removal of fluid will relieve the acute haemodynamic disturbance but right heart pressures will remain high even after pericardial pressure has fallen to zero.

Pericardial aspiration may be from the sub-xiphoid or apical route; most prefer the sub-xiphoid approach. Prior to attempting to drain an effusion it is wise to perform echocardiography to check that there is a sizeable effusion *anteriorly* and not merely a loculated effusion elsewhere. The technique of pericardial aspiration is described in Chapter 5.

OBLITERATIVE CARDIOMYOPATHY

The two conditions included here, endomyocardial fibrosis (EMF) and eosinophillic heart disease (Löffler's endocarditis, hypereosinophillic syndrome) might be included under the restrictive cardiomyopathies as both exhibit abnormalities of diastolic function with impaired filling. However they have peculiar features — notably cavity obliteration. EMF is largely a disease of tropical Africa and affects a young age group. Eosinophilic heart disease affects mainly middle aged Caucasians. Eosinophillia is not a feature of established EMF whereas the hypereosinophillic syndrome is characterised by eosinophil counts of $>1500/mm^3$. Mural thrombus formation is uncommon in EMF but frequently leads of embolism in eosinophillic heart disease. Despite these differences a common aetiology has been proposed. EMF may affect both ventricles or predominantly the right or the left ventricle. In right ventricular EMF the haemodynamics are of restriction with raised filling pressure and square root sign though tricuspid regurgitation, commonly present, will superimpose a large v wave on the right atrial trace. Pulmonary hypertension is absent. Angiography [22] reveals obliteration of the apex of the ventricle (Fig. 16.8); involvement of the subvalve

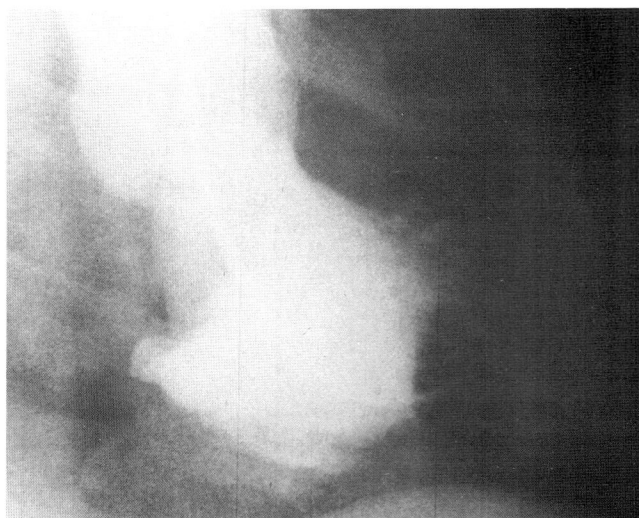

Fig. 16.8 Obliterative cardiomyopathy in a patient from West Africa. There is apical obliteration of the left ventricular cavity suggesting a diagnosis of endomyocardial fibrosis (EMF).

apparatus leads to tricuspid regurgitation and cardiac enlargement is due to a hugely dilated right atrium. Left-sided EMF causes similar apical obliteration but the impaired filling together with mitral regurgitation leads to a high pulmonary venous pressure and pulmonary hypertension.

Similar haemodynamics (impaired filling) and cavity obliteration due to fibrosis and mural thrombus involving the inflow tract and apex are found in eosinophillic heart disease. Atrioventricular valve regurgitation occurs in the same way. Eosinophillic infiltrates may be detected by biopsy in the early, acute, phase but are scanty or absent in the established disease.

ENDOCARDIAL FIBROELASTOSIS

Endocardial fibroelastosis (EFE) is a disease of the neonate and infant. Primary and secondary forms exist; the secondary form being associated with conditions causing increased left ventricular afterload (e.g. aortic stenosis, coarctation). There is diffuse endocardial thickening by fibroelastic tissue — sometimes several millimetres thick. The haemodynamics reflect both impaired diastolic and systolic function. Thus although the ventricle is stiff with high filling pressures it is also greatly dilated with increased end-systolic and end-diastolic volumes and greatly reduced ejection fraction. Angiography reveals a large globular smooth-walled cavity (Fig. 16.9) with increased wall thickness, little change in dimension between systole and diastole and, often, associated mitral regurgitation. The aetiology is unknown [23] and the condition appears to be much less common today than it was 20 years ago.

CARDIAC TUMOURS

Primary tumours of the heart are much less common than are secondary deposits. Of the primary tumours some two-thirds are benign and of these myxomas are by far the commonest, accounting for 30—50% of all primary cardiac tumours (Fig. 16.10). Atrial myxomas usually arise from the fossa ovalis and are much commoner in the left than the right atrium. Rarely myxomas may arise in the right or left ventricle or from cardiac valves. Benign tumours of ventricular myocardium include rhabdomyomas,

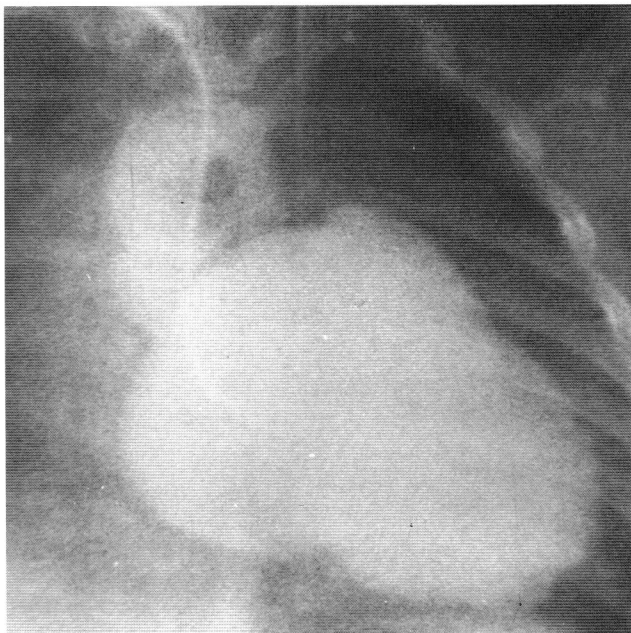

Fig. 16.9 Endocardial fibroelastosis in an infant — gross chamber enlargement (with low ejection fraction) of the left ventricle.

fibromas and hamartomas; all occur predominantly in children. Of these tumours rhabdomyomas are the commonest, the majority being found in neonates and infants — often in association with tuberous sclerosis and often multiple.

Of the malignant tumours almost all are sarcomas; rhabdomyosarcoma, angiosarcoma and fibrosarcoma. They may involve, in order of frequency, the right or left atrium and the right or left ventricle or interventricular septum.

The diagnosis of cardiac tumour is best made by two dimensional echocardiography. If non-invasive techniques fail to demonstrate the tumour then angiography may show the tumour as a filling defect; left atrial tumours being demonstrated by follow-through cine pulmonary arteriography and right atrial myxomas by caval injections. The transseptal technique is contraindicated. Atrial myxomas may prolapse through the mitral or tricuspid valve during ventricular diastole. Ventricular tumours may cause ventricular dysfunction or outflow-tract obstruction. Filling defects due to the tumour may be revealed by ventriculography and a tumour circulation may be revealed by coronary arteriography (Fig. 16.11) though the absence of a pathological circulation does not exclude a cardiac tumour.

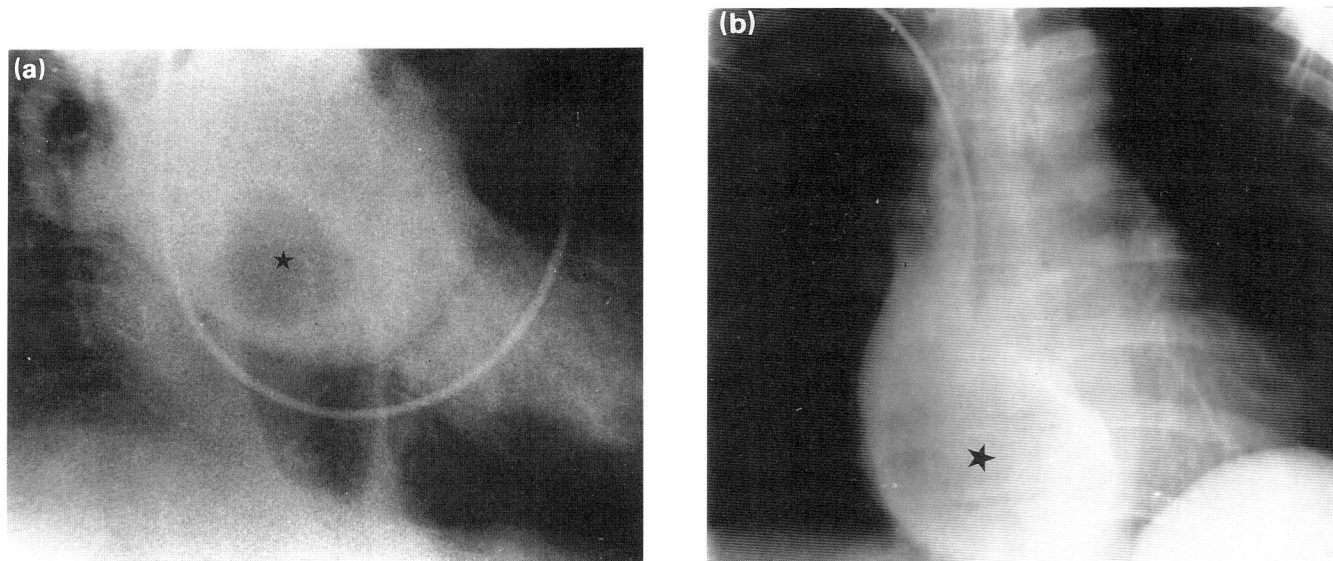

Fig. 16.10 Cardiac tumours — Myxoma. Left (a) and right (b) atrial myxomas producing filling defects (asterisks) within the opacified atria.

ENDOMYOCARDIAL BIOPSY

The technique of transcatheter biopsy has been described elsewhere (Chapter 3). How useful cardiac biopsy is in the investigation of cardiomyopathies is the subject of debate. Although abnormalities are present in biopsies taken from patients with a dilated cardiomayopathy the findings are non-specific, seldom provide information about the aetiology and are unlikely to influence management though there is some evidence that they may be used as a guide to prognosis. Similarly bizarre and disorganised muscle array found in hypertrophic cardiomyopathy can be found in other conditions and even in normal hearts. The diagnosis will have been established clinically and angiographically and will be uninfluenced by the biopsy findings; nor will management be altered. Biopsy has most value in the restrictive cardiomyopathies when, for example, the findings of amyloid deposits may establish the diagnosis even if it does not change the management. Endomyocardial biopsy is of most value, therefore, in:

1 The management of rejection in cardiac transplantation (see Chapter 23).
2 The diagnosis of adriamycin induced cardiomyopathy.
3 The diagnosis of amyloid, haemochromatosis, sarcoid, glycogen storage and Fabry's disease.

It may be of value in myocarditis and in diagnosing cardiac tumours if they are accessible to the bioptome. In endocardial fibroelastosis the diagnosis is obvious clinically and angiographically but biopsy is possible (though difficult) in infants and a myocarditis is a possible differential diagnosis.

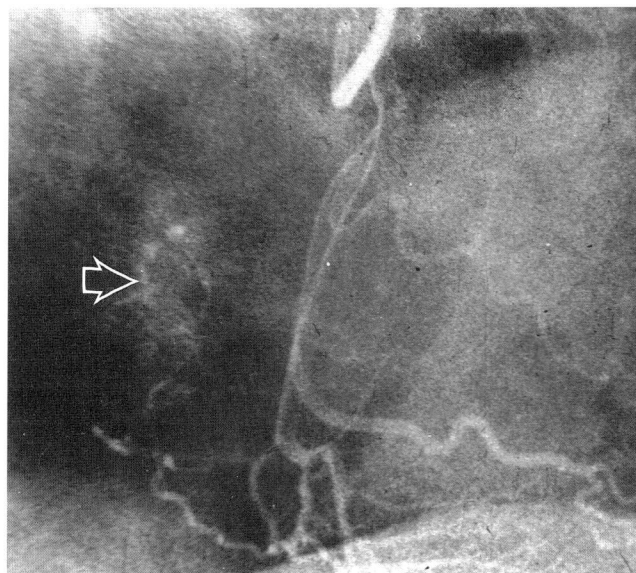

Fig. 16.11 Atrial tumour; a tumour circulation (arrow) is seen following coronary arteriography.

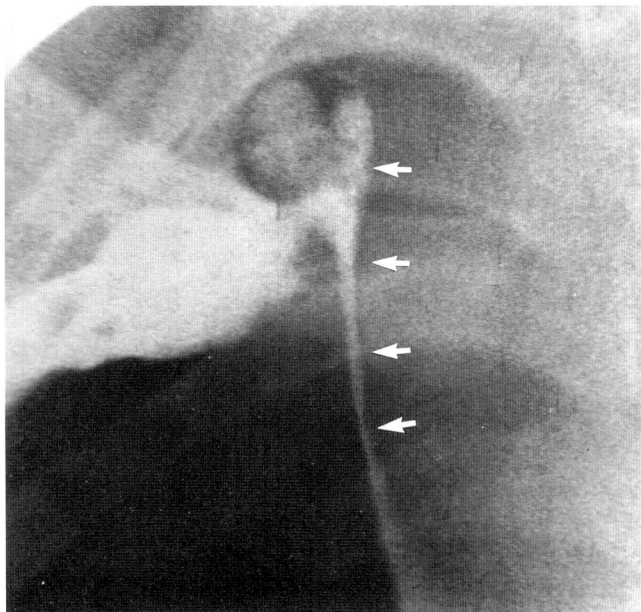

Fig. 16.12 Cardiac tumour. External compression of the SVC can result from neoplasms (which may invade the vein). In this example superior vena caval obstruction has resulted from compression due to a large mediastinal tumour. The SVC is seen as a thin line of contrast medium compressed by the tumour mass (arrows). The grossly elevated superior caval pressure might suggest an (erroneous) diagnosis of cardiac tamponade or constriction.

REFERENCES

1 Kreulen TH, Gorlin R, Herman MV. Ventriculographic patterns and hemodynamics in primary myocardial disease. *Circulation* 1973;**47**:299.

2 Johnson RA, Palacios I. Dilated cardiomyopathy of the adult. *New Engl J Med* 1982;**307**:1051 and 1119.

3 Burch GE, DePasquale NP. Alcoholic cardiomyopathy. *Am J Cardiol* 1969;**23**:723.

4 Bristow MR, Mason JW, Billingham ME, Daniels JR. Doxorubicin cardiomyopathy. Evaluation by phonocardiography, endomyocardial biopsy and cardiac catheterisation. *Ann Int Med* 1978;**88**:168.

5 Mills BA, Roberts RW. Cyclophosphamide induced cardiomyopathy. A report of two cases and a review of the English literature. *Cancer* 1979;**43**:2223.

6 Alexander CS. Cobalt-beer cardiomyopathy. A clinical and pathological study of twenty eight cases. *Am J Med* 1972;**53**:395.

7 Demakis JG, Rahimtoola SH. Peripartum cardiomyopathy. *Circulation* 1971;**44**:964.

8 Braunwald E *et al.* Ideopathic hypertrophic subaortic stenosis. *Circulation* 1964;**29/30** (suppl. IV): 1.

9 Shabetai R. Cardiomyopathy: how far have we come in 25 years, how far yet to go? *J Am Coll Cardiol* 1983;**1**:252.

10 Bush CA, Stang JM, Wooley CF, Kilman JW. Occult constrictive pericardial disease: diagnosis be rapid volume expansion and correction by pericardiectomy. *Circulation* 1977;**56**:924.

11 Chew C, Ziady GM, Raphael MJ, Oakley CM. The functional defect in amyloid heart disease. The "stiff heart" syndrome. *Am J Cardiol* 1975;**36**:438.

12 Buja LM, Khoi NB, Roberts WC. Clinically significant cardiac amyloidosis. *Am J Cardiol* 1970;**26**:394.

13 Buja LM, Roberts WC. Iron in the heart. Etiology and clinical significance. *Am J Med* 1971;**51**:209.

14 Fleming HA. Sarcoid heart disease. *Br Heart J* 1974;**36**:54.

15 Silverman KJ, Hutchins GM, Bulkley BH, Cardiac sarcoid: a clinico pathologic study of 84 unselected patients with systemic sarcoidosis. *Circulation* 1978;**58**:1204.

16 Parrillo JE *et al.* The cardiovascular manifestations of the hypereosinophilic syndrome. Prospective study of 26 patients with review of the literature. *Am J Med* 1979;**67**:573.

17 Desnick RJ *et al.* Cardiac valvular anomalies in Fabry disease. Clinical, morphologic and biochemical studies. *Circulation* 1976;**54**:818.

18 Collucci WS *et al.* Hypertrophic obstructive cardiomyopathy due to Fabry's disease. *New Engl J Med* 1982;**307**:926.

19 Bulkley BH, Hutchins GM. Pompe's disease presenting as hypertrophic cardiomyopathy with Wolff—Parkinson—White syndrome. *Am Heart J* 1978;**96**:246.

20 Meeran MK, Ahmed AH. Parsons FM, Anderson CK. Constrictive pericarditis due to Methysergide therapy. *S Afr Med J* 1976;**50**:1595.

21 Shabetai R, Fowler NO, Guntheroth WG. The hemodynamics of cardiac tamponade and constrictive pericarditis. *Am J Cardiol* 1973;**26**:480.

22 Goebel N, Gander MP, Hess OM. Angiographic aspects of endomyocardial fibrosis. *Ann Radiol* 1978;**21**:475.

23 Schryer MJP, Karnauchow PN. Endocardial fibroelastosis: etiologic and pathogenic considerations in children. *Am Heart J* 1974;**88**:557.

Congenital heart disease

PART I: INTRODUCTION

The indications for catheterisation in neonates and infants have changed dramatically in recent years as the result of developments in echocardiography, particularly cross sectional echocardiography, and the introduction of prostaglandin for maintaining duct patency. Formerly catheterisation was required to establish or confirm the diagnosis and was often needed on an emergency basis in very sick, cyanosed, infants before emergency surgical correction or palliation could be undertaken. Emergency catheterisation is seldom needed today; in the neonate with a duct-dependent pulmonary or systemic circulation prostaglandin restores a stable circulation while cross-sectional echocardiography establishes the diagnosis and, in perhaps the majority of cases, allows corrective or palliative surgery to be performed *without prior catheterisation*. Even balloon atrial septostomy can now be performed under echocardiographic control. Today the indications for catheterisation centre around the need to measure pulmonary flow and resistance, the need to measure valve gradients, the need to demonstrate multiple VSDs and the need to visualise the details of great vessel anatomy. In many instances these questions need answering at the time when a decision about definitive surgical correction is to be made. The patient will present for catheterisation with a firm diagnosis already established by echocardiography and, in all probability, having already had palliative surgery (e.g. systemic-to-pulmonary shunt, pulmonary artery banding).

In many ways these developments have made catheterisation easier; the operator starts with a firm and detailed diagnosis and a clear understanding of the questions which have still to be answered. Echocardiography is superior to angiography in several areas — notably in delineating the anatomy of the atrioventricular junction. Paradoxically patients with congenital heart disease are now coming to catheterisation in increasing numbers not for diag-

nosis but for *treatment* — balloon valvuloplasty for example.

Despite these developments cardiac catheterisation remains an important part of the management of infants and children with congenital heart disease and continues to provide a technical and intellectual challenge.

TECHNIQUES OF CATHETERISATION

Technical problems are related to the need to complete the procedure quickly and safely in a group of patients who may be both very small and very sick. They can be listed as follows:

1 The clinical state is often critical; small errors of technique may have fatal consequences.
2 Both general anaesthesia and sedation have disadvantages and a choice has to be made.
3 Small blood vessels make entry technically difficult.
4 Blood loss can be significant in relation to the small blood volume.
5 The maximum permissable quantity of contrast medium is easily exceeded.
6 Neonates and infants are liable to hypothermia and hypoglycaemia.
7 Delicate blood vessels and myocardium are easily damaged.
8 The patient cannot cooperate — e.g. for measurement of oxygen consumption.

Clinical state

The metabolic consequences of imperiled pulmonary or systemic flow must be corrected *before* transfer to the catheterisation laboratory (and, if necessary, during the study). Thus acid/base imbalance must be corrected (as must hypoglycaemia). An arterial sample for acid/base and blood gas estimation should be obtained as early as possible during the study so that any imbalance can be corrected before complications ensue and hypercapnoea due to inadequate ventilation has lead to increased pulmonary resistance invalidating the haemodynamic study. The amount of sodium bicarbonate (1 mmol/ml) needed to half correct acidosis is calculated as:

$$1/2 \times [\text{wt(kg)}/3] \times \text{base deficit} = \text{mmol sodium bicarbonate needed.}$$

Where there is a history of hypercyanotic attacks due to infundibular spasm (e.g. tetralogy of Fallot) propranalol 0.1 mg/kg should be given intravenously at the start of the study.

Anaesthesia or sedation?

In many laboratories neonates and infants are studied using sedation alone. The following are widely used regimens:
1 Age less than 1 year: no sedation or chloral 50 mg/kg by mouth.
2 Age 1 year or more, no or slight cyanosis: 1 ml/10 kg up to a maximum of 2 ml/10 kg of so-called 'Toronto mixture' containing chlorpromazine (thorazine) 6.25 mg/ml, promethazine (phenergan) 6.25 mg/ml, and pethidine (meperidine, demerol) 25 mg/ml given by deep intramuscular injection.
3 Age 1 year or more, cyanosis moderate or severe: Toronto mixture 1/2 ml/10 kg.
4 Tetralogy of Fallot: morphine 0.1 mg/kg. If further sedation is required during the study diazepam (valium) 0.1 mg/kg can be given intravenously.

The advantage of using sedation alone is, of course, that the cardiac depressant effect of anaesthetic drugs is avoided as are the risks associated with intubation. There are, however, important disadvantages. If sedation is inadequate the baby's struggles make an already difficult dissection impossible. In addition, if the baby's state varies between active crying and deep sleep, the haemodynamic state will also vary widely making it very difficult to compare measurements obtained at different times during the study. If sedation is overdone there is a danger of depressing respiration so that the resulting hypercapnoea leads to a rise in pulmonary vascular resistance and haemodynamic findings which do not reflect the true situation. For all these reasons it is probably preferable to employ general anaesthesia — provided

the services of an anaesthetist skilled in neonatal anaesthesia are available. General anaesthesia and intubation with intermittent positive pressure ventilation using 30% oxygen is our preferred technique.

Small blood vessels

The problem of access in neonates and infants can be a very real one. Only the femoral and axillary vessels will be large enough to accept a catheter of adequate size (no.5F or larger). When a cut-down is used vessel entry is facilitated by using a special introducer of semi-circular section. The choice of catheter and the use of this introducer is discussed in Chapter 2. The techniques of entry are discussed in Chapter 3. The umbilical artery and vein may be used in the first 2—3 days of life but manipulation of a catheter via the umbilical vein is difficult and the umbilical approach introduces the possibility of sepsis.

Heparin 50 u/kg is given if a retrograde arterial approach is used and many centres employ heparinisation routinely for all studies.

Blood loss

It is important to remember that the total blood volume of, for example, a 2 kg neonate is only 160 ml. Thus a mere 16 ml loss from the cut-down and from sampling, trivial in an adult, would represent a significant (10%) loss in a neonate. It follows that meticulous surgical and catheter technique is mandatory. Blood samples must be analysed by an on-line system which allows them to be re-infused or, more usually, by using an oximeter which only requires a very small (0.4 ml) volume of blood.

Haemoglobin should be estimated before catheterisation. Blood group should be known and neonates and small infants may have cross-matched blood available. Significant blood loss should be replaced before the infant leaves the laboratory.

Effects of contrast medium

Most radio-opaque contrast media are hyperosmolar and can result in worsening heart failure. In infants who are polycythaemic they can lead to cerebral venous thrombosis and may cause a (temporary) increase in pulmonary vascular resistance. For these reasons the total volume of contrast medium given during the course of the study should not exceed 4.0 ml/kg. Non-ionic contrast media (see Chapter 7) cause less haemodynamic disturbance and should be used in the very sick patient. The total volume of non-ionic media should probably not exceed 5.0 ml/kg. In a 2.0 kg neonate 4.0 ml/kg is only a total of 8.0 ml including all test injections. This volume is easily exceeded unless the operator keeps a close track of how much has been given throughout the study.

Hypothermia

Neonates and infants are very liable to heat loss and this must be guarded against. All parts of the body that do not need to be exposed for catheter introduction must be covered in woollen clothing or wadding — not forgetting the head. The temperature of the laboratory must be not less than 25°C and some form of heating device will be needed. Radiant heaters cannot be used during fluoroscopy/angiography; a plastic blanket through which warm water circulates can be placed beneath the patient and will not significantly interfere with the quality of the angiograms.

Hypoglycaemia

This is prevented by giving 3.0 ml/kg of 10% dextrose during the study. A 5.0% dextrose solution is used a the flush solution to avoid giving a sodium load.

Avoiding damage to vessels/myocardium

The rules that govern all catheter manipulation are more than ever important. The heart should be explored with a small soft catheter (e.g. Goodale—Lubin) and neither catheter nor guide wire should ever be advanced against resistance. A small test injection should precede angiography to guard against the danger of an intramyocardial injection of contrast medium. Many cardiologists use balloon-tipped catheters for the study of infants and children. The catheters are soft and the inflated balloon spreads the forces at the tip thus reducing the danger of myocardial damage. Such catheters have the added advantage of being flow-guided allowing access to otherwise inaccessible sites within the heart and great vessels. Because of the danger of air em-

bolism following accidental balloon rupture the balloon *must* be inflated with carbon dioxide (not air) whenever these catheters are used in a patient with right-to-left shunting or when there is a possibility of the catheter entering the left heart.

Measured oxygen consumption

The technique for measuring oxygen consumption, and hence cardiac output, in infants and children and applicable both in sedated and anaesthetised patients is described in Chapter 9.

PROFILES OF CONGENITAL HEART DISEASE

Congenital cardiac malformations are found in approximately 8/1000 live births. The six most commonly occurring lesions are, in order of frequency: atrial septal defect, ventricular septal defect, pulmonary stenosis, persistent (patent) ductus, tetralogy of Fallot and coarctation of the aorta. In addition aortic valve anomalies (e.g. bicuspid valve) are probably very common but may not be detected until aortic stenosis develops in adult life at which time it may be impossible to distinguish between a congenital and an acquired lesion. Although the above six lesions are the commonest overall they are not necessarily the commonest lesions in any particular age group. In particular the spectrum of congenital heart lesions presenting in the neonatal period is quite different; in this age group transposition of the great arteries is common together with other lesions causing severe cyanosis (e.g. pulmonary atresia) and including one, aortic atresia, which is only encountered in the first week or so of life (Figs 20.11 and 20.12). The spectrum of congenital heart disease in any given age group depends on (1) the overall frequency of the lesion modified by, (2) its 'survivability', and (3) the effect of physiological changes occurring, particularly, immediately after birth but also throughout life. This is most easily explained by considering specific examples. Thus any malformation in which either the systemic or the pulmonary circulation are dependent on the ductus arteriosus remaining patent will result in distress as soon as the ductus begins to close in the first few hours or days after birth. Examples of such lesions with duct-dependent pulmonary circulation are pulmonary atresia and tricuspid atresia together with extreme tetralogy of Fallot. The systemic circulation is duct-dependent in aortic atresia and aortic interruption. Patients with complete transposition of the great arteries are at no great disadvantage while oxygenation is placental but become severely cyanosed after birth as they become dependant on pulmonary oxygenation.

The effect of lesions with a potential for left-to-right shunting is markedly age-dependant. Thus such lesions rarely cause distress in the first month of life as persistence of the foetal pattern of a high pulmonary vascular resistance prevents the full development of the left-to-right shunt. The pulmonary vascular resistance has usually fallen to normal (low) levels by one month of age and it is at this time that such infants will present with the consequences of a large volume load. If untreated the consequences of a high pulmonary pressure and flow will become manifest at least by early adult life and such patients will present at this time with the Eisenmenger reaction and are unlikely to survive much beyond the third decade of life. Where pulmonary flow is high but pressure is not, as in atrial septal defect, the Eisenmenger reaction is unlikely to develop, if at all, until late adult life so that atrial septal defect, being very 'survivable', becomes almost the only congenital defect encountered in patients over the age of 50.

This very brief summary of the way in which the physiological disturbance determines the time and mode of presentation of patients with congenital heart disease has great importance for the physician undertaking diagnostic catheterisation. Firstly, it explains the timing of the investigation; in the neonate, for example, urgent catheterisation may be required in cyanotic congenital heart disease prior to urgent palliation such as the creation of a systemic-to-pulmonary shunt or, in complete transposition, the creation of an atrial septal defect by balloon septostomy. Alternatively catheterisation may be needed to demonstrate the anatomy in a sick neonate with a downstream lesion such as coarctation prior to urgent surgical repair. In a slightly older age group catheterisation may be needed to measure the magnitude of a left-to-right shunt and to measure the pulmonary arteriolar resistance prior to consideration of surgical correction or palliation (pulmonary artery banding).

Secondly, it is clear that there is an intimate relation between catheterisation and cardiac surgery; catheterisation may be needed when, and if, surgical treatment is being considered. Conversely there is no point in undertaking a potentially dangerous procedure if surgery is not, for the moment, being contemplated or if other investigations, such as echocardiography, can provide all the necessary information.

Finally, although it is the anatomy which determines the physiological derangement, catheterisation, as it proceeds, provides *physiological* information — pressures, saturations and so on. It is by thinking about what anatomical arrangement must be present to explain the physiological findings that the operator obtains a mental picture of the anatomical derangement that must be present. Selective angiography is then performed, with appropriate sites of injection, volumes of contrast medium and radiological projections, to confirm and display the anatomical arrangement of the heart being studied.

PHYSIOLOGICAL CLASSIFICATION OF CONGENITAL HEART DISEASE

A classification of congenital heart disease which is useful clinically and in the catheterisation laboratory starts by recognising four main subgroups:
1 'Simple' left-to-right shunting lesions.
2 'Simple' right-to-left shunting lesions.
3 'Mixing' lesions.
4 'Downstream' and isolated valvar lesions.

Simple left-to-right shunting lesions

The characteristic finding in all these lesions is that a left-to-right shunt (step-up) is detected somewhere in the right side of the heart and *there is no arterial desaturation*. Within this group there are several subgroups depending on whether or not the right ventricular pressure is raised. These will be discussed later.

Simple right-to-left shunting lesions

These lesions are characterised by the presence of (1) arterial desaturation, (2) a raised right ventricular pressure (with a few, very rare, exceptions), and (3) no left-to-right shunt, that is to say pulmonary artery saturation is the same as 'mixed venous' saturation as there is no pulmonary venous contribution to pulmonary artery flow. The preceding statement needs some qualification; when resistance to right ventricular outflow is approximately equal to resistance to left ventricular outflow (the systemic resistance) there may be some bidirectional shunting at, for example, the ventricular septal defect in tetralogy of Fallot.

'Mixing' lesions

These lesions all share the characteristic of having both a left-to-right and a right-to-left shunt. A left-to-right shunt exists when a proportion of pulmonary arterial blood is derived directly from pulmonary vein blood. A right-to-left shunt exists when a proportion of systemic arterial blood is derived directly from systemic venous blood. When this definition of right-to-left and left-to-right shunting is borne in mind it becomes obvious why situations in which there is both left-to-right and right-to-left shunting are termed mixing situations; there is mixing of pulmonary and systemic venous blood in both the pulmonary and systemic circulations. Thus there is both a step-up in saturation from mixed venous saturation to pulmonary artery saturation *and* arterial desaturation. A mixing situation is easily recognised clinically when there is obvious cyanosis and when, at the same time, the plain chest X-ray reveals pulmonary plethora; the hall-mark of a high pulmonary flow due to left-to-right shunting. Unfortunately the diagnosis is not always so simple; when pulmonary flow is very high and mixing is complete the degree of arterial desaturation may be so slight that clinically recognisable cyanosis is absent. At the other extreme there may be marked cyanosis and though pulmonary arterial blood contains an admixture of pulmonary vein blood the left-to-right shunt may be small and total pulmonary flow *reduced* as a result of obstruction to pulmonary flow. There are thus three subgroups of mixing situations. In the first situation the patients appear to have a simple left-to-right shunt and the true situation is only recognised if arterial Po_2 is measured and arterial desaturation thus recognised. Examples include persistent truncus arteriosus and, possibly, double inlet atrioventricular connection with a high pulmonary flow. In the second situation the patients appear to have a simple right-to-left shunting situation with a low pulmonary flow

(oligaemia on the plain chest X-ray) and marked arterial desaturation (cyanosis). Examples include classical tricuspid atresia, pulmonary atresia and any form of univentricular atrioventricular connection with severe obstruction to pulmonary flow. The third group are classical mixing situations with obvious cyanosis and obvious left-to-right shunting and pulmonary plethora. Complete transposition of the great arteries is an example. The ways in which these various forms of mixing lesions are distinguished in the catheterisation laboratory will be discussed later in this chapter.

'Downstream' and isolated valvar lesions

This group includes isolated lesions of cardiac valves and abnormalities of myocardial function — those congenital cardiac lesions in which there is no intra-cardiac shunt. In practice there may be an associated defect which allows some shunting; for example an atrial septal defect or patent foramen ovale associated with pulmonary valve stenosis. In aortic interruption there has to be a right-to-left shunt through the ductus if lower body perfusion is to be preserved. Aortic atresia presents as a severe downstream lesion but is actually a mixing situation by definition as all systemic and pulmonary flow are derived from mixing of pulmonary and systemic venous blood at the level (usually) of the right atrium.

This physiological classification of congenital heart disease is of use in guiding the physician towards the correct diagnosis during cardiac catheterisation. It indicates the questions to be answered by the study which will include:

1 Is there a left-to-right shunt? If so at what level is it first detected?
2 Is there arterial desaturation? If so, why?
3 Is there both left-to-right and right-to-left shunting?
If so there is a mixing situation the anatomical arrangement of which needs to be demonstrated.

Unfortunately the items of information obtained as catheterisation proceeds are not necessarily obtained in the order one would like; some may be unobtainable. One item of information, however, is almost always obtainable and obtained early in the study. This is the level of the right ventricular systolic pressure. Four possibilities exist:

1 Right ventricular pressure is normal (<30 mmHg systolic).

2 Right ventricular pressure is raised but is significantly less than systemic pressure.

3 Right ventricular systolic pressure is the same as left ventricular or systemic pressure.

4 Right ventricular systolic pressure is significantly higher than systemic pressure.

Within each of these four categories, as defined by the right ventricular pressure, there are four possibilities (1) there is a left-to-right shunt with no arterial desaturation, (2) there is a right-to-left shunt (arterial desaturation present) without a significant left-to-right shunt, (3) there is both a left-to-right and a right-to-left shunt (mixing), and (4) there are no shunts. In other words our original four physiological categories of congenital heart disease.

We have now reached the point at which we can look at each of these four-by-four possibilities in terms of the diagnostic possibilities in each subgroup.

Normal right ventricular pressure

The significance of this finding is that:

1 The ventricular septum is intact or that any defect present must be small.

2 There cannot be significant right ventricular outflow tract obstruction (RVOTO) or significant pulmonary vascular disease.

3 The right ventricle (more accurately the systemic venous ventricle) cannot be supporting the systemic circulation.

NORMAL RIGHT VENTRICULAR PRESSURE
WITH A SIMPLE LEFT-TO-RIGHT SHUNTING
LESION

Since right ventricular pressure is normal the only situation which could cause left-to-right shunting at ventricular level would be a *small* VSD or, possibly a coronary-to-right ventricular fistula or ruptured sinus of Valsalva aneurysm. The shunt is more likely to be at caval or right atrial level due to partial anomalous pulmonary venous return, an atrial septal defect or an atrioventricular defect without a significant ventricular component (partial AV canal, 'primum' ASD). If the shunt is detected at pulmonary artery level a (small) patent ductus is the most likely diagnosis. Aortopulmonary septal defect usually results in pulmonary artery pressures near to systemic level. Coronary artery to pulmonary artery fistula is a possibility but is rare.

NORMAL RIGHT VENTRICULAR PRESSURE
WITH A SIMPLE RIGHT-TO-LEFT SHUNTING
LESION

Since right ventricular pressure is normal the shunt can only be at atrial level. There cannot be RVOTO causing right ventricular hypertrophy and reduced ventricular compliance so that the only possible cause for right-to-left shunting is that there is resistance to filling of the right ventricle either because of an anomaly of the tricuspid valve (stenosis, regurgitation) or because of an anomaly of the right ventricle resulting in reduced compliance (congenital hypoplasia or Uhl ' syndrome). Both mechanisms are probably responsible for right-to-left interatrial shunting with normal RV pressure in Ebstein's anomaly of the tricuspid valve.

NORMAL RIGHT VENTRICULAR PRESSURE
WITH RIGHT-TO-LEFT AND LEFT-TO-RIGHT
SHUNTING (MIXING)

As is the case in simple right-to-left shunting, and for the same reasons, the right-to-left shunt can only be at atrial level. Atrial level mixing lesions that can have a normal right ventricular systolic pressure are total anomalous pulmonary venous return and common atrium. Patients with total anomalous pulmonary venous return (TAPVR) may have a normal right ventricular pressure or a raised pressure, on occasion there may even be suprasystemic right ventricular pressure. The level of the right ventricular and pulmonary arterial pressure depends on (1) the degree to which pulmonary arteriolar resistance is increased, (2) whether or not there is obstruction to pulmonary venous return, and (3) the magnitude of the left-to-right shunt. In patients under 1 year of age it is unusual for the right ventricular pressure to be low; in the neonate, in particular, persistence of the foetal pattern of a high pulmonary vascular resistance and the early presentation of those with obstructed pulmonary venous return (notably those with infradiaphragmatic TAPVR) means that high right ventricular and pulmonary arterial pressures are the rule. The hall-mark of TAPVR is that pulmonary arterial saturation tends to be a few percentage points *higher* than systemic saturation. The exception to this rule is infradiaphragmatic TAPVR when streaming of highly saturated IVC blood across the ASD to left atrium and of low saturation SVC blood across the tricuspid valve to RV and PA leads to a lower saturation in PA than in the systemic arteries. The site at which highly saturated blood is sampled provides the clue to the site of drainage; SVC and left innominate vein when drainage is supracardiac, right atrium when it is at cardiac level (directly to right atrium or via the coronary sinus) and IVC when it is infracardiac.

Common atrium is a rare anomaly characterised by almost complete absence of the atrial septum with atrial situs solitus (right-sided morphologic right and left-sided morphologic left atria). The haemodynamic findings resemble those of an ASD with the addition of some arterial desaturation due to mixing at atrial level.

Tricuspid atresia needs to be mentioned in this section. This is a mixing situation in which mixing occurs in the left atrium as all systemic venous return has to cross the atrial septum. The operator cannot reach the right ventricle from the right atrium but instead will reach a *high pressure* ventricle via the mitral valve. In the commonest form of this malformation there *is* a right ventricle which is rudimentary and at low pressure and from which the pulmonary artery arises. If this chamber is reached from the main chamber (morphologic LV) then this arrangement could be classified as belonging to the group of mixing situations with a normal right ventricular pressure; but this is not how the haemodynamic findings strike the operator. Thus tricuspid atresia is best considered along with other examples of abnormal atrioventricular connections which have systemic pressure in the main ventricular chamber and arterial desaturation due to mixing.

NORMAL RIGHT VENTRICULAR PRESSURE AND NO SHUNTS: 'DOWNSTREAM' AND VALVAR LESIONS

The implication of this finding is that (1) all septa must be effectively intact, and (2) that there cannot be RVOTO so that any lesions present must be trivial or on the left side of the heart where they cannot be of sufficient severity to cause much elevation of pulmonary vein (and hence pulmonary artery and right ventricular) pressure. Included in this group are patients who turn out to have no cardiac abnormality. It would be tedious to list all the possible diagnoses that could be included in this group; nor would such a list reflect the real situation since

Table 17.1 Conditions which may exist with normal right ventricular pressure.

With simple left-to-right shunt
Shunt at caval level:
    Partial anomalous pulmonary venous return
    Coronary to superior vena cava fistula
Shunt at atrial level:
    Atrial septal defect, (secundum, partial AV defect, sinus venosus defect)
    Ruptured sinus of Valsalva to RA
    Coronary to RA fistula
Shunt at ventricular level:
    Ventricular septal defect (small)
    Ruptured sinus of Valsalva to RV
    Coronary artery to RV fistula
Shunt at pulmonary artery level:
    Patent ductus arteriosus (small)
    Coronary artery to pulmonary artery fistula

With simple right-to-left shunt
Shunt at atrial level (all with ASD):
    Isolated congenital hypoplasia of the right ventricle
    Ebstein's anomaly of the tricuspid valve
    Tricuspid stenosis
    Dysplastic tricuspid valve

With right-to-right and left-to-right shunt ('mixing')
Shunt at caval level:
    Total anomalous pulmonary venous return (supracardiac)
Shunt at atrial level:
    Total anomalous pulmonary venous return (cardiac)
    Common atrium

With no shunt
    Normal heart
    Left sided anomalies without significant elevation of pulmonary vein pressure

patients are referred for catheterisation with a limited list of diagnostic possibilities in mind. Thus an asymptomatic patient with a systolic murmur, normal right heart pressures and no detectable shunt may have a small ventricular septal defect and only if such a defect is not found and the murmur thought to indicate organic heart disease is there a need to proceed to left heart catheterisation to investigate, for example, the possibility that the murmur is due to aortic stenosis.

Table 17.1 lists those conditions that may exist with a normal right ventricular pressure.

Right ventricular pressure raised but less than systemic

The significance of this finding is much the same as as in the first group of conditions with a normal right ventricular pressure but the lesions are likely to be more severe. Some degree of RVOTO is now a possibility and a normal heart is not. It is now possible that there is a significant ventricular septal defect but such a defect will still be too small to equalise right and left ventricular pressures. A patent ductus is a real possibility too, among the simple left-to-right shunting lesions. Among those with a simple right-to-left shunt the fact that the pressure in the right ventricle is lower than in the left excludes tetralogy of Fallot and all other examples of RVOTO with right-to-left shunting at ventricular level; the shunt must be at atrial level. Similarly the finding excludes all those mixing situations in which mixing takes place at ventricular level.

Table 17.2 is a list of conditions that may exist with moderate elevation of right ventricular pressure.

Right ventricular pressure equal to systemic pressure

Included here are a large and important group of lesions. The significance of equal RV and systemic pressures is that it suggests that either there is free communication between the right and left sides of the heart (e.g. large VSD, 'common ventricle') or that the ventricle (RV) entered from the right atrium is the systemic ventricle (e.g. complete transposition, double-outlet right ventricle).

RIGHT VENTRICULAR PRESSURE AT SYSTEMIC LEVEL AND SIMPLE LEFT-TO-RIGHT SHUNTING LESION

In this group the left-to-right shunt is most likely to be detected at ventricular level and a ventricular septal defect is by far the most likely diagnosis. If a left-to-right shunt is detected at atrial level it is probable that there is a mixing situation (see below) though an atrial septal defect *and* a VSD is a possi-

Table 17.2 Right ventricular pressure raised but less than systemic.

With simple left-to-right shunt	*With no shunts*
Shunt at caval level:	With low pulmonary artery pressure:
As for simple left-to-right shunt but lesions more severe	Mild/moderate pulmonary valve stenosis
Shunt at atrial level:	Mild/moderate infundibular stenosis
As for simple left-to-right shunt but lesions more severe	Anomalous muscle bundle of right ventricle
Shunt at ventricular level:	With raised proximal pulmonary artery pressure:
Ventricular septal defect (moderate)	Supravalve and peripheral pulmonary artery stenosis
Ruptured sinus of Valsalva to RV	Primary pulmonary hypertension
Coronary to RV fistula	Persistent foetal (pulmonary) circulation
Shunt at pulmonary artery level:	With raised pulmonary vein or wedge pressure:
Patent ductus arteriosus	Downstream lesions:
Aortopulmonary septal defect (window)	Cor triatriatum
Coronary to PA fistula	Supravalve stenosing ring of left atrium
	Mitral valve lesions
With simple right-to-left shunt	Left ventricular disease (e.g. cardiomyopathy, endocardial fibro-elastosis)
Shunt at atrial level:	Subaortic stenosis
Mild/moderate pulmonary stenosis and atrial septal defect	Aortic valve and supravalve stenosis
Atrial septal defect with raised pulmonary arteriolar resistance	Aortic regurgitation
	Coarctation
With right-to-left and left-to-right shunt ('mixing')	
Shunt at caval or atrial level:	
Total anomalous pulmonary venous return	
Common atrium	
Cerebral arteriovenous fistula (in the neonate)	
Pulmonary atresia with intact ventricular septum and tricuspid regurgitation (dilated right ventricle)	
(Note also univentricular atrioventricular connections in which outflow chamber (RV) is at low pressure but main chamber is at systemic pressure).	

bility. If the shunt is detected at pulmonary artery level a (large) patent ductus is the most likely diagnosis though aortopulmonary septal defect (window) is a (rare) possibility.

The fact that right ventricular pressure is at systemic level and there is a left-to-right shunt at ventricular level does not exclude some degree of RVOTO; patients with an 'acyanotic tetralogy' or the 'absent pulmonary valve syndrome' have these haemodynamic findings. But for the shunt to be from left-to-right implies that the resistance to right ventricular outflow is still less than the resistance to entry to the systemic circulation. Once the resistance to entry to the pulmonary circulation is greater than, the systemic resistance the shunt will reverse and the situation is that represented by the next category of haemodynamic findings.

RIGHT VENTRICULAR PRESSURE AT SYSTEMIC LEVEL AND A SIMPLE RIGHT-TO-LEFT SHUNTING LESION

The significance of this finding is that there is a free communication between the right and left heart but that there is a high resistance to entry to the pulmonary circulation. This high resistance to entry to the pulmonary circulation must be present since there would otherwise be left-to-right shunting at ventricular level. The site of obstruction ('resistance') may be within the body of the pulmonary ventricle (e.g. infundibular stenosis, tetralogy), at pulmonary valve level (valvar stenosis), above the pulmonary valve (supravalve stenosis, pulmonary artery banding, peripheral pulmonary artery stenosis) or within the pulmonary circulation itself (raised arteriolar resistance, Eisenmenger reaction). In each case there must be an accompanying VSD unless the right-to-left shunt is at atrial level and the two ventricles happen to be at the same pressure by chance and not because of a free communication between them.

There are many conditions other than those listed above in which the ventricles are at the same pressure and there is a right-to-left shunt but they are 'mixing situations' so that there is an additional left-to-right shunt. However there may be some bidirectional shunting (left-to-right or right-to-left) in simple lesions such as tetralogy when the resistance to egress into the pulmonary and systemic circulations is of the same order; this situation must

not be confused with true 'mixing situations' as discribed below.

RIGHT VENTRICULAR PRESSURE AT SYSTEMIC LEVEL AND BOTH LEFT-TO-RIGHT AND RIGHT-TO-LEFT SHUNTING (MIXING SITUATIONS)

Up to now reference to *right* ventricular pressure need cause no confusion; with the exception of 'corrected transposition' the ventricle entered via the right sided atrioventricular valve will be the morphological right ventricle and is also the 'pulmonary' ventricle supplying the pulmonary circulation. But in the group of abnormalities to be discussed here the ventricle entered via the right sided atrioventricular valve may be a morphological *left* ventricle or a right ventricle or even a solitary ventricle of indeterminate morphology. This ventricle may support either the pulmonary circulation or the systemic circulation (or both). In some cases there will be no connection between the systemic venous atrium and the ventricle (tricuspid atresia — absent right atrioventricular connection) and the ventricle can only be entered after the catheter has traversed an interatrial communication and the left sided atrioventricular valve. We are concerned here with the *haemodynamic* characterisation of various forms of congenital heart disease and the term 'right ventricular pressure' is used in the understanding that it refers to the pressure in the ventricle entered from the systemic venous atrium and in the knowledge that it is not necessarily a morphologic right ventricle.

In this group of conditions there are three possible reasons for the 'right' ventricle being at systemic pressure;

1 There are two separate ventricles with a free communication between them (e.g. truncus arteriosus, pulmonary atresia with VSD).

2 There are two separate ventricles but the 'right' ventricle supports the systemic circulation (e.g. complete transposition, double outlet right ventricle).

3 There is only one ventricle or, more commonly, one ventricle is rudimentary (various forms of univentricular atrioventricular connection). The physician performing catheterisation will need to seek the answers to a number of questions which include: (1) at which level is the left-to-right shunt first detected?, (2) how many ventricles are there?, and (3) from where does the pulmonary circulation arise and what is the pressure and resistance within it?

The level at which the left-to-right shunt is first detected

If a left-to-right shunt if detected at the level of the great veins total anomalous pulmonary venous return, with or without other anomalies, is the probable diagnosis but the reason for the systemic pressure in the right ventricle must be sought; TAPVD not infrequently coexists with truncus arteriosus and with aortic interruption. If the shunt is at atrial level TAPVD is again a possibility as is complete transposition of the great vessels with bidirectional interatrial shunting. With a 'right' ventricle at systemic pressure it is perhaps surprising to find left-to-right atrial shunting; one would expect the right ventricular hypertrophy to result in impaired filling and, if anything, right-to-left interatrial shunting. Thus the finding of left-to-right shunting should alert the operator to the possibility that egress from the left atrium is impaired; as in atresia, hypoplasia or stenosis of the left AV value. When mitral atresia coexist with aortic atresia (hypoplastic left heart syndrome) the right ventricular pressure is usually slightly higher than systemic pressure (see next section) but other forms of univentricular atrioventricular connection may have atresia/hypoplasia of the left atrioventricular valve.

The majority of anomalies in this group have a left-to-right shunt first detected at ventricular level including the various forms of univentricular atrioventricular connection, complete transposition with ventricular septal defect, Truncus arteriosus and pulmonary atresia with VSD.

How many ventricles are there?

Before this question can be answered we need a definition of a 'ventricle'. A normal ventricle has three components; an inflow portion, a trabecular portion and an outflow portion. When the inflow and trabecular portions are missing the chamber is referred to as an 'outflow chamber' and is usually of right ventricular morphology. The 'rudimentary' right ventricle found in most examples of tricuspid atresia is a good example. When the inflow and outflow portions are missing and only the trabecular portion is present the chamber is referred to as a 'trabecular pouch' and is usually of left ventricular morphology. Although these chambers can be regarded as ventricles in that they are separate

chambers within the ventricular mass it is simpler to confine the term 'ventricle' to a chamber possessing an inflow (though it may lack an outflow or even a trabecular and outflow portion). The demonstration of two separate ventricles or of a single ventricle (main chamber) with an outflow chamber or trabecular pouch depends on angiography in most instances. In complete transposition with intact ventricular septum, however, the finding of a low pressure chamber entered from the left atrium establishes the presence of two ventricles as well as establishing the diagnosis of 'simple' transposition.

The origin of the pulmonary blood supply

The malformations discussed in this section are unified by having systemic pressure in the right ventricle or 'main chamber' and both left-to-right and right-to-left shunting. In most the left-to-right shunt is first detected at ventricular level and the conditions are differentiated by the origin of the pulmonary circulation. In complete transposition the pulmonary artery arises from a separate, posterior, morphologic left ventricle. In double outlet right ventricle there are two ventricles but more than half of both the aorta and the pulmonary artery arise from the right ventricle. In truncus arteriosus the pulmonary arteries arise from the ascending aorta (strictly the arterial trunk) while in pulmonary atresia with VSD the pulmonary supply is from collaterals arising from the descending aorta. Even in those conditions with but one main chamber (double inlet atrioventricular connection and absent atrioventricular connection) the origin of the pulmonary blood supply is of importance; it may be from an outlet chamber (as in most forms of tricuspid atresia) or from the main chamber. There may be coexisting pulmonary atresia with the pulmonary arteries supplied from a persistent ductus or from a surgically created shunt. Thus catheterisation in this group is incomplete until the origin of the pulmonary supply has been identified and, if possible, the pressure and saturation within the pulmonary circulation determined.

Table 17.3 is a list of conditions characterised by equal right ventricular and systemic pressures.

Table 17.3 Right ventricular pressure equal to systemic pressure.

With simple left-to-right shunt
Shunt at atrial level:
    Atrioventricular defect ('complete AV canal')
Shunt at ventricular level:
    Ventricular septal defect(s) — large
    'Acyanotic tetralogy of Fallot'
    Absent pulmonary valve syndrome
Shunt at pulmonary artery level:
    Aortopulmonary septal defect ('window')

With simple right-to-left shunt
With low pulmonary artery pressure:
    Tetralogy of Fallot
    Other forms of RVOTO with (large) VSD
With equal RV and PA systolic pressures:
    Eisenmenger VSD, PDA

With right-to-left and left-to-right shunt ('mixing')
Shunt at caval or atrial level:
    Total anomalous pulmonary venous return plus a lesion
    equalising ventricular pressures — e.g. truncus
    Complete transposition
Shunt at ventricular level:
    Complete transposition
    Double-outlet right ventricle
    Truncus
    Pulmonary atresia with VSD
    All forms of univentricular atrioventricular connection (e.g.
    Double-inlet and absent atrioventricular connection
    including tricuspid atresia)

With no shunts
Right ventricular pressure at systemic level by chance — no interventricular communication:
    With low pulmonary artery pressure
        Pulmonary valve stenosis — severe
        Isolated infundibular stenosis — severe
    Pulmonary artery systolic pressure the same as right
        ventricular systolic pressure
        With low wedge or LA pressure;
            Primary or thromboembolic pulmonary hypertension
        With high wedge or LA pressure;
            Severe downstream lesion (e.g. mitral stenosis)

Right ventricular pressure higher than systemic pressure

The significance of this finding, as with the group with right ventricular pressure less than systemic, is that there must be two ventricles and the ventricular septum must be intact — or nearly so. In addition the suprasystemic pressure must mean that the resistance to egress from the right ventricle must be very high. The site of this high resistance may be within the body of the right ventricle (infundibular stenosis), at the pulmonary valve (pulmonary valve stenosis), in the main pulmonary arteries (supravalve stenosis, pulmonary artery banding, peripheral pulmonary artery stenosis) or within the micro circulation/pulmonary arterioles as in the Eisenmenger reaction, primary pulmonary hypertension, etc. It is even possible for part, at least, of the high resistance to be downstream, that is at the level of the pulmonary veins (obstructed total anomalous pulmonary venous return), the left atrium (Cor triatriatum) or the mitral valve or left ventricle.

It will be apparent from the above that patients with a high right ventricular pressure fall into two groups: those with a low pulmonary artery pressure and those in whom pulmonary artery systolic pressure is at the same high level as the right ventricular pressure. In the former subgroup we are dealing with some form of right ventricular outflow tract obstruction, in the latter with either a high pulmonary vascular resistance or a high downstream (pulmonary vein) pressure — or both.

The combination of suprasystemic right ventricular pressure and a simple left-to-right shunt is a very unlikely one; if there is an intracardiac defect the shunt will almost inevitably be from right-to-left. Right-to-left shunting in this situation is, however, common. Since the ventricular septum must be nearly intact such shunting is likely to be at atrial level and so-called 'pulmonary stenosis with reversed interatrial shunt' is the obvious example. Isolated infundibular stenosis is rare — there is usually a VSD as well and though this may be too small to equalise pressures and it is a possible source of right-to-left shunting. 'Mixing situations' with suprasystemic right ventricular pressures do occur and four of these deserve mention. Pulmonary atresia with intact ventricular septum presents in the neonatal period; since pulmonary arterial supply is exclusively via the ductus this is, strictly speaking, a 'mixing situation' but, in common with other mixing situations with severe obstruction to pulmonary flow it more closely resembles a simple right-to-left shunting situation with marked pulmonary oligaemia. The second anomaly, critical pulmonary stenosis in the neonate, is very similar from the haemodynamic point of view and again the majority of the pulmonary supply is likely to be via the ductus. The third anomaly, obstructed total anomalous pulmonary venous return, has already been discussed and is suspected when, in the above setting, there is left-to-right shunting detected at atrial level. The fourth condition, aortic and mitral atresia, is also characterised by left-to-right interatrial shunting since there is no other egress from the left atrium. In this instance it is the systemic circulation which is 'duct-dependant' and for the flow across the duct to be from right-to-left the pulmonary vascular resistance must be higher than the systemic resistance. Although right ventricular pressure might, therefore, be at systemic level there is usually a pressure drop across the duct and suprasystemic right ventricular pressure.

Finally there are patients with suprasystemic

pressure in the right ventricle and no shunts. Almost invariably they have infundibular or valvar pulmonary stenosis and, since there is no shunt, intact atrial and ventricular septa. In the adult primary (ideopathic) pulmonary hypertension or chronic thromboembolic pulmonary hypertension can also present with suprasystemic right ventricular pressure and no shunt.

Table 17.4 is a list of conditions in which right ventricular pressure may be suprasystemic.

Table 17.4 Right ventricular pressure higher than systemic pressure.

With simple left-to-right shunt — (almost) impossible

With simple right-to-left shunt
With low pulmonary artery pressure:
    Pulmonary valve stenosis (severe) with 'reversed' interatrial shunt
    Infundibular stenosis with small VSD or interatrial shunt
With high pulmonary artery pressure:
    Primary pulmonary hypertension (and ASD or PFO)
    Peripheral pulmonary artery stenosis, Rubella syndrome, etc. (and ASD)

With right-to-left shunt and left-to-right shunt ('mixing')
    Total anomalous pulmonary venous return (obstructed)
    Pulmonary atresia with intact ventricular septum
    Aortic and mitral atresia — hypoplastic left heart syndrome

With no shunts
    As for simple right-to-left shunt without ASD or PFO

GENERAL READING

1 Freedom RM, Culham JAG, Moes CAF. *Angiocardiography of congenital heart disease.* New York, Macmillan Publishing Company, 1984.
2 Moss AJ, Adams FH, Emmanouilides GC. *Heart disease in infants, children and adolescents.* 2nd edn. Baltimore, Williams and Wilkins Company, 1977.
3 Keith JD, Rowe RD, Vlad P. *Heart disease is infancy and childhood.* 3rd edn. New York, Macmillan Publishing Company, 1978.
4 Miller GAH, Anderson RH, Rigby ML. *The diagnosis of congenital heart disease.* Tunbridge Wells, Castle House Publications Ltd., 1985.
5 Amplatz K, Moller JH, Castaneda-Zuniga WR. *Radiology of congenital heart disease.* Volume 1. New York, Thieme Medical Publishers, 1986.
6 Shinebourne EA, Macartney FJ, Anderson RH. Sequential chamber localisation; the logical approach to diagnosis in congenital heart disease. *Br Heart J* 1976;**38**;327.
7 Tynan MJ *et al.* Nomenclature and classification of congenital heart disease. *Br Heart J* 1979;**41**:544.

Congenital heart disease

PART II: ILLUSTRATIONS

In the following section are illustrated most of the commonly occurring congenital cardiac malformations affecting the systemic and pulmonary veins, the atria, the atrioventricular junction, the ventricles and the ventriculo-arterial junction. Congenital malformations of the pulmonary, systemic and coronary circulations are illustrated in the chapters devoted to these circulations.

Many different diagnostic codes exist for congenital heart disease but it is widely accepted that, to be of practical use, all must be based on a system of *segmental nomenclature* as originally proposed by Van Praagh [1]. Such a system, universally accepted in principle if not in detail, provides a complete description of any heart, however complex, without making use of eponyms or requiring that the user is familiar with a particular complex of lesions. It is self descriptive, one of the desirable attributes of a universal diagnostic code. The system outlined here is that proposed by Shinebourne [2] and used at the Brompton Hospital, London.

The first question that has to be asked is 'Are the *connections* normal?' In the vast majority of cases (and all cases of acquired heart disease) the answer is 'Yes' and only additional lesions need to be described. By normal connections we mean that the right atrium is on the right (and the left atrium on the left) and the two atria connect to their appropriate ventricles by way of two separate atrioventricular valves. The ventricles, in turn, are connected to the appropriate great artery by way of patent ventriculo-arterial valves. The right sided, morphologically right, ventricle connects to the pulmonary artery and the left sided, morphologically left, ventricle connects to the aorta. In such cases all that is needed is to describe the individual lesions (e.g. ventricular septal defect or pulmonary stenosis). But

in some examples of congenital heart disease, including the most complex, this is not so. Such cases have abnormal connections.

Segmental nomenclature demands that each of the three segments, the atria, the ventricles and the great vessels, can be separately identified (by angiography or echocardiography) and that the connections of one with the next can be defined. The first step, in describing any heart, is to decide if the connections are normal — as defined above. If not the abnormal connections that are present must be defined. What follows is a brief summary of the principles of segmental nomenclature; brief because the cases to which it applies form but a small minority of cases coming to cardiac catheterisation in any but a specialised paediatric cardiology unit. A fuller explanation will be found elsewhere [2, 3].

THE ATRIA

The terms 'right atrium' and 'left atrium' describe their morphology and not necessarily their position in the thorax. The morphologic right atrium is characterised by having a blunt-ended appendage with a wide orifice. Normally (but not invariably) it receives the superior and inferior cavae and the coronary sinus. Normally (but not invariably) it lies to the right of the great arteries. The left atrium has a finger-like appendage with a narrow ostium leading into it. Normally (but not invariably) it lies posteriorly and to the left of the great arteries and receives the four pulmonary veins. The possibilities are:

1 Atrial *situs solitus* — morphologic right atrium on the right, morphologic left atrium on the left; the normal arrangement.

2 Atrial *situs inversus* — the opposite of the above.
3 Atrial *situs ambiguus* (atrial isomerism — there are bilateral left atria (L-isomerism) or bilateral right atria (D-isomerism).

Next we have to describe the atrioventricular junction; the connections between the atria and the ventricle(s). The possibilities here are determined both by the atrial arrangement and by the ventricular morphology. The atria may be lateralised (*solitus* or *inversus*) or isomeric (*ambiguus*). The connection may be *biventricular* or *univentricular*. By a biventricular atrioventricular connection we mean that there are two chambers within the ventricular mass *each of which receives (or potentially receives) an atrioventricular valve or the major part of a valve*. By a univentricular atrioventricular connection we mean that *only one chamber in the ventricular mass receives the atrioventricular valves, or valve*. The possibilities are:
1 For lateralised atria with a biventricular AV connection; *concordant atrioventricular connection*. The morphologic right atrium connects to the morphologic right ventricle and the morphologic left atrium to the morphologic left ventricle. The normal situation.
Discordant atrioventricular connection. The reverse of the above (left atrium to right ventricle, right atrium to left ventricle).
2 For lateralised atria with a univentricular atrioventricular connection; *absent (right or left) atrioventricular connection, double-inlet atrioventricular connection*.
For each of these three possibilities there are three subdivisions; the connection may be to a right ventricle, to a left ventricle or to a 'solitary, indeterminate, ventricle' (see section on ventricles below).

By absent atrioventricular connection we mean that there is no connection, or potential connection, between one atrium and a ventricle. This is the situation in most cases of 'tricuspid atresia' where sulcus tissue intervenes between the floor of the atrium and the ventricular cavity. By double inlet we mean that both AV valves, or the major portion of them (the 50% rule) connect to one ventricle. There may be, and usually is, a second 'ventricle' present but it does not receive an AV valve or receives less than 50% of one. This, rudimentary, ventricle may, however, have an outlet.
3 For isomeric (*ambiguus*) atria with a biventricular atrioventricular connection there is only one possibility; *ambiguus atrioventricular connection*. This is

because one atrium will always connect to an inappropriate ventricle. When isomeric atria connect to two separate ventricles it is necessary to describe the topology of the right ventricle (see section on ventricles below) since either right-hand or left-hand topology may be present and which is present is not, otherwise, self evident. In almost all cases with lateralised atria the topology is appropriate for the connection and need only be separately described in those (rare) cases where it is not.

For isomeric atria with a univentricular atrioventricular connection the same possibilities exist as those for lateralised atria with a univentricular atrioventricular connection (above); *double inlet, absent right or absent left (sided) atrioventricular connection*.

THE VENTRICLES

The normal right ventricle has three components; an inflow portion, an apical trabecular portion which is *coarsely* trabeculated and a smoother outflow portion. The coarse trabeculations are the angiographic hallmark of a morphologic right ventricle. In the normal heart the right ventricle can be represented by *right hand* grasping the left ventricle with the palm against the right ventricular septum. The extended thumb represents the inflow portion, the dorsum of the hand represents the trabecular portion and the fingers extend into the outflow. This pattern is referred to as right-hand topology. In some cases there is left-hand topology in which the ventricle is arranged so that a left hand with the palm against the septum will have the left thumb extended towards the inflow and the fingers towards the outflow.

A left ventricle also has an inflow, an apical trabecular and an outflow portion. The angiographic hall-mark of a left ventricle are the much finer trabeculations.

There has been much debate about what is, or is not, a ventricle [4, 5]. The debate is more concerned with definitions than disagreement about the observed facts. In the over whelming majority of cases there are two chambers within the ventricular mass but one of these chambers may lack its inflow portion, its apical trabecular portion or its outflow portion. This rudimentary chamber is most commonly of right ventricular morphology but lacks an inflow portion. In such cases the main chamber will be of left ventricular morphology and receives the

AV valve, or valves. A rudimentary right ventricle is almost always situated anteriorly but may lie to the right or the left. In a few cases the rudimentary ventricle is of left ventricular morphology and the main chamber will be a coarsely trabeculated, morphologic right, ventricle. Rudimentary left ventricles usually lack both an inflow and an outflow portion (and have therefore been termed 'a trabecular pouch'). They lie posteriorly but may be very small and difficult to detect angiographically. Rarely there may be but a single chamber of indeterminate morphology ('solitary indeterminate ventricle').

Having determined the atrial arrangement, the atrioventricular connection and the ventricular morphology the final step is to determine the ventriculo-arterial connection. The possibilities are:

1 Concordant ventriculo-arterial connection.
2 Discordant ventriculo-arterial connection.
3 Double outlet ventricle.
4 Single outlet heart.

A concordant ventriculo-arterial connection exists when the pulmonary artery arises, entirely or mostly, from the morphologic right ventricle and the aorta from the morphologic left ventricle. A discordant connection describes the opposite situation (pulmonary artery from the morphologic left ventricle, aorta from the right). Double outlet ventricle describes the situation when both, or the major portion(s) of both, great arteries arise from one ventricle. Single outlet heart is deemed to exist when only one great artery can be traced back to a ventricle. Persistent truncus arteriosus is the obvious example but in some cases of pulmonary atresia it is impossible to trace the (atretic) pulmonary artery back to one or other ventricle. In almost all cases of aortic atresia it is possible to trace a potential connection between the left ventricle and the aorta though the aortic valve is atretic. It will be seen, from the foregoing, that that atresia of a valve does not necessarily imply 'single outlet heart' or, indeed, absent atrioventricular connection. This aspect of segmental nomenclature will be discussed below.

Modes of connection

By themselves the terms concordant, discordant, double outlet and single outlet as applied to the ventriculo-arterial junction do not describe, completely, the ventriculo-arterial connection. There are a number of subsets. Thus if there are two ventricles present, each giving rise to its own great artery the connection must be concordant or discordant. If double outlet is present we have to state if the arrangement is double outlet right ventricle, double outlet left ventricle or double outlet solitary, indeterminate ventricle. Where there is override the 50% rule is invoked. The situation that obtains when there is a single outlet is more complex; theoretically there are 16 possibilities depending on whether the single great vessel is a common (aortic and pulmonary) trunk, an aortic trunk with pulmonary atresia, a pulmonary trunk with aortic atresia or a solitary trunk which cannot be identified as aortic or pulmonary (when there are no intrapericardial pulmonary arteries). To these possibilities we must add whether the trunk arises from a right, a left or a solitary ventricle or has a balanced connection to both right and left ventricles.

As if the situation were not already complex enough (though once mastered the system actually provides the simplicity inherent in any logical approach) we have yet to describe the *modes of connection* and the *spatial relationships of the heart and its component parts*.

At the atrioventricular junction there may be two patent valves, a common atrioventricular valve or an imperforate valve (right or left). In addition the valve, or valves, may straddle or override the septum. Straddling valves have a tensor apparatus (chordae) arising from both sides of the septum. This is seldom detectable by angiography (but is by echocardiography).

At the ventriculo-arterial junction the possible modes of connection are (1) two perforate valves, or (2) an imperforate (aortic or pulmonary) valve. In addition either valve may override the septum.

The flow chart (Appendix 17.1) summarises the steps involved in describing hearts with abnormal connections.

THE GREAT VEINS (Figs 17.1 to 17.22)

Normal anatomy

In the normal (*solitus*) arrangement the superior caval vein—superior vena cava—lies on the right of the spine and is formed by the junction of the two innominate veins. The left innominate (brachiocephalic) vein courses inferiorly and to the right (Fig. 17.4). The superior vena cava (SVC) receives the azygos vein from its medial and posterior aspect (Figs 17.1 and 17.2) and enters the posterior aspect of the high right atrium. The hemi-azygos vein enters the left SVC. The inferior vena cava (IVC) lies to the right of the spine and receives the hepatic veins. It has a very short intrathoracic segment before entering the posterior aspect of the low right atrium.

Congenital anomalies

In mirror-image situations (*situs inversus*) the superior and inferior caval veins lie to the left of the spine. Anomalies of systemic venous drainage are common in atrial isomerism. Interruption of the IVC with azygos continuation is characteristic of left atrial isomerism (Fig. 17.3) but interruption of the IVC can occur with lateralised atria.

The lower body may drain via a left IVC which crosses the midline to join with the hepatic veins and suprahepatic portion of the right IVC. Alternatively the IVC may continue as the azygos vein (azygos continuation) and enter the right SVC while the hepatic veins enter the right atrium directly.

Azygos continuation poses problems when right heart catheterisation has been attempted from the leg.

A 'persistent left SVC' draining to the coronary sinus is common (Fig. 17.7), there may be a right SVC as well which may (Fig. 17.8), or may not, communicate via an innominate vein. Alternatively the right SVC may be absent. A persistent left SVC must be excluded if certain corrective operations (e.g. Fontan's operation for tricuspid atresia) are being considered.

Drainage of both SVC and IVC to the left atrium occurs and, again, anomalies are common with isometric atria.

Acquired anomalies

SVC and/or IVC obstruction can result from contraction or malposition of atrial baffles (Mustard's operation for correction of transposition) and the azygos circulation may open up to allow drainage of upper or lower body blood (Figs 17.1 and 17.2).

Thrombosis of iliac veins may follow previous catheterisation and frustrate a subsequent approach from the leg (Fig. 17.2).

ATLAS-CONGENITAL CORONARY ANOMALIES

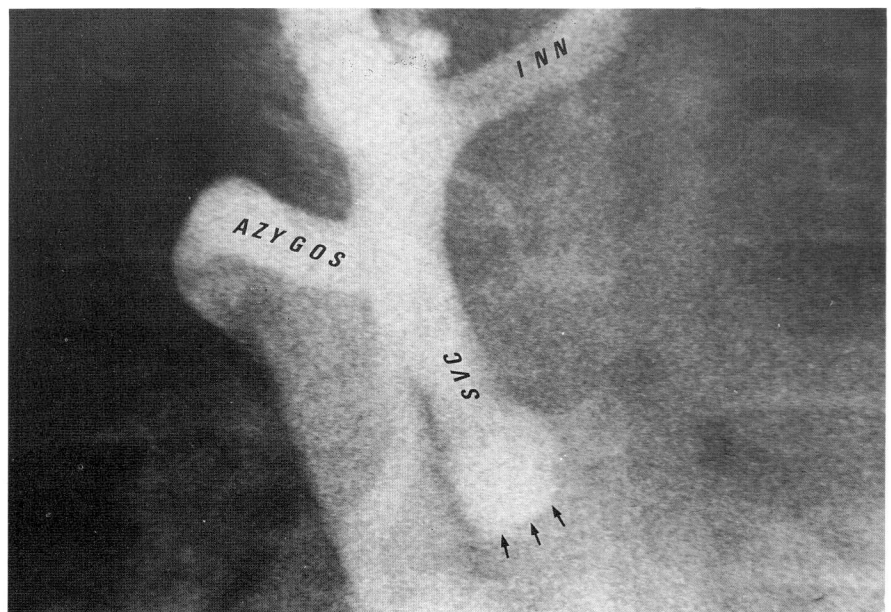

Fig. 17.1 *The systemic veins.* An injection into the Rt. subclavian vein in a patient with total occlusion of the superior vena cava following Mustard's operation (arrows) serves to show the normal arrangement of innominate vein (INN), superior vena cava (SVC) and the junction of the azygos vein with the superior vena cava. The azygos vein is dilated as it is carrying all upper-body venous return.

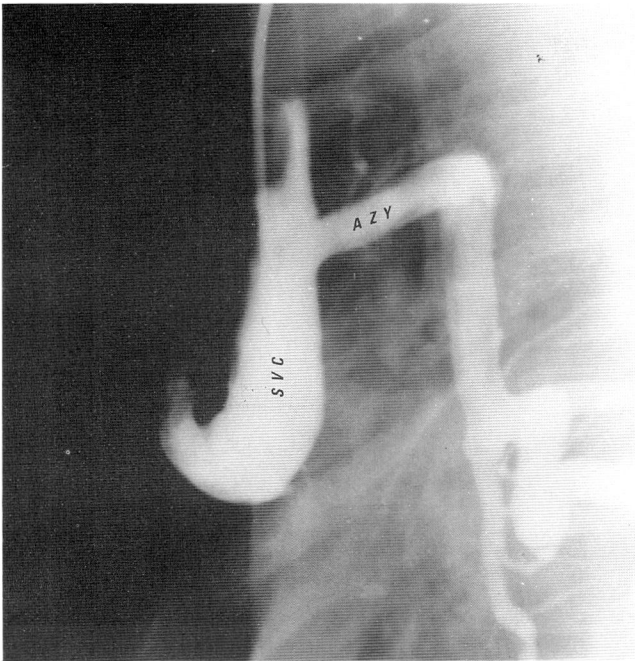

Fig. 17.2 *The systemic veins*. In another patient with superior vena caval obstruction following Mustard's operation a lateral projection demonstrates the dilated azygos vein entering the posterior aspect of the superior vena cava.

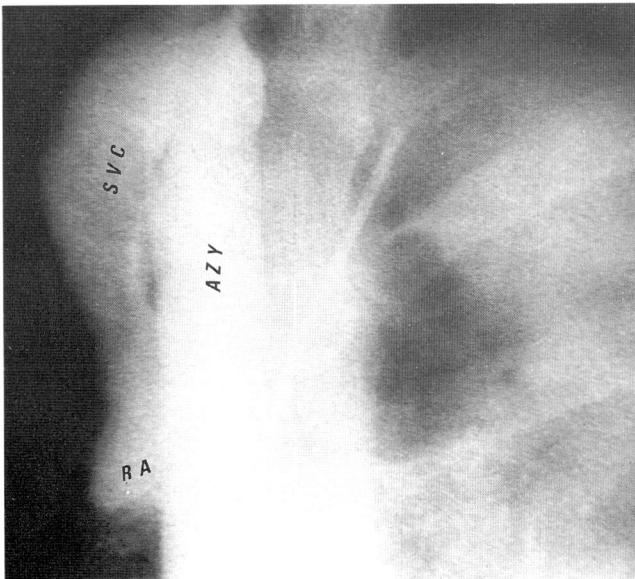

Fig. 17.3 *The systemic veins*. Azygos continuation of the inferior vena cava to the superior vena cava (SVC) (RA: right atrium). This anomaly can make right heart catheterisation difficult if the approach has been from the femoral or saphenous vein.

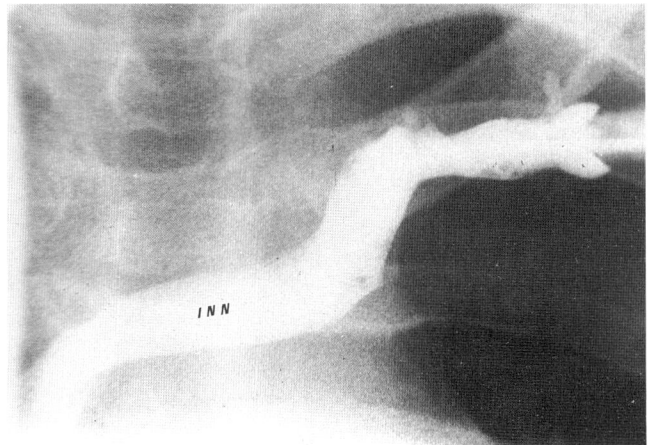

Fig. 17.4 *The systemic veins*. The normal (left) innominate vein. A venous valve is well seen.

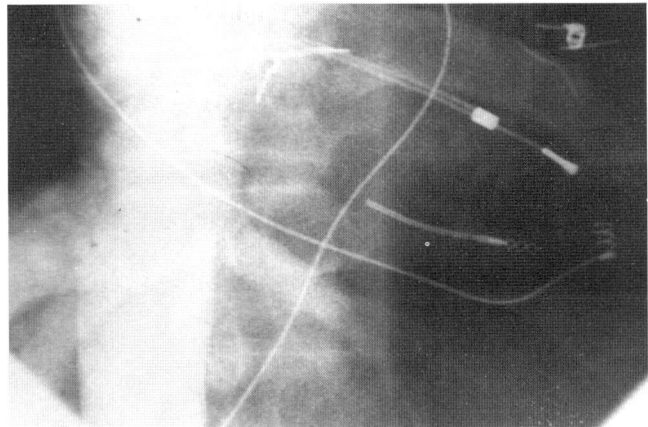

Fig. 17.5 *The systemic veins*. Normal inferior vena cava showing reflux into the hepatic veins.

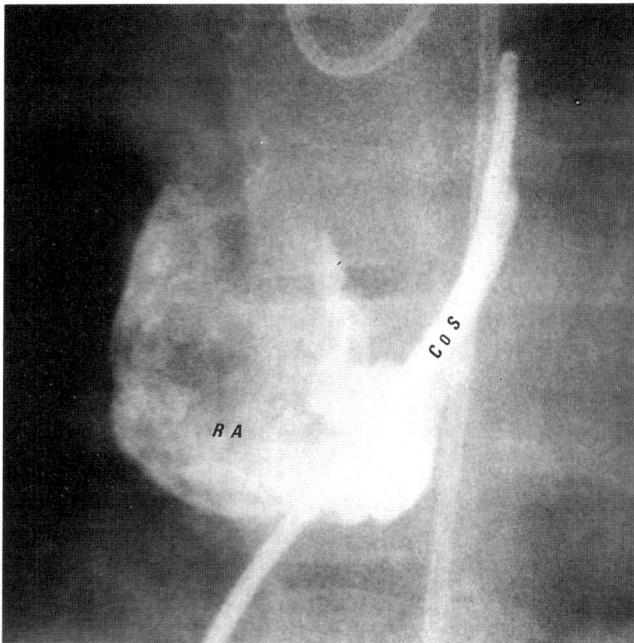

Fig. 17.6 *The systemic veins*. The normal coronary sinus (CoS) draining to the right atrium (RA).

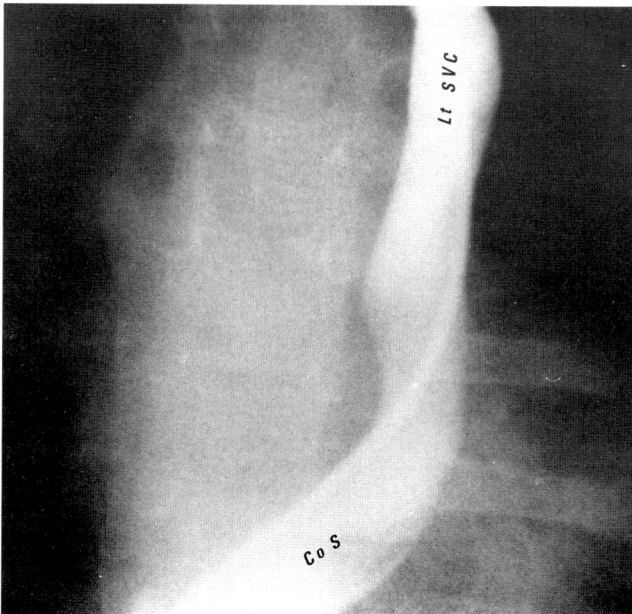

Fig. 17.8 *The systemic veins*. When both the right and left superior vena cava persist they may, as in this case, or may not be joined by an innominate vein (INN).

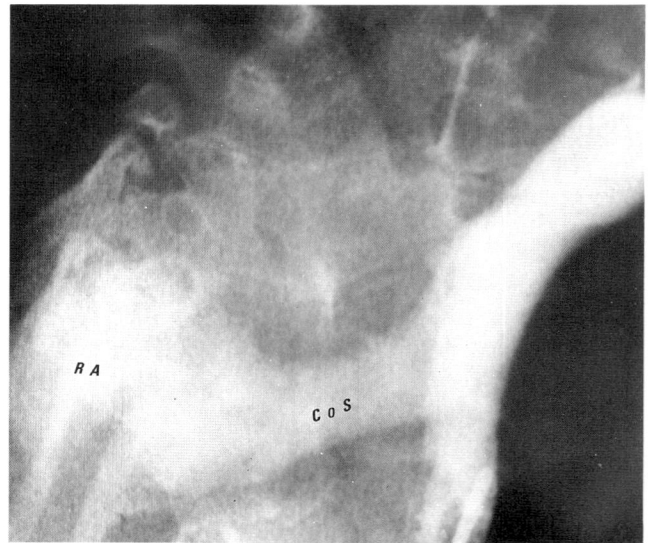

Fig. 17.7 *The systemic veins*. Persistent left superior vena cava (Lt. SVC) draining to the coronary sinus (CoS). The anomaly is not uncommon. A catheter may enter the dilated coronary sinus instead of traversing the tricuspid valve.

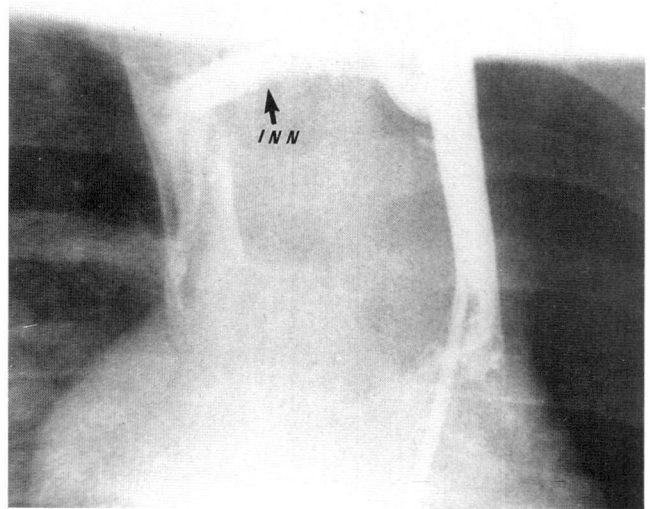

Fig. 17.9 *The systemic veins*. In this patient, with dextrocardia, a left-sided azygos vein connects with the left SVC and drains to the right atrium (RA) via the coronary sinus (CoS).

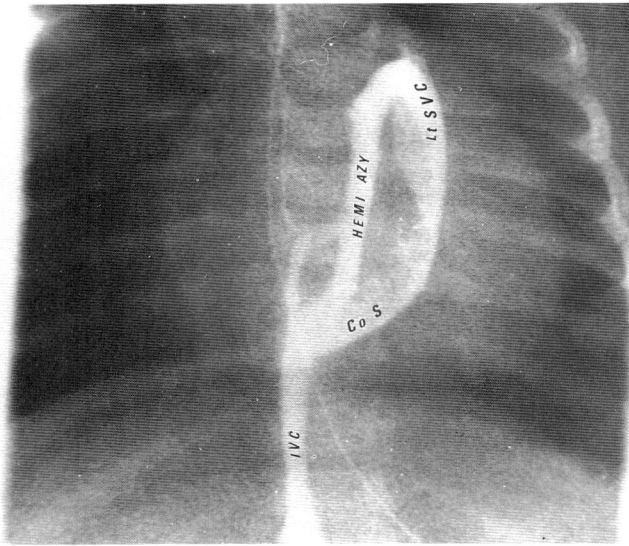

Fig. 17.10 *The systemic veins.* In this patient the inferior vena cava (IVC) crosses the midline to continue as a (left-sided) hemiazygos vein (HEMIAZY) which drains to a persistent left SVC and thence to the right atrium via the coronary sinus (CoS).

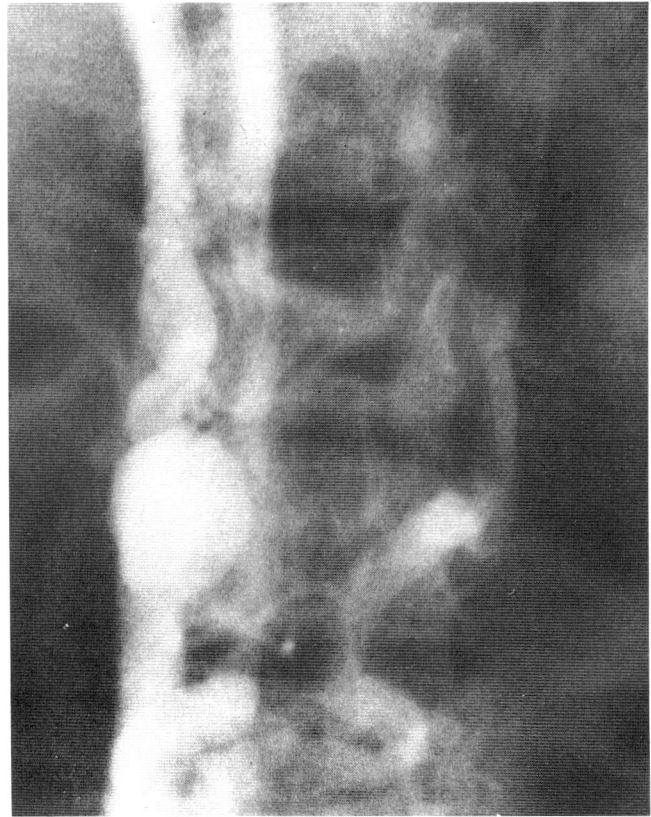

Fig. 17.12 *The systemic veins.* Obstruction to systemic venous drainage. Inferior vena caval obstruction. Lower-body systemic venous return is continued via a leash of collateral veins.

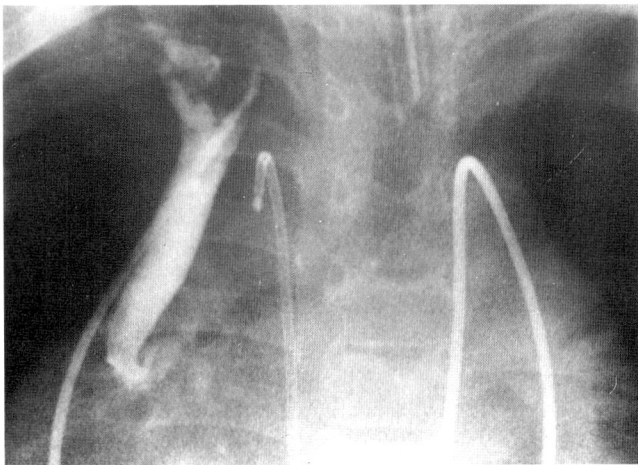

Fig. 17.11 *The systemic veins.* Anomalies of systemic venous drainage are common in cases of atrial isomerism. In this patient, with left atrial isomerism, a right-sided SVC drains to a right-sided, morphologic left, atrium. Long bilateral left bronchi — 'hyparterial bronchi' — can be seen.

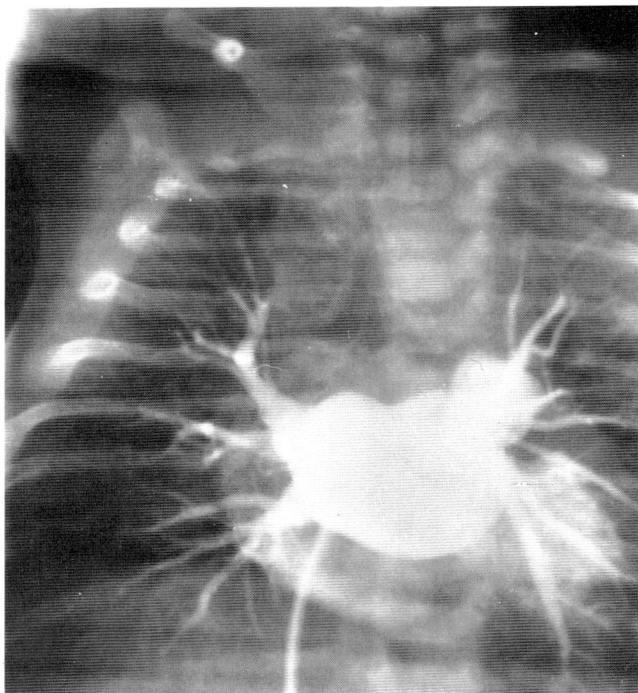

Fig. 17.13 *The pulmonary veins.* In the normal heart four pulmonary veins (right upper and lower and left upper and lower) join the posterior aspect of the left atrium — seen here as a result of reflux into the veins following injection of contrast medium into the left atrium.

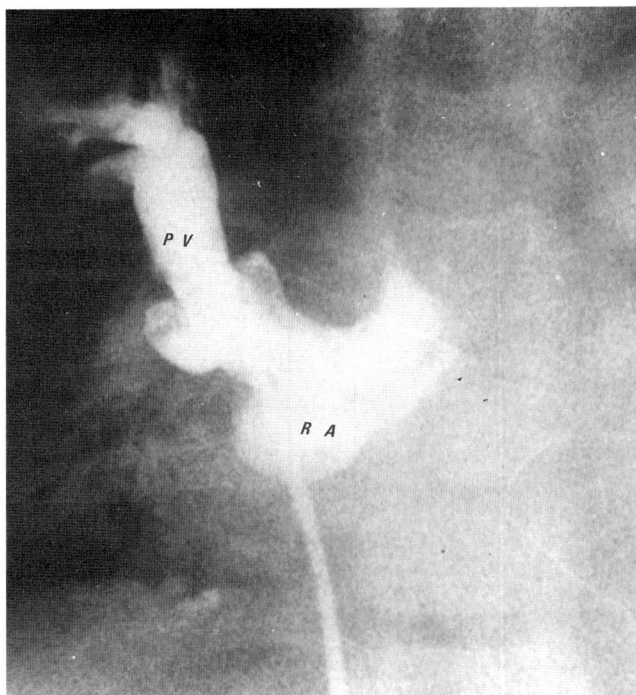

Fig. 17.14 *The pulmonary veins.* Partial anomalous pulmonary venous drainage; injection into the right upper pulmonary vein which drains to the right atrium. Commonly associated with a 'sinus venosus' type of atrial septal defect.

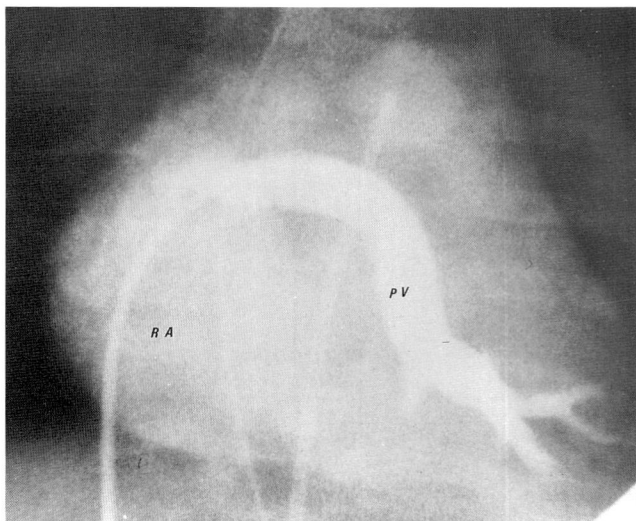

Fig. 17.15 *The pulmonary veins.* Partial anomalous pulmonary venous drainage; the left lower pulmonary vein drains to the right atrium.

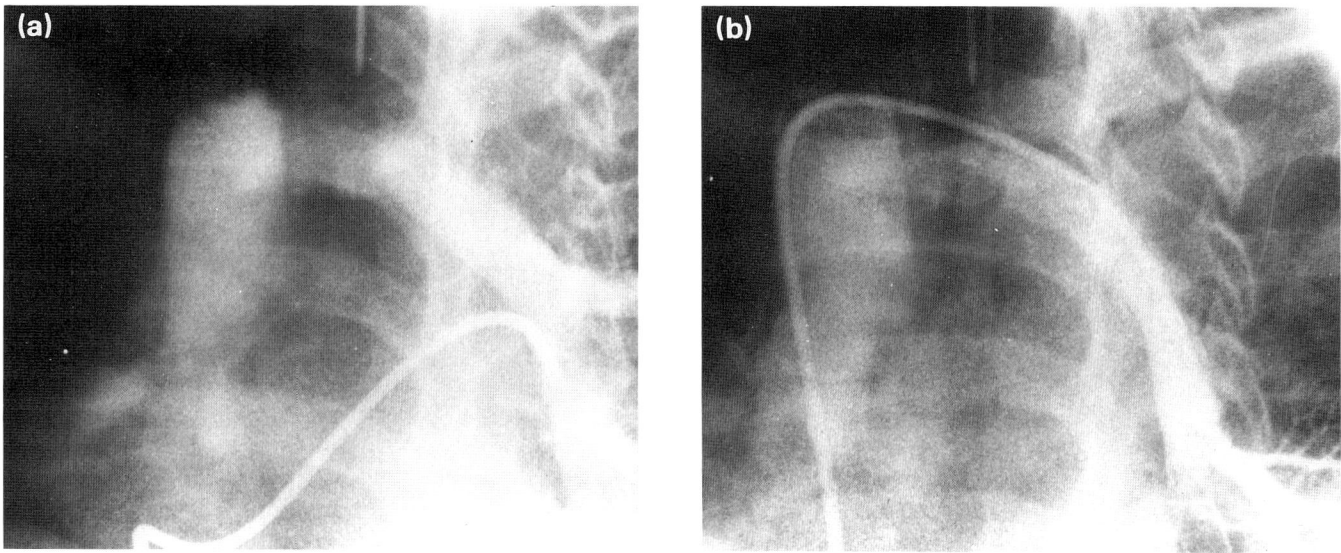

Fig. 17.16 (a) *The pulmonary veins.* When all the veins from one lung drain anomalously the condition is termed 'hemi-anomalous pulmonary venous drainage'. In this patient hemi-anomalous drainage from the left lung to the SVC is demonstrated following the injection of contrast medium into the left pulmonary artery. (b) The anomalously draining veins may also be demonstrated by injecting contrast medium into the veins directly.

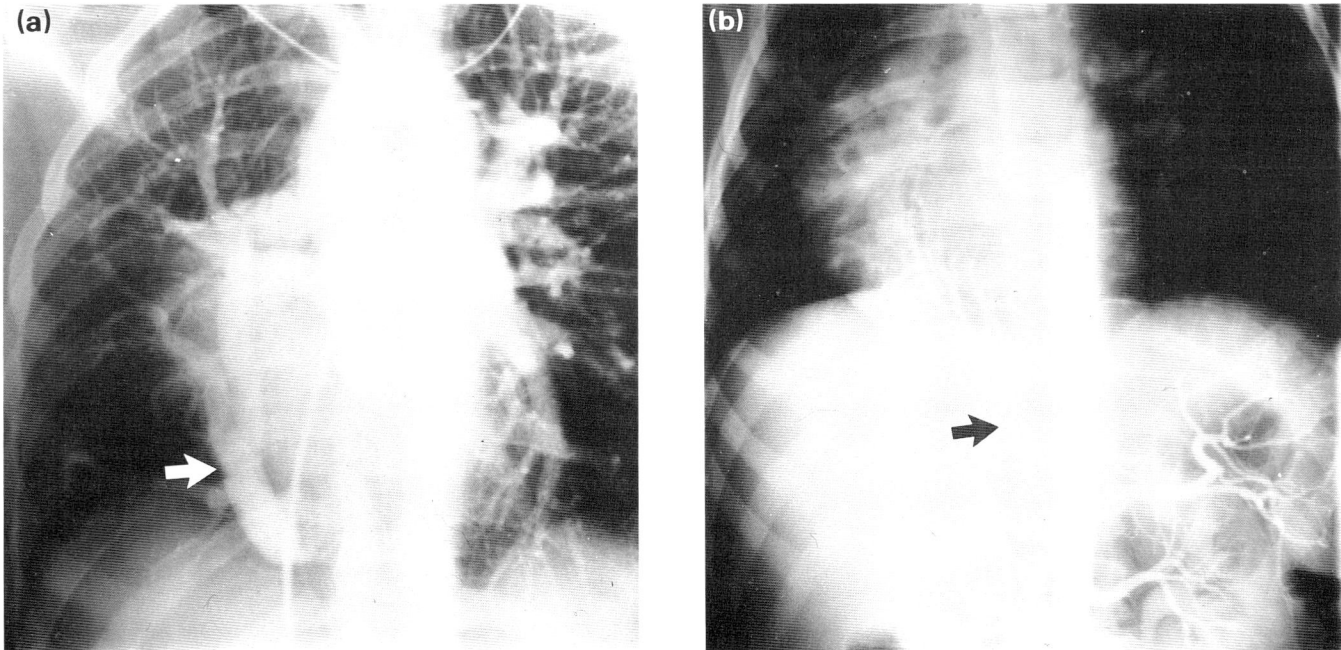

Fig. 17.17 (a) *The pulmonary veins.* So-called 'scimitar syndrome'. The right pulmonary veins (arrow) drain to the inferior vena cava making a scimitar shape which may be seen on the plain chest X-ray. (b) The scimitar syndrome is frequently associated with sequestration of a segment of lung. In the same patient an aortogram demonstrates an anomalous systemic arterial supply (arrow) to the sequestered segment.

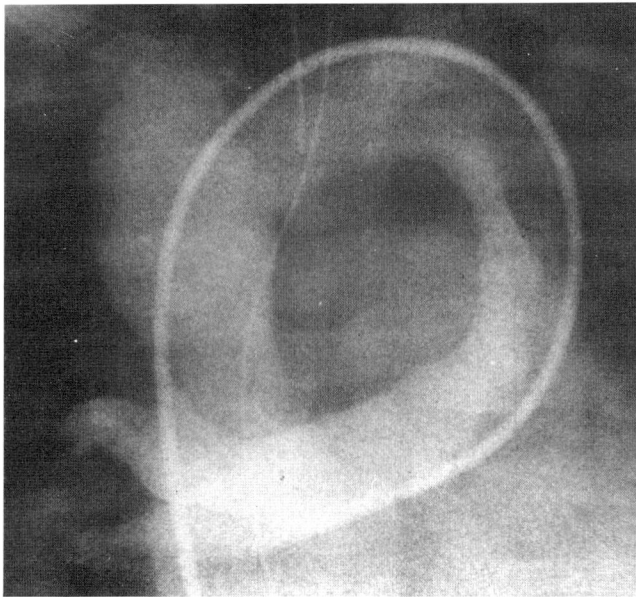

Fig. 17.18 *The pulmonary veins.* When all the veins from both lungs drain to the right side of the heart the condition is known as 'total anomalous pulmonary venous drainage' (or 'return') — TAPVD (or TAPVR). In this example of 'supracardiac TAPVD' the veins from both lungs join to form a 'vertical vein' which communicates with the left innominate vein and thence to the SVC and right atrium. The anomalously draining veins may be demonstrated by injecting them directly or following an injection of contrast medium into the pulmonary artery.

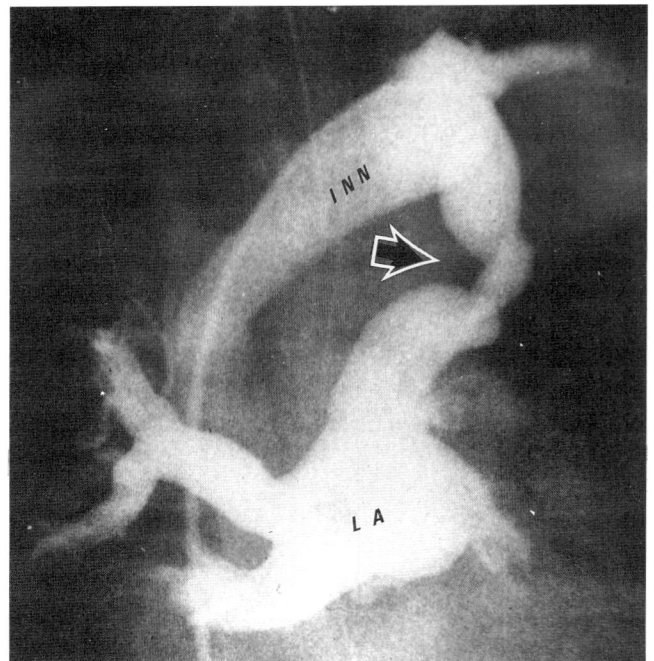

Fig. 17.19 *The pulmonary veins.* An unusual example of 'supracardiac TAPVD'. The catheter has traversed the innominate (INN) and vertical veins but the injection has been made into the left atrium (LA). There is mitral atresia and the vertical vein provides the only route of egress of pulmonary vein blood from the left atrium. Obstruction to pulmonary venous return can occur at the point where the left main bronchus crosses the vertical vein (arrow).

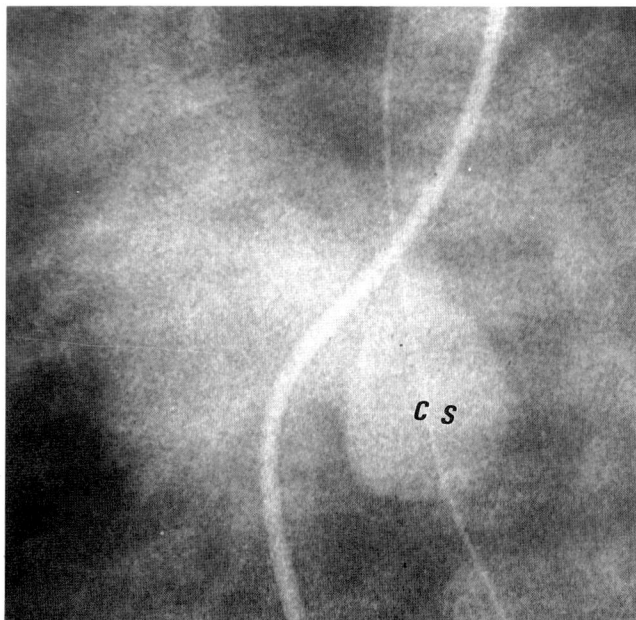

Fig. 17.20 *The pulmonary veins.* Total anomalous pulmonary venous drainage may be at 'cardiac level' — the veins drain directly to the right atrium or to the coronary sinus. In this patient the venous phase of a pulmonary arteriogram has resulted in opacification of a dilated coronary sinus (CS); the site of pulmonary venous drainage.

Fig. 17.21 *The pulmonary veins.* Anomalous pulmonary venous drainage may be 'mixed'. In this patient some of the pulmonary veins drain directly to the right atrium but a large coronary sinus (CS) has also opacified as other veins drain to this site.

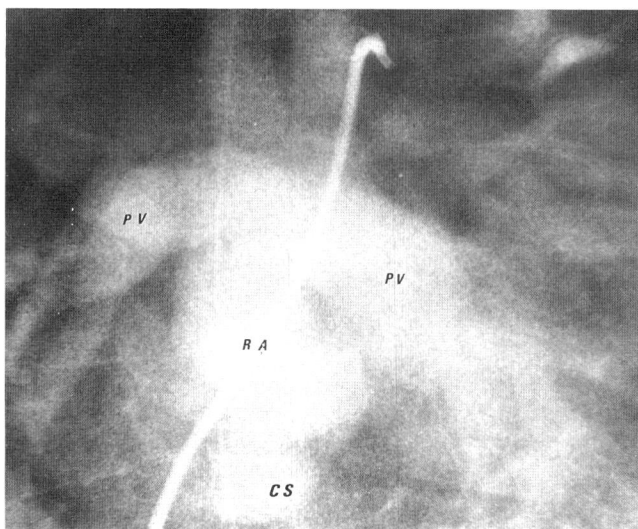

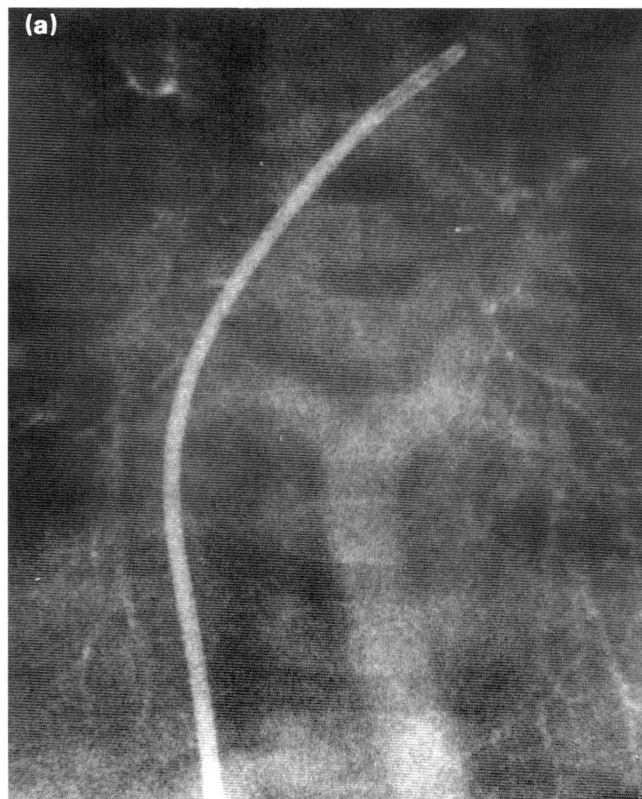

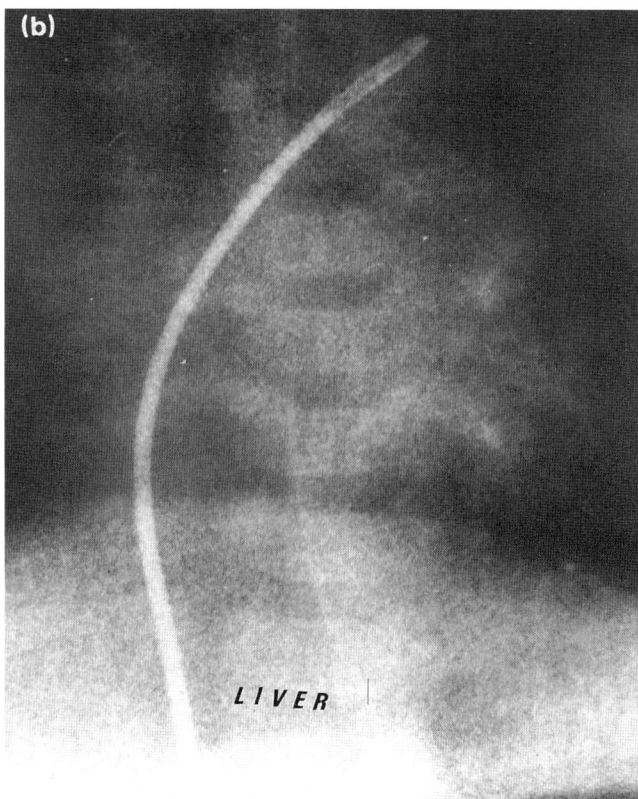

Fig. 17.22 (a) *The pulmonary veins.* Obstructed pulmonary venous drainage is the rule when all the veins drain below the diaphragm ('infradiaphragmatic TAPVD') and join the hepatic or portal veins. The injection has been made into the pulmonary artery. As a result of obstruction to pulmonary venous return flow is slow and filming has to continue for several seconds until the anomalously draining vein is seen forming a Y-shaped shadow and draining below the diaphragm. In the same patient later films (b) show diffuse opacification of the liver indicating that pulmonary venous drainage was to the portal system. Compare with (a) in which the liver is not yet opacified.

THE ATRIA (Figs 17.23 to 17.31)

In most patients atrial position (*situs*) reflects the position of the abdominal organs; the right atrium and liver on the right and the left atrium and stomach air bubble on the left in normal *situs* (*situs solitus*) and the reverse in *situs inversus*. But this is not always the case; moreover in patients with atrial isomerism there is visceral symmetry and the position of the abdominal organs is of little help in determining atrial situs. Fortunately atrial situs almost always reflects bronchial morphology [6, 7]. The morphologically *left* main bronchus is much longer than the *right* and passes *beneath* the artery to the lower lobe (so-called 'hyparterial bronchus') while the *right* main bronchus is shorter and courses *above* the lower lobe artery ('eparterial bronchus').

Bronchial morphology may be determined from the plain chest X-ray but is more easily determined from a penetrated chest X-ray [8] or (in case of doubt) from bronchial tomography.

In left atrial isomerism there will be bilateral left (long, hyparterial), bronchi (Fig. 17.11) and bilateral right (short, eparterial) bronchi in right atrial isomerism. In *situs inversus* atrial and bronchial *situs* is reversed.

The morphologic right atrium is distinguished from the left atrium by having a triangular appendage with a broad base (Fig. 17.23); the left atrial appendage has a narrow ostium and is angulated first superiorly and then inferiorly (Figs 17.24 and 17.25). In a normal right atrial angiogram the hepatic veins will be filled.

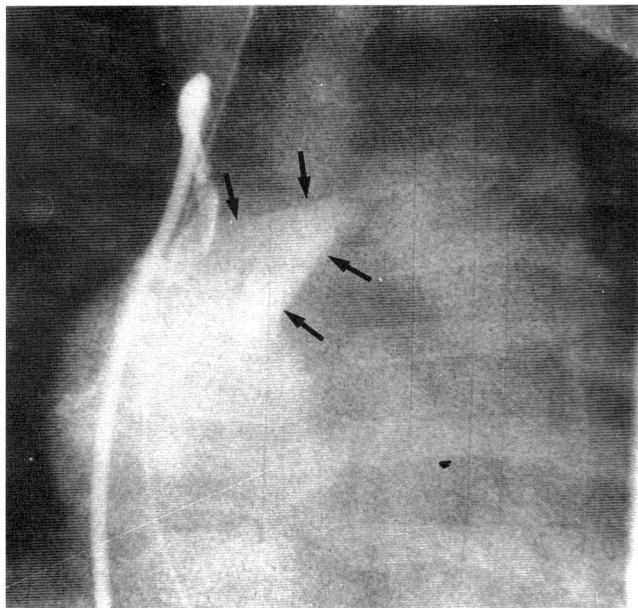

Fig. 17.23 *The atria.* Right atrial appendage (arrows). A triangular structure with a wide base and a wide opening into the atrium.

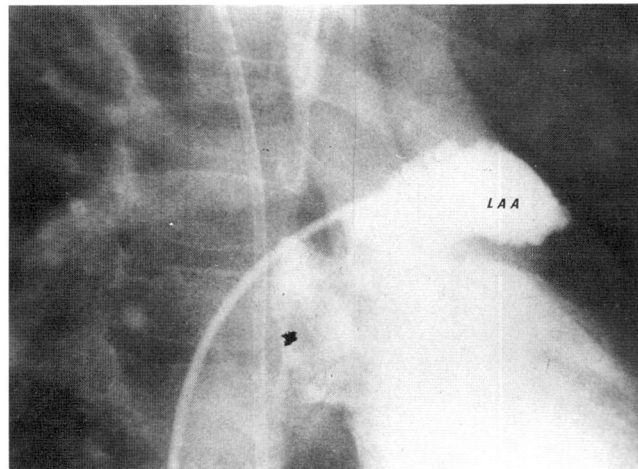

Fig. 17.24 *The atria.* The left atrial appendage (LAA) is a finger-like extension with a narrow opening into the atrium.

Fig. 17.25 *The atria.* The morphology of the atrial appendages allows the atria to be identified even when their position is abnormal. In this patient the morphologic left atrium is to the right and there is complex congenital heart disease and dextrocardia (apex to the right); nonetheless the finger-like left atrial appendage is easily identified and establishes the site of injection as being into a morphologic left atrium.

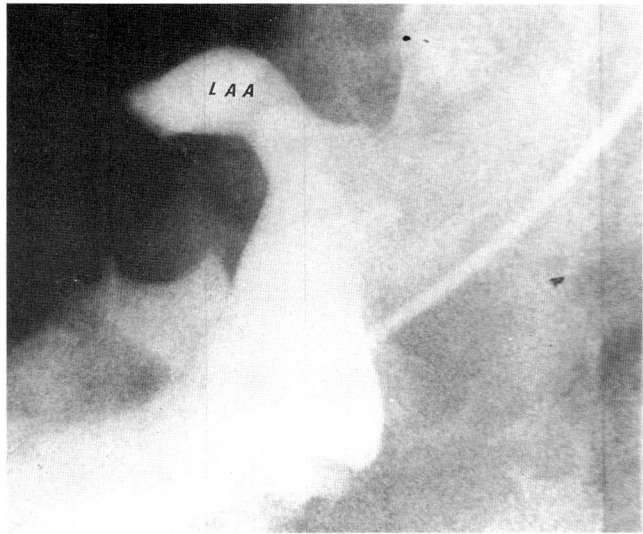

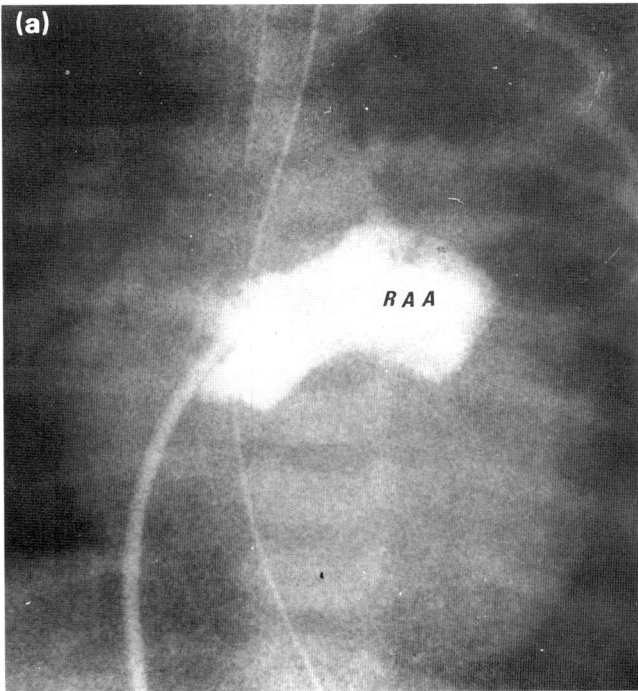

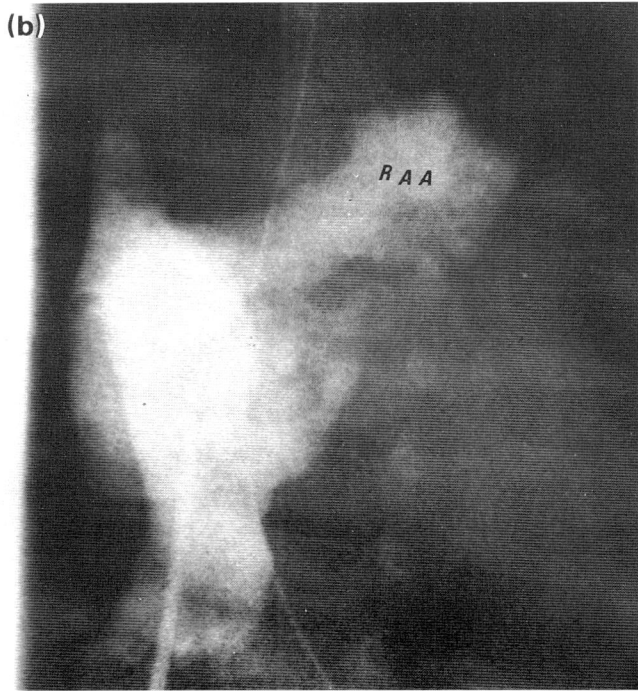

Fig. 17.26 (a) *The atria.* Rarely both atrial appendages may lie to the same side of the great vessels — juxtaposition of the atrial appendages. In these two examples the right atrial appendage lies to the left ('left juxtaposition') and beside the left atrial appendage (not seen). Right juxtaposition also occurs but is very rare. Juxtaposition of the atrial appendages is often associated with other congenital cardiac anomalies as in (b) where there is also tricuspid atresia.

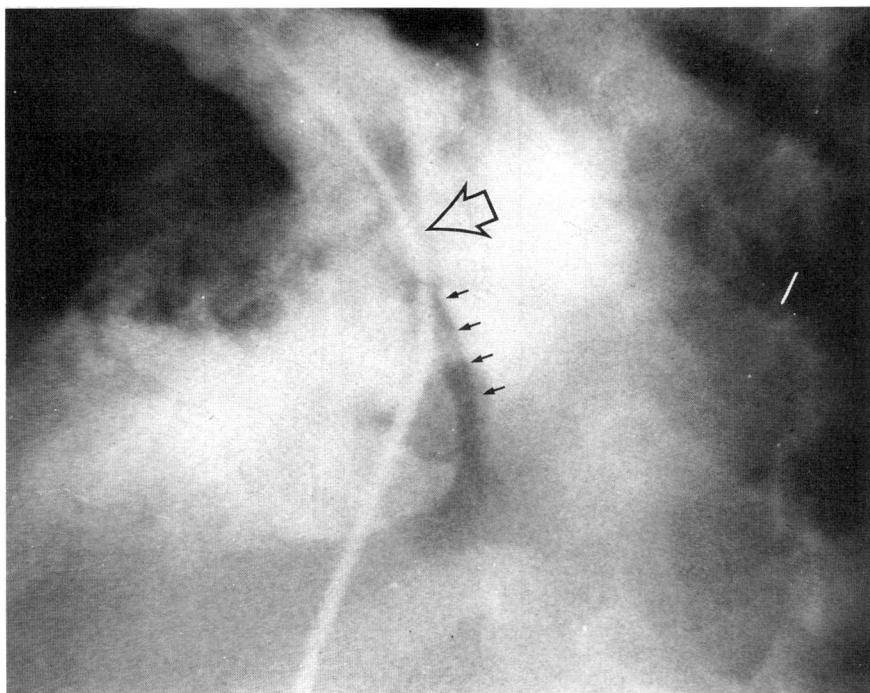

Fig. 17.27 *Atrial septal defects*. An injection into the right upper pulmonary vein while filming in the four chamber projection will profile the atrial septum. In this patient contrast medium has crossed a septum secundum defect (large arrow) — as has the catheter. The lower portion of the atrial septum is profiled (small arrows) and is intact thus establishing the fact that the defect is of a secundum type and excluding a septum primum defect.

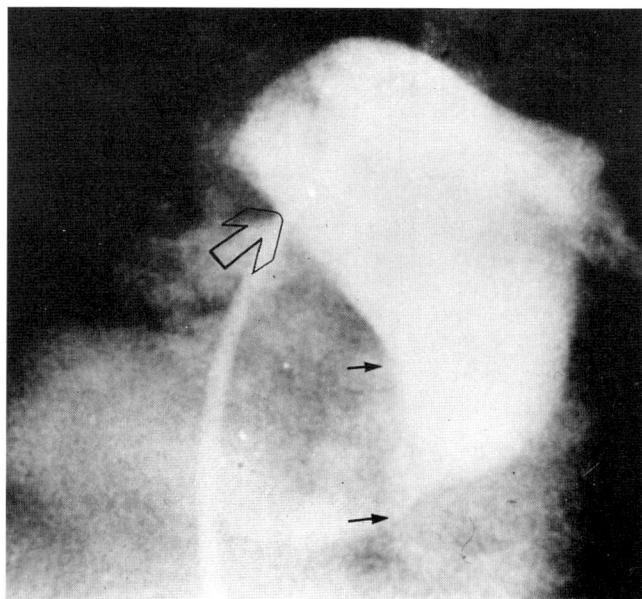

Fig. 17.28 *The atria*. The catheter has crossed a small septum secundum defect (large arrow) and contrast medium injected into the left atrium. Contrast medium is seen crossing the lower part of the atrial septum between the two small arrows and there is no atrial septum visible below. The appearances are those of a septum primum defect (atrioventricular septal defect); the patient has both a secundum and a primum defect.

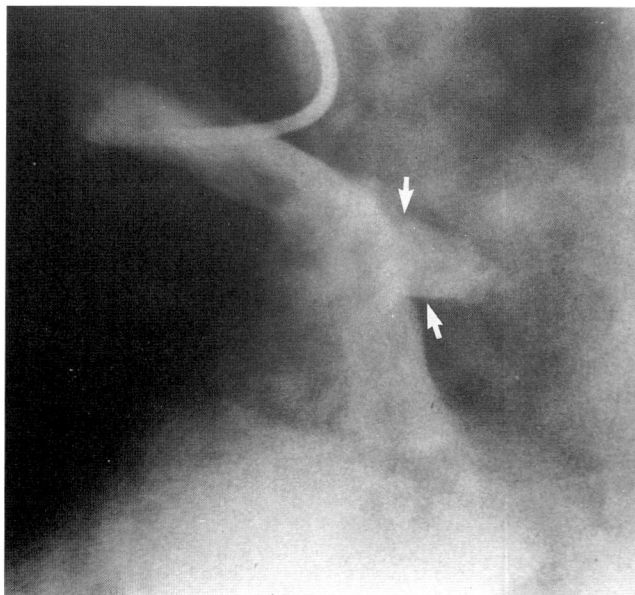

Fig. 17.29 *Atrial septal defects*. Contrast medium has been injected into the right upper pulmonary vein which drains anomalously to the right atrium. A little contrast medium has outlined a high defect — sinus venosus atrial septal defect (arrows). Anomalous drainage of the right upper pulmonary vein and sinus venosus defect are commonly associated.

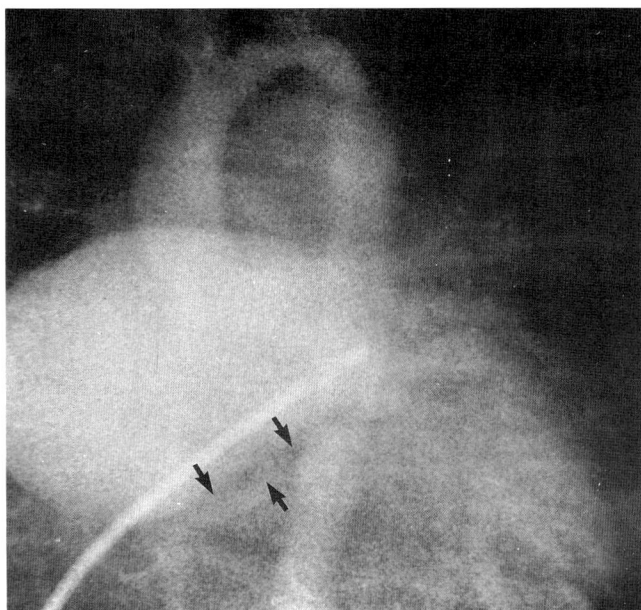

Fig. 17.30 *The atria.* Supravalve stenosing ring of the left atrium seen as a linear filling defect between the arrows. The appearances of Cor triatriatum are similar.

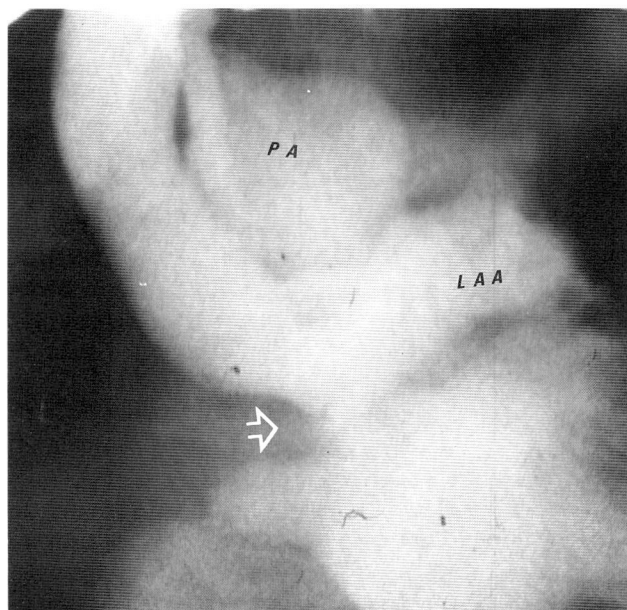

Fig. 17.31 *The atria.* Mustard's operation for complete transposition of the great arteries. Contrast medium has been injected into the superior vena cava. There is opacification of the left atrial appendage (LAA) and left atrium as well as the left ventricle and pulmonary artery (PA). The filling defect due to the baffle (arrow) is seen and there is some reflux of contrast medium into the inferior vena cava.

THE ATRIOVENTRICULAR JUNCTION AND VALVES (Figs 17.32 to 17.42)

The atrioventricular connection — concordant, discordant, ambiguus, absence of one connection or double-inlet ventricle — together with the *mode* of connection — straddling and overriding valves and so on — is most easily determined by cross-sectional echocardiography. Angiographically the atrioventricular connection may be demonstrated following an injection of contrast medium into the atria or by seeing unopacified blood washing out contrast medium from a ventricular injection during diastole. Only a few of the many possible abnormalities of the atrioventricular junction can be illustrated in this, non-specialised atlas.

The angiographic study of atrioventricular septal defects involves answering several questions:

1 Are there separate right and left atrioventricular valve orifices or is there a common atrioventricular valve orifice? The difference depends on whether there is or is not a connecting tongue between the anterior and posterior bridging leaflets (see Fig. 17.38).

2 Is there an interventricular defect (VSD)? The deficiency in the upper part of the ventricular septum is present in all patients with atrioventricular septal defects whether or not there is a VSD. If the atrioventricular valves are attached directly to the crest of the septum there will be no interventricular component to the defect. If the valves are free-floating or attached by chordae to the crest of the septum there will be an interventricular component which may be seen to be crossed by chordae. Since the defect is in the posterior, inlet, portion of the ventricular septum the presence, or absence, of a VSD is best determined by left ventriculography in the 'four chamber' view (Fig. 17.41).

3 Is the (partitioned or common) AV valve equally committed to the right and left ventricle or does it communicate mainly with one or other ventricle? If the valve(s) communicate mainly with one ventricle

(e.g. the right) the other ventricle will be hypoplastic (e.g. 'right dominance').

4 Is there AV valve regurgitation? Mitral regurgitation may occur — often at the site of the cleft between the anterior and posterior bridging leaflets. A left ventriculogram may result in opacification of the left atrium but the regurgitant jet is frequently directed through the cleft into the lower part of the right atrium; best seen in the four chamber view.

5 Finally there may be subaortic stenosis and atrioventricular septal defects can exist in association with other congenital cardiac malformations (e.g. tetralogy of Fallot).

The defect in the lower part of the atrial septum can be visualised in the four chamber view if contrast medium is injected into the left atrium or right upper pulmonary vein (see Fig. 17.28).

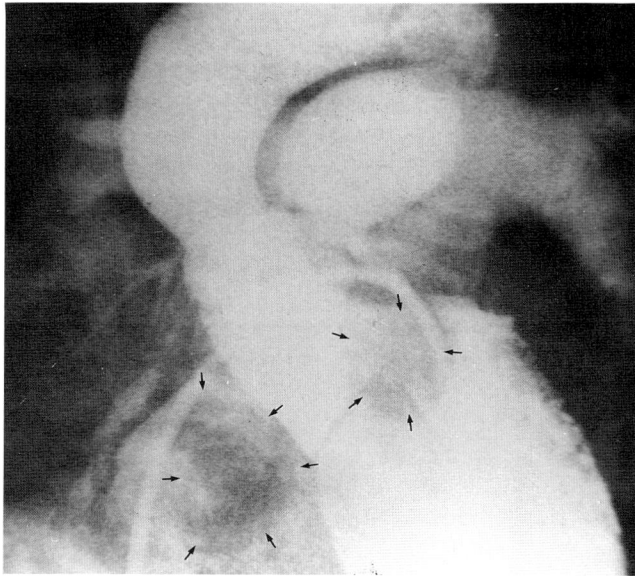

Fig. 17.32 *The AV junction and valves.* Left ventricular angiogram (four chamber view) in a patient with a ventricular septal defect resulting in opacification of both right and left ventricles. Normally connected (concordant) right (tricuspid) and left (mitral) AV valves are outlined by unopacified blood (arrows) during ventricular diastole.

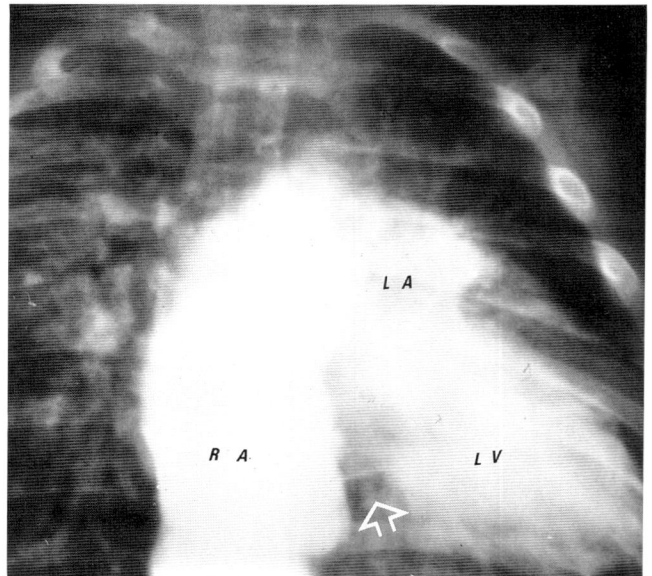

Fig. 17.33 *The AV junction and valves.* Absent (right) atrioventricular connection (tricuspid atresia). Contrast medium injected into the right atrium (RA) has opacified, in turn, the left atrium (LA) and left ventricle (LV). There is no potential communication between the right atrium and ventricle resulting in a filling defect (window) in the position normally occupied by the tricuspid valve (arrow).

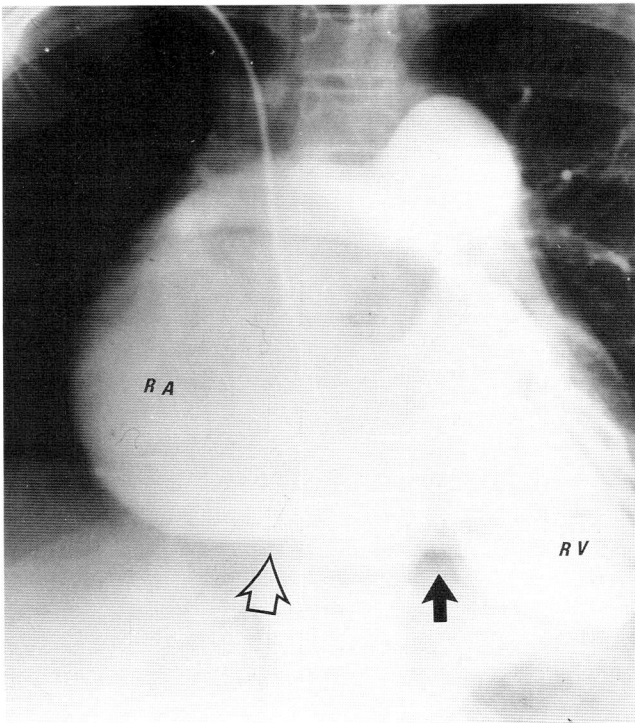

Fig. 17.34 *The AV junction and valves.* Ebstein's anomaly of the tricuspid valve. The true atrioventricular junction is marked by an inferior indentation (open arrow). A second, more distal, indentation marks the point of attachment of the tricuspid valve (solid arrow) which is displaced into the right ventricle. The area between is smoothly trabeculated and represents the 'atrialised' portion of the right ventricle. Often a thin, linear filling defect is seen crossing the ventricle and representing the valve leaflets. In this patient the right atrium has opacified following injection of contrast medium into the ventricle indicating severe AV (tricuspid) valve regurgitation.

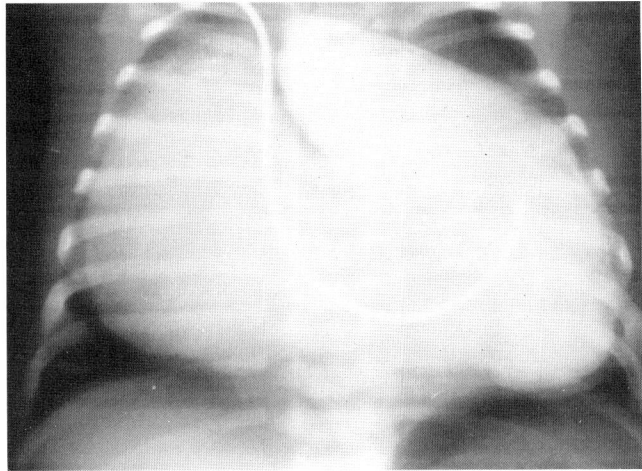

Fig. 17.35 *The AV junction and valves.* Congenital anomalies of the right atrioventricular valve can produce gross cardiac enlargement. In this neonate there is right ventricular outflow atresia and a dysplastic tricuspid valve with gross tricuspid regurgitation.

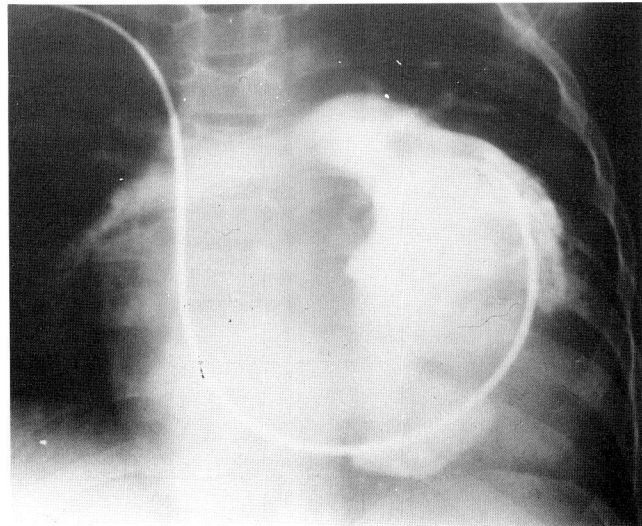

Fig. 17.36 *The AV junction and valves.* A similar appearance to that shown in Fig. 17.35 produced by congenital absence of the tricuspid valve. (In this case there is a patent pulmonary valve and right ventricular — pulmonary arterial continuity.)

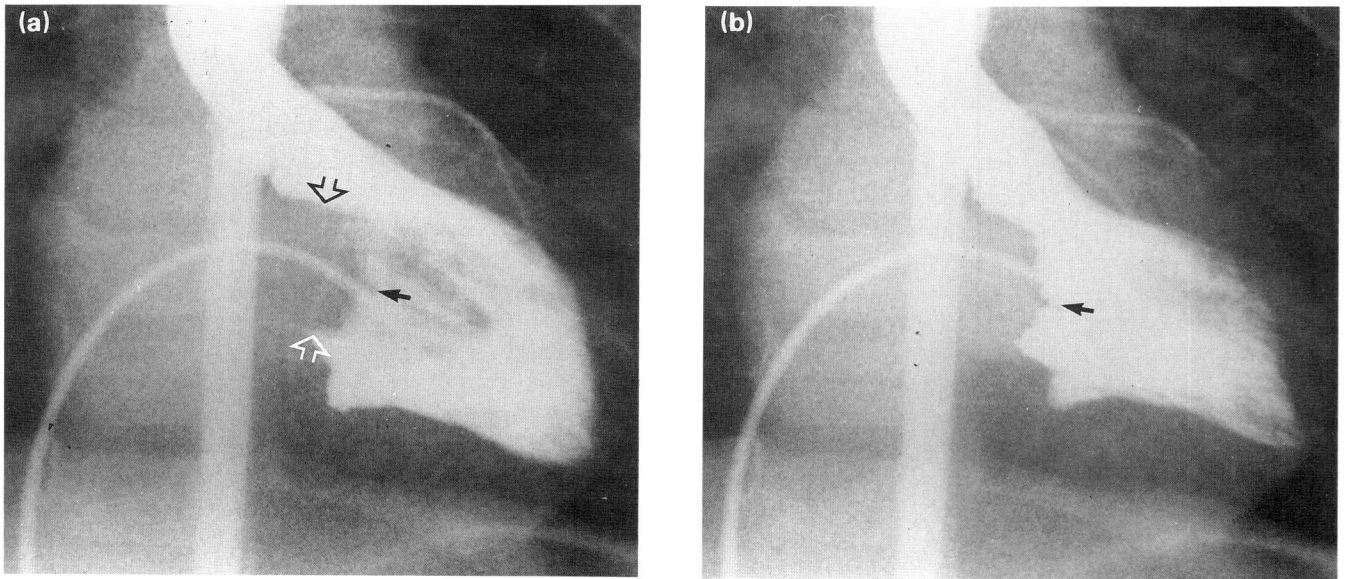

Fig. 17.37 *AV septal defects.* The angiographic hall-mark of atrioventricular septal defects ('primum ASD', 'endocardial cushion defects', 'partial' and 'complete AV canal') is the goose-neck deformity of the left ventricle. This is best seen in an anteroposterior projection. This appearance results from the abnormal insertion of the left AV valve and a disparity between the lengths of the inlet and outlet septa. In the normal heart the distance from the mitral valve insertion to the apex is roughly the same as that from the aortic valve to the apex. In atrioventricular septal defects the length of the inlet septum from the AV valve insertion to the apex is less than that of the outlet septum from the apex to the aortic valve. The left ventricular outlet thus appears elongated. (a) During ventricular diastole unopacified blood is entering the ventricle between the superior (or anterior) bridging leaflet (black open arrow) and the inferior (or posterior) bridging leaflet (white open arrow). The elongated outlet and the disproportion between inlet and outlet septa resulting in the gooseneck deformity is well seen. (b) Ventricular systole. The valve presents a 'scalloped' appearance between points of chordal attachment to the crest of the septum. The so-called cleft is indicated by a small arrow in both figures and represents the point of apposition between the anterior and posterior bridging leaflets.

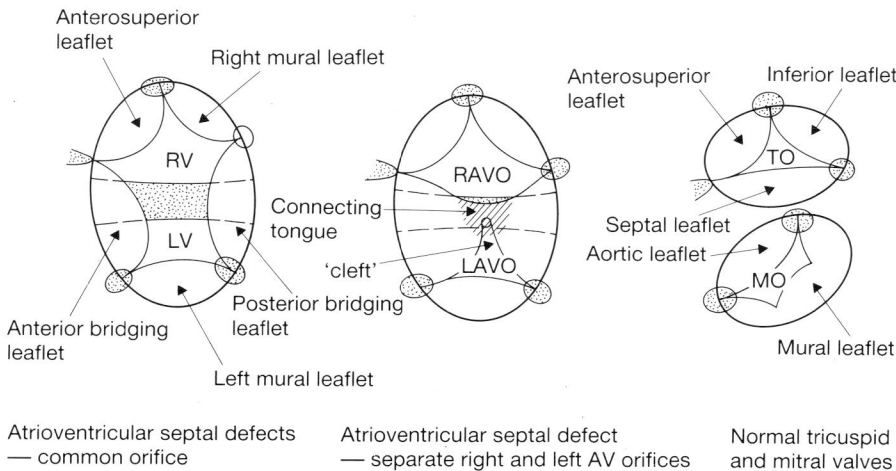

Atrioventricular septal defects — common orifice

Atrioventricular septal defect — separate right and left AV orifices

Normal tricuspid and mitral valves

Fig. 17.38 *AV septal defects.* The morphology of the atrioventricular valves is illustrated in this diagram. (Reproduced with permission from Becker AE, Anderson RH. Atrioventricular septal defects: what's in a name? *J. Thoracic Cardiovasc Surg* 1982;**83**:461). RAVO: right atrioventricular orifice; LAVO: left atrioventricular orifice; TO: tricuspid orifice; MO: mitral orifice.

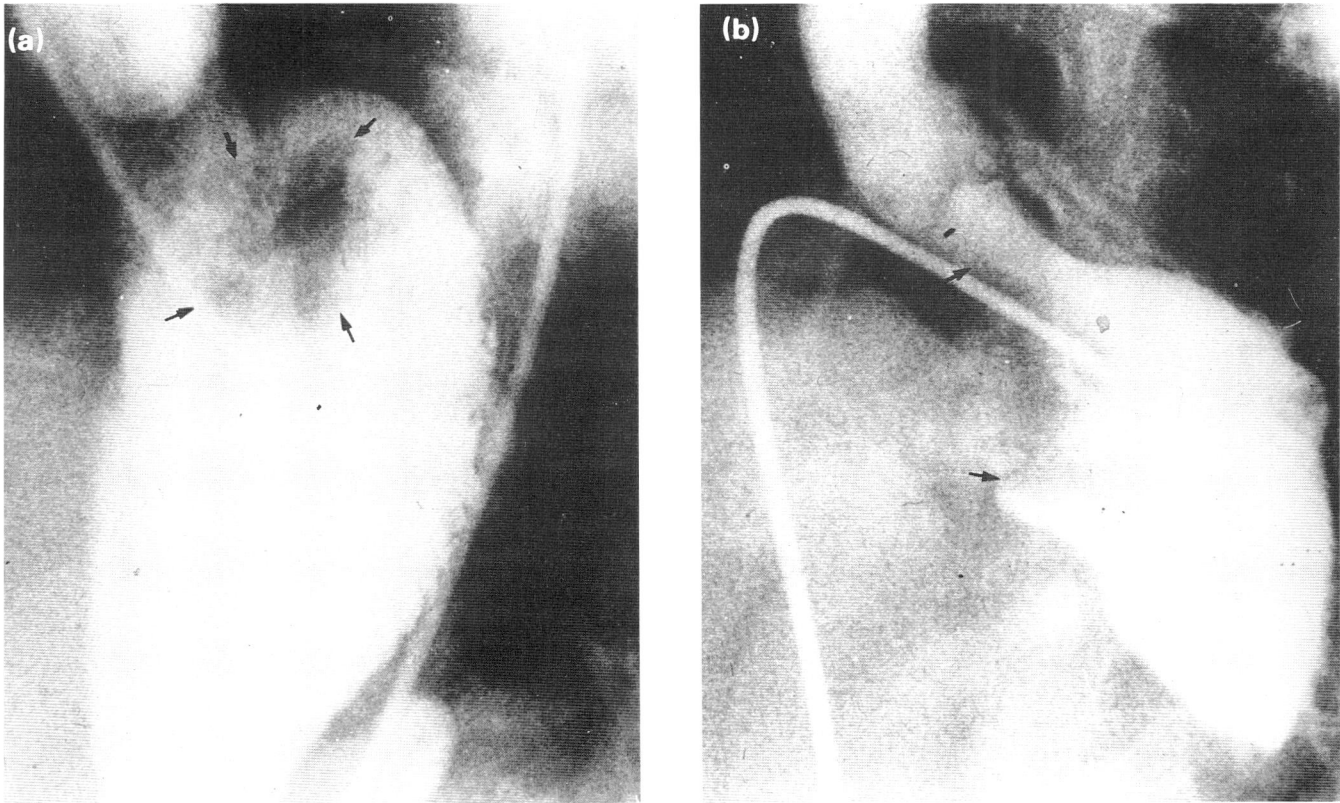

Fig. 17.39 Elongated left oblique view of a left ventriculogram in a normal heart (a) compared with a patient with an atrioventricular septal defect (b). The left atrioventricular valve is outlined by unopacified blood entering the ventricle during diastole (arrows). In (b) the abnormal insertion of the mitral valve results in unopacified blood entering the ventricle from above and *in front* instead of from above and *behind* as in the normal heart.

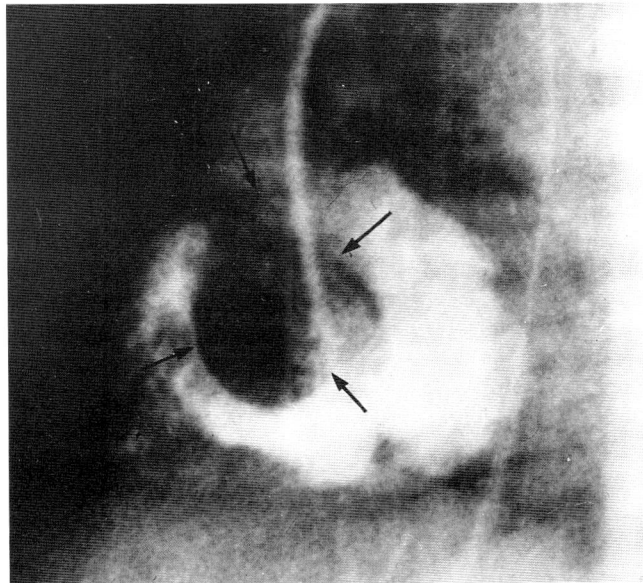

Fig. 17.40 A common atrioventricular valve is most easily recognised by left ventriculography in the long axis or four chamber view. The valve is outlined by unopacified blood (arrows).

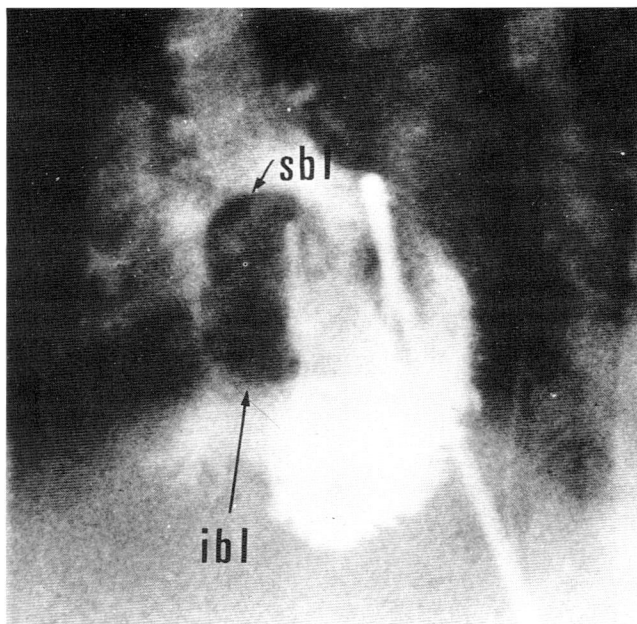

Fig. 17.41 *AV septal defect.* Complete AV canal. Left ventriculogram in four chamber view. A ventricular septal defect is seen beneath the inferior bridging leaflet (ibl).

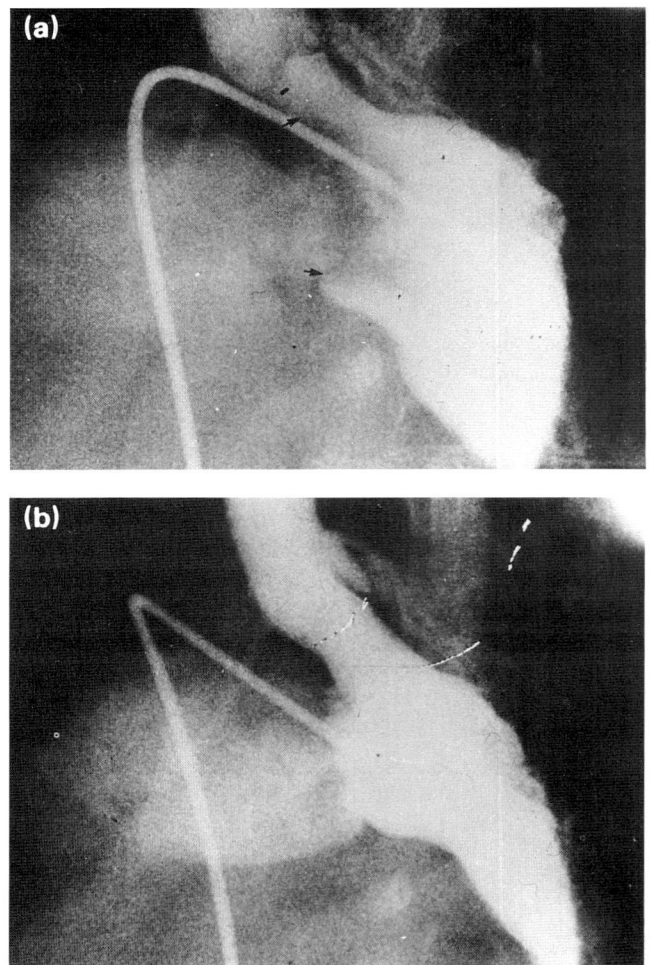

Fig. 17.42 Left ventriculogram in a patient with atrioventricular septal defect: (a) diastole, and (b) systole. Atrial opacification has occurred in (b) indicating left atrioventricular (mitral) valve regurgitation.

THE VENTRICLES (Figs 17.43 to 17.78)

The left and right ventricles are most easily distinguised by their trabeculation; left ventricular trabeculation is fine giving it a smooth outline while the right ventricle is coarsely trabeculated.

The *left* ventricle is hypoplastic in mitral atresia; since this condition is usually seen in conjunction with aortic atresia (see the section on the aorta; Figs 20.11 and 20.12) as part of the hypoplastic left heart syndrome the slit-like left ventricle is not demonstrable angiographically.

Ventricular septal defect

The ventricular septum is composed of a small membranous and a large muscular component. The muscular septum can be divided into inlet, trabecular and outlet portions. Ventricular septal defects (Fig. 17.55) may be:

1 Perimembranous; defects related to the central fibrous body and roofed by the aortic valve but which may extend into the inlet, trabecular or outlet septa. Some 80% of ventricular septal defects are of this type.

2 Muscular; defects which are completely surrounded by muscle and which may be found in the inlet, trabecular or outlet septa.

3 Subarterial; defects due to a defect in the infundibular septum and roofed by the pulmonary and aortic valves ('doubly-committed').

The angiographic demonstration of ventricular septal defects

1 Left ventriculography must be performed using a cranially orientated projection to avoid foreshortening of the ventricular septum which is directed anteriorly as well as to the left, (see Chapter 7).

2 Defects which lie posteriorly, in the inlet septum, require steep (45°) cranial angulation but only a shallow (25°) left oblique projection (the fourchamber view). Perimembranous defects extending into the more anterior trabecular and outlet septa are profiled using a less steep cranial angulation (25°) but require a steeper (75°) left oblique projection (the long axis view). Subarterial defects are the most anterior of all and may be profiled by a left lateral or elongated right oblique projection.

3 Perimembranous defects will be seen to be roofed, to a greater or lesser degree, by the right and non-coronary aortic valve cusps. Muscular defects will be separated from the arterial valves by a portion of the ventricular septum. Subarterial defects are roofed by the aortic and pulmonary valves.

4 The sequence of opacification of the right ventricle provides a clue to the position of a ventricular septal defect. When the defect extends into the inlet septum contrast medium first opacifies the inlet portion of the right ventricle beneath the septal leaflet of the tricuspid valve. Defects involving the trabecular septum will first opacify the trabecular portion of the right ventricle and not, initially, the region of the tricuspid valve. Subarterial defects first opacify the outlet portion of the right ventricle beneath the pulmonary valve.

Left ventricular outflow tract obstruction (subaortic stenosis) is illustrated with aortic valve lesions in Chapter 15. Hypertrophic cardiomyopathy is discussed in Chapter 16.

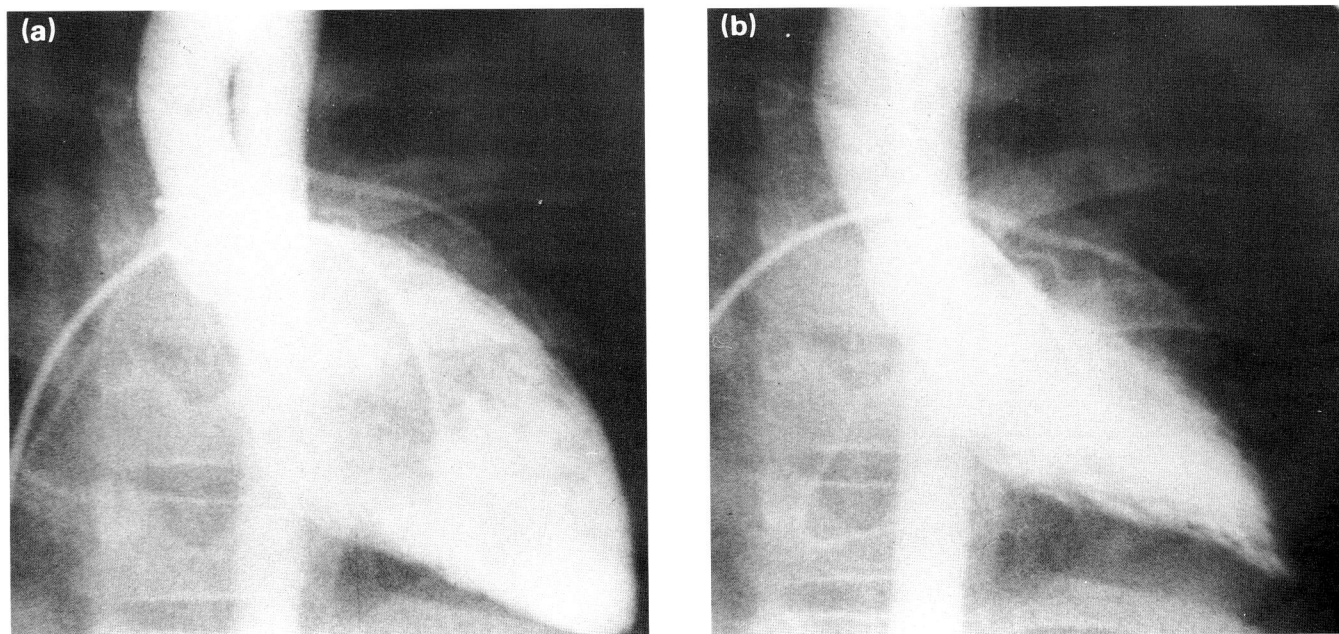

Fig. 17.43 The normal left ventricle in (a) diastole, and (b) systole. The ventricle is *smoothly* trabeculated.

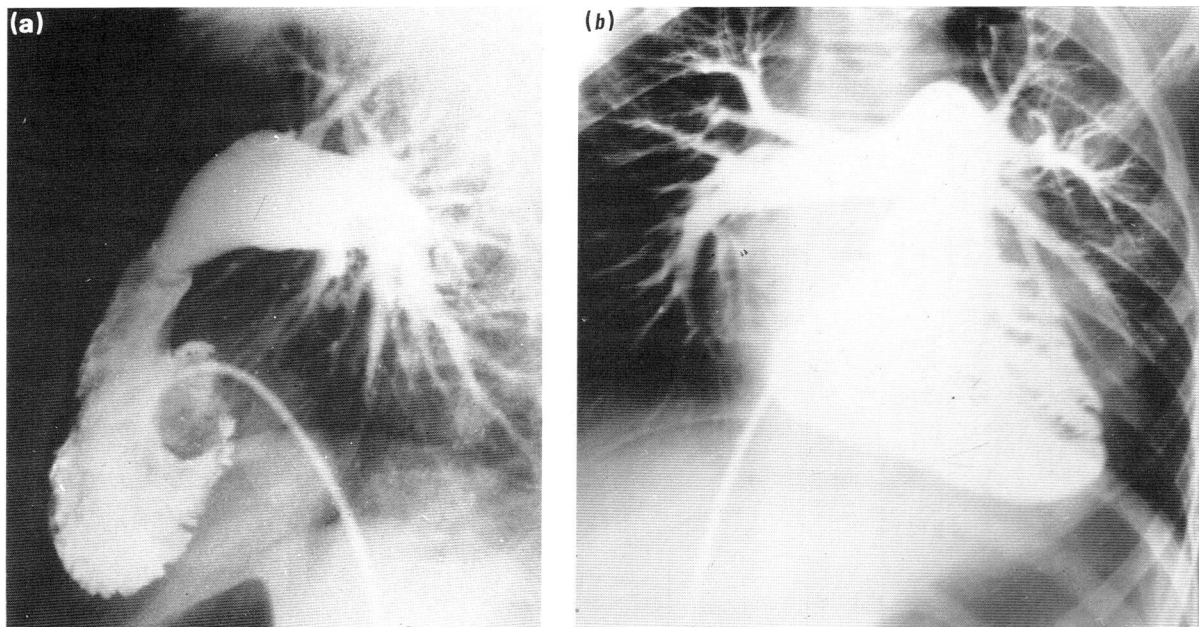

Fig. 17.44 The normal right ventricle; (b) anteroposterior projection, and (a) lateral projection. The tricuspid valve is outlined by unopacified blood entering the ventricle during diastole. The trabecular pattern is coarser than that of a morphologic left ventricle (compare with Figs 17.43a and b). The normal pulmonary arterial tree is also well seen.

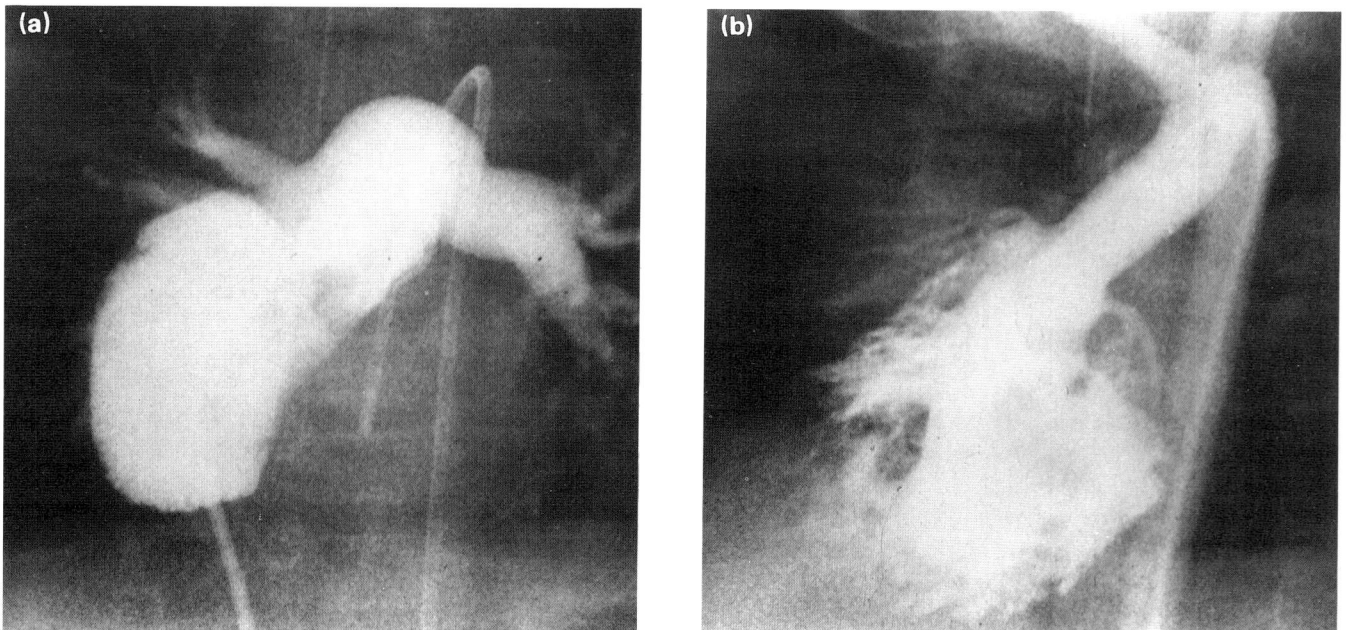

Fig. 17.45 The trabeculation of the ventricles allows them to be identified even when abnormally positioned or connected. In (a) a smoothly trabeculated, morphologic left, ventricle is right-sided and connects with the pulmonary artery. In the same patient (b) the coarse trabeculations allow the right ventricle to be identified even though it lies to the left of the morphologic left ventricle and is connected to the aorta.

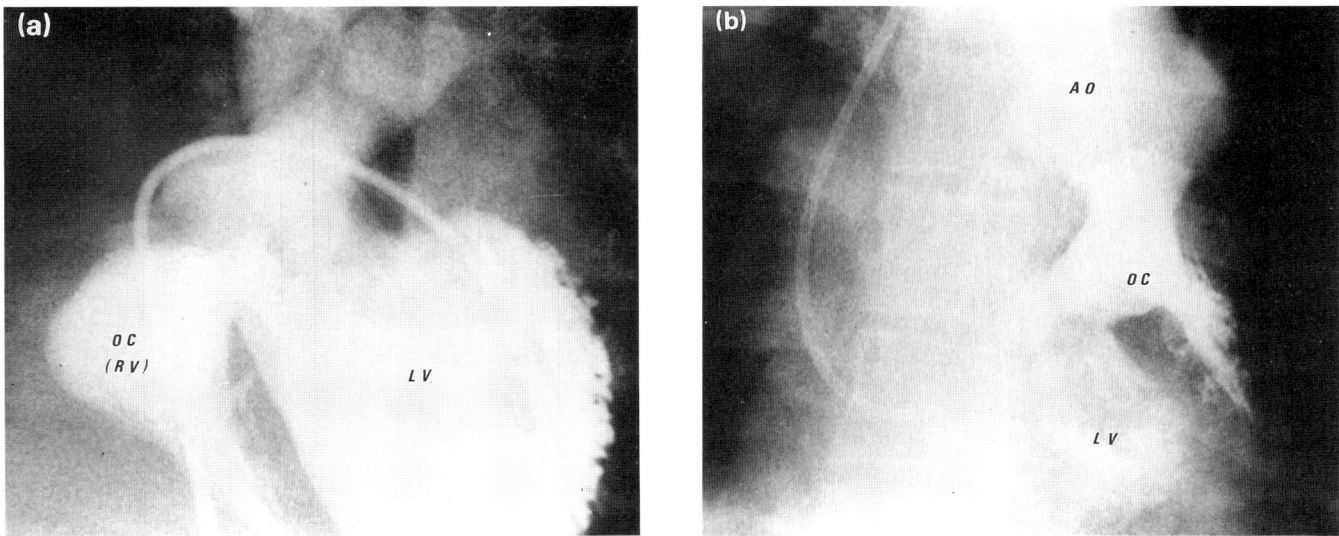

Fig. 17.46 Ventricles can be regarded as having an inlet, an apical trabecular and an outlet portion. When a ventricle lacks its inlet portion but retains its trabecular and outlet portions it may be termed an 'outlet chamber'. In this patient the main chamber is smoothly trabeculated and is therefore identifiable as a morphologic *left* ventricle (LV). The outlet chamber (OC) is more coarsely trabeculated and is a morphologic *right* ventricle (RV). Such 'rudimentary' right ventricles are almost always anterior in position but may lie to the right, as in this example, or (b) to the left. The coarse trabeculations of this left-sided outlet chamber identify it as a right ventricle even though it gives origin to the aorta (and lacks an inlet portion).

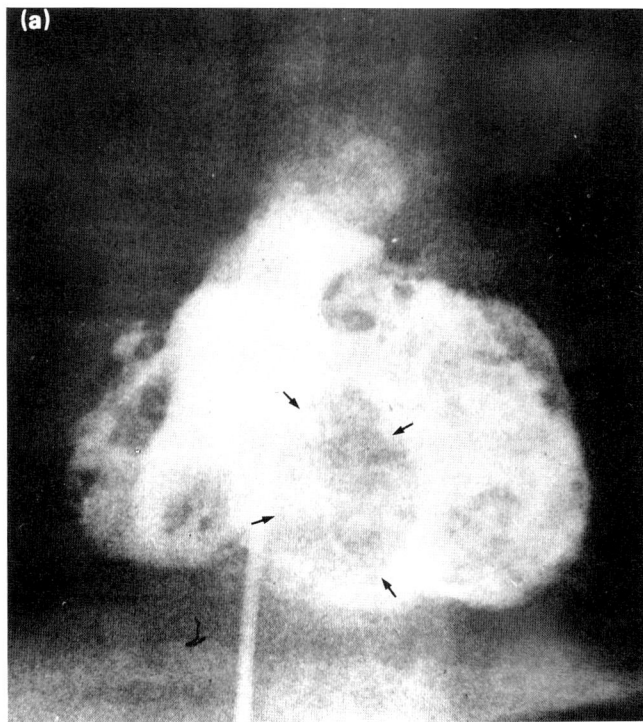

Fig. 17.47 When a ventricle lacks both an inlet and an outlet portion it may be termed a 'trabecular pouch'. In this example the coarse trabeculations of the main chamber (a) make it clear that it is a morphologic *right* ventricle and its inlet valve is visible due to the entry of unopacified blood (arrows).

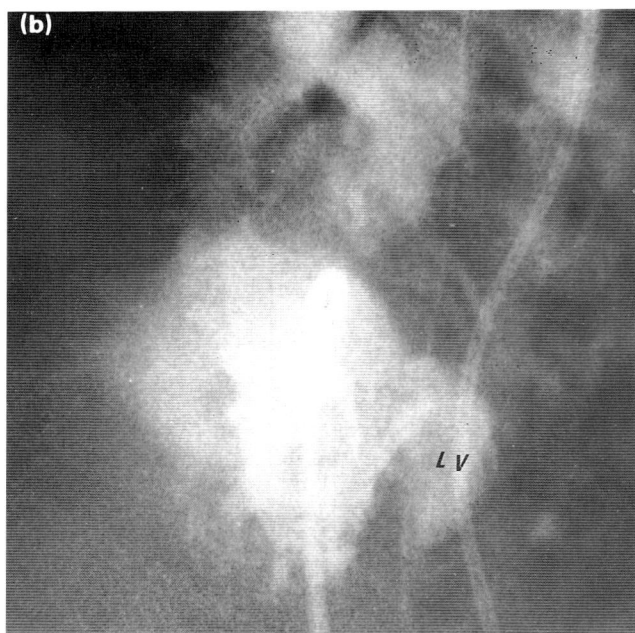

Fig. 17.47 *cont.* Only in the lateral projection (b) is the other ventricle seen since it lies posteriorly and is the rudimentary *left* ventricle (LV). Such small, rudimentary, left ventricles are easily overlooked unless deliberately searched for. Since both atrioventricular valves or, as in this example, a single atrioventricular valve, enter one ventricle only this is an example of a 'univentricular atrioventricular connection' — in this case 'absent left atrioventricular connection, double outlet *right* ventricle'.

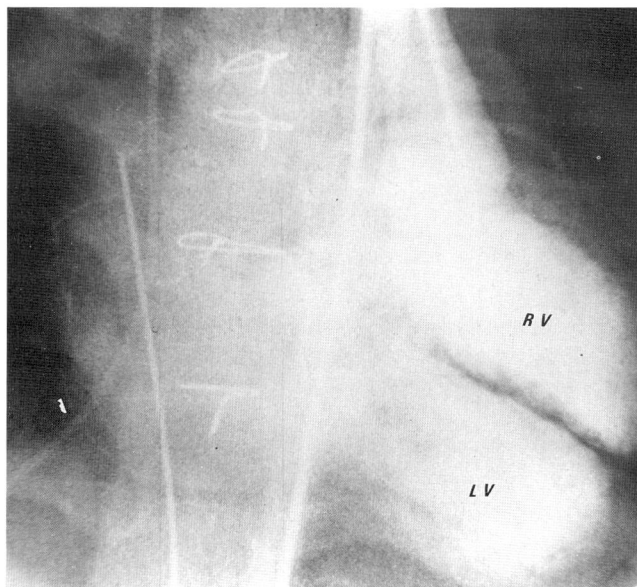

Fig. 17.48 The ventricles are not always easy to identify. In this example the trabecular pattern is similar in each though, in fact, this is an example of atrioventricular and ventriculo-arterial *discordance* ('corrected transposition') in which the right ventricle (RV) gives rise to the aorta and is superiorly positioned in relation to the left ventricle (LV). This superior/inferior relationship of the ventricles is commonly seen in this condition and the appearances have been compared to a 'hamburger'.

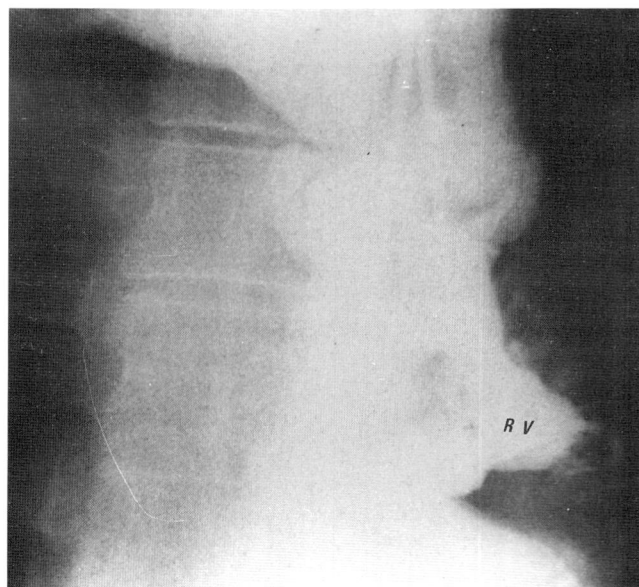

Fig. 17.49 Ventricular *dominance*. In this example the right, and much of the left, atrioventricular valve are committed to the main chamber. As a result the right ventricle (RV) is hypoplastic.

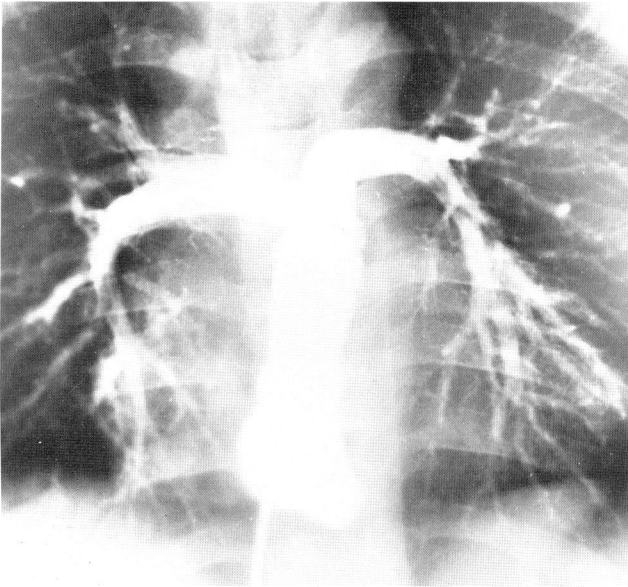

Fig. 17.50 Rarely the right ventricle may be hypoplastic despite being normally connected. In this example of 'isolated congenital hypoplasia of the right ventricle' the trabecular portion of the ventricle is absent or hypoplastic but the inflow and outflow portions are present.

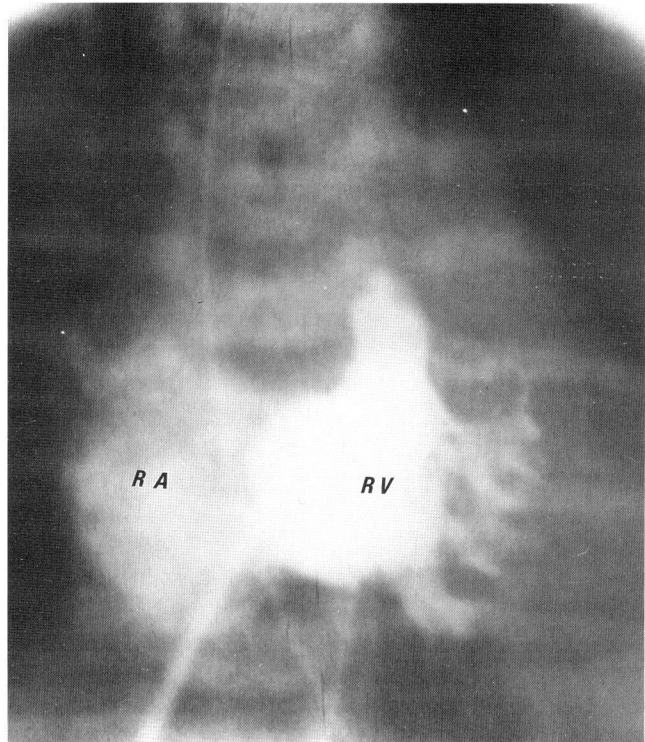

Fig. 17.51 A much more common cause of right ventricular hypoplasia with normal connections is the condition illustrated here — 'pulmonary atresia with intact ventricular septum'. Since the pulmonary valve is atretic there is no flow through the ventricle during foetal life; the right ventricle and tricuspid valve are hypoplastic. This hypoplasia may affect all portions of the right ventricle, as here, where inlet, trabecular and outflow portions are all present and the outflow portion ends blindly at the level of the atretic pulmonary valve. Alternatively, in this condition, the ventricle may lack its outflow portion or both outflow and trabecular portions.

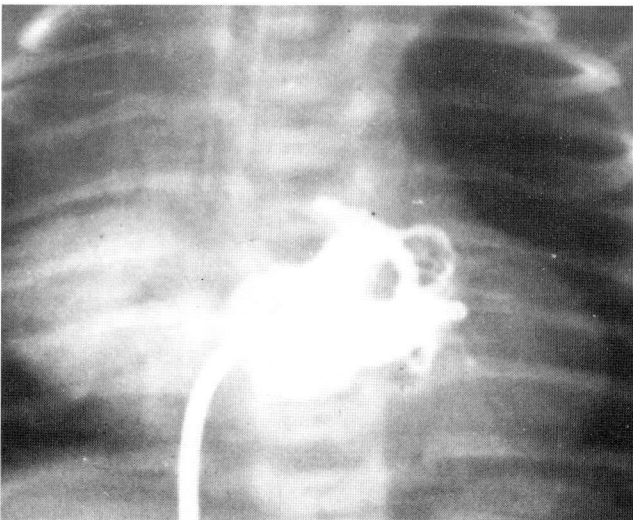

Fig. 17.52 *The ventricles* — pulmonary atresia with intact ventricular septum. Another example of pulmonary atresia with intact ventricular septum. An injection into the hypoplastic right ventricle has resulted in filling of myocardial 'sinusoids' — a feature of this condition.

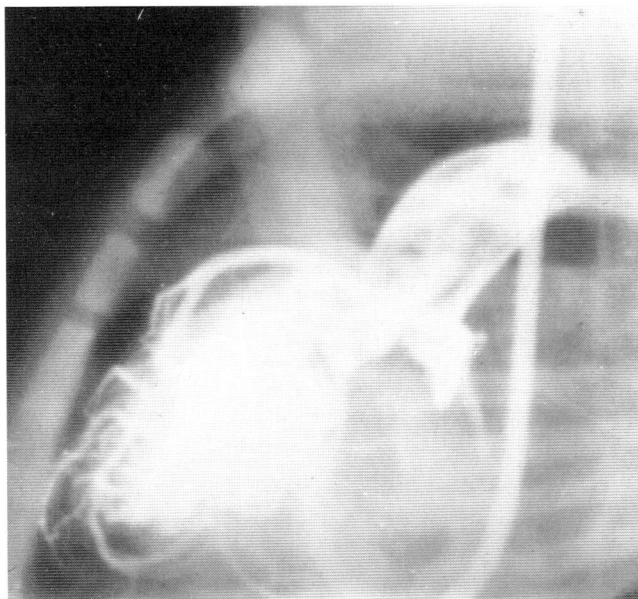

Fig. 17.53 In this patient with pulmonary atresia and intact ventricular septum the myocardial sinusoids communicate with the coronary circulation and retrograde flow of contrast through the coronary arteries has forced contrast medium to enter the aorta which is densely opacified following a right ventricular injection! (Lateral projection).

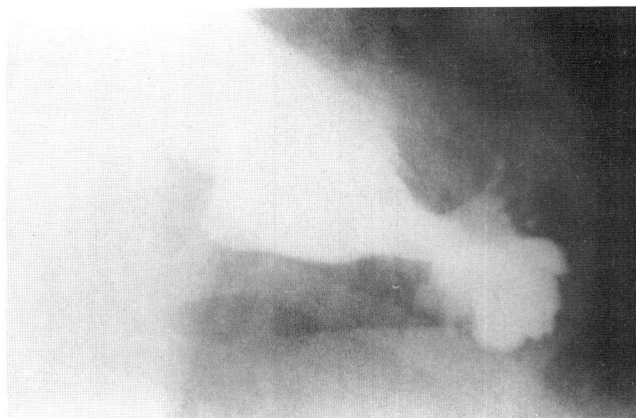

Fig. 17.54 *The ventricles.* Congenital diverticulum or aneurysm of the left ventricle. This rare anomaly may be associated with midline thoraco-abdominal defects when the diverticulum presents as a pulsatile mass in the epigastrium. In this patient the diverticulum was an isolated anomaly and was not associated with a midline defect.

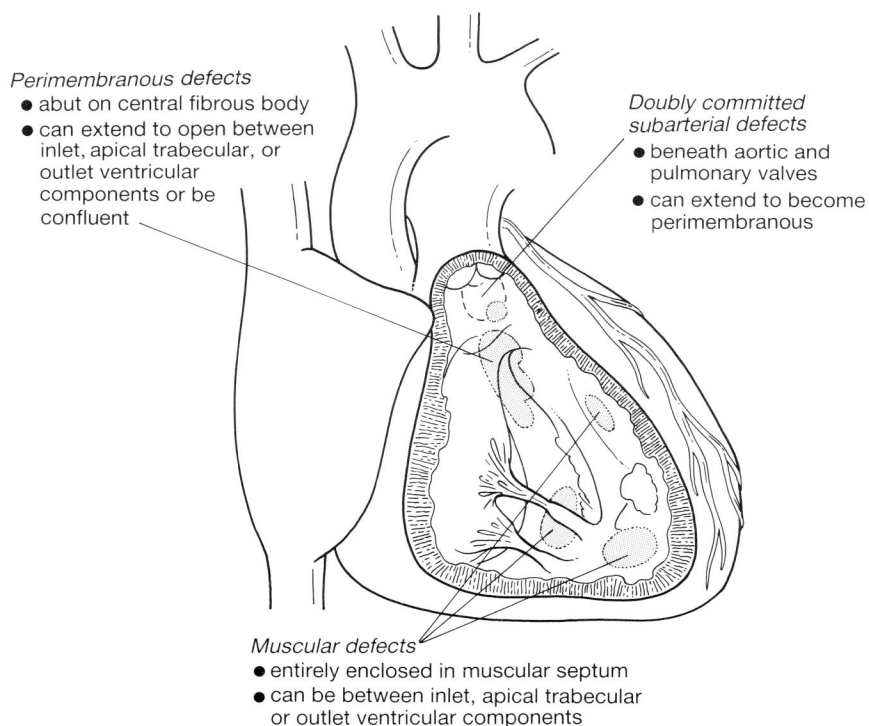

Perimembranous defects
● abut on central fibrous body
● can extend to open between inlet, apical trabecular, or outlet ventricular components or be confluent

Doubly committed subarterial defects
● beneath aortic and pulmonary valves
● can extend to become perimembranous

Muscular defects
● entirely enclosed in muscular septum
● can be between inlet, apical trabecular or outlet ventricular components

Fig. 17.55 Ventricular septal defects (reproduced from Miller GAH, Rigby M, Anderson RH. *The diagnosis of congenital heart disease*, Castle House, 1985, with permission).

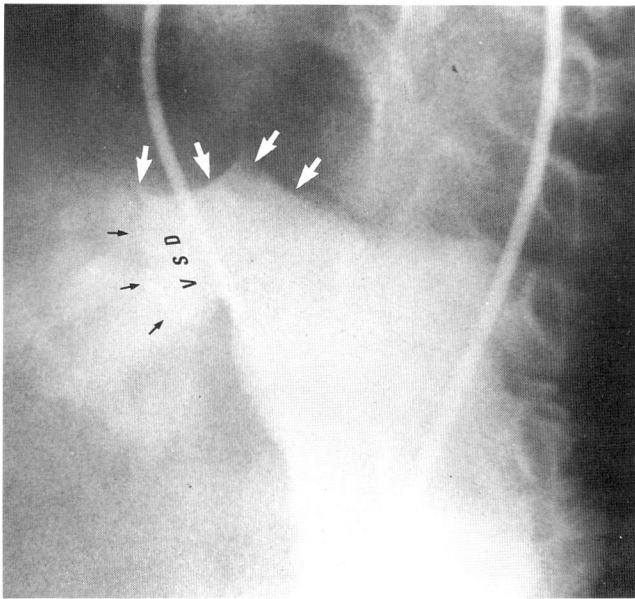

Fig. 17.56 *The ventricles* — ventricular septal defect. Perimembranous VSD. The defect lies immediately beneath, and is roofed by, the aortic valve (white arrows). The defect extends into the inlet septum and contrast medium has accumulated beneath the septal leaflet of the tricuspid valve (small black arrows).

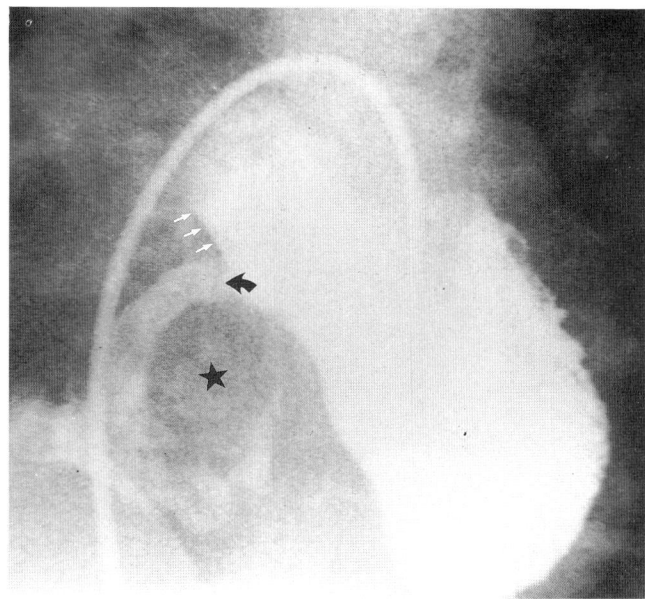

Fig. 17.57 Muscular VSD (curved arrow) involving the inlet septum. Contrast medium is seen outlining the tricuspid valve (asterisk). The membranous septum (small arrows) is intact and separates the defect from the aortic valve.

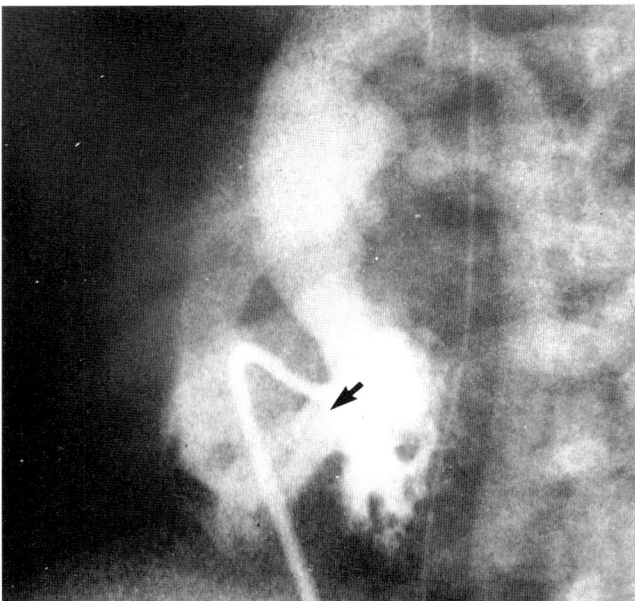

Fig. 17.58 Muscular ventricular septal defect (arrow) involving the trabecular portion of the muscular septum. The trabecular portion of the right ventricle opacifies first following injection into the left ventricle. The catheter has crossed the defect from the right to the left ventricle.

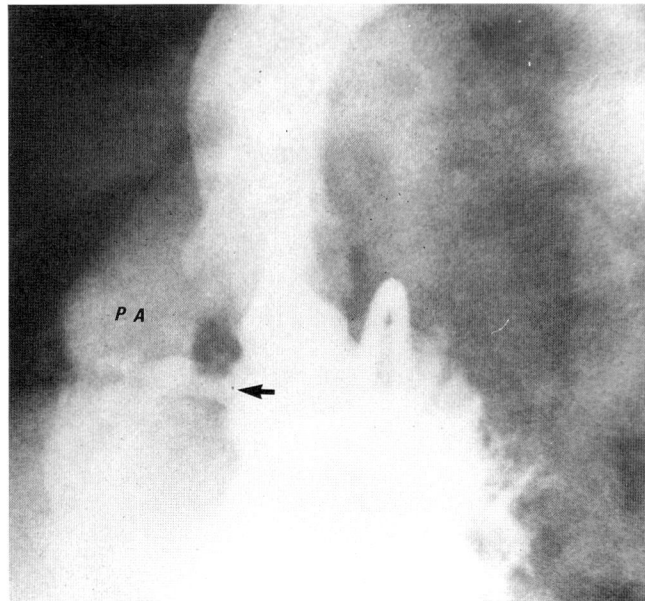

Fig. 17.59 Muscular VSD involving the outlet septum. The outlet portion of the right ventricle and pulmonary artery opacify first. The membranous septum is intact and separates the defect from the aortic valve.

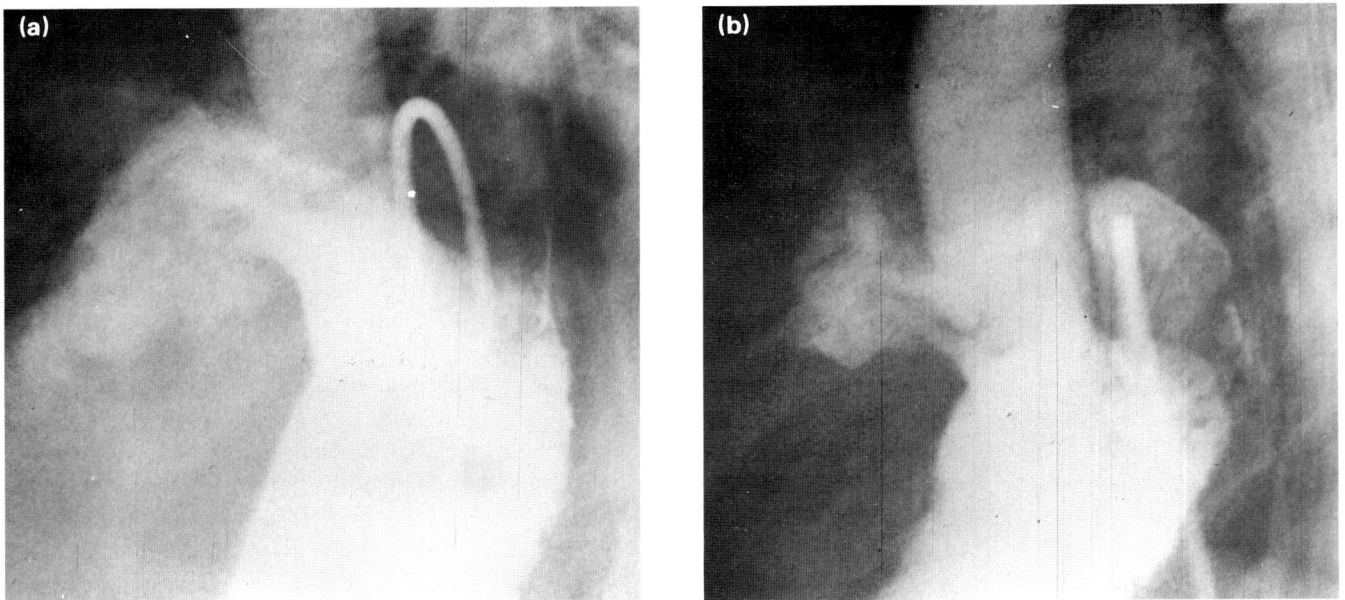

Fig. 17.60 *The ventricles* — ventricular septal defect. Perimembranous outlet VSD. In (a) contrast medium has been injected into the left ventricle and has opacified the *outlet* portion of the right ventricle. Defects in the outlet septum are the most anterior of all and the defect is not well profiled in this long axis view. In (b) a lateral projection has profiled this anterior defect which is seen to be immediately beneath the aortic valve.

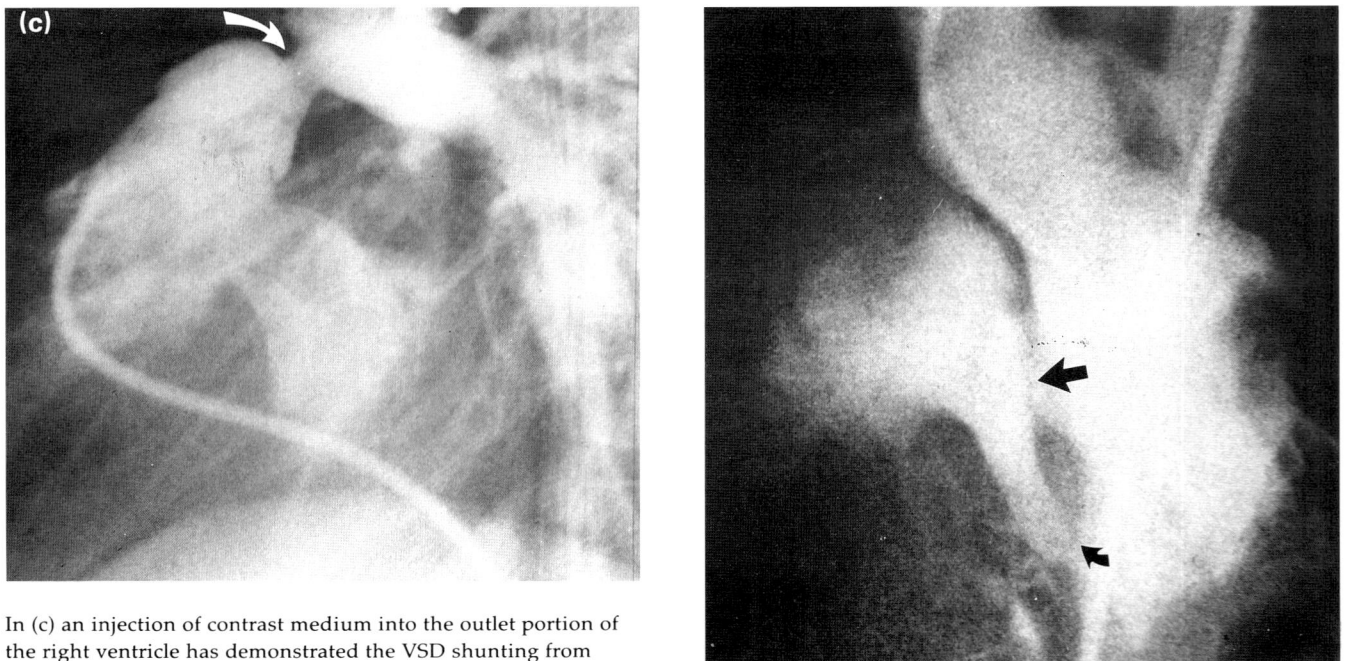

In (c) an injection of contrast medium into the outlet portion of the right ventricle has demonstrated the VSD shunting from right-to-left as a result of previous pulmonary artery banding (the band is indicated by the arrow).

Fig. 17.61 *The ventricles* — ventricular septal defect. Multiple muscular VSDs. At least two, moderately sized, muscular VSDs are seen (arrows).

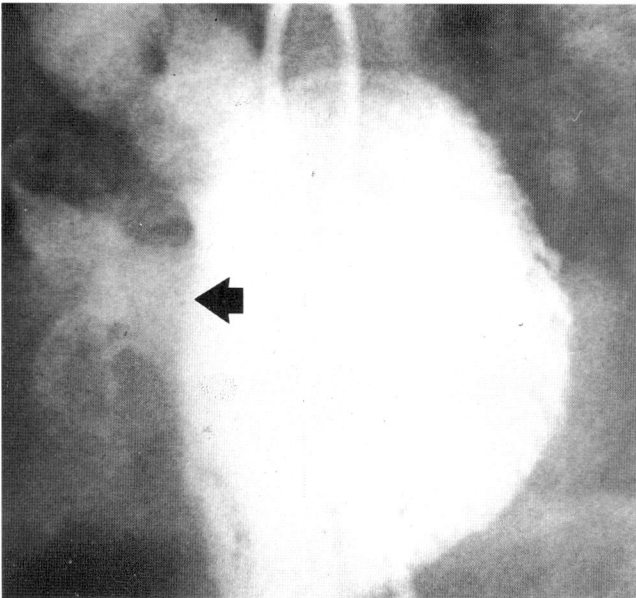

Fig. 17.62 Large single muscular VSD. There is also a perimembranous defect (not well seen).

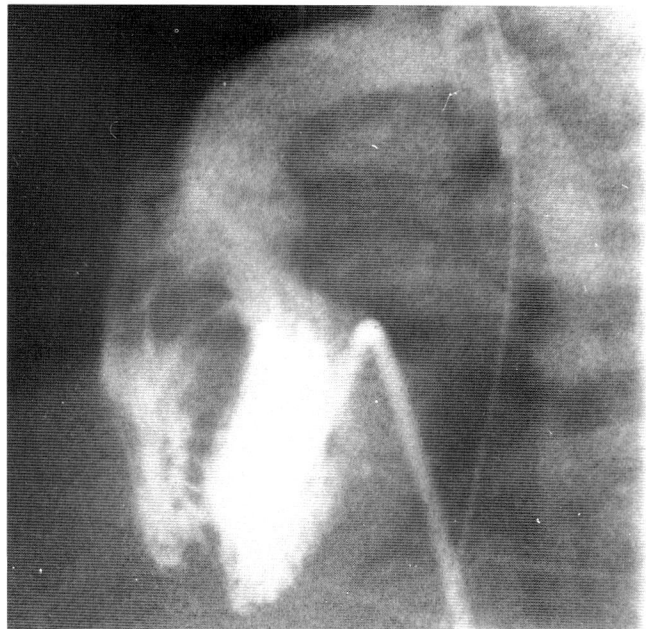

Fig. 17.63 *The ventricles* — ventricular septal defect. Multiple small defects in the apical part of the muscular septum.

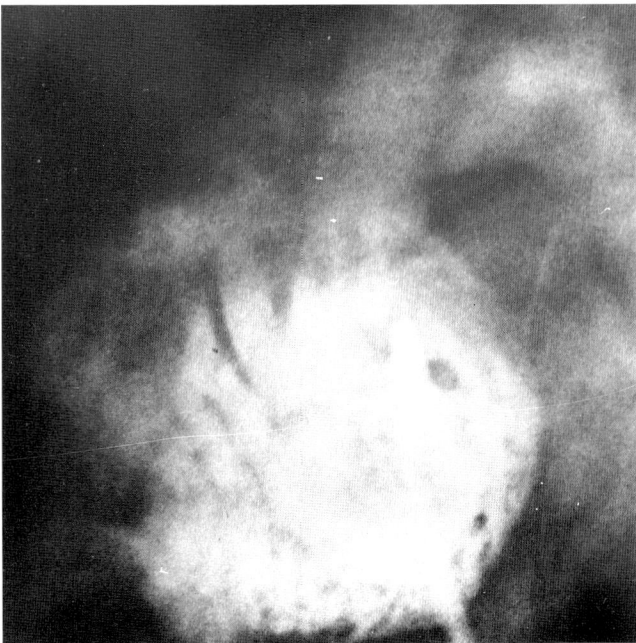

Fig. 17.64 Multiple muscular defects of the so-called 'Swiss cheese' variety.

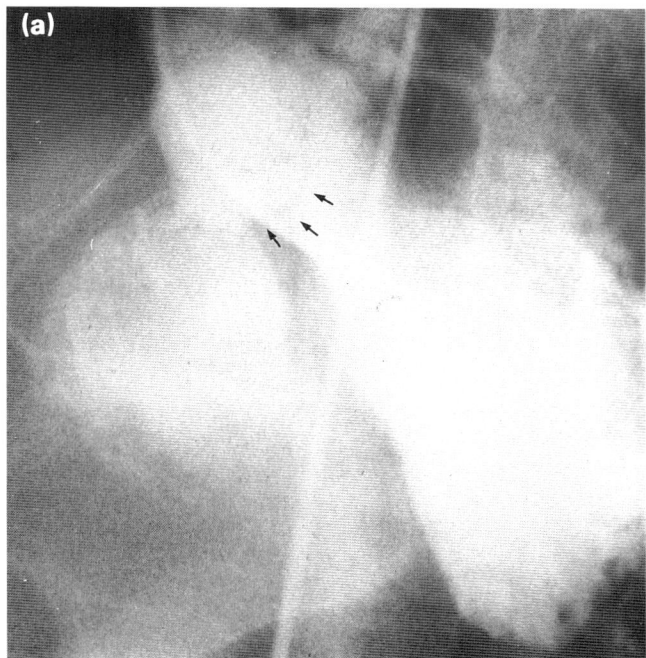

Fig. 17.65 *The ventricles* — ventricular septal defect. (a) Defect in the infundibular septum ('supracristal VSD') with prolapsing aortic valve cusp (arrows) partially occluding the defect.

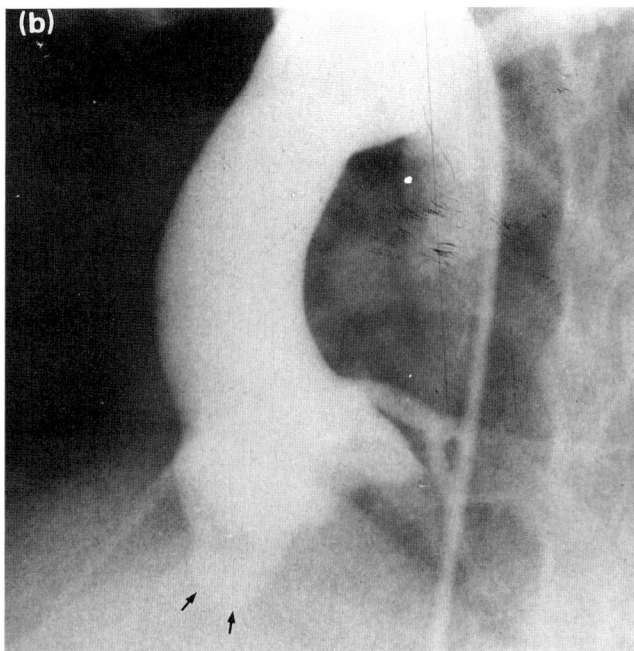

Fig. 17.65 *cont.* (b) In the same patient an aortogram demonstrates the prolapsed aortic cusp.

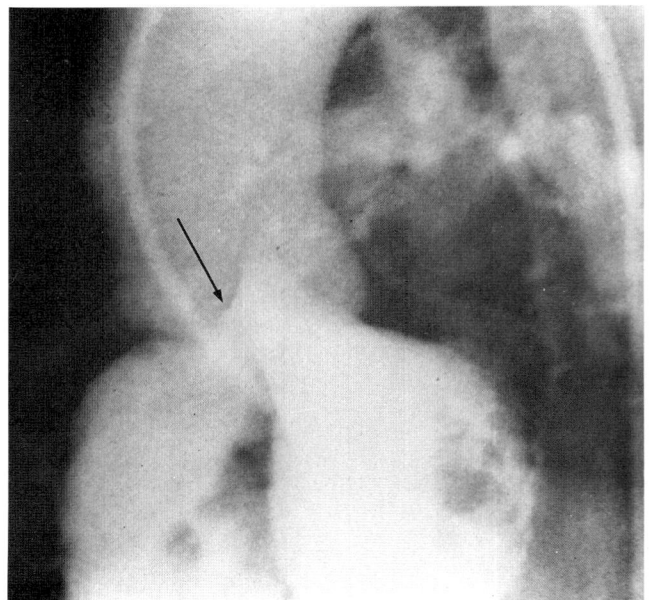

Fig. 17.66 *The ventricles* — ventricular septal defect with 'aortic override'. The plane of the ventricular septum is indicated by the long arrow. About one-third of the aortic valve overrides the ventricular septum.

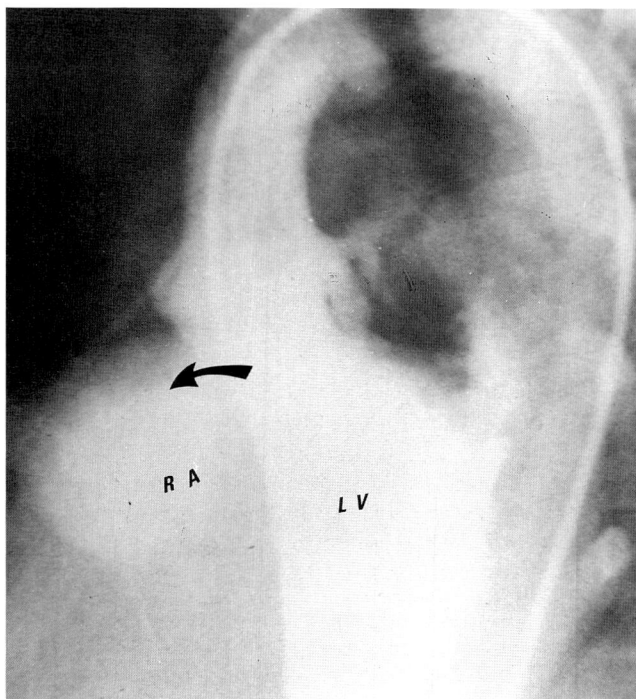

Fig. 17.67 Shunting from the left ventricle to the right atrium (arrow). This may be due to a defect in that portion of the septum which, because of the lower insertion of the tricuspid than the mitral valve, separates the right atrium from the left ventricle ('Gerbode defect'). Similar appearances can result from a ventricular septal defect with associated tricuspid regurgitation or shunting through a cleft in the tricuspid valve. Contrast medium injected into the left ventricle (LV) has opacified the right atrium (RA) *before* there has been any opacification of the right ventricle.

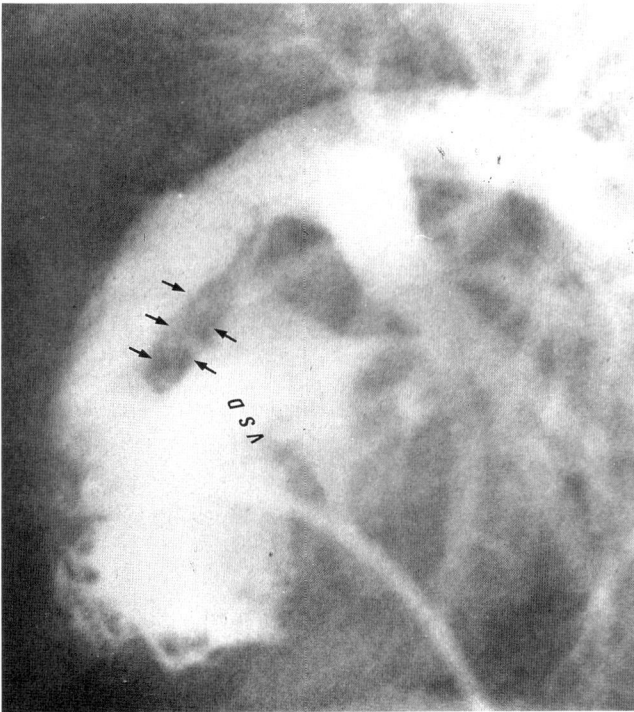

Fig. 17.68 *The ventricles* — ventricular septal defect.
'Malalignment VSD'. In this patient, with the anatomy of
tetralogy of Fallot, there is anterior deviation of the infundibular
septum (arrows). As a result there is malalignment between the
infundibular septum and muscular septum resulting in a defect
(VSD) which lies *beneath* the malaligned infundibular septum.

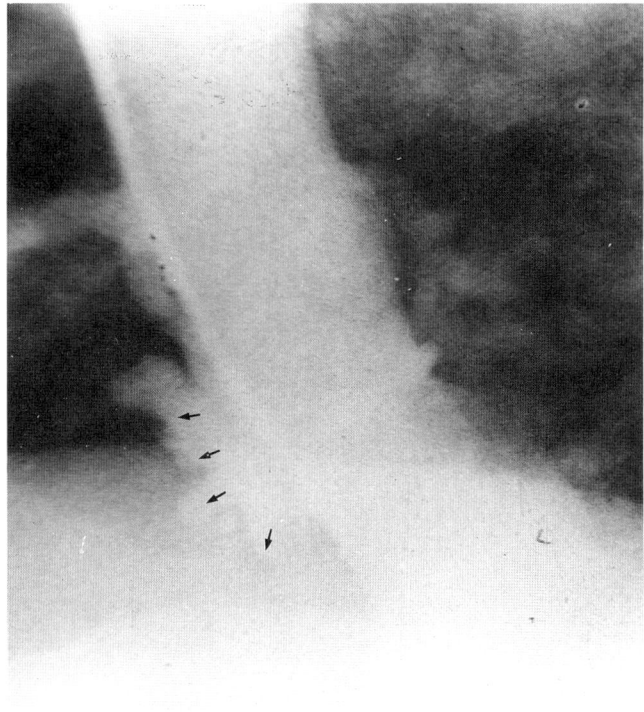

Fig. 17.69 So-called 'aneurysm of the ventricular septum'
(arrows). In fact more usually due to the apposition of tricuspid
valve tissue resulting in the closure of a ventricular septal defect.

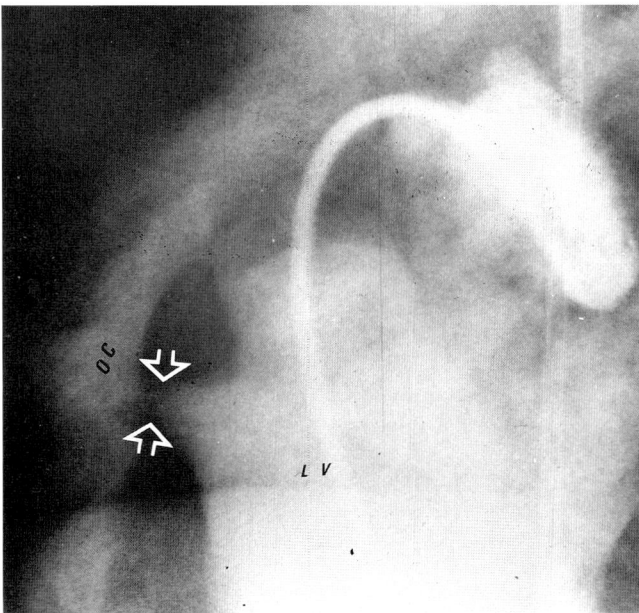

Fig. 17.70 In so-called 'classical tricuspid atresia' with ventriculo-
arterial concordance blood reaches the pulmonary circulation
from the left ventricle by way of a ventricular septal defect (or
'outlet foramen') and via the hypoplastic right ventricle to the
pulmonary artery. Obstruction to pulmonary flow is the rule; this
obstruction may be at the pulmonary valve (pulmonary stenosis),
as a result of the small size of the outlet chamber (RV) or because
the VSD is restrictive. In this example the VSD — between the
two white open arrows — is restrictive, pulmonary flow is
reduced and the pulmonary artery and outlet chamber (OC) are
small.

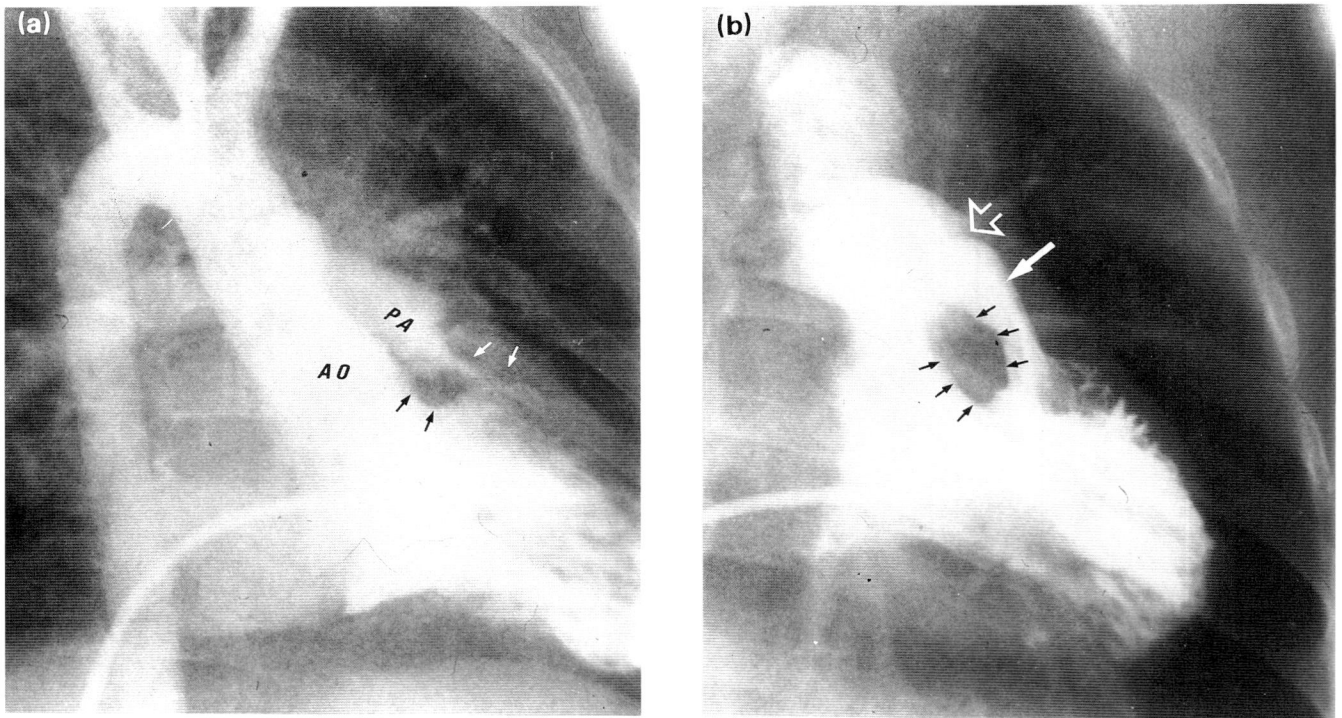

Fig. 17.71 *The ventricles* — outflow tract obstruction. Right ventricular outflow tract obstruction in the tetralogy of Fallot is due to anterior deviation and leftward rotation of the infundibular septum. The right ventricular outflow tract is narrowed between the deviated septum: black arrows in (a) and hypertrophied muscle bundles of the right ventricular free wall (white arrows) producing severe infundibular stenosis. The aortic arch is right sided in 20–30% of cases — as here. (b) Hypertrophy of the infundibular septum may contribute to right ventricular outflow obstruction in the tetralogy of Fallot. In this example there is considerable hypertrophy of the infundibular septum (black arrows) and an elongated, narrow, hypoplastic infundibulum (solid white arrow) beneath the pulmonary valve (open white arrow). The pulmonary valve ring may be small and the valve stenotic. Right ventricular outflow tract anatomy in the tetralogy of Fallot is best seen in the right oblique projection — as used in these two examples.

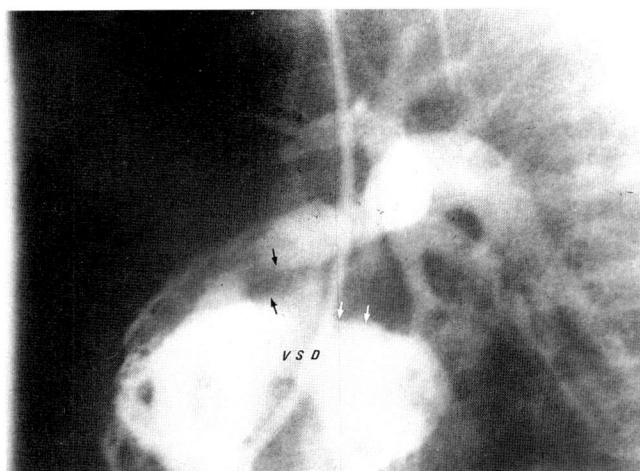

VSD

Fig. 17.72 *Tetralogy of Fallot.* Deviation of the infundibular septum results in malalignment between it and the trabecular septum thus creating a so-called 'malalignment ventricular septal defect'. The VSD is beneath the aortic valve (white arrows) and beneath the infundibular septum (between the two black arrows). The aorta overrides the trabecular septum by a variable amount (see also Figs 17.66 and 17.68); when more than 50% of the aorta arises from the right ventricle the ventriculo-arterial connection is termed 'double-outlet right ventricle' but the anatomy that results from deviation of the infundibular septum may still be that of tetralogy of Fallot. Thus 'tetralogy anatomy' can coexist with other lesions — with an atrioventricular septal defect, for example.

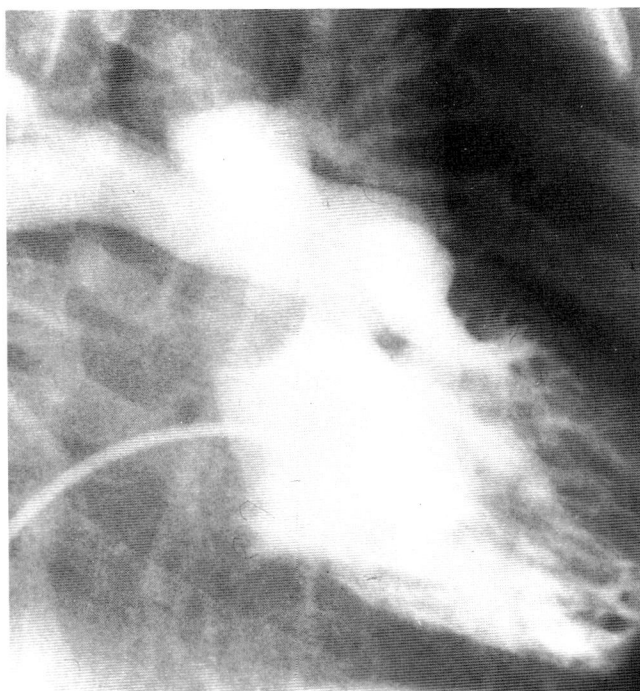

Fig. 17.73 Where there is a lesser degree of anterior deviation of the infundibular septum and leftward rotation predominates outflow obstruction may be minimal and arterial desaturation absent — so-called 'acyanotic tetralogy'. The great arteries tend to be in side-by-side relationship and the relatively high pulmonary flow is reflected in the larger pulmonary arteries — as in this example.

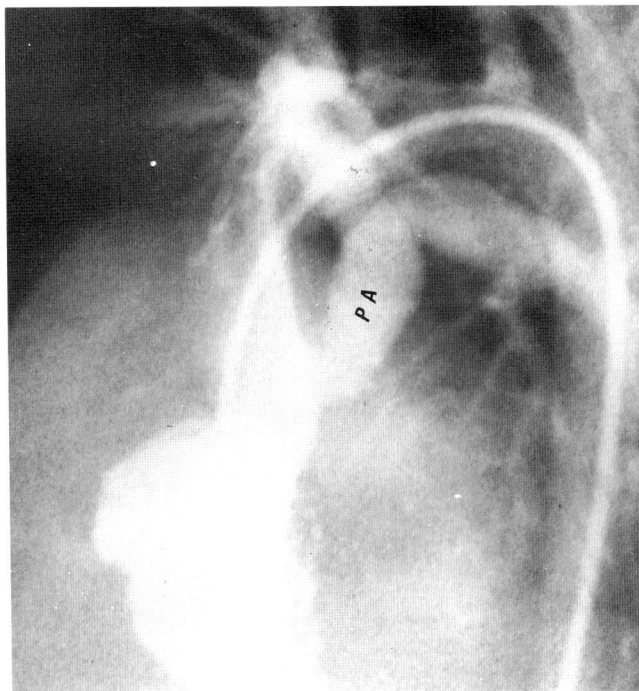

PA

Fig. 17.74 *Tetralogy of Fallot.* It is important to display the anatomy of the pulmonary arteries in tetralogy; hypoplasia, branch stenosis and unilateral absence all occur and the anatomy may have become distorted by a previous shunt operation. The four chamber projection (as in this example) is ideal for this purpose.

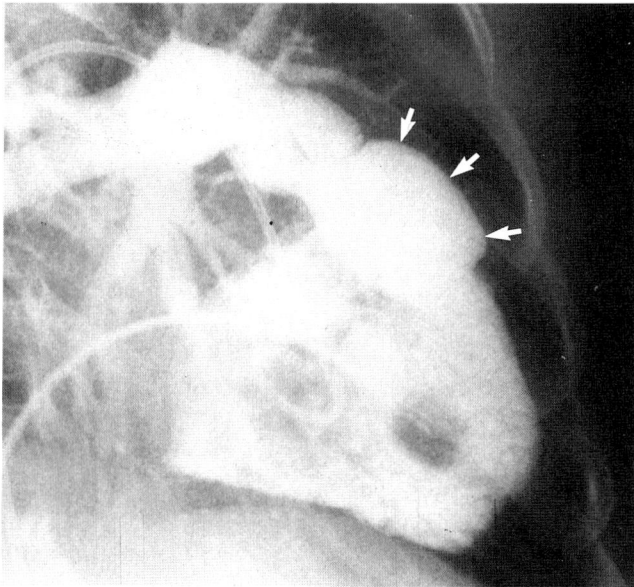

Fig. 17.75 Surgical correction of right ventricular outflow tract obstruction may require the insertion of an outflow patch. A bulge on the outflow tract may result as in this postoperative example (white arrows). If the outflow tract patch has been constructed of pericardium then calcification may occur — as may aneurysmal dilatation.

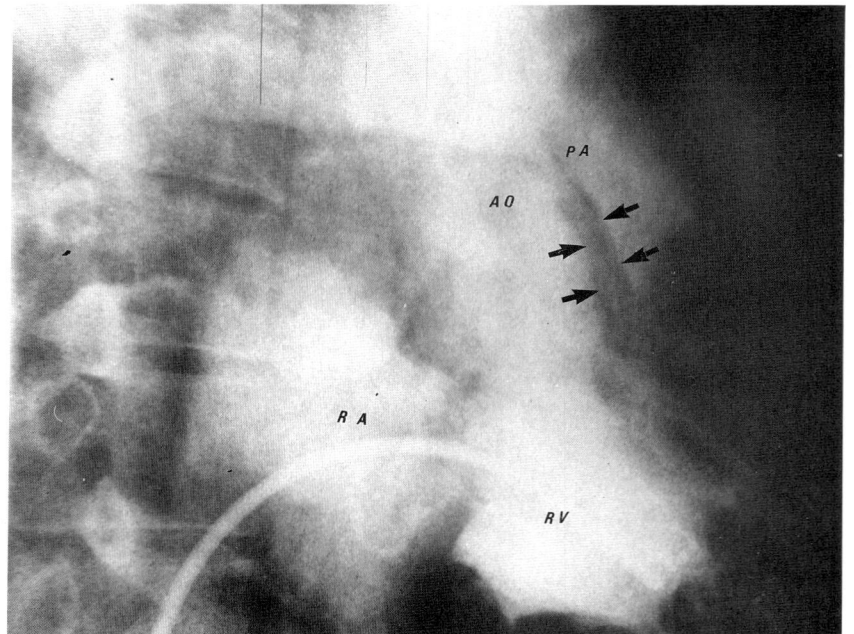

Fig. 17.76 *Tetralogy of Fallot.* A variant of the tetralogy exists in which there is a deficiency of the infundibular septum. In this case the ventricular septal defect is beneath the pulmonary and aortic valves (so-called 'doubly committed defect'). The lack of an infundibular septum results in the close apposition of the posterior aspect of the pulmonary artery and the anterior aspect of the aorta (arrows).

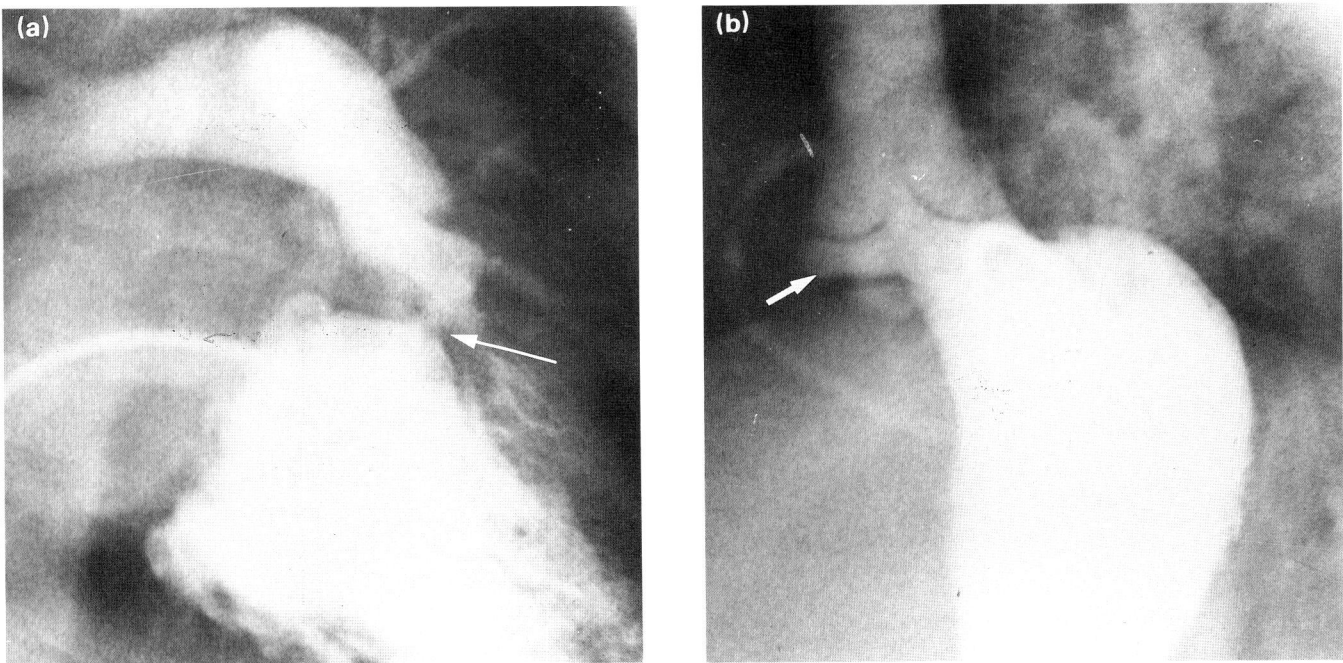

Fig. 17.77 *The ventricles* — outflow tract obstruction. Isolated infundibular stenosis occurs but many examples have, in reality, an associated VSD though this may be small or have closed. In this example (a) there appears to be severe, isolated, infundibular stenosis (arrow) but in (b) a long axis view of the left ventricle reveals an 'aneurysm of the membranous septum' (arrow) representing a VSD that has closed.

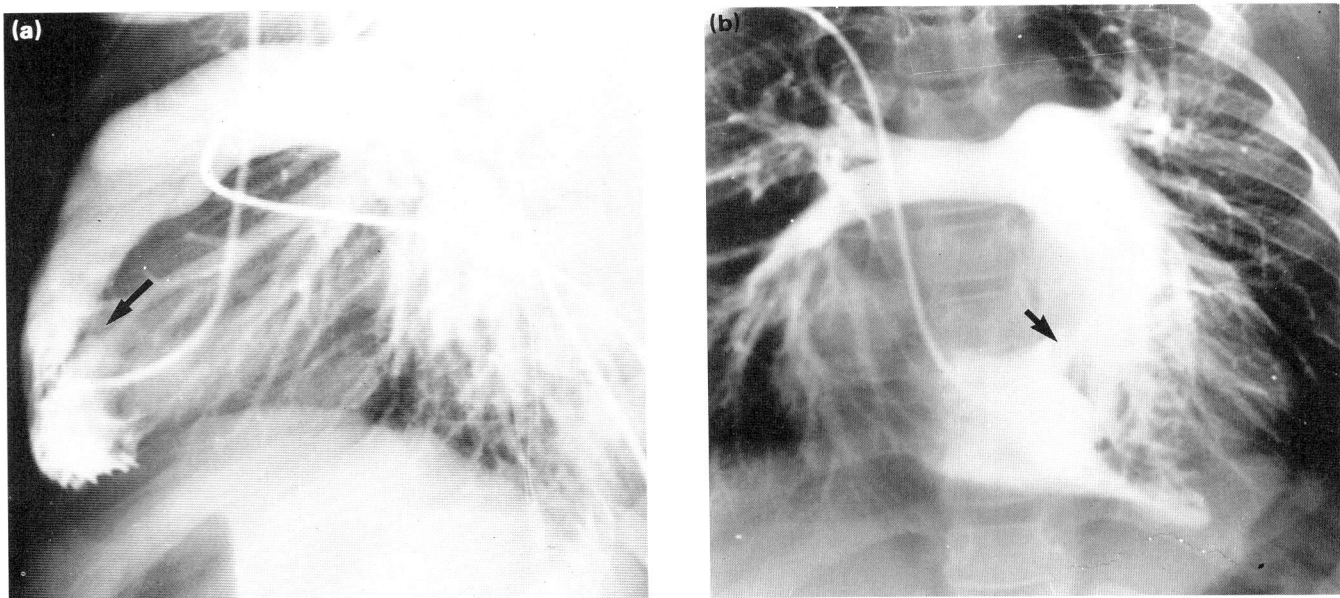

Fig. 17.78 *The ventricles* — outflow tract obstruction. Right ventricular outflow tract obstruction may be due to anomalous muscle bundles seen here (arrows) in the PA and lateral projections. Two-thirds of patients have an associated VSD and subaortic obstruction may also occur so that left ventriculography should form part of the investigation.

THE VENTRICULO-ARTERIAL JUNCTION (Figs 17.79 to 17.85)

The ventriculo-arterial connection may be concordant or discordant, or double outlet ventricle or single outlet heart. Single outlet heart refers to the situation in which only one great vessel can be traced back to the ventricular mass. Persistent truncus arteriosus is the obvious example and is illustrated in the section devoted to anomalies of the aorta. In almost all examples of aortic atresia it is the aortic *valve* which is atretic; a minute ascending aorta *can* be traced back to its potential communication with the left ventricle. This condition is also illustrated in the section devoted to aortic anomalies. The classification of pulmonary atresia poses problems. In many examples the atretic pulmonary trunk can be traced back to its (potential) origin from the right or left ventricle. This is true of pulmonary atresia with intact ven-

tricular septum, in many cases of pulmonary atresia with VSD and in patients with acquired pulmonary atresia (e.g. extreme tetralogy of Fallot), In other cases no pulmonary trunk can be identified and such cases can be classified as single outlet heart. In pulmonary atresia it is better, therefore, simply to describe the pulmonary arterial supply; are there true right and left intrapericardial pulmonary arteries; are they in continuity and is there an atretic pulmonary trunk? Examples of pulmonary atresia are illustrated below and in Chapter 20 since aortography is required to demonstrate the pulmonary arterial supply in this condition.

When the pulmonary artery arises from the right ventricle and the aorta from the left ventricle the ventriculo-arterial connection is said to be *concordant* — as in the normal heart. The opposite situation, ventriculo-arterial *discordance* is illustrated here (Fig. 17.81).

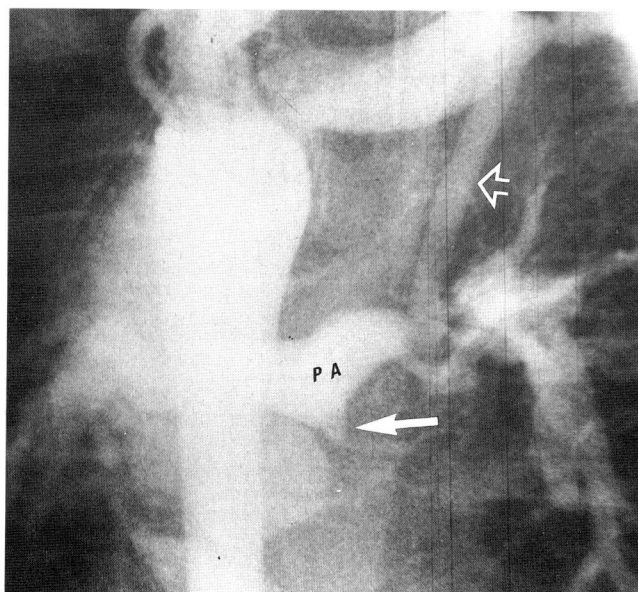

Fig. 17.79 *The ventriculo-arterial junction.* Pulmonary atresia. An aortogram has resulted in opacification of the right and left pulmonary arteries through a left subclavian-to-pulmonary shunt (interposition graft) indicated by the open arrow. A remanent of the main pulmonary artery can be seen pointing towards the right ventricular outflow (solid arrow).

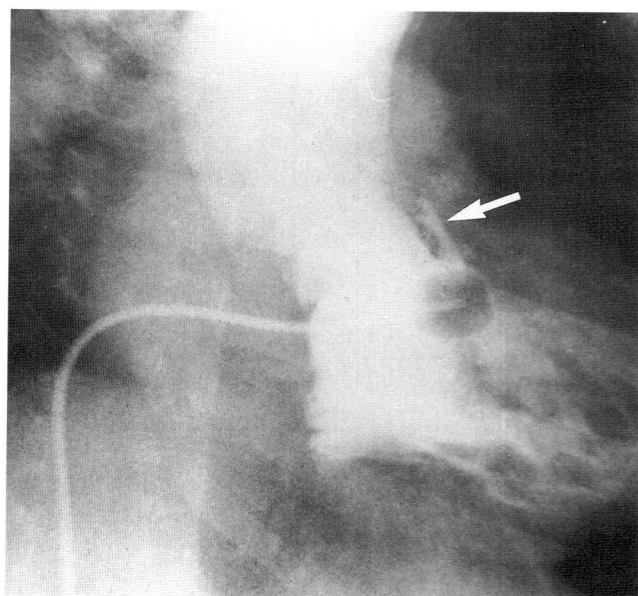

Fig. 17.80 Pulmonary atresia with VSD. A right ventriculogram has demonstrated a small atretic outflow tract (arrow) strongly suggesting that there is potential communication with pulmonary trunk. Contrast medium has also crossed a VSD to opacify the aorta.

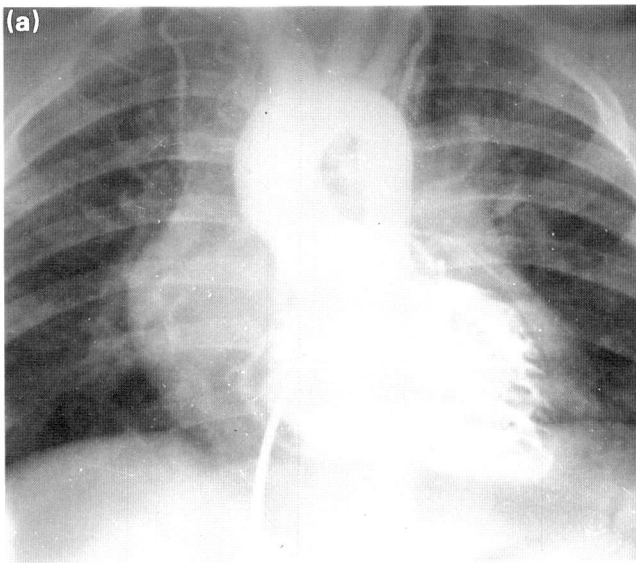

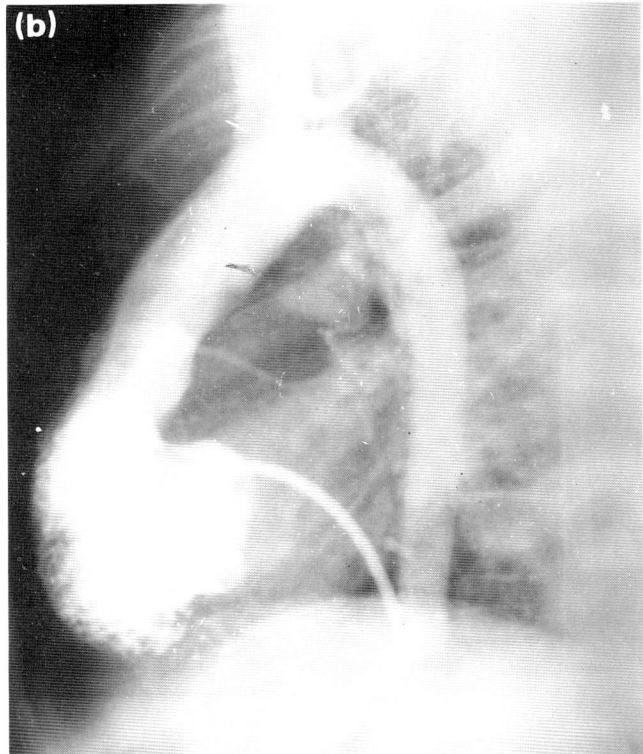

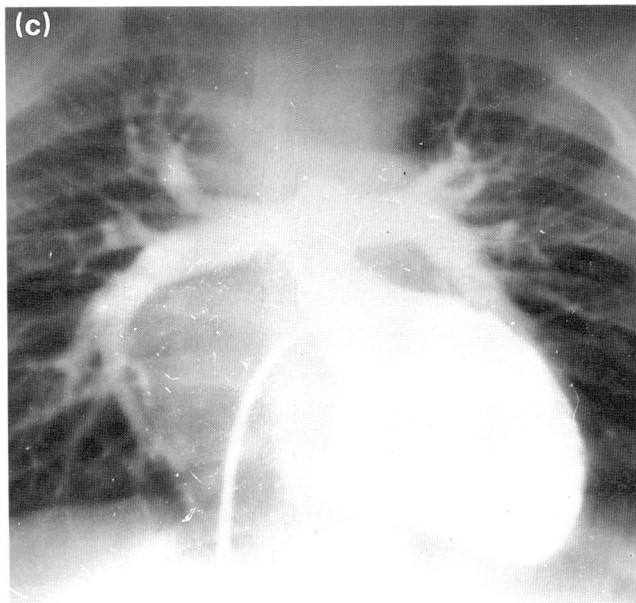

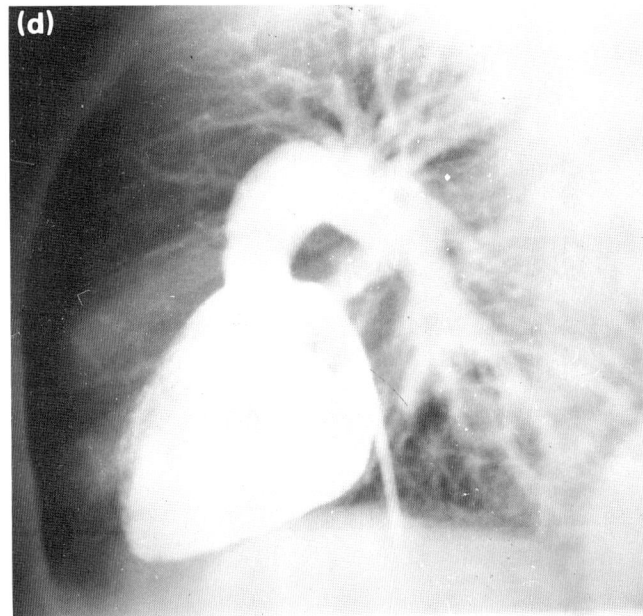

Fig. 17.81 Complete transposition (ventriculo-arterial discordance) of the great arteries. (a and b) Right ventriculogram in anteroposterior and lateral projections. An anteriorly placed aorta arises from the coarsely trabeculated right ventricle. (c and d) A posteriorly positioned pulmonary artery arises from the smoothly trabeculated left ventricle. There is no VSD — so-called 'simple' transposition.

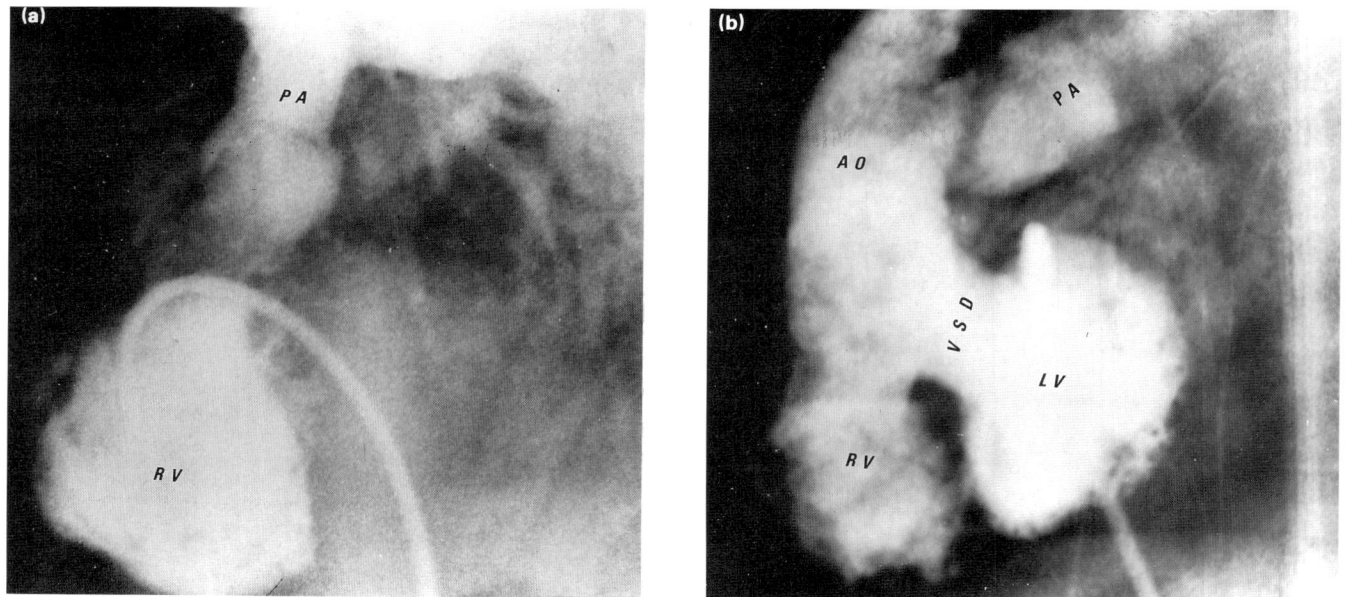

Fig. 17.82 *The ventriculo-arterial junction.* Double outlet right ventricle with subaortic VSD. (b) Left ventriculogram. The VSD provides the only exit from the left ventricle. The anterior, right ventricular, origin of the aorta is clearly seen. The VSD is beneath the aortic valve. There is subpulmonary obstruction and the haemodynamic findings resemble those found in the tetralogy of Fallot. (a) In the same patient a right ventricular injection has resulted in opacification of the pulmonary artery which also arises from the right ventricle.

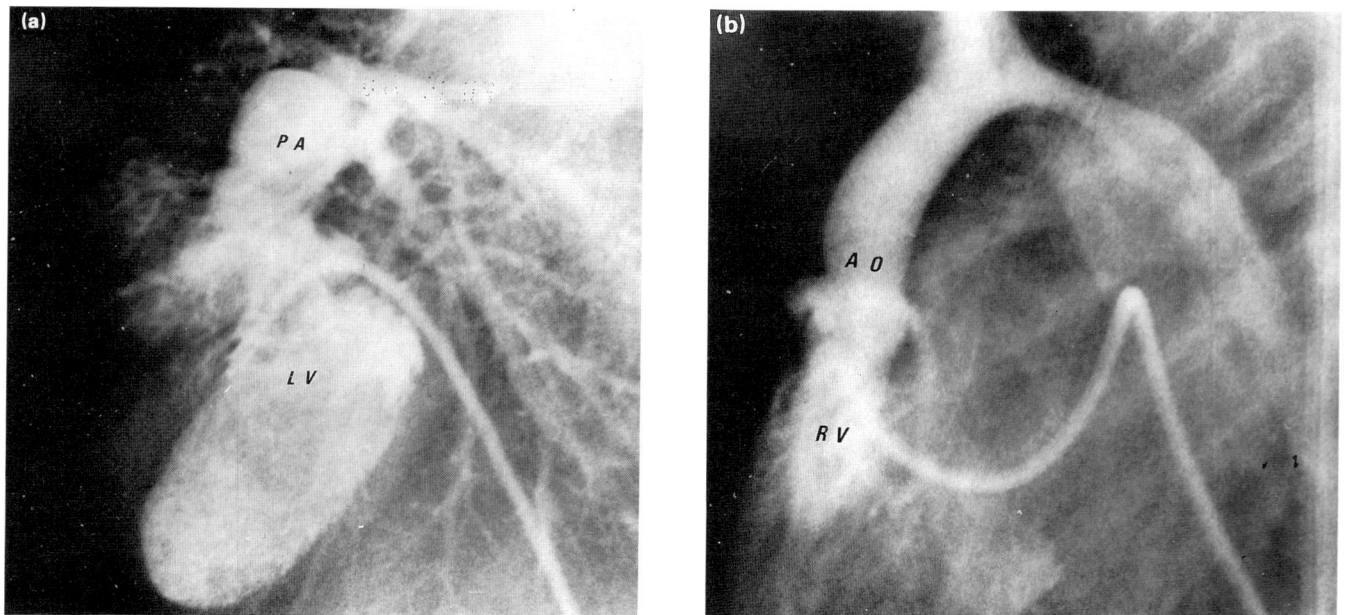

Fig. 17.83 *The ventriculo-arterial junction.* Double outlet right ventricle with subpulmonary VSD. (a) Left ventriculogram. The VSD provides the only exit from the left ventricle but in this case the VSD is beneath the pulmonary artery (PA). (b) In the same patient an injection into the outflow portion of the right ventricle has opacified an anteriorly placed aorta. Both great arteries arise from the right ventricle (double outlet right ventricle) but with a subpulmonary VSD the haemodynamics resemble those of complete transposition in that the saturation of pulmonary arterial blood tends to be higher than that of blood in the aorta.

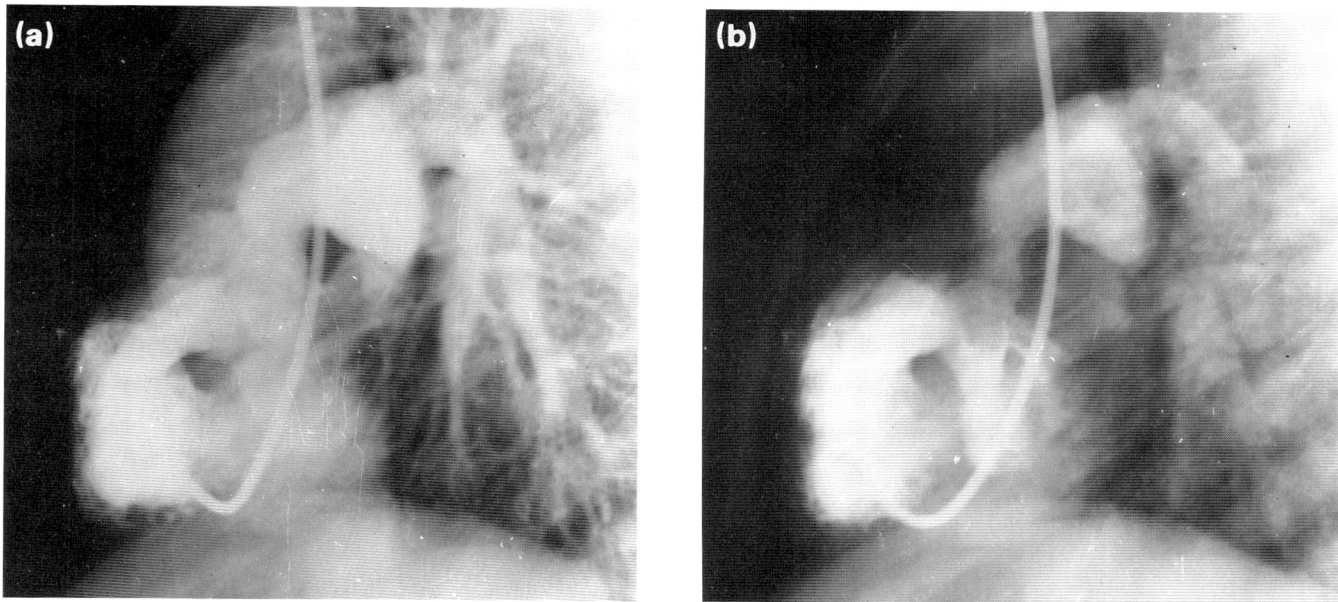

Fig. 17.84 (a and b) *The ventriculo-arterial junction.* Double outlet left ventricle, illustrated here, is very rare. In this example there is atrioventricular concordance and double outlet from the left ventricle with an anterior aorta and subaortic VSD and a posterior pulmonary artery. Other varieties exist.

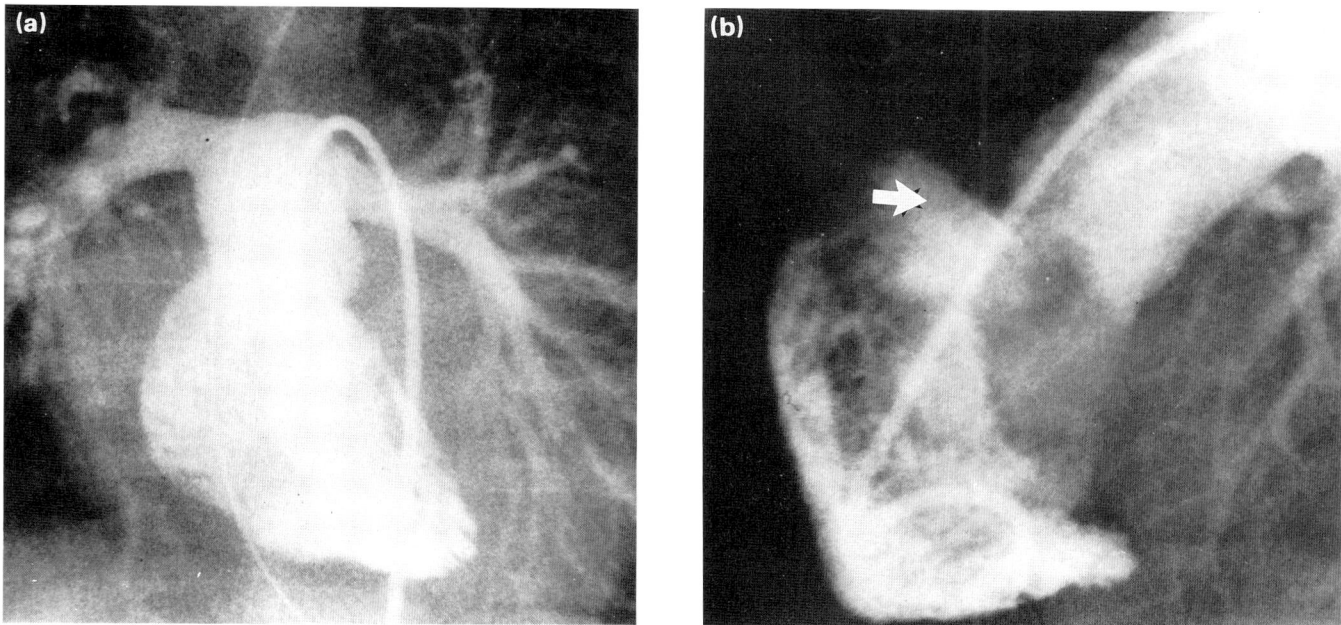

Fig. 17.85 *The ventriculo-arterial junction.* 'Corrected transposition'. The atrioventricular connection is discordant in this patient and so is the ventriculo-arterial connection. (a) Contrast medium injected into a smoothly trabeculated, morphologic left, ventricle has opacified the pulmonary arteries. (b) The lateral projection of the same ventriculogram shows how the pulmonary artery arises more posteriorly (and medially) than in the normal heart. There is an anterior 'pouch' (arrow) which tends to trap the tip of the catheter so that entry to the pulmonary artery can be difficult in this situation. The origin of the aorta from the morphologic *right* ventricle is illustrated in Fig. 17.45b in the section devoted to the ventricles.

REFERENCES

1 Van Praagh R. The sequential approach to diagnosis in congenital heart disease *Birth Defects* 1972;**8**:4.
2 Shinebourne EA, Macartney FJ, Anderson RH. Sequential chamber localisation: the logical approach to diagnosis in congenital heart disease. *Br Heart J* 1976;*38*:327.
3 Miller GAH, Anderson RH, Rigby ML. *The diagnosis of congenital heart disease*. Tunbridge Wells, Castle House Publications Ltd. 1985.
4 Van Praagh R, David I, Van Praagh S. What is a ventricle? The single ventricle trap. *Pediatr Cardiol* 1982;**2**:79.

5 Tynan MJ *et al*. Nomenclature and classification of congenital heart disease. *Br Heart J* 1979;**41**:544.
6 Van Mierop LHS, Eisen S, Schiebler GL. The radiographic appearances of the tracheobronchial tree as an indicator of visceral situs. *Am J Cardiol* 1970;**26**:432.
7 Partridge JB, Scott O, Deverall PB, Macartney FJ. Visualisation and measurement of the main bronchi by tomography as an objective indicator of thoracic situs in congenital heart disease. *Circulation* 1975;**51**:188.
8 Deanfield JE *et al*. Use of high kilovoltage filtered beam radiographs for detection of bronchial situs in infants and young children. *Br Heart J* 1980;**44**:577.

Coding of connections

☆ STEP 1
No abnormality

Abnormal connections

Normal connections

☆ STEP 2
Associated lesions present

☆ STEP 3: determine atrial arrangement

Lateralised atria		Isomeric atria	
Usual	Mirror-image	Right isomerism	Left isomerism

☆ STEP 4: determine atrioventricular connections

Bivent. AV connection			Univent. AV connection			Bivent. AV connection	
Concordant	Discordant		Double Inlet	Absent RAVC	Absent LAVC	Ambiguous connection	
		to RV				Right-hand topology	Left-hand topology
		to LV					
		to Indet. Vent.					

☆ STEP 5: determine ventriculo-arterial connections

Two ventricles present

One ventricle present

DORV
DOLV
DO Ind. Vent.

Concordant
Discordant

Single outlet of the heart			
Common trunk	Aorta	Pulm. trunk	Sol. trunk
Balanced connection			
from RV			
from LV			
from Ind. Vent.			

Describe 'associated lesions'
as in ☆ STEP 2

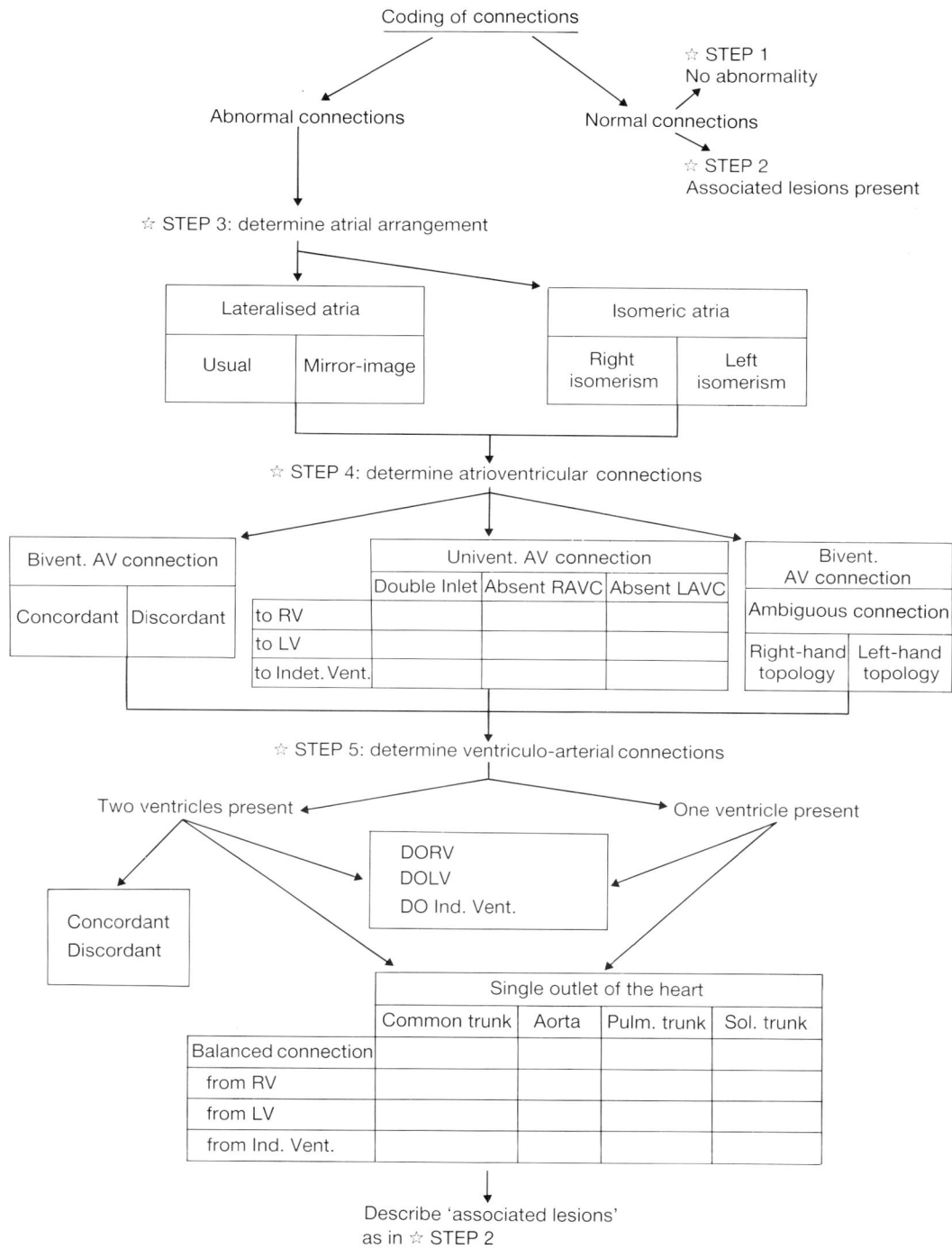

Appendix 17.1 Flowchart for the diagnosis of congenitally malformed hearts. Modified from Miller, Anderson & Rigby [3].

Congenital heart disease in the adult

Some of the most difficult catheterisation studies to perform are in adults with congenital heart disease. Access may be difficult as a result of past arterial and venous cut-downs; there is often gross chamber enlargement so that catheter manipulation is difficult and angiographic opacification is poor; 'cross-fogging' due to X-ray scatter makes biplane angiography unrewarding and previous surgery may have complicated the original anatomy. Most importantly long-standing disease may have introduced complications — notably myocardial dysfunction, dysrhythmias (Fig. 18.1), valve regurgitation and pulmonary vascular disease. Yet it is certain that, as a result of advances in the surgery of infants and children with congenital heart disease, the catheterisation laboratory will see increasing numbers of adults with congenital cardiac defects [1].

The spectrum of congenital heart disease seen in adult life includes; (1) conditions whose presentation is commonly delayed until adulthood, (2) conditions presenting in childhood in which the natural history can include survival into adult life, and (3) conditions in which surgical correction or palliation has allowed survival into adult life.

CONDITIONS COMMONLY PRESENTING IN ADULT LIFE

When presentation is delayed until adult life it is usually because the lesion is one which causes little haemodynamic disturbance until some complication draws attention to its presence. Examples include the development of stenosis at a congenitally bicuspid valve, the development of arrhythmias in association with atrial septal defect and aortic dissection in Marfan disease. Alternatively a benign congenital cardiac anomaly may be discovered by chance — perhaps at a routine examination or during the investigation of another illness. The following is

a list of conditions whose presentation is commonly delayed until adult life:

1 Bicuspid aortic valve.
2 Atrial septal defect.
3 'Floppy' mitral valve and mitral prolapse.
4 Marfan disease of aorta — aneurysm and dissection.
5 Coarctation of the aorta.
6 Aneurysm of the sinus of Valsalva.
7 Coronary-cameral fistula.
8 Patent ductus arteriosus.
9 Pulmonary valve and infundibular stenosis.
10 Ideopathic dilatation of the pulmonary trunk.
11 Pulmonary arteriovenous fistula.
12 Partial anomalous pulmonary venous return.
13 'Corrected transposition'.
14 Congenital complete heart block.

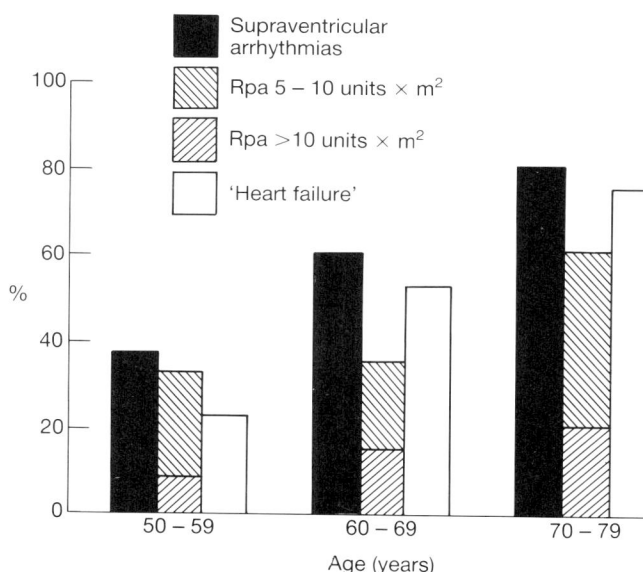

Fig. 18.1 Atrial septal defect first presenting in adult life. The increasing prevalence of complications present in patients first presenting in the decades from 50 to 79. (From Paolillo V, Dawkins KD, Miller GAH. Atrial septal defect in patients over the age of 50. *Int J Cardiol* 1985;9:139.

15 Congenital coronary anomalies.
16 Hypertrophic cardiomyopathy.
17 Ebstein's malformation of the tricuspid valve.
(See also Table 18.1.)

Bicuspid (and unicuspid) aortic valve

It is probable that congenitally bicuspid aortic valve is the commonest congenital cardiac anomaly; its incidence has been estimated as between 0.7 and 2.0% [2]. The condition may be associated with coarctation [3], with pulmonary stenosis and with a syndrome of short left main stem coronary artery with left coronary dominance [4]. Although common the lesion usually does not cause a haemodynamic disturbance until progressive stenosis has occurred. Perhaps one-third of those born with a bicuspid valve will develop progressive stenosis and calcification [5]. The incidence of stenosis increases with age; in developed countries bicuspid valve is the leading cause of isolated calcific aortic stenosis in adults. In the child without severe stenosis and without valve calcification the bicuspid morphology can be detected by aortography or ventriculography. Calcification is rare until adult life but when present the bicuspid nature of the valve may have become obscured. Cardiac catheterisation is required to estimate the severity of stenosis; significant stenosis is present when the peak systolic gradient is 50 mmHg or more and the calculated orifice area less than $0.7 \, \text{cm}^2/\text{m}^2$. Severe stenosis is indicated by gradient of 75 mmHg or more and orifice area $<0.5 \, \text{cm}^2/\text{m}^2$. [6]. Valve regurgitation is uncommon unless due to valve destruction by infective endocarditis.

Atrial septal defect

With the probable exception of bicuspid aortic valve atrial septal defect is by far the commonest lesion presenting in adult life. Although well tolerated for many years atrial septal defect is not a benign lesion; in those aged 50 or more about half will develop a supraventricular arrhythmia and about a third will have some increase in pulmonary vascular resistance which will be severe enough to preclude surgery in about 12% [7] (Fig. 18.2). The catheterisation protocol does not differ from that employed in children; an increase in saturation is detected at atrial level and the defect can be visualised angiographically by right upper lobe pulmonary vein injection with filming in the 'four chamber' projection. Catheterisation should be by the percutaneous femoral vein approach and the defect will be crossed by the catheter. Accurate measurement of pulmonary arteriolar resistance is of crucial importance (see Chapter 9); above 10 units $\times$ m^2 the patients are certainly inoperable, between 5 and 10 units represents significant pulmonary vascular disease but such patients may still be operable. Whether or not to advise closure of the defect in the elderly is controversial [8–10]. Patients with atrial septal defect present in late adult life with the onset of supraventricular dys-

Lesion	Age (years)						Total	%
	20–29	30–39	40–49	50–59	60–69	70–79		
ASD	50	38	41	24	20	5	178	45
VSD	24	13	6	2	1	0	46	12
PS	20	10	6	4	0	0	40	10
Coarctation	14	4	4	0	2	0	24	6
PDA	6	3	4	6	4	0	23	6
Fallot	9	8	2	1	0	0	20	5
AV defects	8	3	2	2	0	0	15	4
Complex cyanotic	6	1	4	0	0	0	11	3
AV dis	5	2	0	1	0	0	8	2
Infundibular stenosis	5	2	1	0	0	0	8	2
PAPVR	2	1	1	1	1	0	6	2
AV fistulae	1	2	2	1	0	0	6	2
Ebstein's malformation	3	0	1	0	0	0	4	1
Other	4	1	2	0	0	0	7	2
Total	157	88	76	42	28	5	396	100

Table 18.1 The incidence of specific lesions in each decade among 396 patients with congenital heart disease who first presented in adult life (aged 20 years or more). Brompton Hospital figures, unpublished data.

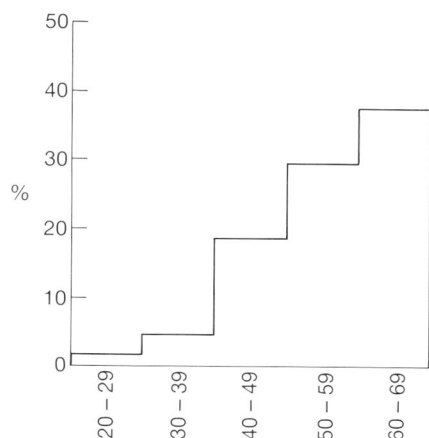

Fig. 18.2 The increasing prevalence of supraventricular dysrhythmias with age in a group of 212 patients with congenital heart disease first presenting in adult life (excluding patients with atrial septal defect or with coexisting rheumatic heart disease). Vertical axis: percentage of patients first presenting in each decade who had developed a supraventricular dysrhythmia by the time of first presentation. Horizontal axis: age at first presentation (decades).

rhythmias or 'heart failure'. Closure of the defect certainly does not prevent the development of a dysrhythmia and impaired ventricular function is unlikely to be improved by surgery. Surgery is of doubtful benefit in patients over the age of 70. Left ventriculography should be part of the investigation; ventricular function can be assessed and other abnormalities such as mitral cusp prolapse detected.

SEPTUM PRIMUM DEFECTS

In *septum primum defects (atrioventricular defects)* ventriculography reveals a 'goose-neck' deformity of the left ventricle [11] with the inlet septum shorter than the outlet septum [12, 13]. A right upper lobe pulmonary vein or left atrial injection in the 'four chamber' projection reveals absence of the lower part of the septum.

Atrioventricular defects occasionally present in adult life and are a common finding in Down syndrome. The probability of significant pulmonary vascular disease is increased if there is a significant ventricular component or significant incompetence of the left AV valve. Severe pulmonary vascular disease is the rule in Down syndrome — probably due to the superadded effect of chronic upper airways obstruction.

'COMMON ATRIUM'

Common atrium is characterised by complete, or almost complete, absence of the interatrial septum with preservation of right and left atrial morphology. The condition is thus distinguished from isomeric atria (bilateral right or left atria) with absence of the atrial septum. As in atrioventricular defects the defect involves the atrioventricular septum and left ventricular angiography reveals a goose-neck deformity. In addition to a large left-to-right shunt there is some mixing at atrial level so that some arterial desaturation is the rule in common atrium. There is an association between common atrium and the Ellis—van Creveld syndrome (Fig. 18.3) [14] characterised by short stature and polydactyly.

Prolapsing mitral leaflet, floppy mitral valve

The clinical syndrome — click, late systolic murmur, etc. [15—16] — is accompanied by a recognisable angiographic abnormality. Left ventricular angio-

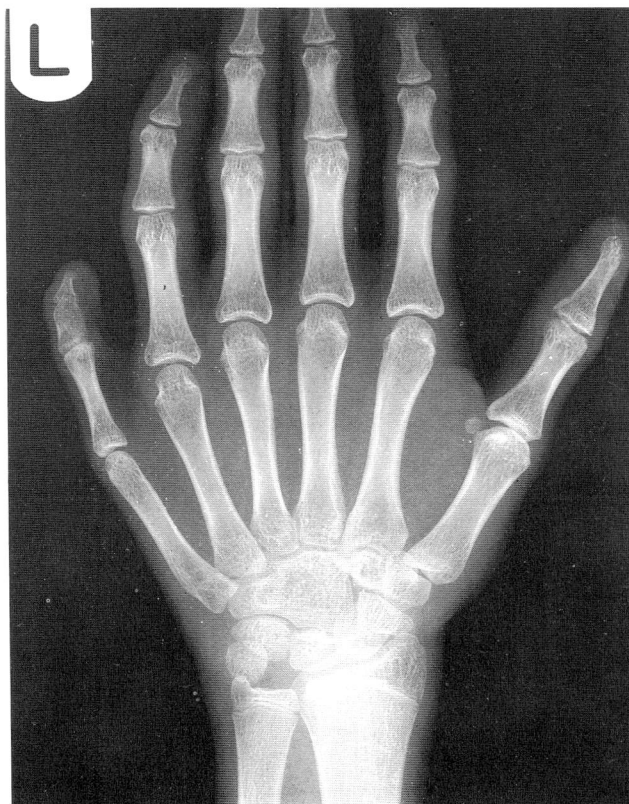

Fig. 18.3 Polydactyly in a patient with the Ellis—van Creveld syndrome and common atrium presenting in adult life.

graphy in the 45° RAO projection will demonstrate posterior bulging of the leaflet beyond the plane of the mitral annulus (Fig. 15.5). The ventriculographic appearance has been described as a 'ballerina's foot' [17]. When there is associated mitral incompetence a jet of contrast will be seen which is often directed inferiorly towards the floor of the atrium and the timing of which may be obviously late systolic. Minor degrees of cusp prolapse are so common as to be virtually a normal variant and the angiographer should avoid over diagnosing the condition. Mitral regurgitation may result from stretching or rupture of the chordae tendinae — especially as a complication of infective endocarditis [18]. Annular calcification may occur and may be gross (Fig. 15.5). Floppy mitral valve occurs in the Marfan syndrome and other connective tissue disorders and mild degrees of mitral prolapse are a common finding in septum secundum atrial septal defects.

Marfan disease of the aorta

The characteristic and unmistakable feature of Marfan disease of the aorta is that the gross dilatation is confined to the ascending aorta with an abrupt reduction to normal calibre before the origins of the head and neck vessels (Fig. 20.47). Aortic rupture and dissection occur; dissection need not be preceded by aneurysm formation. Aortic regurgitation may result from dilatation of the valve ring [19]. The disease is most likely to be detected in early adult life — the age at which dissection can occur. The cardiac manifestations of Marfan disease are most often seen in patients without other stigmata of the syndrome. Investigation requires aortography and left ventriculography; mitral regurgitation due to a 'floppy valve' is a common finding.

Coarctation

Coarctation of the aorta, present at birth, may not be detected until adult life; perhaps as a result of the discovery of (upper body) hypertension, because of endocarditis at the coarctation site or on an associated bicuspid aortic valve or because of bleeding from a berry aneurysm [20–22]. Aortography, using a left oblique projection, should be performed from the brachial approach as it may be impossible to traverse the coarctation from the descending aorta. Not infrequently the coarctation may be so severe as

to create an aortic interruption with lower body circulation preserved by large intercostal collateral vessels (Fig. 20.15). The severity of the coarctation may be assessed angiographically and by measuring the gradient across the coarcted segment. The gradient may be obtained by catheter passage or by simultaneous recording of ascending aortic and femoral arterial pressures. Femoral arterial pressure will appear damped with a lower systolic pressure and delayed peak pressure.

'Parachute mitral valve' with a single, large, papillary muscle is an occasional association; left ventriculography in the right oblique projection may reveal a filling defect due to the single papillary muscle.

Aneurysm of the sinus of Valsalva [23]

Sinus of Valsalva aneurysm, though due to congenital deficiency of the aortic media, rarely presents before adult life (Fig. 20.35). Of our cases only one presented in childhood (aged 12); the remaining eight cases presented between 23 and 49 years of age (mean: 33 years). There is a male preponderance. Presentation is usually due to rupture of the aneurysm. In two-thirds of the cases the right coronary sinus is involved and usually ruptures into the right ventricle. In one-third of cases the noncoronary sinus is involved and may rupture to the right atrium. Aneurysm of the left sinus is very rare.

Three other conditions are characterised by a communication between the aorta and a cardiac chamber; coronary-cameral fistula, aortico-left ventricular tunnel and the combination of ventricular septal defect and aortic regurgitation.

Coronary-cameral fistula

Coronary-cameral fistula is compatible with long survival. Two forms are seen; the classical coronary-cameral fistula produces a large shunt, usually to the right atrium or ventricle, and is associated with enormous dilatation and tortuosity of the affected coronary artery (Fig. 13.37). A second form is usually detected in adult life, often as a chance finding during coronary arteriography, and consists of a small fistulous communication — usually communicating with the pulmonary artery (Fig. 13.38). Similar small fistulae are found between a coronary and pulmonary artery in long standing cyanotic heart disease with low pulmonary flow and in patients with bronchiectasis.

Aortico-left ventricular tunnel [24-25]

Aortico-left ventricular tunnel is distinguished from ruptured sinus of Valsalva since the tunnel originates *above* the sinus. Taking origin above the right sinus the tunnel bypasses the aortic valve (where it may displace the infundibular septum anteriorly causing right ventricular outflow obstruction) and enters the ventricle a short distance below the valve. There may be marked dilatation of the ascending aorta and all three sinuses but there is not the localised dilatation of one sinus as in sinus of Valsalva aneurysm. Aortic root dilatation may result in severe aortic regurgitation. Aortography reveals these features and a left oblique projection will demonstrate the anterosuperior course of the tunnel.

Aortico-left ventricular tunnel is very rare and there are only isolated case reports of the similar conditions of aortico-right ventricular tunnel [26] and the even rarer aortico-left atrial tunnel [27].

It may be difficult to distinguish between ruptured sinus of Valsalva and ventricular septal defect with aortic regurgitation [28]. In both there may be aortic regurgitation resulting in left ventricular opacification following aortography. Aortic regurgitation is due to deformation of the valve cusps and in VSD/AI is often due to cusp prolapse in association with a supracristal VSD. The prominent prolapsed cusp (usually the right) resembles a sinus aneurysm and aortography fills the right ventricle across the VSD. VSD/AI tends to occur more in children than adults while the reverse is true of ruptured sinus of Valsalva aneurysms.

Patent ductus arteriosus

Patent ductus has a bimodal presentation; the majority of symptomatic patients present in infancy or childhood with a large left-to-right shunt. In asymptomatic children the chance discovery of the typical murmur may result in referral. However some cases are discovered for the first time in adult life and the condition is compatible with long survival though most patients will have had the defect corrected in childhood. Apart from chance discovery adults may present as a result of a complication of PDA; infective arteritis, supraventricular arrhythmia, congestive

heart failure or the development of pulmonary vascular disease. Aortic regurgitation may also develop — presumably as a result of aortic root dilatation. When pulmonary vascular disease results from a PDA it does so in patients aged between 20 and 40 — not, apparently, in older patients. This observation may be explained if we think of a PDA as being either large or small. A patient with a large PDA, if he escapes notice because of heart failure in infancy, is liable to develop the Eisenmenger reaction in the teens or early adulthood — as do patients with a high pressure/high flow pulmonary circulation due to a ventricular septal defect. Survival much beyond the age of 30 is unlikely. The patient with a small PDA behaves like those with an atrial septal defect. Presentation is likely to be due to the onset of a supraventricular arrhythmia — of 23 patients with PDA first presenting to us at age 20 or more arrhythmias were confined to those aged 40 or more in whom there was a 43% incidence of supraventricular arrhythmias. Severe pulmonary vascular disease (pulmonary arteriolar resistance >10 units × m^2) was confined to patients aged between 20 and 43. As with patients with an atrial septal defect some elevation of pulmonary arteriolar resistance (between 5 and 10 units) was present in five patients aged between 50 and 60 but the fully developed Eisenmenger reaction was not present. None the less these patients had pulmonary artery systolic pressures between 50 and 60 mmHg.

Pulmonary valve and infundibular stenosis

Pulmonary valve stenosis also has a bimodal pattern of presentation; critical pulmonary stenosis presents in the neonate, less severe stenosis may be detected at any age and frequently not until adult life. Breathlessness is the commonest symptom but many patients are asymptomatic; late onset supraventricular arrhythmias occur uncommonly and infective endocarditis is very rare. Even severe degrees of stenosis are well tolerated for years; in our series of 40 patients with valvar pulmonary stenosis who first presented over the age of 20 there were roughly the same proportion of patients with mild, moderate and severe stenosis presenting in all age groups up to the oldest at age 50-60. In the past, treatment has been by pulmonary valvotomy in any patient with a valve gradient in excess of 75 mmHg and probably in any with a gradient in excess of 50 mmHg. Today the treatment of choice is by balloon pulmonary valvuloplasty performed during cardiac catheterisation. The technique is described in Chapter 5. Since balloon valvuloplasty is simple, safe, and avoids the complications of surgery it is probably that any significant degree of valve stenosis merits treatment. Although early experience was in children experience is now accumulating which suggests that balloon pulmonary valvuloplasty can be equally successful in adults with long standing valvar pulmonary stenosis. Residual gradients may be due to infundibular hypertrophy and such gradients diminish with time as the hypertrophy regresses. Pulmonary regurgitation might be expected to result from the procedure though it is unusual to hear a pulmonary diastolic murmur in treated patients. Pulmonary regurgitation is, in any case, well tolerated as a complication of surgical valvotomy. Balloon valvuloplasty is effective in 'typical' valvar stenosis with thin leaflets which 'dome' during systole; it is ineffective when the valve cusps are thickened and dysplastic. Pulmonary stenosis due to a dysplastic valve is a feature of Noonan syndrome [29].

Cardiac catheterisation allows the diagnosis to be confirmed and the gradient measured prior to valvuloplasty. Right ventricular angiography may demonstrate secondary infundibular stenosis and an associated ASD or patent foramen ovale may be found. Right-to-left shunting across an interatrial communication can occur as a result of right ventricular hypertrophy and reduced compliance. Such shunting can cause marked cyanosis and paradoxical embolism; right-to-left shunting can persist after valvotomy as ventricular hypertrophy regresses slowly. It may be that patients who exhibit these features should still be treated surgically so that an interatrial communication can be closed and, if necessary, infundibular resection performed.

Isolated infundibular stenosis

Isolated infundibular stenosis is much less common than valvar stenosis at any age. Occasional patients present in adult life — our oldest patient first presented at 43 years with a right ventricular systolic pressure of 134 mmHg. One other patient had a pressure of 220 mmHg in the right ventricle. Although termed 'isolated' infundibular stenosis is often accompanied by a small ventricular septal

defect — present in three of our eight patients presenting over the age of 20. When right ventricular pressure is suprasystemic such a VSD can allow right-to-left shunting and arterial desaturation.

Ideopathic dilatation of the pulmonary trunk

On occasion adult patients are found — perhaps as a result of a routine chest X-ray — to have dilatation of the pulmonary trunk and at catheterisation no other abnormality is found. The only importance of the condition is that other causes, such as atrial septal defect and valvar pulmonary stenosis, have to be excluded, by catheterisation, before the patient can be reassured.

Congenital absence of the pulmonary valve
[30, 31]

This is a rare condition characterised by enormous dilatation of the pulmonary trunk *and* the proximal right and left pulmonary arteries with abrupt diminution in calibre thereafter (Fig. 19.18). The roof of the left atrium may be flattened by the dilated left pulmonary artery and there may be bronchial compression. Although the pulmonary valve is represented only by a ridge of tissue (Fig. 19.19) there is a gradient between the right ventricle and the pulmonary artery. A ventricular septal defect is almost always present and right ventricular systolic pressure is at, or near, systemic levels. There is left-to-right shunting so that the haemodynamic findings resemble those of 'acyanotic Fallot'. Of the cases seen at the Brompton Hospital one first presented at 25 years of age.

Pulmonary arteriovenous fistula

Pulmonary arteriovenous fistula [32] may present at any age; very large fistulae may cause heart failure in infancy or cause severe arterial desaturation in childhood. Most cases present in adult life either because an opacity is seen on a plain chest X-ray or because of unexplained arterial desaturation or the occurrence of a cerebrovascular accident or cerebral abcess. In about half of the cases there are arteriovenous malformations elsewhere — hereditary haemorrhagic telangectasia, Rendu–Osler–Weber syndrome. The lesions are frequently multiple and may exist anywhere in the lung though the lower lobes are most commonly affected (Figs 19.21 to 19.23). Even when the chest X-ray has suggested a single lesion it is common for pulmonary angiography to reveal other, smaller, arteriovenous malformations. Treatment includes the possibility of transcatheter embolisation (Fig. 5.12) but the subsequent enlargement of other, undetected, malformations may result in the re-appearance of cyanosis. Selective pulmonary arteriograms will be required to delineate the feeding vessels if embolisation is being planned; the feeding vessels are often large so that there is a danger of systemic migration of the detachable balloon or spring coil unless great care is taken to select a large enough device for the vessel involved [33].

One other, very rare, cause of unexplained arterial desaturation deserves mention — connection of the superior or inferior vena cava to the left atrium [34—35].

Partial anomalous pulmonary venous return

Since the haemodynamic derangement is essentially the same as in atrial septal defect it is not surprising that presentation may be delayed until adult life or that the complications include late onset supraventricular dysrhythmias and, sometimes, late onset pulmonary vascular disease. The anomalously draining vein(s) are most commonly those from the right lung (Figs 17.14 and 17.15) but almost any pattern may occur including drainage of left sided veins to the inferior vena cava. In the commonest form the right vein(s) drain to the superior vena cava/right atrial junction and there is a sinus venosus atrial septal defect (Fig. 17.29). The detection of a 'step-up' at atrial level together with the demonstration of an atrial septal defect may lead to an erroneous diagnosis of atrial septal defect (alone). This is of little consequence if the anomalously draining vein is seen (at operation) close to a large sinus venosus defect. However the atrial defect crossed by the catheter may be no more than a patent foramen ovale and the shunt due to hemianomalous drainage to SVC (for example). This situation can be missed at operation since the entry point of the anomalously draining vein can be occluded by superior caval cannulation for bypass. Catheterisation of suspected PAPVR therefore involves selective right and left pulmonary arteriograms and, if possible, selective pulmonary vein injections — all in the four chamber projection which

separates the atria and profiles the interatrial septum.

The 'scimitar syndrome' (Fig 17.17) is but one of various combinations of abnormalities of tracheobronchial connection, of arterial supply, of venous drainage and of parenchyma of a lung segment. Many patients present in infancy but some present in adult life. In the scimitar syndrome the right pulmonary vein(s) drain to the inferior vena cava above or below the diaphragm (producing the scimitar-shaped shadow on the chest X-ray) and there may be hypoplasia of the right lung with resulting dextrocardia. In some patients there will be an anomalous arterial supply from the descending aorta. This anomalous artery may be single or there may be several and there may be a dual (pulmonary and systemic) blood supply to at least part of the lung segment. Transcatheter embolisation has been used as part of the management — clearly the preliminary angiographic study must include aortography and pulmonary arteriography and may require selective injections to fully describe the arterial supply and venous drainage of the affected segment.

'Corrected transposition'

Corrected transposition (Fig. 17.45) (more properly *physiologically* corrected transposition) is a convenient name for the segmental abnormality of atrioventricular and ventriculo-arterial discordance. Although the anomaly may be compatible with a normal life span associated anomalies occur which may cause a haemodynamic disturbance. Thus an associated ventricular septal defect may be present and the natural history includes the development of complete AV dissociation (heart block). In this condition the morphologic left ventricle is the pulmonary ventricle while the morphologic right ventricle supports the systemic circulation. Since the atrioventricular valves 'go with the ventricles' the left AV valve is a morphologic tricuspid valve but has to support systemic pressures. Either because this valve is less able to stand up to high pressure than is a morphologic mitral valve or because an Ebstein-like malformation of the valve is not uncommon, left AV valve incompetence is a frequent complication of corrected transposition. Failure of the systemic (morphologic right) ventricle in middle age has been described [36].

Catheterising the pulmonary artery in such hearts

can be difficult; the aorta lies anteriorly and to the left while the pulmonary artery lies medially and more posterior than usual. The catheter position which normally leads to the pulmonary artery does not do so — instead there is a blind-ending pouch anteriorly and the catheter has to be manipulated medially and posteriorly (Fig. 17.85b). Use of a balloon-tipped, flow-guided, catheter will overcome this problem.

Congenital complete heart block

Mentioned as a complication of corrected transposition above, congenital heart block also occurs as an isolated anomaly — frequently presenting in adult life [37]. The heart rate is not as slow as in acquired AV dissociation and the ventricular complexes less abnormal. Catheterisation may be performed to exclude other infrequent, defects, and left ventriculography will reveal a large chamber, reflecting the large stroke volume, with a normal or increased ejection fraction.

Congenital coronary anomalies

These have been discussed and illustrated in Chapter 14. Patients with anomalous origin of the left coronary from the pulmonary artery have survived into adulthood — often with surprisingly little disability in view of the gross left ventricular dysfunction present. Anomalous aortic origin is usually of academic interest only though a few forms have been associated with sudden death in young adults.

Hypertrophic cardiomyopathy

Included here because of it's probable congenital origin and its presentation in adult life; the condition is discussed in Chapter 16.

Ebstein's anomaly of the tricuspid valve

This rare condition can present at any age [38]; severe forms causing death in the neonate and mild forms compatible with a normal life-span. Presentation in the adult is likely to be because of tricuspid incompetence, right heart failure and cyanosis or because of an arrhythmia (supraventricular or ventricular tachycardia; WPW type B is a common finding). The malformation consists of displacement of the tricuspid valve attachment from the valve annulus into the right ventricle. As a result the right ventricle is divided into two parts; a smooth 'atrialised' portion between the tricuspid annulus and the displaced tricuspid leaflets and a trabecular and outlet portion which is smaller than normal. The angiographic appearance are unmistakable. The medial and septal leaflets may not be seen but the large anterior leaflet can be seen as a thin linear translucency separating the atrialised portion of the ventricle from the trabecular and outflow portions. The position of the true tricuspid annulus is marked by an indentation on the inferior surface and separates the true right atrium from the atrialised portion of the ventricle (Fig. 17.34). The atrialised ventricle contracts synchronously with the rest of the ventricle and asynchronously with the true atrium. The valve is often incompetent so that the right atrium may be greatly dilated. A secundum atrial septal defect is often present and impaired filling of the small residual right ventricle together with tricuspid regurgitation may result in right-to-left shunting across the defect and arterial desaturation. Right atrial and/ or right ventricular angiograms in the anteroposterior projection will establish the diagnosis. In the past, catheterisation has been thought to be dangerous in Ebstein's disease because of the danger of precipitating an arrhythmia; this has not been our experience and, in any case, D/C cardioversion is now available in all catheterisation laboratories.

Isolated congenital hypoplasia of the right ventricle

This is a very rare condition with similar haemodynamics [39–40]. We have experience of one patient with the condition who first presented at the age of 45 and died 2 years later. The trabecular portion of the ventricle is absent or hypoplastic and only the smooth inflow and outflow portions are seen giving a characteristic tubular appearance to the ventricle (Fig. 17.50). Right ventricular pressure is low — often indistinguishable from right atrial pressure. Filling of the small volume ventricle is impaired and, as a result, there is right-to-left shunting across an atrial septal defect if one is present. Ebstein's anomaly and isolated hypoplasia of the right ventricle are among the few conditions causing right-to-left interatrial shunting with normal right ventricular pressure [40].

CONDITIONS PRESENTING IN CHILDHOOD WITH SURVIVAL INTO ADULT LIFE

Under this heading are also considered the third category of 'adult congenital heart disease' — those conditions in which corrective or palliative surgery in childhood has allowed survival into adulthood.

In conditions with a central shunt, either right-to-left or left-to-right, the secret of survival is for there to be enough resistance to entry to the pulmonary circulation to protect against the development of the Eisenmenger reaction (protected pulmonary circulation) without it being so extreme as to cause severe arterial desaturation. It is also necessary, in 'mixing situations' (Chapter 17), for there to be good mixing of pulmonary venous and systemic venous blood. The possible sites of obstruction to entry to the pulmonary circulation can be listed:

1 Within the ventricle e.g. infundibular stenosis, anomalous muscle bundle, muscular subpulmonary stenosis.
2 At the pulmonary valve e.g. pulmonary valve stenosis.
3 Above the pulmonary valve e.g. surgical 'banding'.
4 At the outlet of a main chamber e.g. at the outlet foramen in tricuspid atresia with subpulmonary outlet chamber (VA concordance).
5 At the origin of a systemic artery to pulmonary artery supply e.g. systemic to pulmonary collaterals in pulmonary atresia with VSD, at the origin of the pulmonary arteries in truncus arteriosus (rarely), surgically created systemic to pulmonary shunts.

When the pulmonary circulation is unprotected the penalties are heart failure and repeated chest infections in childhood followed by the development of pulmonary vascular disease (Fig. 18.4). At this stage there is a period of apparent clinical improvement but this is followed by shunt reversal and increasing cyanosis. Survival is unlikely much beyond the age of 40. The complications of long standing right-to-left shunting, arterial desaturation and polycythaemia include cerebrovascular accidents (thrombosis, embolism) and cerebral abcess and gout. Pregnancy carries a very high risk in the Eisenmenger situation [41].

There are thus two groups of patients with central shunts who may survive into adult life; one group has a protected pulmonary circulation but are likely to have severe arterial desaturation, the other

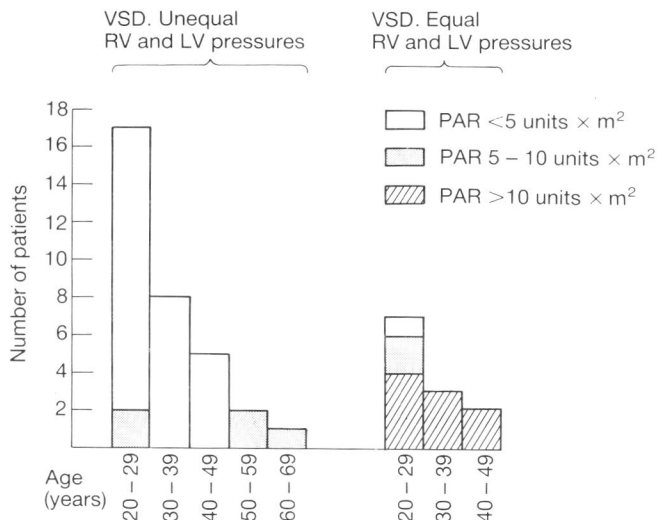

Fig. 18.4 Pulmonary vascular disease and ventricular septal defect in adult life. *Left-hand panel*: 33 patients with isolated ventricular septal defect who first presented over the age of 20 years and who had unequal right and left ventricular systolic pressures ('small VSD'). None have a value for pulmonary arteriolar resistance (PAR) greater than 10 units × m². *Right-hand panel*: 12 patients with isolated ventricular septal defect who first presented over the age of 20 years and who were found to have equal right and left ventricular pressures ('large VSD'). Only three patients, all presenting in the decade 20–29 years, had escaped the development of severe pulmonary vascular disease (PAR > 10 units × m²). No patients with VSD and equal ventricular pressures presented after the age of 49 years. (Brompton Hospital figures, unpublished data.)

have developed the Eisenmenger reaction and are inoperable.

A third group of patients with congenital heart disease encountered in adult life are those whose condition was detected in childhood but was, *or has become*, a mild lesion which is not life-threatening. The obvious example is ventricular septal defect. Small ventricular septal defects with normal or near-normal right heart pressures pose no threat of developing pulmonary vascular disease (Fig. 18.4); the only important risk is of infective endocarditis. We might expect to see many such patients in adult life but in fact such patients are rare; the probable reason is that the majority of small ventricular septal defects close spontaneously — one of the few *beneficial* changes that occur with time [42]. One mechanism of closure results in a so-called 'aneurysm of the membranous septum' — though many such aneurysms are, in reality, the result of apposition of tricuspid valve tissue [43–44] (Fig. 17.69).

A second beneficial change that can occur in association with ventricular septal defect is the development of subpulmonary (infundibular) stenosis so that the pulmonary circulation becomes 'protected' [45].

With the above discussion in mind we can list the conditions in which adult survival is possible:

1 Conditions with protected pulmonary circulation

Tetralogy of Fallot and VSD with acquired infundibular stenosis.
Double outlet right ventricle with subaortic VSD and pulmonary stenosis.
Tricuspid atresia with subpulmonary outlet chamber.
Double inlet ventricle with pulmonary or subpulmonary stenosis.
Pulmonary atresia with VSD and systemic-to-pulmonary collaterals.
Persistent truncus with stenotic origin(s) of pulmonary artery.
Plus the above conditions with low pulmonary flow palliated by a Blalock-type shunt in childhood together with conditions with a high pulmonary flow (see 2 below) palliated by pulmonary artery banding.

2 Conditions with unprotected pulmonary circulation (pulmonary vascular disease likely)

Large ventricular septal defect.
Most of the conditions listed above *without* pulmonary or subpulmonary stenosis, e.g. truncus arteriosus; double outlet right ventricle with subpulmonary VSD and no PS (Taussig—Bing anomaly); tricuspid atresia with double outlet left ventricle; double inlet ventricle with double outlet and no pulmonary stenosis; aortopulmonary septal defect (window).
Plus conditions with (originally) a low pulmonary flow palliated by a Potts or Waterston—Cooley type shunt.

3 Conditions with trivial lesions

Small ventricular septal defect and most of those conditions discussed earlier as 'conditions commonly presenting in adult life'.

It follows from the above that cardiac catheterisation in adults with congenital heart disease is concerned with:
1 The measurement of pulmonary vascular (arteriolar) resistance.
2 Describing the (often complex) anatomy.
3 The assessment of ventricular function.
4 Demonstrating acquired AV valve incompetence.
5 Investigating the consequences of previous palliative or corrective surgery.

The complications of previous surgery that are frequently encountered include developing stenosis of homograft and xenograft valves, calcification of conduits fashioned of biological material, false aneurysm formation at the site of outflow tract enlargement, pulmonary vascular disease developing following a 'too-large' shunt (especially Potts and Waterston—Cooley shunts), distortion and possible occlusion of a pulmonary artery at the site of shunt insertion, fibrosis and stenosis of interatrial baffles, residual stenosis of the pulmonary artery following banding, occlusion or stenosis of systemic-to-pulmonary shunts, recoarctation, patch dehiscence, myocardial dysfunction following cardiopulmonary bypass and ventriculotomy and, no doubt, many more.

GENERAL READING

Roberts WC (ed.) *Congenital heart disease in adults.* Philadelphia, FA Davis Company, 1979.
Freedom RM, Culham JAG, Moes CA. *Angiocardiography of congenital heart disease.* New York, Macmillan Publishing Company, 1984.
Perloff JK. Pediatric congenital becomes a postoperative adult. The changing population of congenital heart disease. *Circulation* 1973;**47**:606.

REFERENCES

1 Flanagan MF *et al.* Changing trends of congenital heart disease in adults: a catheterization laboratory perspective *Cathet Cardiovasc Diagn* 1986;**12**:215.
2 Roberts WC. The congenitally bicuspid aortic valve — a study of 85 autopsy cases. *Am J Cardiol* 1970;**26**:72.
3 Tawes RL, Berry CL, Aberdeen E. Congenital bicuspid aortic valve associated with coarctation of the aorta in children. *Br Heart J* 1969;**31**:127.

4 Higgins EB, Wexler L. Reversal of dominance of the coronary arterial system in isolated aortic stenosis and bicuspid aortic valve. *Circulation* 1975;**52**:292.

5 Fenoglio JJ *et al.* Congenital bicuspid aortic valve after age 20. *Am J Cardiol* 1977;**39**:164.

6 Friedman WF, Kirkpatrick SE. Congenital aortic stenosis and supravalvular. In: Moss AJ, Adams FH, Emmanouilides GC (eds.) *Heart disease in infants, children and adolescents* 2nd edn. Baltimore, Williams & Wilkins Co, 1977; 178.

7 Paolillo V, Dawkins KD, Miller GAH. Atrial septal defect in patients over the age of 50. *Int J Cardiol* 1985; **9**:139.

8 Diacoff GR, Brandenburg RO, Kirklin JW. Results of operation for atrial septal defect in patients 45 years of age and older. *Circulation* 1967;**35** (suppl 1):143.

9 Wolf PS, Vogel JHK, Prior R, Blount SG. Atrial septal defect in patients over 45 years of age. *Br Heart J* 1968;**30**:115.

10 St John Sutton MG, Tajik AJ, McGoon DC. Atrial septal defect in patients aged 60 years or older; operative results and long-term follow up. *Circulation* 1981;**64**:402.

11 Baron MG, Wolf BS, Steinfeld L, Van Mierop LHS. Endocardial cushion defects. Specific diagnosis by angiocardiography. *Am J Cardiol* 1964;**13**:162.

12 Blieden LC *et al.* The 'Goose-Neck' of the endocardial cushion defect: anatomic basis. *Chest* 1974;**65**:13.

13 Becker AE, Anderson RH. Atrioventricular septal defects: whats in a name? *J Thorac Cardiovasc Surg* 1982; **83**:461.

14 Giknis FL. Single atrium and the Ellis–van Creveld syndrome. *J Pediatr* 1963;**62**:558.

15 Barlow JB, Bosman CK. Aneurysmal protrusion of the posterior leaflet of the mitral valve. An auscultatory-electrocardiographic syndrome. *Am Heart J* 1965;**71**:166.

16 Criley JM *et al.* Prolapse of the mitral valve: clinical and cineangiographic findings. *Br Heart J* 1966;**28**:488.

17 Scampardonis G *et al.* Left ventricular abnormalities in prolapsed mitral leaflet syndrome. *Circulation* 1973; **48**:287.

18 Rose JD *et al.* Long term prognosis of mitral valve prolapse — 53 patients followed for 10–22 years (mean 14 years). *Am J Cardiol* 1977;**39**:272.

19 Lemon DK, White CW. Annuloaortic ectasia: angiographic, hemodynamic and clinical comparison with aortic valve insufficiency. *Am J Cardiol* 1978;**41**:482.

20 Presbitero P *et al.* Long term results (15–30 years) of surgical repair of aortic coarctation. *Br Heart J* 1987; **57**:462.

21 Clarkson PM *et al.* Results after repair of coarctation of the aorta beyond infancy: a 10 to 28 years follow-up with particular reference to late systemic hypertension. *Am J Cardiol* 1983;**51**:1481.

22 Fraser TS *et al.* Coarctation of the aorta in adults. *Can Med Ass J* 1976;**115**:415.

23 Sakakibara S, Konno S. Congenital aneurysm of the sinus of valsalva. Anatomy and classification. *Am Heart J* 1962;**63**:405.

24 Levy MJ *et al.* Aortico-left ventricular tunnel. *Circulation* 1963;**27**:841.

25 Sung CS *et al.* Aortico-left ventricular tunnel. *Am Heart J* 1979;**98**:87.

26 Saylam A *et al.* Aorto-right ventricular tunnel. *Ann Thorac Surg* 1974;**18**:643.

27 Yu LC *et al.* Congenital aortico-left atrial tunnel. *Pediatr Cardiol* 1979/80;**1**:153.

28 Keane JF, Plauth WH, Nadas AS. Ventricular septal defect with aortic regurgitation. *Circulation* 1977;**56** (suppl 1):72.

29 Noonan JA, Emke DA. Associated non-cardiac malformations in children with congenital heart disease. *J Pediatr* 1963;**63**:468.

30 Buendia A *et al.* Congenital absence of the pulmonary valve leaflets. *Br Heart J* 1983;**50**:31.

31 Macartney FJ, Miller GAH. Congenital absence of the pulmonary valve. *Br Heart J* 1970;**32**:483.

32 Dines DE, Arms RA, Bernatz PE, Gomez MR. Pulmonary arteriovenous fistulas. *Mayo Clin Proc* 1974;**49**:460.

33 White RI *et al.* Angioarchitecture of pulmonary arteriovenous malformations: an important consideration before embolotherapy. *Am J Roentgenol* 1983;**140**:681.

34 Meadows WR, Bergstrand I, Sharp JT. Isolated anomalous connection of a great vein to the left atrium. *Circulation* 1961;**24**:669.

35 Miller GAH, Ongley PA, Rastelli GC, Kirklin JW. Surgical correction of total anomalous systemic venous connection. *Proc Staff Meet Mayo Clin* 1965;**40**:532.

36 Nagle JP, Cheitlen MD, McCarty RJ. Corrected transposition of the great vessels without associated anomalies: report of a case with congestive failure at age 45. *Chest* 1971;**60**:367.

37 McHenry MM. Factors influencing longevity in adults with congenital complete heart block. *Am J Cardiol* 1972; **29**:416.

38 Genton E, Blount SG. The spectrum of Ebstein's anomaly. *Am Heart J* 1967;**73**:395.

39 Van der Hauwaert LG, Michaelsson M. Isolated right ventricular hypoplasia. *Circulation* 1971;**44**:466.

40 Haworth SG, Shinebourne EA, Miller GAH. Right-to-left interatrial shunting with normal right ventricular pressure. A puzzling haemodynamic picture associated with some rare congenital malformations of the right ventricle and tricuspid valve. *Br Heart J* 1975;**37**:386.

41 Mark H, Young D. Congenital heart disease in the adult. *Am J Cardiol* 1965;**15**:293.

42 Weidman WH, DuShane JW, Ellison RC. Clinical course in adults with ventricular septal defect. *Circulation* 1977; **56** (suppl 1):178.

43 Nugent EW *et al.* Aneurysm of the membranous septum in ventricular septal defect. *Circulation* 1977;**56** (suppl 1):82.

44 Hoeffel JC *et al.* Radiologic patterns of aneurysms of the membranous septum. *Am Heart J* 1976;**91**:450.

45 Gasul BM, Dillon RJ, Vela V. The natural transformation of ventricular septal defects into ventricular septal defects with pulmonary stenosis. *Am J Dis Child* 1957; **94**:424.

Pulmonary arteriography, pulmonary embolism

Pulmonary arteriography allows visualisation of the whole of the pulmonary circulation — veins as well as arteries — and, with somewhat reduced clarity, the left heart and systemic circulation. This chapter will describe those conditions in which pulmonary arteriography is the investigation of choice.

TECHNIQUES

The angiographic techniques that can be employed for investigating the pulmonary circulation are:
1 'Conventional' pulmonary arteriography.
2 Balloon-occlusion pulmonary angiography.
3 Pulmonary (artery) wedge angiography.
4 Pulmonary vein wedge angiography.

'Conventional' pulmonary arteriography

Most pulmonary arteriograms are of this type; contrast medium is injected into the pulmonary trunk or selectively into the right or left pulmonary arteries or their branches. An angiographic catheter is used and the approach may be from the arm or the leg. Catheters of the NIH or Eppendorf type are commonly used but the Grollman angled pigtail catheter is an alternative and is more easily advanced through the right ventricle, when the approach is from the leg, than are conventional catheters. If the Grollman catheter is used the patient should be heparinised since thrombus formation is liable to occur in the tip of all pigtail catheters. Care is necessary when the Grollman catheter is withdrawn since the curled tip may catch in the chordae of the tricuspid valve; if resistance is felt at this point the catheter should be re-advanced and withdrawal repeated with a different orientation of the catheter [1].

The amount of contrast medium injected depends on the condition studied and the site of injection. Pulmonary arteriography can be hazardous in conditions characterised by a high pulmonary vascular resistance ('primary' pulmonary hypertension, pulmonary embolism) and the amount of contrast given should be limited to no more than 0.5 ml/kg and a non-ionic medium used. Similarly selective injections into segmental arteries call for reduced amounts of contrast. For other conditions and for injections into the pulmonary trunk 0.5 to 1.0 mg/kg are required. If the aim is to opacify the pulmonary veins and there is a high pulmonary flow (e.g. total anomalous pulmonary venous return) 1.5 to 2.0 ml/kg are likely to be needed.

Filming may employ large format, serial, films or cine film. There is no doubt that large format films provide the most exquisite detail and are ideal for many purposes — if available. A preliminary, scout film must be taken to check that the field has been correctly selected and that the exposure is optimal. The operator has to decide how best to time filming. The programmes available vary among different makes of equipment. Most are capable of filming rates between 1 and 4 or 6 per second. Some are capable of filming at three different rates consecutively. In the normal pulmonary circulation contrast medium, injected in the pulmonary trunk, will appear in the pulmonary veins and left atrium 4–6 seconds later. A programme of, say, 4 films/second for 4 seconds followed by 1/second for 4 seconds will provide a number of films during the pulmonary arterial phase (and allow for the duration of injection — say 2 seconds) while covering the laevophase so as to visualise the left heart and aorta. In conditions such as massive pulmonary embolism, where pulmonary resistance is high and cardiac output is low, pulmonary flow is slow and a slower rate of filming is indicated.

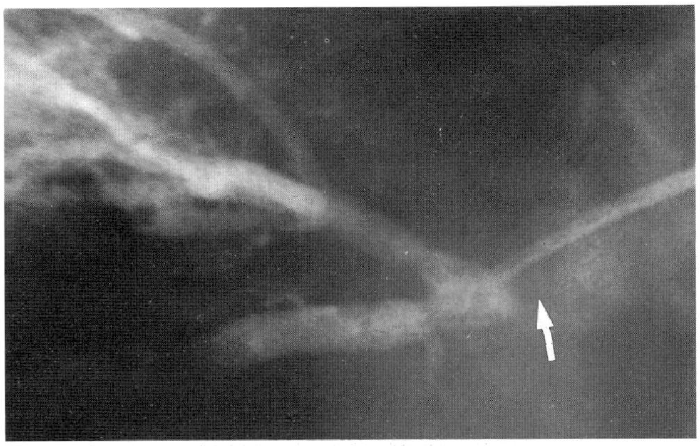

Fig. 19.1 Balloon occlusion pulmonary arteriography. In this example a catheter with an end-hole distal to the balloon (arrow) has been used. Pulmonary flow is arrested by the inflated balloon providing enhanced opacification of the distal pulmonary artery.

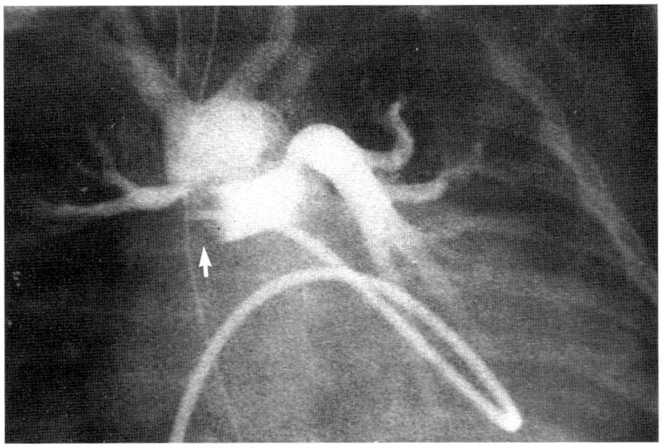

Fig. 19.2 Balloon occlusion pulmonary arteriography. In this example the side-holes of the catheter are proximal to the balloon so that no contrast medium can enter the right pulmonary artery which is occluded by the inflated balloon (arrow), as a result there is selective opacification of the left pulmonary artery (and some opacification of the aorta in this patient with persistent truncus arteriosus).

Cine angiography, besides being more widely available, has the advantage that structures are often more easily detected on a dynamic than on a static image. The immediate playback capability (using video recording) provided by cine angiography is also an advantage; serial, large format, films have to be developed and fixed before diagnostic information is available.

The anteroposterior projection is often used in pulmonary arteriography but is not necessarily the best projection for all anomalies. The projections

that should be used are described for the individual lesions in the sections that follow.

Balloon occlusion pulmonary angiography (Figs 19.1 and 19.2)

This technique can be used to detect pulmonary emboli in segmental, or subsegmental, pulmonary arteries [2–4]. Conventional pulmonary angiography, excellent for visualising large, central, emboli, may fail to demonstrate small, peripheral, emboli, A 7F, balloon-tipped end-hole catheter, is inflated and allowed to occlude a segmental artery in the area of interest. A hand injection of less than 10 ml of contrast medium over 2–4 seconds serves to opacify the whole of the vascular segment distal to the occlusion. Filming continues during slow deflation of the balloon and further information may be gained as flow recommences around the filling defects.

Pulmonary (artery) wedge angiography

This technique has been used to confirm that a catheter is in the true wedge position — there should be no forward movement of a hand injection of 2–5 ml of contrast medium over several seconds [5] — and, more importantly, to assess pulmonary vascular disease [6–7]. In the presence of pulmonary vascular disease the morphology of the pulmonary vascular tree changes; the number of small branches is decreased ('pruning') and the larger vessels become dilated and tortuous. These changes can be appreciated on conventional pulmonary arteriography but magnification wedge angiography allows quantification. With an end-hole catheter in the wedge position a slow, hand injection of 0.5–3.0 ml of contrast medium is followed by a 5–10 ml flush with 5% dextrose solution. Magnification is achieved using a 15 cm (6 inch) intensifier positioned 52.5 cm (21 inch) from the table top. Further magnification to a total of 7.5 × actual size is obtained by projection onto a screen at a distance of 1.80–2.4 m (6–8 feet) [7].

Pulmonary vein wedge angiography (Fig. 19.3)

This important technique is used to opacify the

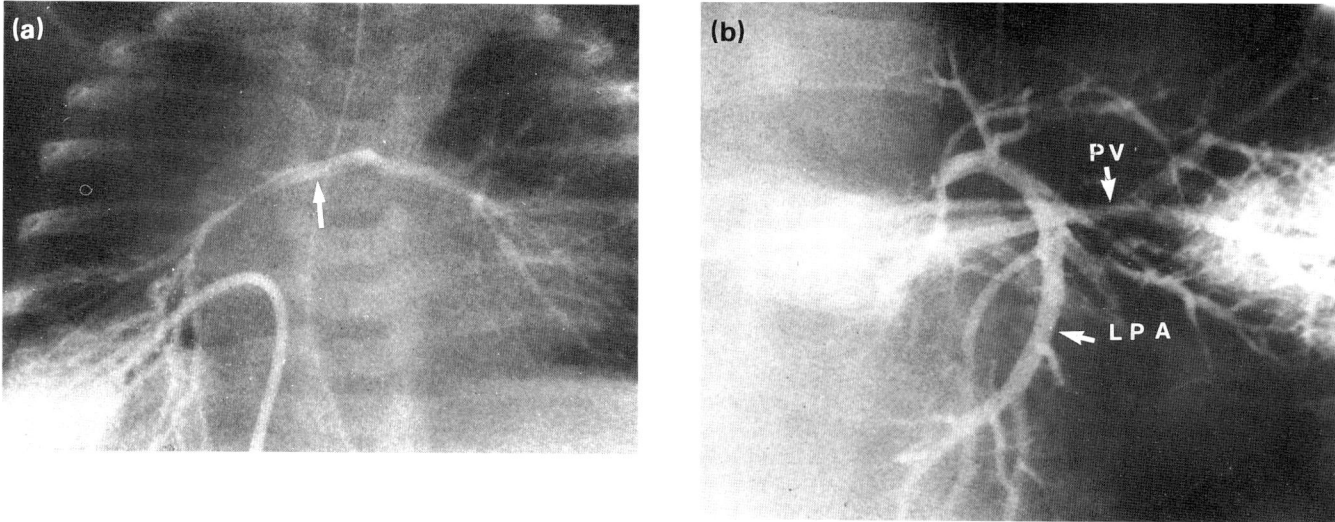

Fig. 19.3 (a) Pulmonary vein wedge angiography. Injection of contrast medium in the 'wedged pulmonary vein' position in the right lower lobe has resulted in filling of very hypoplastic right and left pulmonary arteries (arrow) in a patient with pulmonary atresia. (b) Another example of pulmonary vein wedge angiography. An injection in a left pulmonary vein (PV) has resulted in filling of a small left pulmonary artery (LPA) which had no connection to either ventricle or to the aorta.

pulmonary arteries when they cannot be opacified antegradely or through a systemic-to-pulmonary communication. Classically the technique is used in pulmonary atresia with ventricular septal defect in order to determine the presence or absence of intra-pericardial pulmonary arteries [8–9]. An end-hole catheter is used (side-holes may predispose to extra-vasation of contrast) and a slow (2–3 second), hand injection, of 0.4–0.8 ml/kg of contrast medium made with the catheter wedged in a pulmonary vein. Complications are rare but extravasation into the bronchi with resulting severe bronchospasm has been reported in a case where a pressure injection of 0.3 ml/kg at 20 ml/second was used [10].

segmental arteries and continues as the 'pars inter-lobaris' until the origin of the middle lobe and apical upper lobe segmental arteries. From this point the artery continues as the 'pars basalis' and gives rise to four segmental arteries of the lower lobe.

The left pulmonary artery is smaller than the right and has no large upper lobe branch. Instead it arches backwards over the left main bronchus as the 'pars superior' and supplies the upper lobe from a variable number of small branches arising from its outer aspect. The left pulmonary artery then descends as the 'pars interlobaris' and 'pars basalis' and supplies segmental branches to the lingula and lower lobe [11].

THE ANATOMY OF THE PULMONARY ARTERIES

The right pulmonary artery passes behind the ascending aorta and superior vena cava and reaches the lung passing in front of the right descending bronchus and between the upper and middle lobe bronchi. It gives off a large branch ('truncus an-terior') to the upper lobe from which arise three

INDICATIONS FOR PULMONARY ANGIOGRAPHY

Pulmonary arteriography is performed (1) to demonstrate congenital or acquired anomalies of the pulmonary circulation, or (2) to opacify the left heart — left atrium and ventricle and aorta — when direct access to these chambers is impossible or undesirable.

Acquired diseases of the pulmonary circulation in which pulmonary arteriography is indicated are:

1 Pulmonary thromboembolic disease — acute minor or acute massive pulmonary embolism, chronic thromboembolic pulmonary hypertension.

2 'Primary' or 'ideopathic' pulmonary hypertension.

3 Pulmonary arteriography can be used to visualise the left heart chambers; left atrial myxomas, cor triatriatum and supravalve stenosing ring of the left atrium can all be visualised in this way though echocardiography has largely replaced angiography for diagnosing these conditions. Pulmonary arteriography with 'follow-through' has been advocated as a low-risk procedure for demonstrating aortic dissections. The risk may not be significantly lower and the poor definition obtained more than outweighs any possible benefit. However the technique of digital subtraction angiography may introduce a new era of non-selective angiography. Aortic dissections can also be demonstrated non-invasively by computerised axial tomography or magnetic resonance imaging.

PULMONARY THROMBOEMBOLISM

Pulmonary embolism results in a number of distinct syndromes; failure to distinguish between these syndromes has resulted in much confusion and many inaccuracies in the voluminous literature devoted to the subject. Terms such as 'symptomatic embolism' are meaningless; minor embolism may be symptomatic in that it results in pleuritic pain and massive embolism symptomatic in that it causes syncope (or sudden death!); the two conditions have a totally different symptomatology, haemodynamic profile and prognosis.

The presentation, physical signs, haemodynamic abnormalities, treatment and prognosis of pulmonary embolic disease are determined by (1) the size of the emboli, (2) the time for which they have been present, and (3) the presence or absence of additional cardiorespiratory disease. A classification which recognises the importance of severity and duration is; (1) acute minor pulmonary embolism, (2) acute massive pulmonary embolism, (3) subacute massive pulmonary embolism, and (4) chronic thromboembolic pulmonary hypertension [12–13].

Syndromes of pulmonary embolism

ACUTE MINOR PULMONARY EMBOLISM

Patients with minor pulmonary embolism may present with an episode of pleuritic pain though it is probable that embolism is 'silent' in the majority of cases. There may be an audible pleural friction rub or crepitations. The plain chest X-ray may show infarct shadows, loss of lung volume or patchy oligaemia but is often normal. There are no abnormal cardiovascular findings and the ECG is normal.

In minor pulmonary embolism there is involvement of less than half of the pulmonary arterial tree. The normal pulmonary circulation can accommodate at least twice the normal flow without an increase of pressure. As a result in minor pulmonary embolism there is no haemodynamic disturbance; right heart and pulmonary artery pressures are normal. Pulmonary arteriography will demonstrate emboli involving less than half of the pulmonary arterial tree.

The angiographic features of pulmonary embolism have been well described by Dalen *et al.* [14] and are:

1 Intraluminal filling defects.
2 Vessel occlusion — arterial 'cut-offs'.
3 Areas of oligaemia.
4 Asymmetry of flow.

These findings may be present in all forms of pulmonary embolic disease though there are differences of detail.

Intraluminal filling defects

Recent emboli produce filling defects which bulge into the contrast-filled pulmonary artery. They may occlude a branch of a pulmonary artery, producing *'arterial cut-offs'* or contrast medium may get past the emboli which are then seen as filling defects within the lumen of the artery giving a 'pipe stem' appearance. Frequently emboli lodge at a bifurcation — narrowing or occluding each of the two pulmonary artery branches — often at the point of origin of the right upper lobe pulmonary artery. When an artery is narrowed or occluded there will be an area of *oligaemia* distally and, since emboli are not evenly distributed, there will be *asymmetry of flow.* Occasionally, in massive embolism, there will actually be areas of uninvolved lung which exhibit 'compensatory hyperaemia'. Infarct shadows and/or loss of lung volume may be, present on the plain chest X-ray and also visible on arteriograms; they are due to previous pulmonary infarction; it follows that they may be present, as a result of prior embolism, but are not necessary accompaniments of any form of embolism.

All these findings may be present in minor embolism but small, peripheral, emboli may be difficult, or impossible to detect. Under these circumstances selective injections (using oblique projections) and balloon occlusion angiography provide the best chance making a positive angiographic diagnosis.

ACUTE MASSIVE PULMONARY EMBOLISM
(Figs 19.4 to 19.9)

Patients with massive embolism present with sudden syncope/cardiac arrest and acute onset dyspnoea. Chest pain, present in about one-third of patients, may be pleuritic (due to minor, premonitory embolism), but is typically central and oppressive in character. Examination of the cardiovascular system may reveal a 'gallop' at the left sternal edge (summation gallop due to third and fourth heart sounds) — a very important physical sign — and a raised central venous pressure. Pulmonary valve closure sound (P2) is delayed or inaudible; it is *not* accentuated unless there is pre-existing cardiorespiratory disease. There is a sinus tachycardia and, often, shock. A mild degree of cyanosis is detectable in some two-thirds of patients and arterial desaturation measurable in almost all.

The radiographic hall-mark of massive embolism is patchy oligaemia. The pulmonary trunk is not obviously dilated but the hilar shadow may be prominent with an abrupt cut-off resulting in a 'pear-shaped hilum'; most easily detected on the right. The ECG can be normal but more usually reveals one of the recognised patterns such as an S wave in standard lead 1 and a Q wave with T wave inversion in standard lead 3 — with or without T wave inversion in the anterior chest leads ('S1 Q3 T3' pattern). Partial or complete right bundle branch block is another commonly seen pattern.

In this condition more than half of the pulmonary arterial tree is involved and, as a result, there is a profound haemodynamic disturbance. The normal right ventricle, faced with a sudden increase in

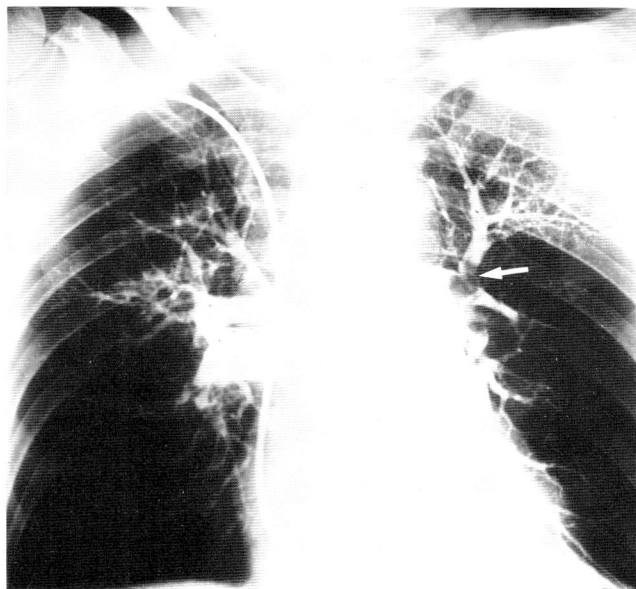

Fig. 19.4 Acute massive pulmonary embolism. There is embolic occlusion of most of the pulmonary arterial tree; only the left upper zone is spared and even here a filling defect due to emboli is seen at the origin of the left upper lobe artery (arrow).

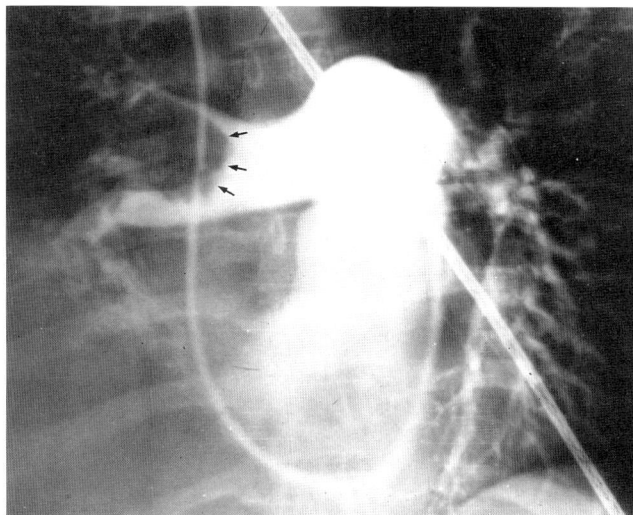

Fig. 19.5 The hall-mark of recent embolism. An embolus has lodged at the bifurcation of the right pulmonary artery (arrows) and *bulges into the contrast-filled pulmonary artery*. Compare with the appearances of chronic thromboembolism illustrated in Fig. 19.11.

afterload, cannot generate a systolic pressure much higher than 40–50 mmHg and, in so doing, becomes acutely dilated with impaired filling. The haemodynamic findings are, therefore:

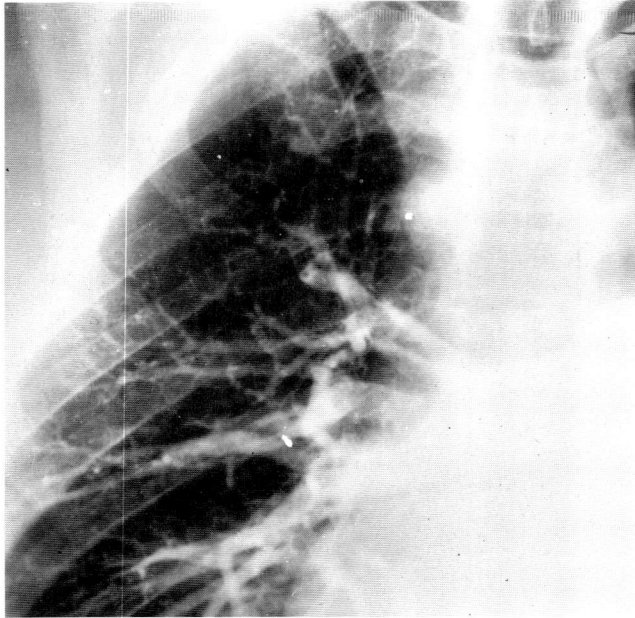

Fig. 19.6 Another angiographic sign of recent (massive) pulmonary embolism; filling defects are seen within the lumens of several branches to the right mid and lower zones. The resulting appearances have been likened to a 'pipe stem'.

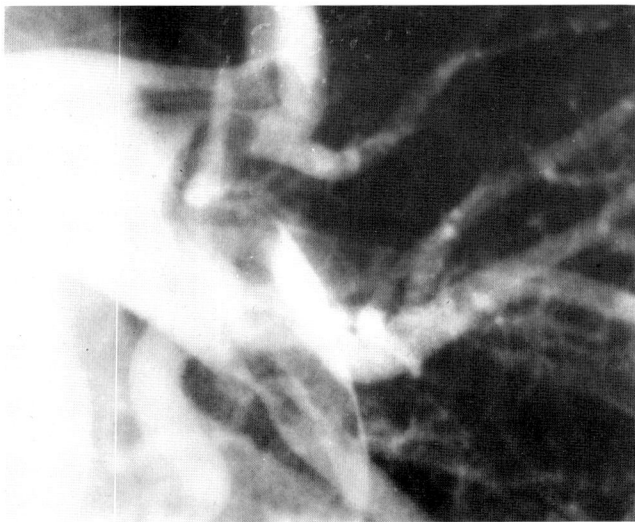

Fig. 19.7 A magnified view demonstrates intraluminal filling defects characteristic of recent embolism.

1 Right ventricular and pulmonary artery systolic pressures of no more than 40–50 mmHg.
2 Raised right ventricular end-diastolic pressure which may approximate to pulmonary diastolic — hence a 'soft P2'.

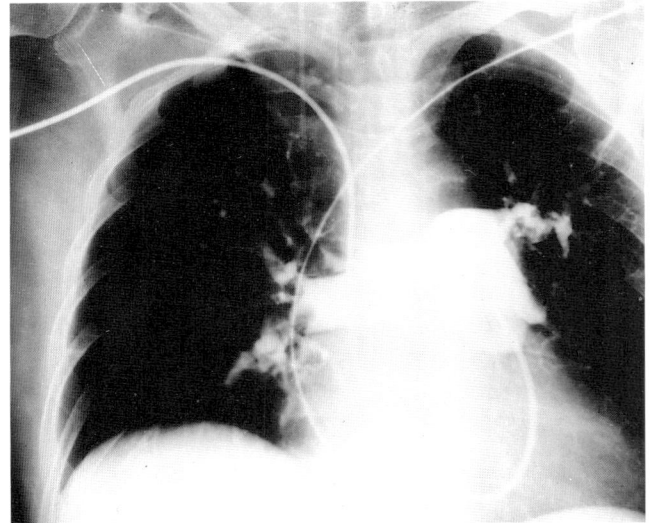

Fig. 19.8 'Supramassive' pulmonary embolism. Despite the near-total occlusion of the pulmonary arterial tree this patient survived following emergency pulmonary embolectomy.

3 Raised right atrial pressure — often with a dominant a wave.
4 A low cardiac output as evidenced by a mixed venous (pulmonary arterial) saturation averaging 40% and an arterial waveform which has a sharp upstroke (vasoconstriction) and a small area beneath the curve. Other signs of shock may be present; low or absent urine flow, hypotension, sweating, mental confusion and so on.
5 Arterial blood gases reveal low values for both Po_2 (average 7 kPa 50 mmHg) and Pco_2 (average 5 kPa 35 mmHg) [15].

All the symptoms and signs of massive pulmonary embolism can be explained as being the result of (1) acute right ventricular failure, (2) acute disturbance of pulmonary ventilation and perfusion, and (3) acute reduction in cardiac output.

Pulmonary arteriography provides the 'gold standard' for the diagnosis of pulmonary embolism. Both false-positive and false-negative findings can occur with perfusion scans and while the accuracy of scintillation scanning can be improved by using ventilation-perfusion scanning the technique is still less accurate than angiography [16]. However massive embolism is incompatible with a normal lung scan; in a patient with shock an alternative diagnosis must be sought if this is the finding. Rather than discuss the indications for pulmonary arteriography

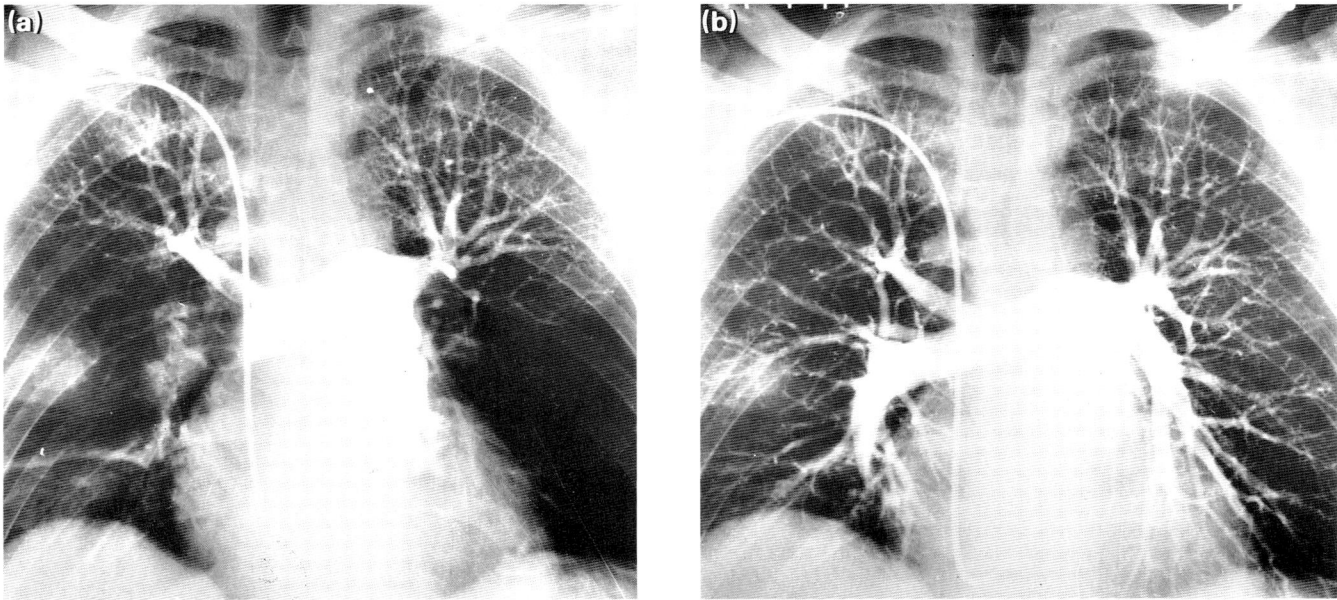

Fig. 19.9 Thrombolytic therapy in acute massive pulmonary embolism. (a) Pulmonary arteriogram obtained on admission to hospital demonstrating massive pulmonary emboli . (b) In the same patient treatment with streptokinase has resulted in almost complete resolution of the emboli after 72 hours.

or scanning it is more worth while emphasising that massive pulmonary embolism is a medical emergency. The above discussion should indicate that the clinical diagnosis of massive embolism, in the absence of other cardiorespiratory disease, is based on very specific findings. If the diagnosis is suspected it is essential that it is confirmed (or excluded) *immediately*. There is no place for delay; death can occur suddenly even in patients who appear haemodynamically stable.

The arteriographic appearances are essentially the same as in minor embolism but the filling defects are much more extensive. There may be such extensive involvement that the patient's survival is dependent on perfusion of but a single lobe or part of a lobe. Catheterisation should be via an arm vein since an approach from the femoral vein carries the risk of dislodging further emboli. An Eppendorf catheter is less rigid than the NIH type and may be preferred since catheter-induced perforation of the right ventricle has been reported in massive embolism.

The effect of contrast medium is to cause some transient increase in pulmonary vascular resistance and a fall in systemic resistance due to a short-lived vasodilatation. Both effects could be fatal in a patient with massive embolism; pulmonary vascular resistance is already high and limiting forward flow so that such patients cannot increase their cardiac output to compensate for contrast medium-induced vasodilatation. A profound fall in arterial pressure can follow angiography in such patients. In practice we have seen no complications or deaths following angiography in over 100 patients with massive embolism. Since the remaining pulmonary vascular tree is so reduced in volume and the flow so low the amount of contrast medium needed to provide good opacification is also much less than would normally be required — 0.5 or 0.3 ml/kg of a non-ionic medium is all that should be given.

Large format serial films provide excellent detail and allow comparison between different patients and different treatments. A single injection in the pulmonary trunk will opacify the whole of the pulmonary arterial tree and the large format films cover both lung fields. Cine angiography will require at least two separate injections since the field size is too small to cover more than one lung field — at best. If cine angiography is used the probability is that multiple selective injections will be required and, under these circumstances, it is logical to use oblique projections selected to provide optimal visualisation of the artery being studied. A left oblique or lateral projection is used for the left lung and an anteroposterior or right oblique for the right [16].

Cine angiograms may, on occasion, reveal emboli extending through the foramen ovale and posing a risk of paradoxical embolism. Such left-sided abnormalities may be less easily appreciated on serial films.

In order to compare the results of different treatments there is a need for an objective method of quantifying the severity of embolism as judged by angiography. Two methods are in common use; that developed for the 'Urokinase Pulmonary Embolism Trial' [17] and that developed for our own use [18]. The latter has the merit of simplicity, since it does not require measurement of the size of emboli which are often difficult to see in their entirety, and provides reasonably consistent results [19]. The system tends, however, to underestimate improvement. In this system the right pulmonary artery is regarded as having nine major segmental branches (three to the upper lobe, two to the middle lobe and four to the lower lobe) and the left pulmonary artery as

having seven major branches (two to the upper lobe, two to the lingula and three to the lower lobe). The presence of a filling defect or defects in any one of these branches scores 1 point so that involvement by emboli of all the branches on the right scores a maximum of 9 and on the left 7 points for 'involvement'. A filling defect or defects proximal to segmental branches scores a value equal to the number of segmental branches arising distally; thus a filling defect in the main right pulmonary artery would score 9 points for 'involvement'. Clearly these scores by themselves could give a totally false picture; a filling defect causing little obstruction and little reduction in flow would score the same as one causing complete occlusion. To allow for this a second score is added which requires that the degree of reduction of flow be assessed for the upper, middle and lower zones of each lung. Absent flow scores 3 points, severe reduction 2 points, mild reduction 1 point and normal flow 0 points. The maximum score for reduction in pulmonary artery flow is therefore 9 points for each lung (maximum theoretical total for flow reduction is 18 points) and this score is added to the score for involvement so that the maximum possible score would be 34 points (Fig. 19.10).

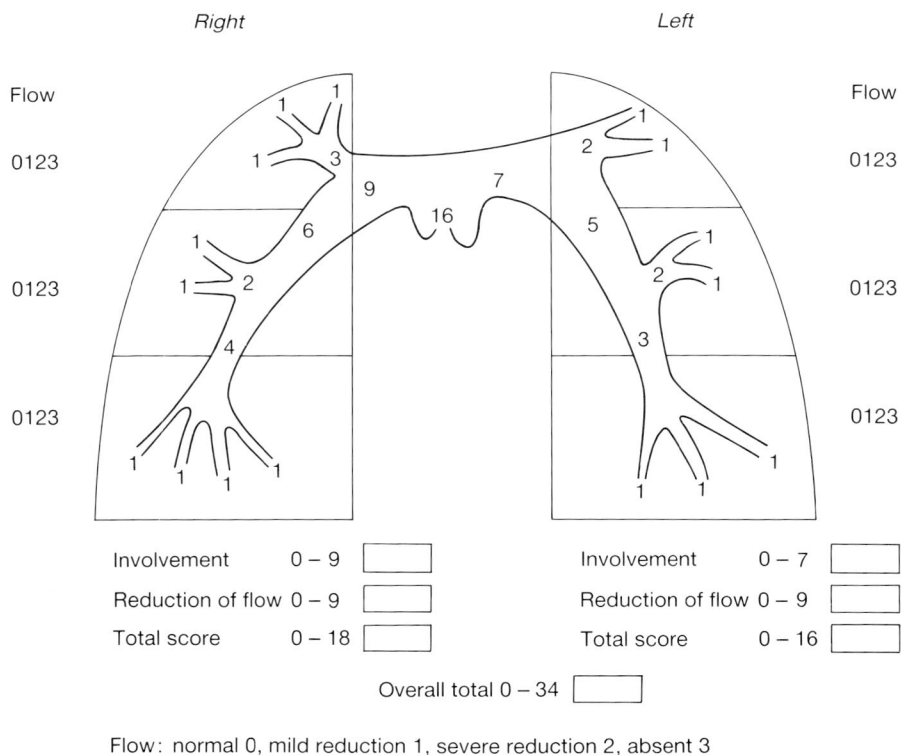

Fig. 19.10 A scoring system which allows numerical coding of the severity of embolism and which can be used to compare the angiographic effects of different treatments (see text).

SUBACUTE MASSIVE PULMONARY EMBOLISM

Although there are some clinical features which separate these patients from those with acute massive embolism they are, essentially, patients who have survived massive embolism for a period of weeks but in whom embolism has not resolved and thrombolytic or surgical treatment not been used. There are some haemodynamic and angiographic differences. Pulmonary artery and right ventricular systolic pressures tend to be higher averaging 54 mmHg as against 41 mmHg for patients with acute massive embolism [12]. Angiographically the filling defects are less sharply defined and no longer bulge into the contrast-filled pulmonary artery — though the more recent emboli may still do so when there have been repeated episodes. These altered appearances are probably due to organisation of the emboli and the effect of naturally occurring partial lysis. The response to thrombolitic agents and to embolectomy is less satisfactory than when embolism is recent and such patients have a higher mortality.

CHRONIC THROMBOEMBOLIC PULMONARY HYPERTENSION

Patients with this condition present with increasing breathlessness and sometimes exertional syncope. As a rule there is no antecedent history suggestive of pulmonary embolism. As a result of long standing disease there is considerable right ventricular hypertrophy and the hypertrophied ventricle *can* generate a high pressure — averaging 85 mmHg (systolic) in our series of patients. In keeping with this finding pulmonary valve closure is accentuated and the plain chest X-ray reveals marked dilatation of the pulmonary trunk as well as patchy oligaemia. The ECG reveals right ventricular hypertrophy and not the 'strain' pattern of acute embolism.

The angiographic appearances differ from those of acute embolism; the central pulmonary arteries are obviously dilated and filling defects are not seen (Figs 19.11 and 19.12). Perfusion is preserved in some zones and absent, or reduced (oligaemia), in others. The vessels are enlarged and tortuous as is seen in patients with severe pulmonary vascular disease. The fact that perfusion is *asymmetrical* suggests a thromboembolic aetiology in contrast to the

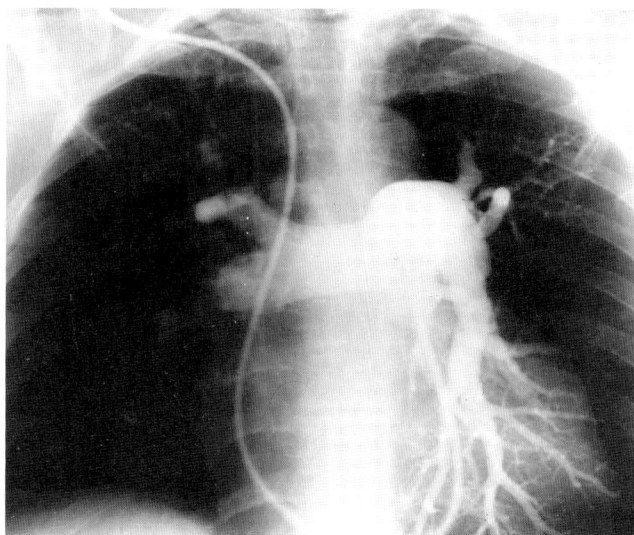

Fig. 19.11 Chronic thromboembolic pulmonary hypertension. The embolic origin of this condition is presumed from the typically assymmetrical involvement of the pulmonary arteries. There is almost no perfusion of the right lung whereas the left lower lobe has been spared. In this chronic situation there is severe pulmonary hypertension reflected in the obvious enlargement of the main and right pulmonary arteries. Note that filling defects are no longer seen and the contrast-filled pulmonary artery has a convex leading edge (compare with Fig. 19.5).

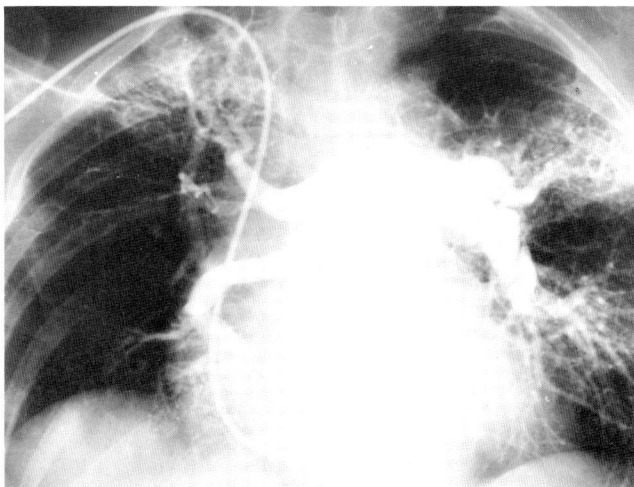

Fig. 19.12 Another example of assymmetrical involvement and tortuous pulmonary arteries in chronic thromboembolic pulmonary hypertension.

uniform changes seen in primary pulmonary hypertension and the Eisenmenger reaction.

Organised emboli/thrombi at bifurcations may cause narrowing of pulmonary artery branches. Occluded vessels present a *concave* edge to the contrast-filled artery as might be explained by organisation and partial lysis of old emboli.

Primary pulmonary hypertension

Although there are suggestive features, such as a tendency to affect females in their 20s and 30s, the diagnosis of primary pulmonary hypertension is largely one of exclusion. Pulmonary arteriography reveals dilated and *tortuous* central pulmonary arteries with a marked reduction in calibre of the smaller, peripheral, vessels ('pruning'). A thromboembolic aetiology is excluded by the fact that the changes are uniform throughout the pulmonary arterial tree.

Dilated and tortuous vessels with peripheral pruning is an angiographic appearance common to severe pulmonary vascular disease from many causes; for example in the Eisenmenger reaction or in pulmonary vascular disease secondary to parenchymal lung disease (cor pulmonale). The Eisenmenger reaction as a cause is excluded if there is no central shunt or septal defect. However some right-to-left shunting across a patent foramen ovale is common in primary pulmonary hypertension. Points of differentiation from an 'Eisenmenger atrial septal defect' are that pulmonary artery systolic pressures are rarely above 50 mmHg in 'Eisenmenger ASD' while in primary pulmonary hypertension pulmonary artery pressure is frequently near to, or even higher than, systemic pressure. The Eisenmenger reaction, if it occurs at all, seldom occurs before late middle age in ASD (at least in Western countries); primary pulmonary hypertension commonly occurs in young adults. Finally it may be possible to demonstrate the absence of a *large* interatrial defect by echocardiography or right atrial angiography — though at these levels of pulmonary hypertension the distinction is academic since treatment is ineffective in both conditions.

In patients with the Eisenmenger reaction secondary to a defect at ventricular or great vessel level (e.g. VSD, truncus arteriosus) right ventricular pressure will be identical to left ventricular pressure and the defect likely to be demonstrable by angiography or indicator dilution techniques.

It is important to exclude a downstream lesion (e.g. mitral stenosis, cor triatriatum) as a cause of pulmonary hypertension. In primary pulmonary hypertension the left atrial or wedge pressure is low; unfortunately it is often difficult, or impossible, to obtain a satisfactory wedge pressure in anyone with severe pulmonary vascular disease. In practice such lesions are likely to have been excluded on clinical or echocardiographic grounds.

Pulmonary arteriography is hazardous in primary pulmonary hypertension; the temporary increase in pulmonary vascular resistance and the systemic vasodilation due to contrast media without the possibility of a compensatory increase in cardiac output may lead to profound hypotension and death. If pulmonary arteriography is performed 0.5 to 0.3 ml/kg of non-ionic contrast medium is all that should be given.

Finally among acquired abnormalities of the pulmonary circulation causing pulmonary hypertension mention must be made of Takayasu disease. Pulmonary involvement is common in this rare disease but affects the larger branch pulmonary arteries and is almost always accompanied by systemic arterial involvement [20].

Indications for pulmonary arteriography in congenital heart disease

1 To demonstrate the size (adequacy) of the pulmonary arteries in tetralogy of Fallot and allied conditions when deciding between complete correction or a preliminary shunt operation. Blackstone and associates [21–22] have shown that it is possible to predict the postoperative RV/LV pressure ratio (*P* RV/LV) from measurements of pulmonary artery and aortic diameters taken from preoperative angiocardiograms. The measurements used are the maximal systolic diameter of the right pulmonary artery (DRPA) and left pulmonary artery (DLPA) just before the origins of their first branches. These values are normalised by dividing by the maximal systolic diameter of the descending aorta just above the diaphragm (Desc. Th. Ao.). The formula is:

$$P \text{ RV/LV} = 0.484 \text{ (DRPA/Desc. Th. Ao.} + \text{DLPA/Desc. Th. Ao.)} + 0.2007.$$

Further allowance can be made for the adverse effect

of a branch pulmonary artery stenosis or a small valve annulus. Depending on the predicted RV/LV pressure ratio the decision can be made as to whether complete correction as a first stage procedure is possible or a preliminary shunt is required to promote pulmonary artery growth.

2 To demonstrate absence or stenosis of a pulmonary artery. In tetralogy and related conditions there may be stenosis of the origin of a pulmonary artery (Fig. 19.17). Absence of one pulmonary artery (Fig. 19.13) can occur and an acquired stenosis or occlusion can follow a previous shunt operation. The pulmonary trunk passes backwards from its origin and is thus foreshortened in the anteroposterior projection. In order to visualise the trunk and its bifurcation a projection is needed which looks down on the pulmonary arteries; a view with 30—45° cranial angulation and, possibly, some left oblique angulation provides this [23].

When one pulmonary artery appears to be absent there may, in reality be an 'isolated pulmonary artery'; that is the pulmonary artery (right or left) may arise from the aorta. In this situation it is usually the pulmonary artery contralateral to the aortic arch which is isolated (i.e. left PA with right aortic arch)

and supply is from a persistent ductus. When the ipsilateral pulmonary artery is isolated it may arise from beneath the aortic arch (Fig. 20.10). If the ductus has closed angiographic demonstration of the artery will depend on opacification via collateral vessels.

3 To demonstrate other primary anomalies of the pulmonary circulation, e.g. hypoplasia in the rubella syndrome (Fig. 19.14) peripheral stenoses in infantile hypercalcaemia (Williams syndrome Fig. 19.15), dilatation in congenital absence of the pulmonary valve (Figs 19.16 to 19.19).

4 To demonstrate the extent of the pulmonary arterial supply to a sequestered lobe with dual supply. So-called pulmonary sequestration includes a spectrum of anomalies of the bronchial tree, the pulmonary and systemic arterial supply and the pulmonary veins [24]. The arterial supply may be from the pulmonary artery alone, from a systemic vessel(s) arising below the diaphragm or from both. Anomalies of pulmonary venous drainage may, or may not, be associated. In one pattern, the 'scimitar syndrome' the veins from the right lung (rarely the left) drain to the inferior cava below the diaphragm resulting in the characteristic scimitar-shaped shadow seen on the chest X-ray. Investigation of pulmonary sequestration must include a pulmonary arteriogram and an aortogram (or selective injection of the anomalous systemic artery) (Fig. 17.17).

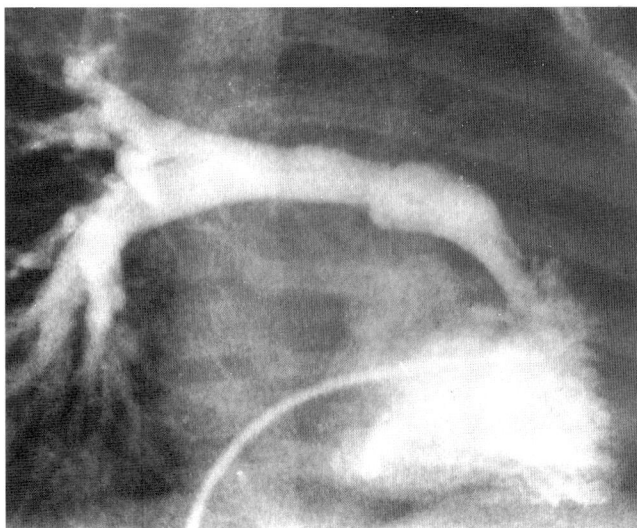

Fig. 19.13 Congenital absence of the left pulmonary artery; only the right pulmonary artery has opacified following the injection of contrast medium into the right ventricle. An aortic origin of the left pulmonary artery must be sought by aortography. In this patient no such aortic origin could be demonstrated. Wedge pulmonary vein angiography is the only remaining way of demonstrating the presence of a left pulmonary artery.

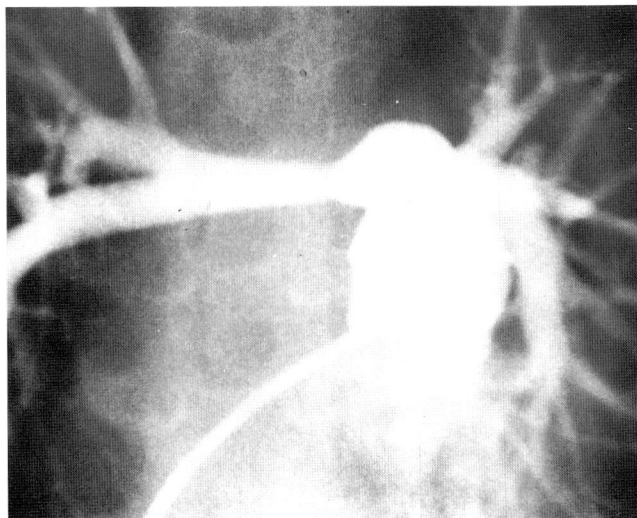

Fig. 19.14 Generalised hypoplasia of the pulmonary arteries in the rubella syndrome.

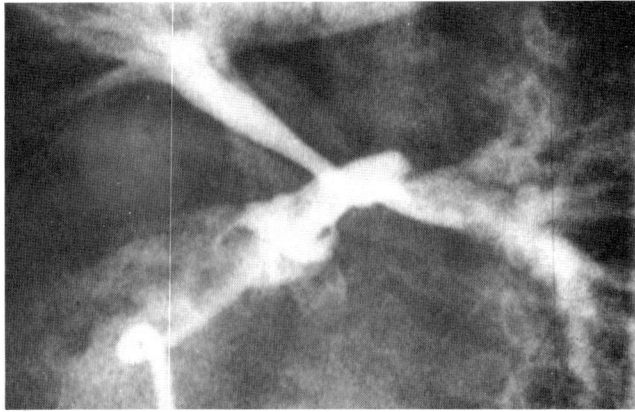

Fig. 19.15 Severe hypoplasia and branch stenosis of the pulmonary arteries in an infant with infantile hypercalcaemia — Williams syndrome. Associated supravalve aortic stenosis is also present in this patient — see aortic anomalies, Figs 20.32 and 20.33.

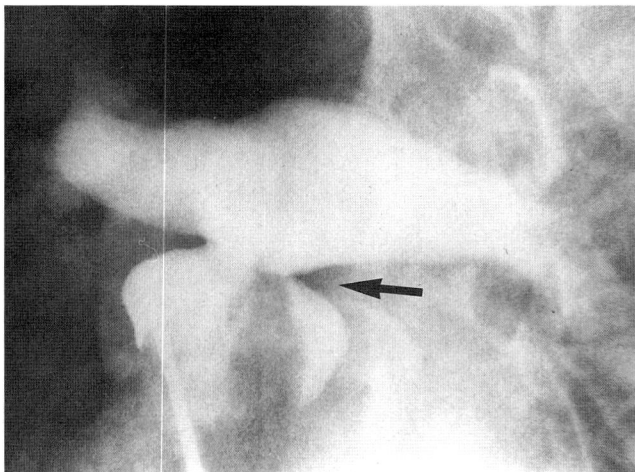

Fig. 19.16 Surgical banding causing supravalve stenosis of the pulmonary artery (arrow).

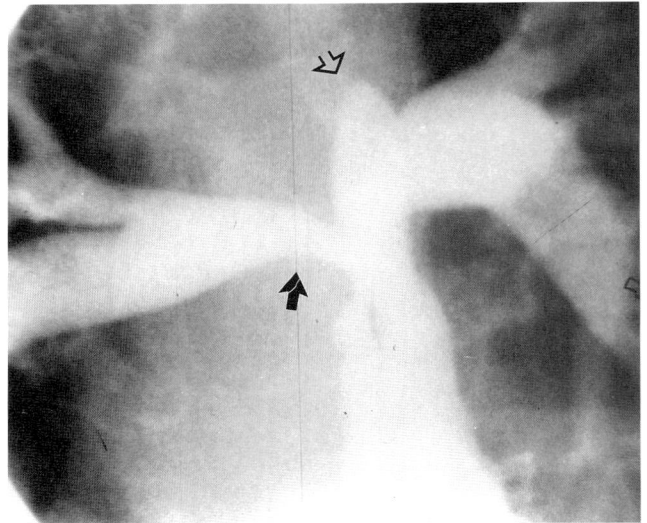

Fig. 19.17 Stenosis of the origin of the right pulmonary artery. Cranial angulation of the X-ray beam together with some left oblique orientation (i.e. the four chamber view) is required to display the origins of the right and left pulmonary arteries. This view is required to display the pulmonary arteries in the tetralogy of Fallot. In this patient there is also a ductus diverticulum (open arrow); frequently seen at the pulmonary arterial end of a (closed) ductus in patients with malformations resulting in reduced pulmonary arterial flow — often, therefore, in the tetralogy of Fallot.

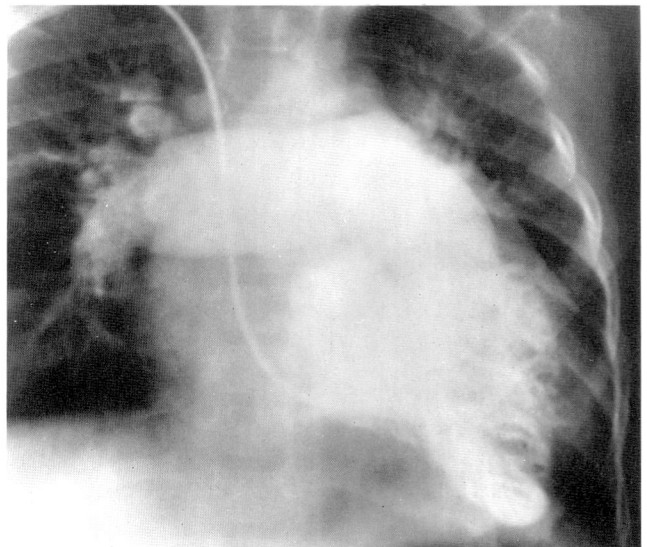

Fig. 19.18 The 'absent pulmonary valve syndrome'. Gross dilatation of the pulmonary arteries with abrupt diminution in calibre at their branches is characteristic of this syndrome. There is usually an associated VSD and a pressure gradient between the right ventricle and pulmonary artery so that the haemodynamic findings resemble those of 'acyanotic tetralogy of Fallot'.

5 In pulmonary atresia with VSD there may be areas of lung with no pulmonary arterial supply and only a supply from systemic-to-pulmonary collaterals or there may be a dual supply [25]. The details of the pulmonary arterial supply need to be elucidated prior to correction by both pulmonary arteriography (if possible) and selective injections into each of the systemic-to-pulmonary collaterals. A previous shunt procedure may allow the catheter to be passed to the pulmonary artery for arteriography. When there is no access to the pulmonary artery a wedge pulmonary

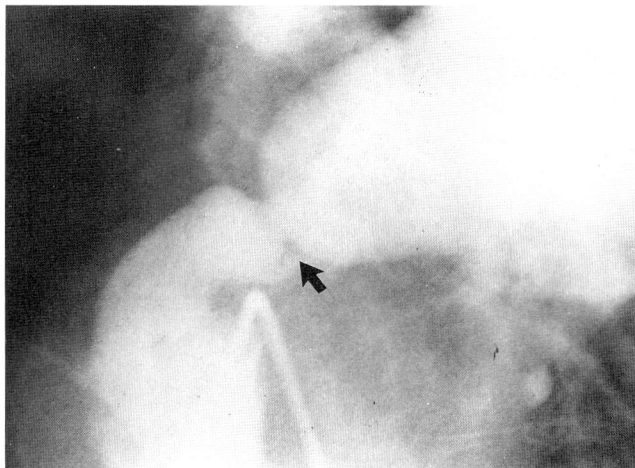

Fig. 19.19 Although the pulmonary valve is absent it is represented by a narrowed ring which is the site of right ventricular outflow obstruction — seen here (arrow) in a lateral projection in another patient with the absent pulmonary valve syndrome.

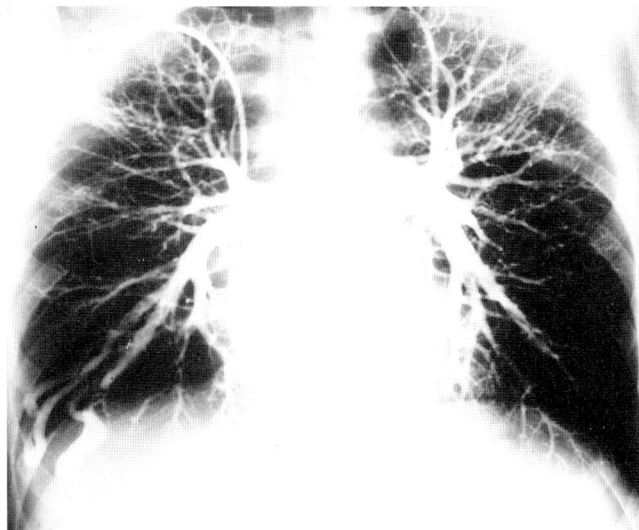

Fig. 19.21 Pulmonary arteriovenous fistulae in the right lower lobe. Although the appearances are similar to Fig. 19.20 there was early filling of the veins draining the malformation.

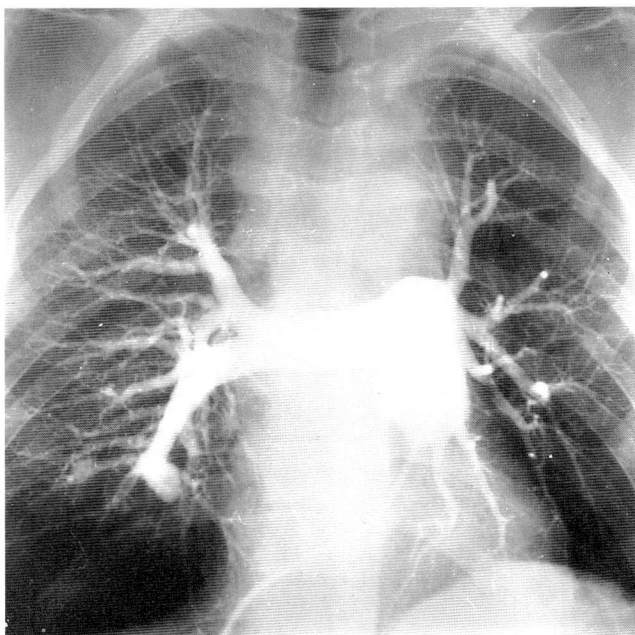

Fig. 19.20 Aneurysm(s) of the pulmonary artery. There is an aneurysm of a branch of the basal artery to the right lower lobe. Absence of early filling of pulmonary veins excluded an arteriovenous fistula. A right ventricular tumour was present and the aneurysm may have resulted from tumour embolism. (A left upper lobectomy has been performed).

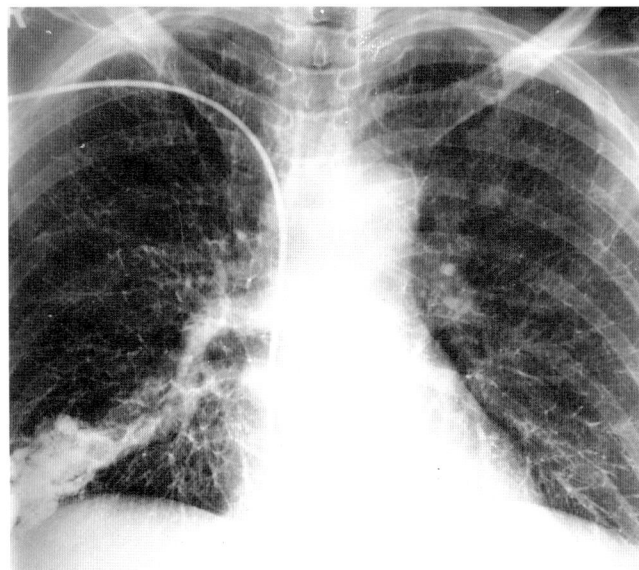

Fig. 19.22 Large 'solitary' pulmonary arteriovenous fistula in the right lower lobe. This malformation might be suitable for treatment by transcatheter embolisation.

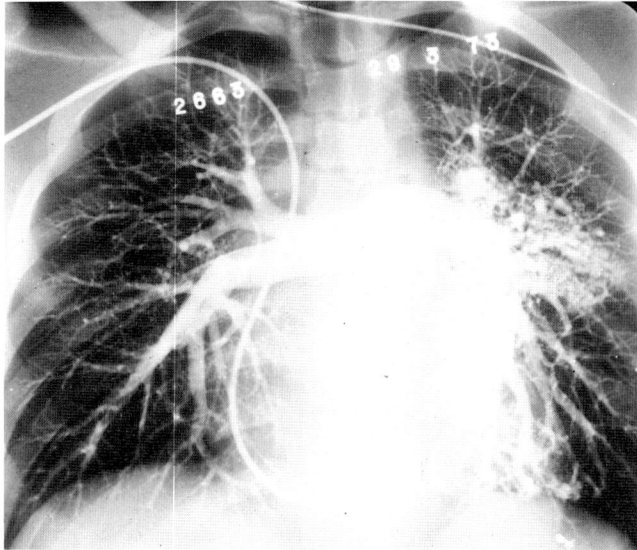

Fig. 19.23 Multiple arteriovenous fistulae of the left lung — clearly unsuitable for embolisation therapy.

vein injection may produce filling of the central pulmonary arteries (Fig. 19.3).

6 To demonstrate pulmonary arteriovenous fistulae [26–28]. These may be single but are often multiple and may be associated with hereditary haemorrhagic telangectasia. Often a pulmonary arteriogram will demonstrate a large arteriovenous (malformation (Figs 19.21 to 19.23) and its draining vein and also demonstrate smaller, unsuspected, lesions. Some lesions are amenable to transcatheter embolisation (Chapter 5).

7 To demonstrate anomalies of pulmonary venous return. These may be difficult to visualise. As noted above a large volume of contrast medium is needed and separate right and left pulmonary artery injections will help to elucidate the abnormal anatomy. There may be a place for balloon occlusion angiography.

8 Pulmonary artery 'sling' is a condition in which the left pulmonary artery arises from the right and passes behind the trachea and in front of the oesophagus. There may be narrowing of the right bronchus with a hyperinflated right lung and dysphagia.

9 The presence of a small ventricular septal defect can be confirmed angiographically by pulmonary arteriography followed through to the left heart. This technique may be indicated when a normal right ventricular pressure excludes the need for surgery

and the (small) risk of a retrograde arterial approach is thought to be unjustified. The injection should be made into the left pulmonary artery to avoid obscuring the plane of the ventricular septum and filming should be in the long axis projection. For most instances of congenital anomalies of the pulmonary artery filming should be with a 45° cranial angulation and usually about 45° left oblique.

REFERENCES

1 Grollman JH. Pigtail catheters in pulmonary angiography. *Cathet Cardiovasc Diagn* 1984;**10**:389.
2 Benotti JR, Ockene IS, Alpert JS, Dalen JE. Balloon-occlusion pulmonary cineangiography for diagnosing pulmonary embolism. *Cathet Cardiovasc Diagn* 1984;**10**:519.
3 Bynum LJ, Wilson JE, Christensen EE, Sorensen C. Radiographic techniques for balloon occlusion pulmonary cineangiography. *Radiology* 1978;**133**:518.
4 Ferris EJ *et al*. Angiography of pulmonary emboli: digital studies and balloon-occlusion cine angiography. *Am J Roentgenol* 1984;**142**:369.
5 Smucker ML, Lipscomb K. A fluoroscopic method to confirm proper catheter position to measure pulmonary artery wedge pressure. *Cathet Cardiovasc Diagn* 1982;**8**:83.
6 Bell ALL *et al*. Pulmonary wedge angiography for the evaluation of pulmonary vascular bed in congenital heart disease. *Radiology* 1959;**73**:566.
7 Nihill MR, McNamara DG. Magnification pulmonary wedge angiography in the evaluation of children with congenital heart disease and pulmonary hypertension. *Circulation* 1978;**58**:1094.
8 Singh SP, Rigby ML, Astley R. Demonstration of pulmonary artery by contrast injection into pulmonary vein. *Br Heart J* 1978;**40**:55.
9 Nihill MR, Mullins CE, McNamara DG. Visualisation of the pulmonary arteries in pseudotruncus by pulmonary vein wedge angiography. *Circulation* 1978;**58**:140.
10 Alpert BS, Culham JAG. A severe complication of pulmonary vein angiography. *Br Heart J* 1979;**41**:727.
11 Kerr IH. Vascular changes in the lungs on the plain radiograph of the chest. *Postgrad Med J* 1970;**46**:3.
12 Sutton GC, Hall RJC, Kerr IH. Clinical course and late prognosis of treated subacute, acute minor, and chronic pulmonary thromboembolism. *Br Heart J* 1977;**39**:1135.
13 Miller GAH, Sutton GC. Acute massive pulmonary embolism. Clinical and haemodynamic findings in 23 patients studied by cardiac catheterisation and pulmonary arteriography. *Br Med J* 1970;**32**:518.

14 Dalen JE *et al*. Pulmonary angiography in acute pulmonary embolism: indications, techniques, and results in 367 patients. *Am Heart J* 1971;**81**:175.

15 Marsh JD, Glynn M, Torman HA. Pulmonary angiography. Application in a new spectrum of patients. *Am J Med* 1983;**75**:763.

16 Gomes AS, Grollman JH, Mink J. Pulmonary angiography for pulmonary emboli: rational selection of oblique views. *Am J Roentgenol* 1977;**129**:1019.

17 Walsh PN *et al*. Angiographic severity index for pulmonary embolism. *Circulation* 1973;**47** and **48** (suppl 2): 101.

18 Miller GAH *et al*. Comparison of streptokinase and heparin in treatment of isolated acute massive pulmonary embolism. *Br Med J* 1971;**2**:681.

19 Tibbutt DA *et al*. Evaluation of a method for quantifying the angiographic severity of major pulmonary embolism. *Am J Roentgenol* 1975;**125**:895.

20 Lande A, Rossi P. The value of total aortography in the diagnosis of Takayasu's arteritis. *Radiology* 1975;**114**: 287.

21 Blackstone EH, Kirklin JW, Pacifico AD. Decision-making in repair of tetralogy of Fallot based on intra-operative measurements of pulmonary arterial outflow tract. *J Thoracic Cardiovasc Surg* 1979;**77**:526.

22 Blackstone EH *et al*. Preoperative prediction from cine angiograms of post repair right ventricular pressure in tetralogy of Fallot. *J Thoracic Cardiovasc Surg* 1979;**78**: 542.

23 Freedom R, Olley PM. Pulmonary arteriography in congenital heart disease. *Cathet Cardiovasc Diagn* 1976; **2**:309.

24 Thilenius OG *et al*. Spectrum of pulmonary sequestration: association with anomalous pulmonary venous drainage in infants. *Pediatr Cardiol* 1983;**4**:97.

25 Macartney FJ, Scott O, Deverall PB. Haemodynamic and anatomical characteristics of pulmonary blood supply in pulmonary atresia with ventricular septal defect — including a case of persistent fifth aortic arch. *Br Heart J* 1974;**36**:1049.

26 Sloan RD, Cooley RN. Congenital pulmonary arteriovenous aneurysm. *Am J Roentgenol* 1953;**70**:183.

27 Moyer JH, Glantz S, Brest AN. Pulmonary arteriovenous fistulas. *Am J Med* 1962;**32**:417.

28 Dines DE, Arms RA, Bernatz PE, Gomez MR. Pulmonary arteriovenous fistulas. *Mayo Clin Proc*, 1974;**49**:460.

Aortography: anomalies of the thoracic aorta

Aortography may be employed to demonstrate anomalies of the thoracic aorta but also serves to demonstrate aortic valve anomalies — notably to assess the severity of aortic regurgitation. The aorta may be entered retrogradely via an approach from the brachial or axillary arteries or femoral artery but in many cases of congenital heart disease it may be entered antegradely — for example via a ventricular septal defect during right heart catheterisation. In infants and children selective aortograms can be obtained from a transvenous approach by using a flow-directed, balloon-tipped, catheter. After crossing the foramen ovale the balloon is inflated with carbon dioxide and allowed to traverse the left ventricle so as to reach the aorta. The distal few centimetres of the catheter may have to be heat-moulded to form a 180° curve; without this modification the balloon tends to become lodged in the apex of the left ventricle instead of turning superiorly towards the outflow tract. A balloon-tipped catheter allows 'balloon occlusion angiography' to be performed (Fig. 20.1). The balloon is inflated (with CO_2) so as to occlude, temporarily, all distal flow while contrast is injected. If an end-hole balloon-tipped catheter is used there will be good opacification of the aorta and branch vessels distal to the occluding balloon. Alternatively a catheter with side-holes proximal to the occluding balloon will provide better opacification of proximal structures such as coarctation or a patent ductus arteriosus than is obtained when the contrast medium is diluted and dispersed by continuing blood flow [1].

Finally aortic anomalies may be visualised following ventriculography without the need for a selective aortogram. In this chapter, therefore, the lesions that will be described are those affecting the thoracic aorta, however visualised.

CONGENITAL ANOMALIES OF THE THORACIC AORTA

Congenital anomalies are numerous and, though many are rare, need to be described in some detail so that they may be recognised if they *are* encountered. The congenital aortic anomalies that will be described are:

1 Double aortic arch, vascular rings and related anomalies.

2 Aortic interruption.

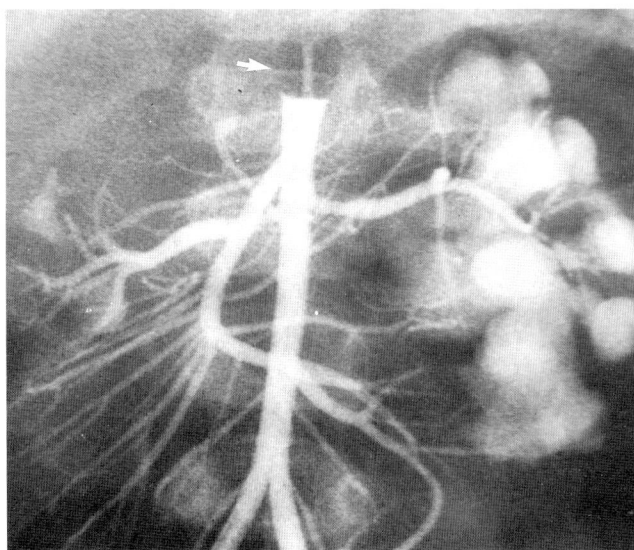

Fig. 20.1 Balloon occlusion aortography. An end-hole catheter has been used to inject contrast medium beyond the occluding balloon (arrow). With no antegrade flow to dilute the contrast medium it is possible to obtain exquisite detail of distal vessels. An alternative technique is to use a catheter with side-holes *proximal* to the balloon; opacification of the aortic arch using a catheter which has traversed a patent ductus is an example of how this, second, technique can be of value.

3 'Hemitruncus' and isolated pulmonary artery.
4 Aortic atresia.
5 Coarctation, 'pseudocoarctation' and isthmal hypoplasia.
6 Patent ductus arteriosus.
7 Aortopulmonary septal defect ('window').
8 Truncus arteriosus.
9 Aortopulmonary collaterals in pulmonary atresia with VSD.
10 Supravalve aortic stenosis.
11 Sinus of Valsalva aneurysms.
Coronary-cameral fistula are described in Chapter 13 and illustrated in Fig. 13.37.

Double aortic arch, vascular rings and associated anomalies

The most satisfactory classification of these anomalies is based on Edward's hypothetical 'double-arch' system [2–3]. A further simplification of this system as applied to 'right aortic arch' was proposed by Garti *et al.* [4] and the classification suggested here is an amplification of the system proposed by Garti. It is envisaged that the hypothetical double aortic arch can undergo involution at a number of different sites or at several of these sites (see Fig. 20.2) (A) proximal to the (left or right) common carotid; (B) between the common carotid and subclavian (left or right); (C) between the subclavian and the ductus (left or right); and (D) the dorsal arch distal to the ductus (left or right).

By postulating various combinations of sites at which involution has taken place and persistence of other parts of the hypothetical double arch it is possible to reproduce all the known patterns of aortic arch anomalies. These are illustrated in the accompanying diagrams. For each there are two forms — with a persistent right arch and with a persistent left arch.

1 *No involution at any site.* This produces a 'double aortic arch with both arches patent'. A vascular ring is formed with oesophageal and tracheal compression (Figs 20.2a and 20.4).

2 *Involution at site A* (proximal to the left or right common carotid). This produces an 'aberrant (left or right) innominate' (Fig. 20.2b). For a persistent right arch the branches are, in order, R common carotid, R subclavian, (R ductus) and finally, the L

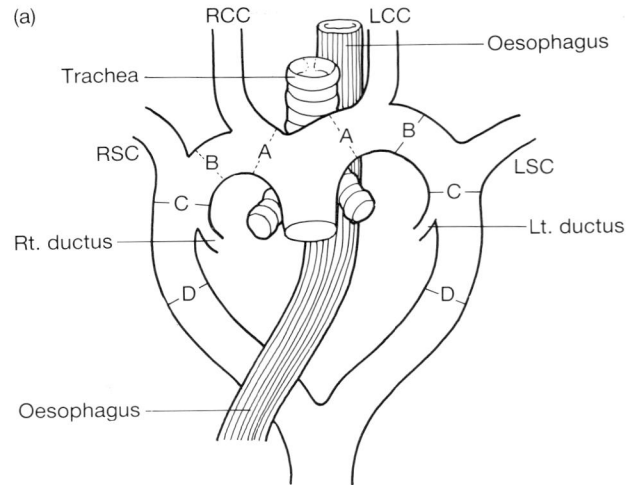

Fig. 20.2 Double aortic arch and related anomalies. (a) The hypothetical double arch system (see Fig. 20.4). Possible sites of involution: A: proximal to the common carotid; B: between the common carotid and subclavian arteries; C: between the subclavian artery and the ductus arteriosus; D: dorsal arch distal to the ductus.

innominate which is actually formed by the distal portion of the left dorsal arch supplying the left common carotid and subclavian arteries. When the left arch is the one that persists a mirror image malformation results. A vascular ring is formed.

3 *Involution at site B* (between the common carotid and subclavian arteries). For a persistent right arch the branches are, in order, L common carotid, R common carotid, R subclavian, (R ductus) and finally, the L subclavian which arises from the descending aorta via a diverticulum (diverticulum of Kommerell) which represents persistence of the distal portion of the left dorsal aorta. When the ductus persists on the same side as the 'aberrant subclavian' a vascular ring is formed. With no ductus there is simply posterior compression of the oesophagus. With a persistent left arch the mirror image malformation is referred to as 'aberrant right subclavian' and is not uncommon (Figs 20.2c and 20.5).

4 *Involution at site C* (between the subclavian and ductus). This produces 'retro-oesophageal ductus from descending aorta'. When the right arch persists the branches are, in order, L innominate, R common carotid, R subclavian, (R ductus) and finally, the L ductus which arises from a retro-oesophageal

(bi)

(bii)

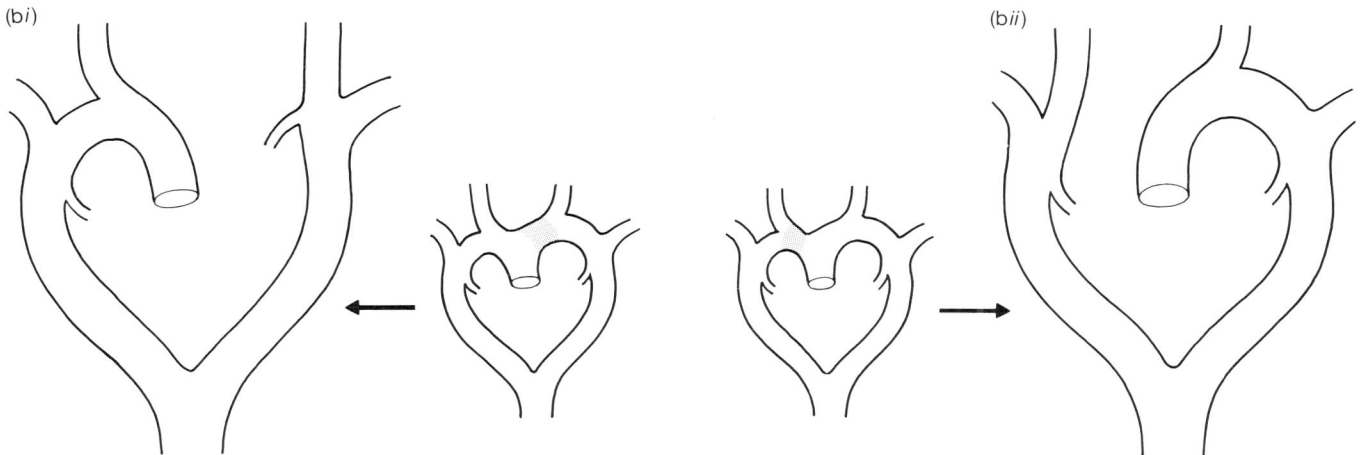

(b) *Involution at one site: A.* (*i*) Persistent right arch with 'aberrant Lt. innominate' = ring. (*ii*) Persistent left arch with 'aberrant Rt. innominate' = ring.

(ci)

(cii)

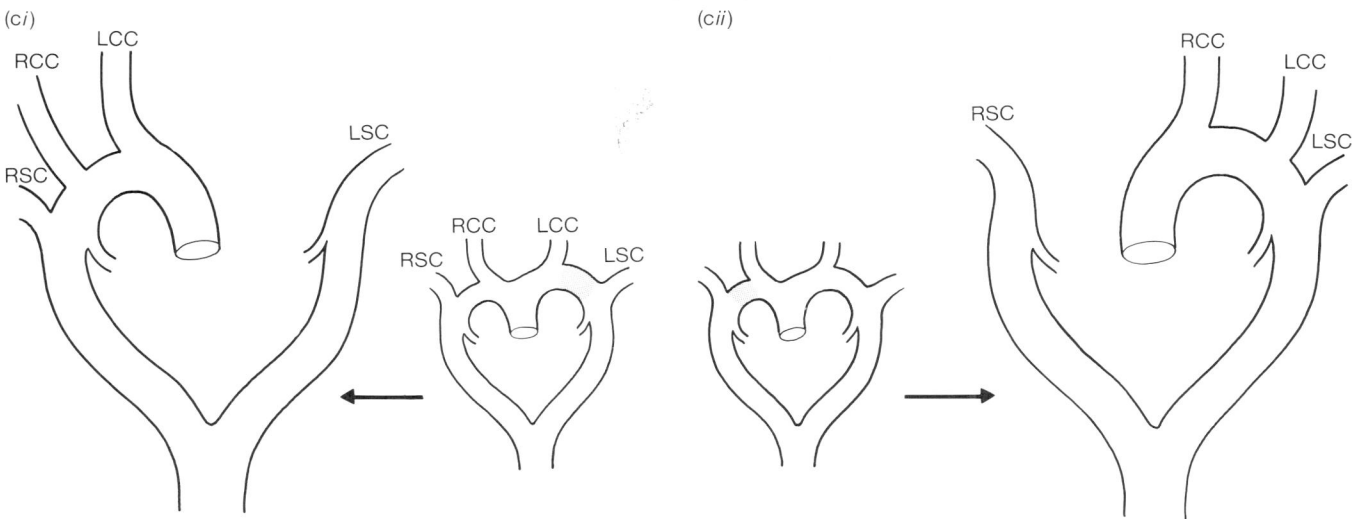

(c) *Involution at one site: B.* (see Fig. 20.5) (*i*) Rt. arch with 'aberrant Lt. subclavian. With Lt. ductus = ring. With Rt. ductus only = oesophageal compression. (Also called Rt. arch with Lt. ductus, 'posterior type'). (*ii*) Lt. arch with 'aberrant Rt. subclavian'. With Rt. ductus = ring. With Lt. ductus only = oesophageal compression.

diverticulum (of Kommerell) which represents the distal portion of the left dorsal aorta. A vascular ring is formed (Fig. 20.2d).

5 *Involution at site D* (dorsal arch distal to the ductus). When the right arch persists this forms 'right arch with mirror image branching' (Fig. 20.3). When there is a contralateral ductus the anomaly is referred to as 'right arch with left ductus — anterior

type'. When the left arch persists the result is a normal left arch with normal branching. No vascular ring is formed (Figs 20.2e and 20.3).

Interruption at two (or more sites)

6 *Involution at sites B and D* (between the common carotid and subclavian and of the dorsal aorta distal to the ductus). This produces 'isolated subclavian'.

(d*i*)

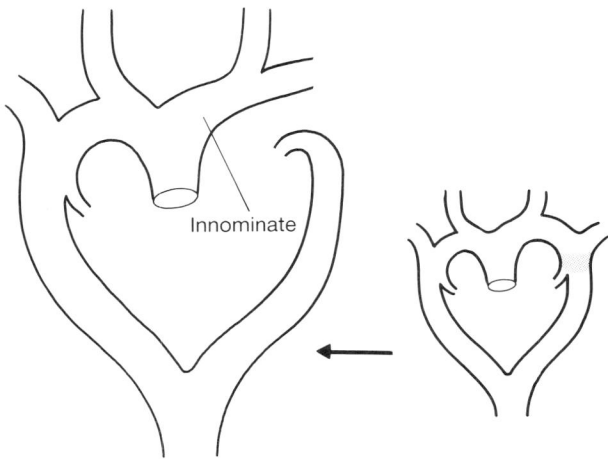

(d*ii*)

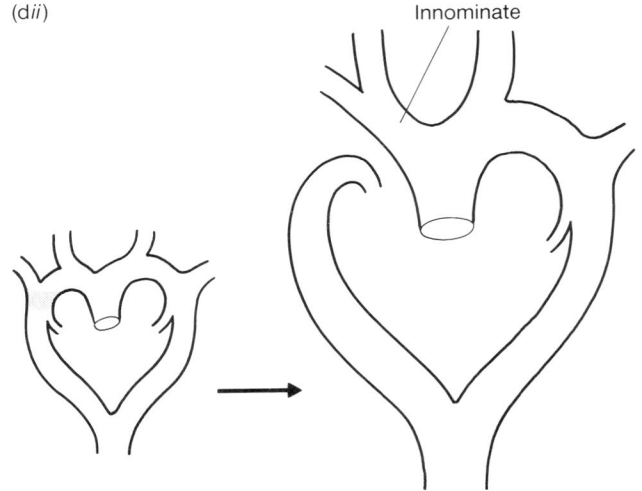

(d) *Involution at one site: C.* (*i*) Rt. arch with Lt. retro-oesophageal ductus = ring. (*ii*) Normal branching with Rt. ductus from descending aorta = ring.

(e*i*)

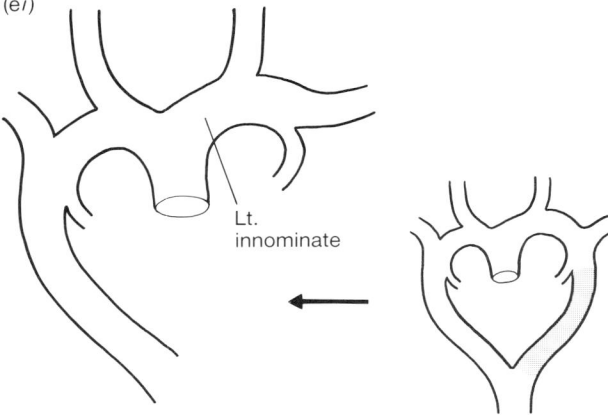

(e*ii*)

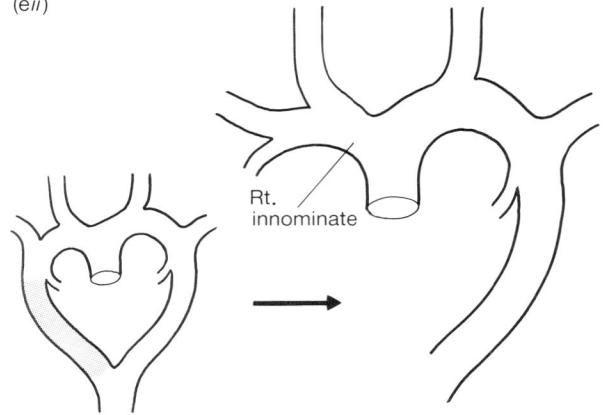

(e) *Involution at one site: D.* (see Fig. 20.3) (*i*) Rt. arch with mirror image branching. No Ring. If Lt. ductus present = Rt. arch with Lt. ductus, 'anterior type'. (*ii*) Normal Lt. arch normal branching. No ring.

The subclavian on the side contralateral to the arch is attached to the pulmonary artery via a duct or ductus ligament but has no direct communication with the aortic arch. There is no vascular ring but there may be a 'subclavian steal' (Fig. 20.2f).

7 *Involution at sites A and D* (proximal to the common carotid and of the dorsal aorta distal to the duct). This produces an 'isolated innominate and ductus'. Again inspection of the figures shows that the isolated innominate and duct will be contralat-

eral to the aortic arch. No vascular ring is formed (Fig. 20.2g).

'Aortic interruption'

This anomaly can also be explained by assuming involution of the hypothetical double arch at two sites — one at each arch.

8 *Involution at site C (right) and site C (left).* This produces 'aortic interruption type A' [5]. The arch is

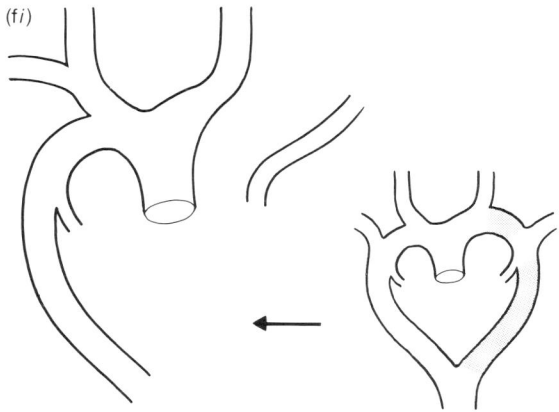

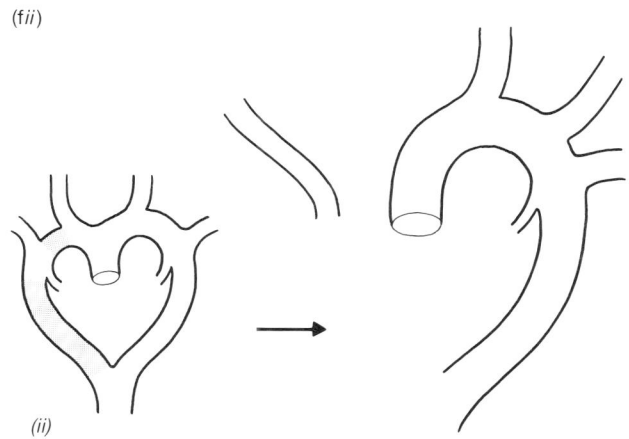

(f) *Involution at two sites: B and D.* (*i*) 'Isolated Lt. subclavian'. No ring. (*ii*) 'Isolated Rt. subclavian'. No ring.

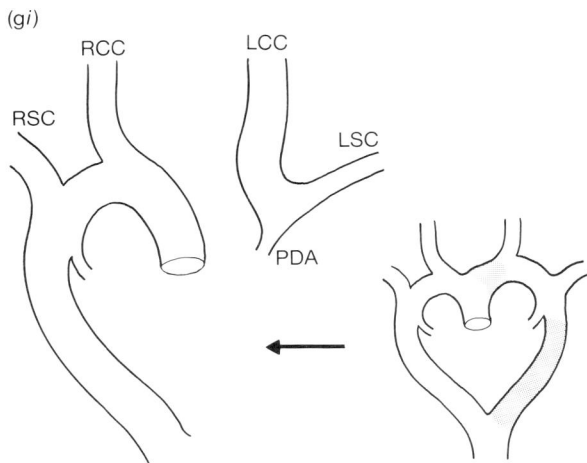

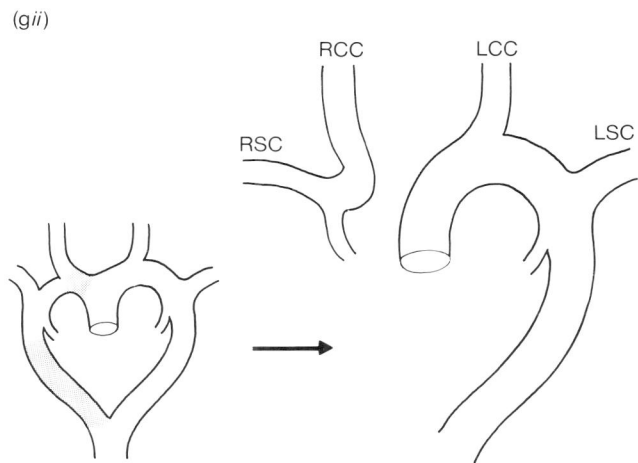

(g) *Involution at two sites: A and D.* (*i*) 'Isolated Lt. innominate and Lt. ductus'. No ring. (*ii*) 'Isolated Rt. innominate and Rt. ductus'. No ring.

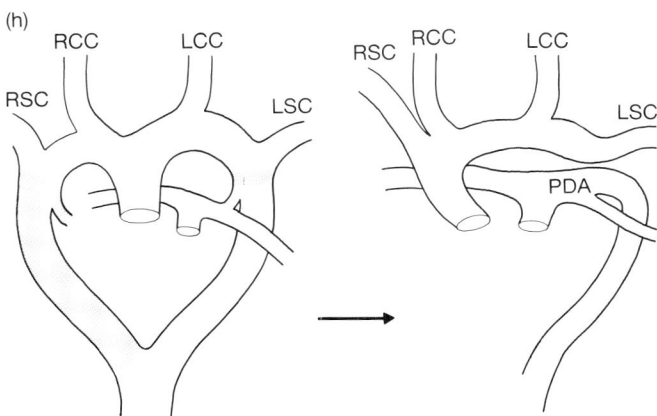

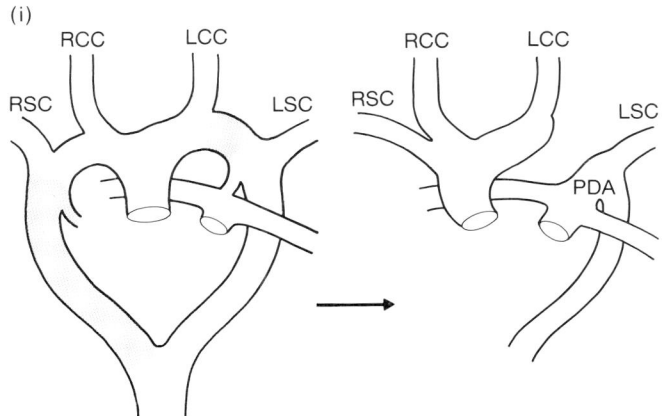

(h) *Involution at two sites: C left and C right* (see Fig. 20.7). 'Aortic interruption type A' (distal to Lt. subclavian).

(i) *Involution at two sites: B left and C right* (see Fig. 20.6). 'Aortic interruption type B' (between innominate and left common carotid).

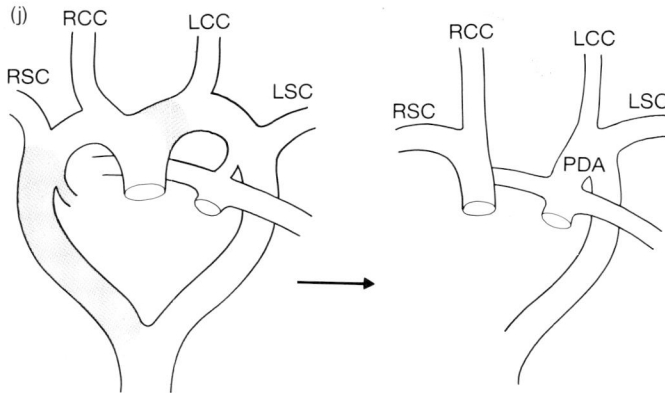

(j) *Involution at two sites: A left and C right.* 'Aortic interruption type C' (between innominate and left common carotid).

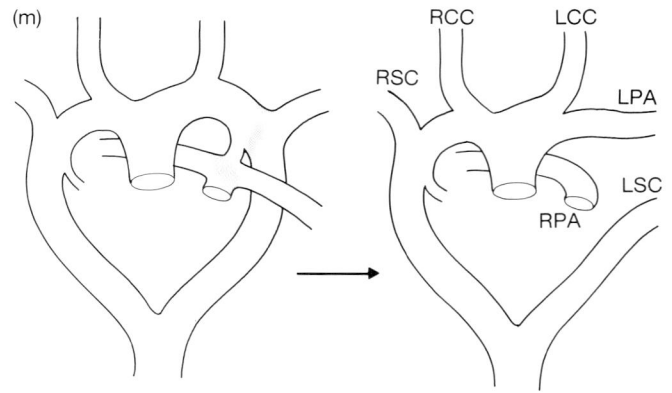

(k) *Involution at two sites: C left and B right* (see Fig. 20.8). 'Aortic interruption type A with aberrant contralateral subclavian'.

(m) 'Origin of left pulmonary artery from the aorta: anterior type' (see Fig. 20.9). RPA from aorta more common than LPA but usually LPA from aorta in association with tetralogy of Fallot. Anomalous PA and subclavian always contralateral to the aortic arch.

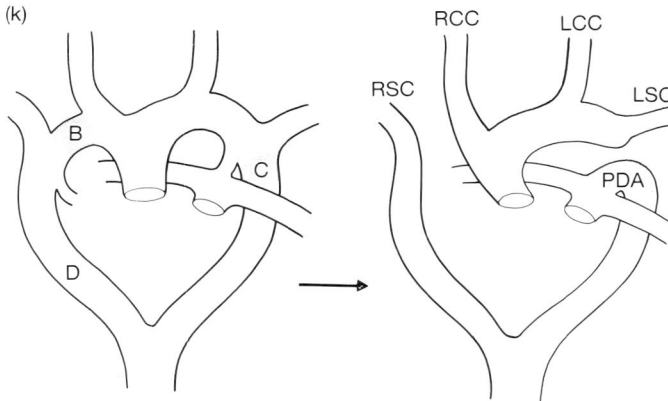

interrupted distal to the left subclavian (Figs 20.2h and 20.7). The right arch regresses and a patent ductus supplies the left dorsal arch (descending aorta).

9 *Involution at site C (right) and site B (left).* This produces 'aortic interruption type B' (between the left common carotid and the left subclavian) (Figs 20.2i and 20.6).

10 *Involution at site C (right) and site A (left).* This produces 'aortic interruption type C' (between the innominate and the left common carotid). Note that in this scheme what we call the 'innominate' (with a

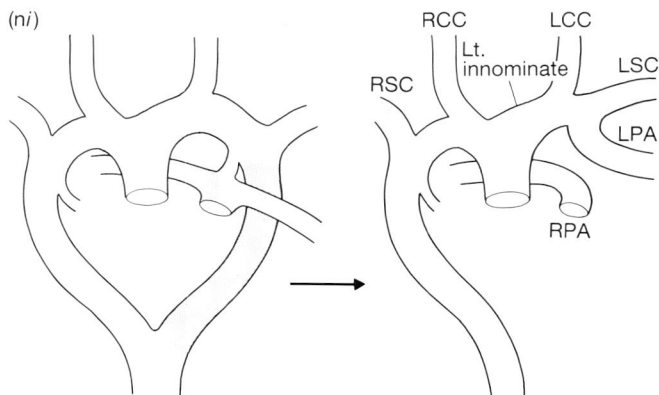

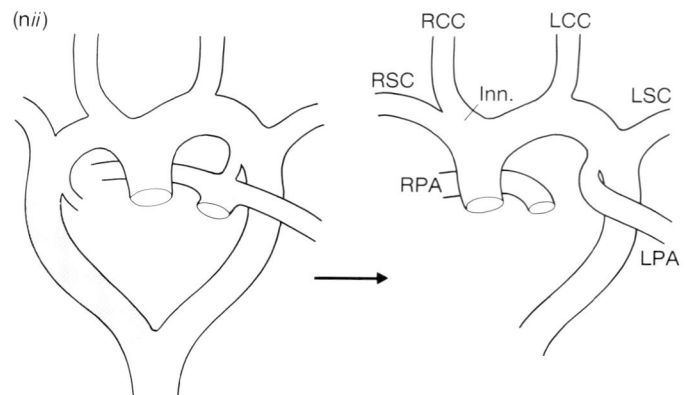

(n) Origin of one pulmonary artery from the aortic arch or ductus (see Fig. 20.10) (*i*) right arch, (*ii*) left arch.

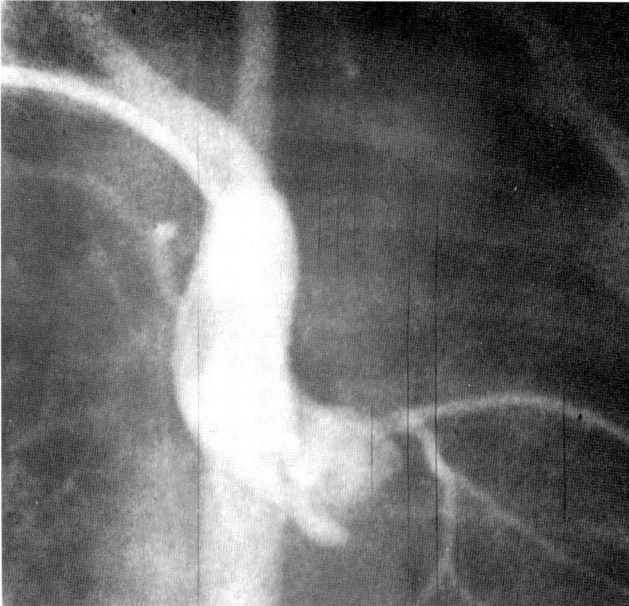

Fig. 20.3 Right aortic arch; the anomaly is not uncommon and occurs, for example, in 30% of patients with the tetralogy of Fallot.

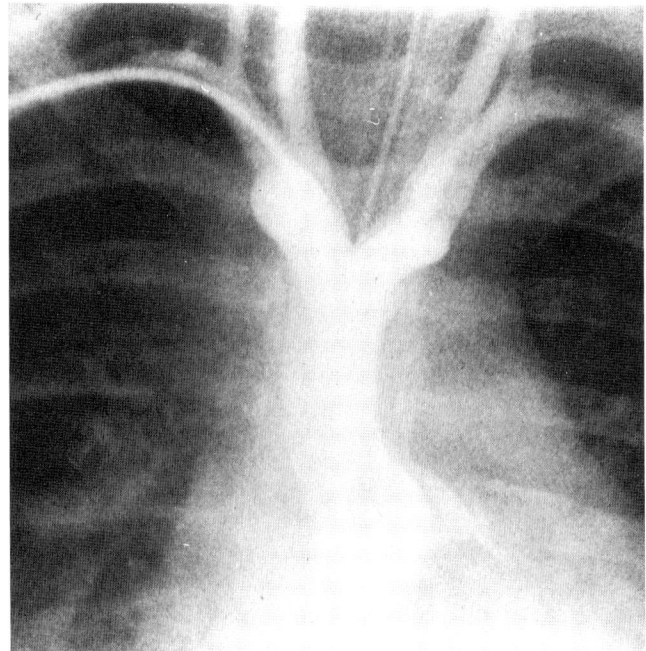

Fig. 20.4 Double aortic arch with both arches patent. This is an example of the basic 'template' — the hypothetical 'double arch system' of Edwards (see text) from which other varieties of 'double arch' can be derived by assuming interruption of one or other arch at one (or more) sites.

left arch) is really the proximal portion of the right dorsal arch — and vice versa for right arch with mirror image branching (Fig. 20.2j).

Based on this hypothetical scheme it is not surprising that 'aberrant subclavian' may be associated with aortic interruption — or that it is *contralateral* subclavian that is 'aberrant'. This malformation can be explained as:

11 *Involution at site C (left) and site B (right).* This produces 'aortic interruption type A with aberrant contralateral subclavian'. The arch is interrupted distal to the left subclavian and the descending aorta (left dorsal arch) is supplied by the ductus and gives rise to a right subclavian arising as the last branch of the aorta from a diverticulum (of Kommerell) which represents persistence of the distal portion of the right dorsal arch (Figs 20.2k and 20.8).

Presumably mirror images of these malformations can be similarly explained by persistence of the *right* arch though aortic interruption with right arch is very rare.

'CERVICAL AORTA'

In this condition the aortic arch extends further into

the neck than is usual (to the level of the second cervical vertebra). The condition has been classified into five types by Haughton [6]. All appear to be examples of right or left arch with interruption at B (between common carotid and subclavian) resulting in aberrant subclavian contralateral to the arch. In addition there are various patterns of origin of the carotid arteries (bicarotid trunk, separate aortic origins of the internal and external carotids).

Anomalous pulmonary artery, isolated pulmonary artery, 'hemitruncus'

These conditions are clearly related to anomalies of the aortic arch and can also be explained with reference to the hypothetical double arch system of Edwards. For this reason they are described here rather than in the chapter devoted to pulmonary arteriography; indeed their demonstration requires aortography. Two forms exist; anomalous origin from the ascending aorta and anomalous origin from the arch or ductus.

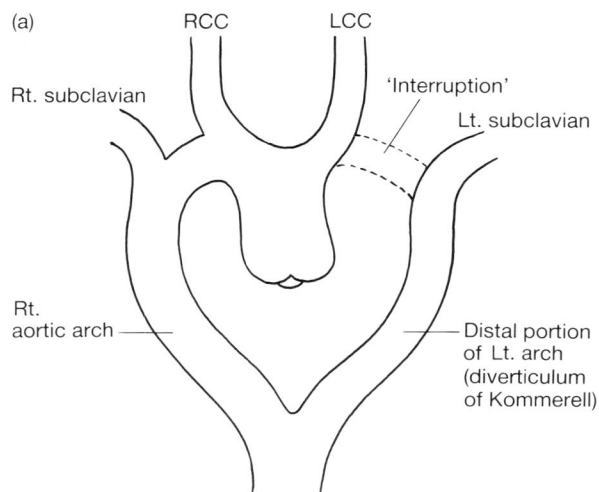

(a)

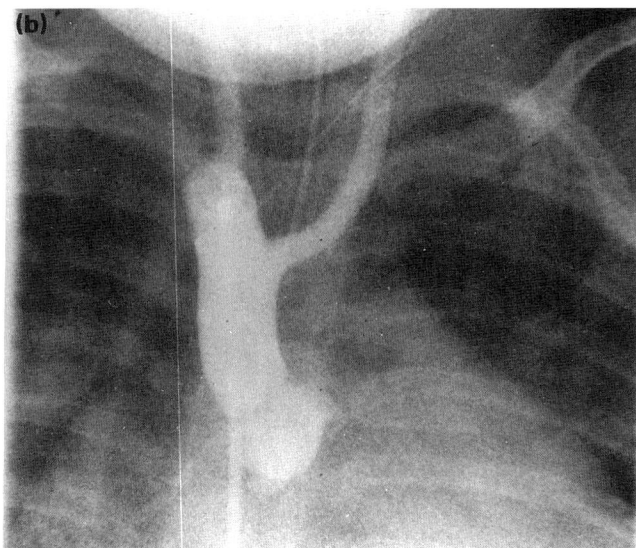

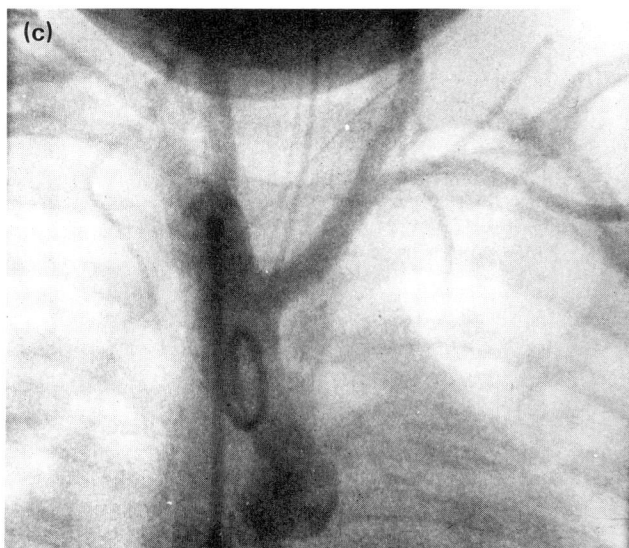

(b) Early film. The left and right common carotid arteries have filled but not the left subclavian. (c) Later film. The left subclavian artery has now filled from the descending aorta via the distal portion of the left arch.

1 Anomalous origin from the ascending aorta (Figs 20.2m and 20.9). Most commonly it is the right pulmonary artery which arises from the ascending aorta just above the aortic sinuses. There is an 'aberrant subclavian' and both this vessel and the anomalous pulmonary artery are contralateral to the aortic arch. The condition can be explained by assuming involution of one arch before the origin of the subclavian (point B) together with interruption of the ipsilateral pulmonary artery at its origin from the pulmonary trunk. The attachment of the pulmonary artery to the ascending aorta is unexplained.

2 Anomalous origin of the pulmonary artery from the arch or ductus (Figs 20.2n and 20.10). In this condition the arch may be right or left sided. The two pulmonary arteries are not in continuity — one arises from the position of the ductus (right or left) while the main trunk continues as the contralateral pulmonary artery. If the ductus is closed the anomalous pulmonary artery becomes 'isolated' and may

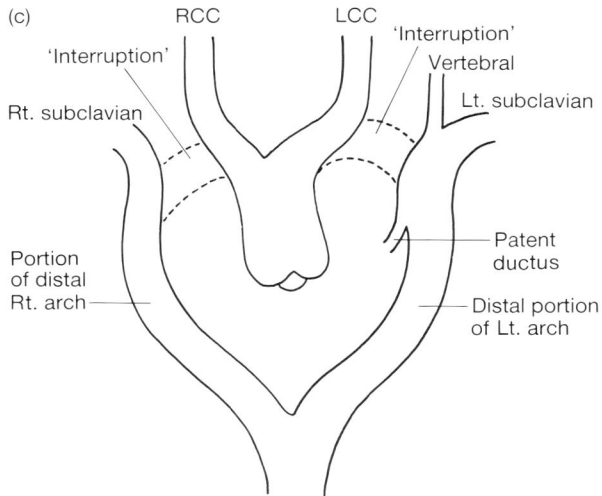

(c)

'Interruption' RCC LCC 'Interruption'
Vertebral
Rt. subclavian Lt. subclavian
Portion of distal Rt. arch
Patent ductus
Distal portion of Lt. arch

Fig. 20.6 (a) Aortic interruption/double-aortic arch. This infant had the DiGeorge syndrome — commonly associated with aortic interruption.

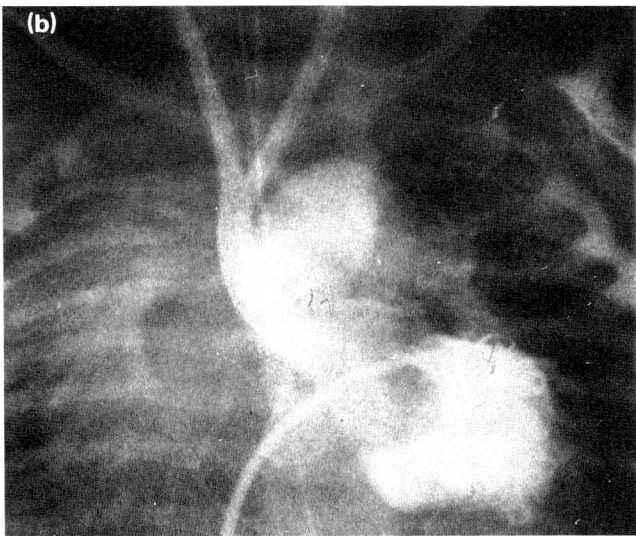

(b)

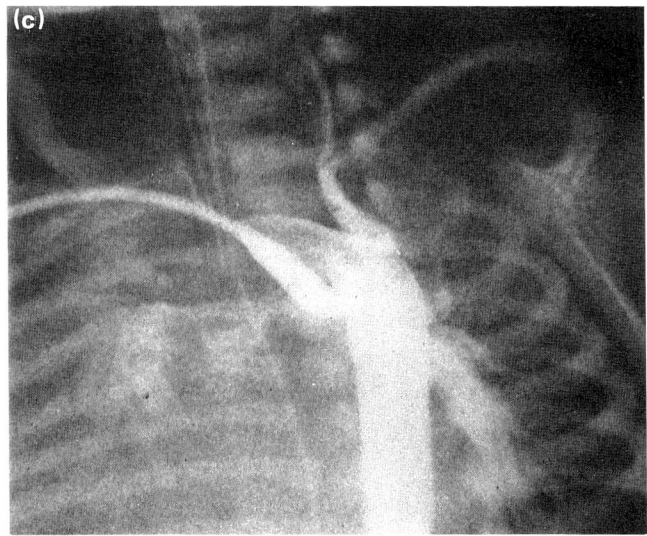

(c)

(b and c) Aortic interruption/double aortic arch. The left arch is patent but is interrupted between the left common carotid and the left subclavian; only the two carotid arteries fill following injection of contrast into the left ventricle. That this can be regarded as a variety of double aortic arch with, in addition, interruption of the right arch between the right common carotid and the right subclavian is demonstrated in (c). An injection has been made into the descending aorta via the right subclavian artery. The right subclavian arises from the descending aorta via the distal portion of the primitive right arch. The left subclavian and vertebral arteries have filled and there is also contrast medium in the pulmonary artery as there is a patent ductus.

fill via systemic-to-pulmonary collaterals or be impossible to demonstrate angiographically.

PULMONARY ARTERY 'SLING'

In this condition the left pulmonary artery arises from the right PA and courses over the right main bronchus (which may be compressed) and then *between* the trachea and the oesophagus to reach the left lung. Note that a vascular ring compresses the oesophagus from the sides and from behind and compresses the trachea from in front. A 'vascular sling' is unique in that it indents the oesophagus from the front.

Aortic (valve) atresia (Figs 20.11 and 20.12)

This condition is only seen in the first week or two of life as it is incompatible with longer survival. The aortic valve is atretic; unless there is a VSD the

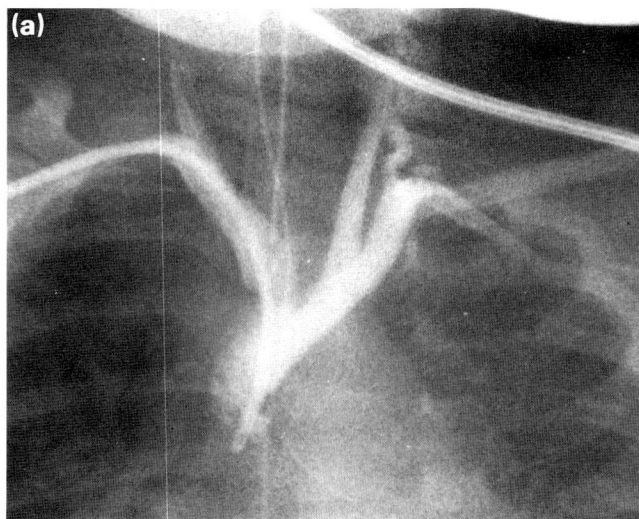

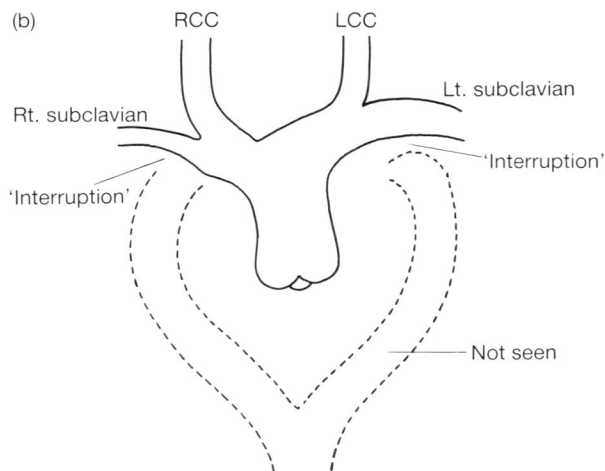

Fig. 20.7 (a and b) Aortic interruption distal to the left subclavian artery (so-called 'Type A'). This can also be regarded as an example of double aortic arch interrupted at two sites. The right arch is interrupted at the usual site — distal to the right subclavian — and the left arch is interrupted distal to the left subclavian (see diagram b).

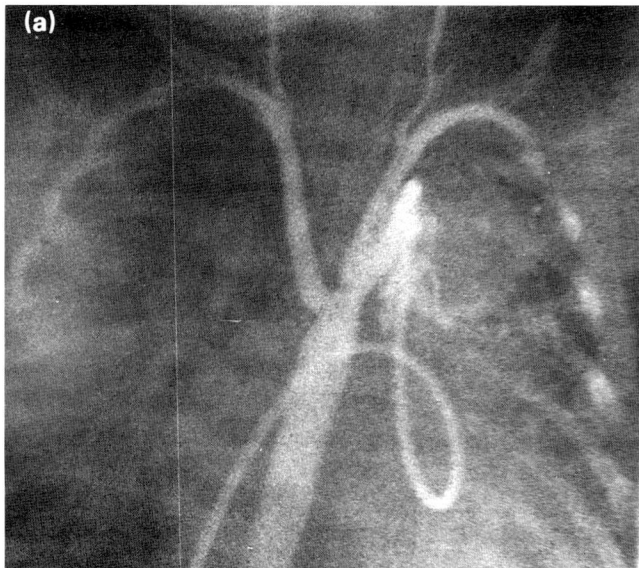

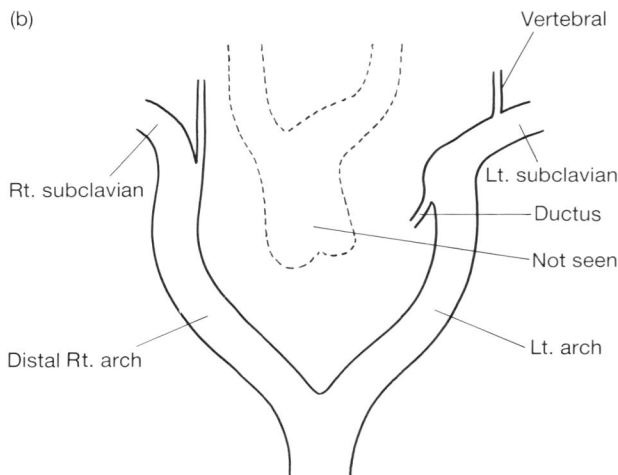

Fig. 20.8 (a and b) That aortic interruption can be viewed as part of the spectrum of double aortic arch is illustrated by this patient. The catheter has entered the descending aorta via a (left) ductus. The aorta is interrupted between the left common carotid and the left subclavian. But the right arch is also interrupted distal to the right common carotid artery and the right subclavian arises from the descending aorta via the distal part of the primitive right arch.

result is that there is no egress from the left ventricle and the left ventricle and mitral valve are very small. The mitral valve may be atretic and the left ventricle merely a slit-like structure. The term 'hypoplastic left heart syndrome' is often used to include cases of mitral and aortic atresia. The only egress from the left atrium is via the foramen ovale or an ASD and there is, therefore, a left-to-right shunt at atrial level. The only way that blood can reach the aorta is via a PDA — and this is only possible so long as the

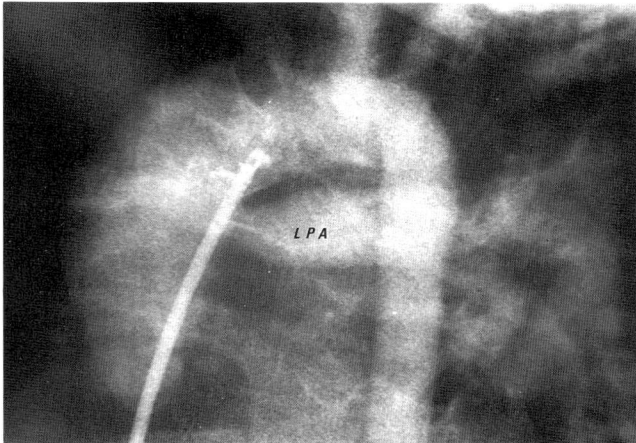

Fig. 20.9 *Aortopulmonary communications.* Origin of one or other pulmonary artery from the aorta, sometimes called 'hemi-truncus'. In this case the left pulmonary artery (LPA) arises from the ascending aorta.

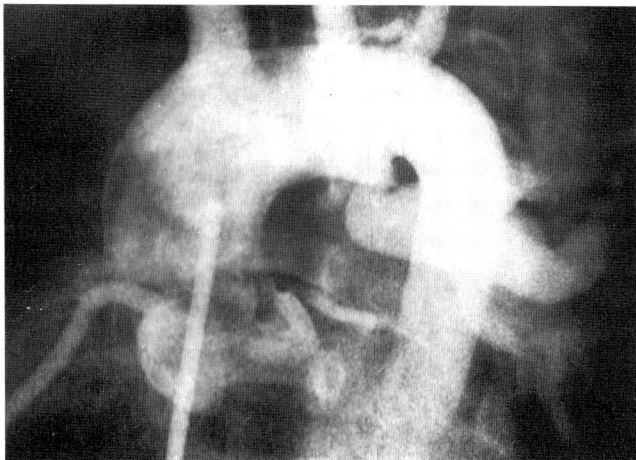

Fig. 20.10 *Aortopulmonary communications.* In this example the left pulmonary artery arises from a left ductus.

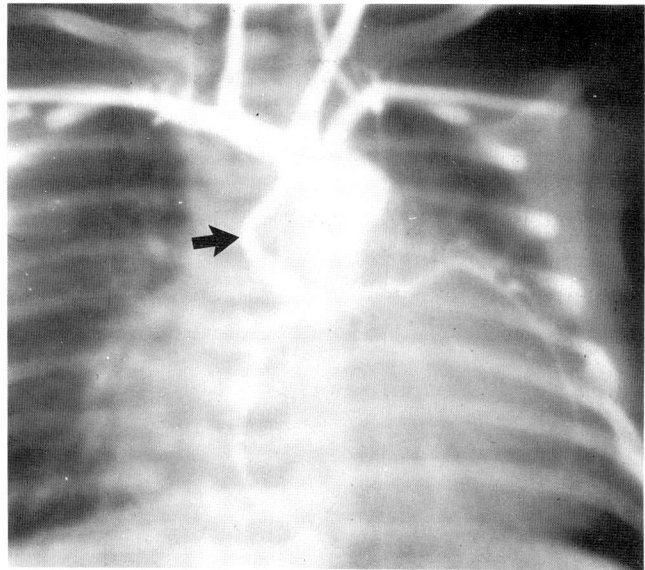

Fig. 20.11 *Aortic (valve) atresia.* The systemic circulation is maintained (poorly) as long as the ductus remains open and the pulmonary resistance remains high. Flow through the ascending aorta is in retrograde direction and supplies the coronary circulation only. As a result the ascending aorta (arrow) is small; beyond the ductus the aorta is of normal calibre.

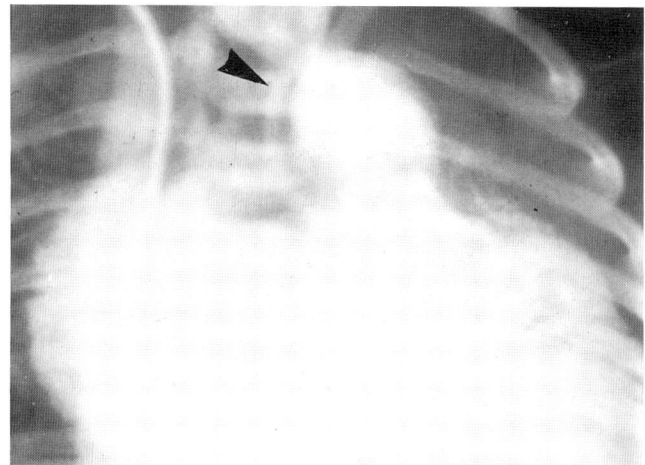

Fig. 20.12 *Aortic atresia.* The characteristic, minute, ascending aorta (arrow) may also be visualised following right-sided injections. Contrast medium opacifies the ascending aorta via the patent ductus.

pulmonary vascular resistance is higher than the systemic vascular resistance. So long as this is the case there will be mild arterial desaturation; as pulmonary resistance falls systemic flow will be reduced and death will result — as it will if the duct closes. Flow round the aortic arch is retrograde and the ascending aorta is only required to transmit the coronary flow; as a result the aorta tapers from the duct towards the aortic valve and the ascending aorta is a minute structure. The diagnosis is likely to

be made clinically and by echocardiography but if catheterisation is requested the findings are: (1) A left-to-right shunt at atrial level, (2) right ventricular and pulmonary artery systolic pressures at or, more commonly, above systemic level, and (3) mild arterial desaturation.

The angiographic diagnosis may be made by injecting in the pulmonary artery or right ventricle but the clearest picture of the anatomy is obtained by aortography. Balloon occlusion aortography should provide an alternative method of demonstrating the anatomy with clarity. The diagnosis is made when the thread-like ascending aorta is displayed. The operator should beware that crossing the duct with the catheter or advancing the catheter to ascending aorta can result in bradycardia and death as coronary flow is jeopardised when the catheter occludes the ascending aorta and all systemic flow is jeopardised if the catheter occludes the ductus.

Coarctation of the aorta, isthmal hypoplasia

Aortic coarctation (Figs 20.13 to 20.16) is due to an infolding of the posterior wall of the aorta at the level of the ductus arteriosus ('juxtaductal coarctation'). Isthmal hypoplasia (Fig. 20.17) consists of a narrowed segment of the aorta proximal to the ductus and extending a variable distance proximally –

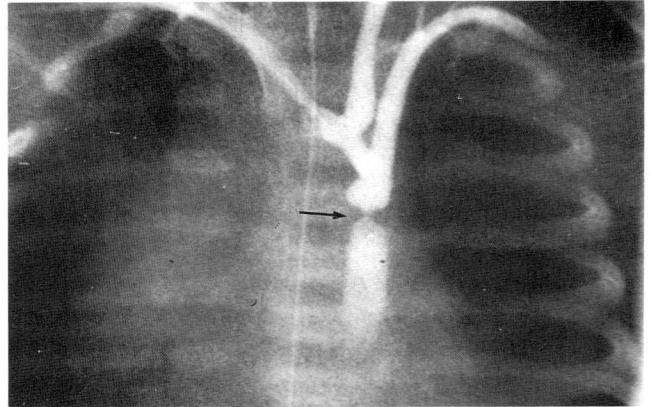

Fig. 20.13 Localised, juxtaductal, coarctation (arrow) in an infant.

sometimes to the origin of the innominate. Isthmal narrowing is a normal finding in the neonate and is explained by the intrauterine flow pattern when only some 16% of the cardiac output traverses the isthmus while some 46% traverses the ductus to enter the descending aorta. An hypothesis which explains many of the findings in coarctation suggests

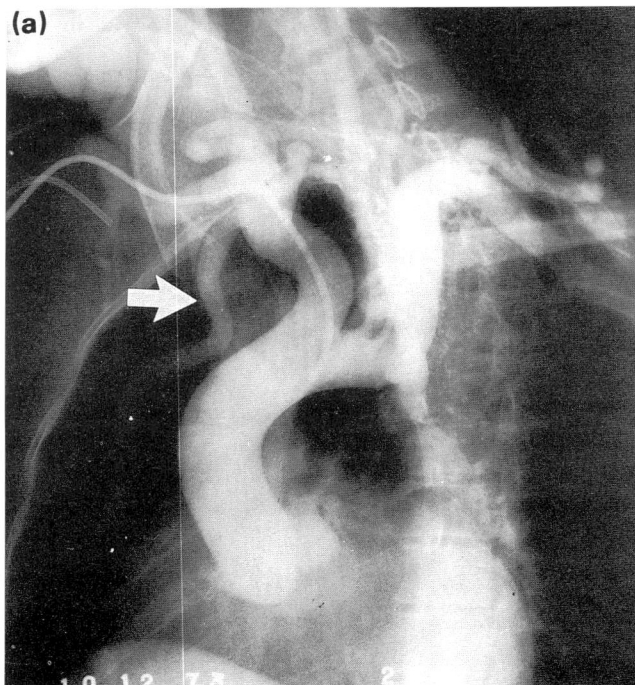

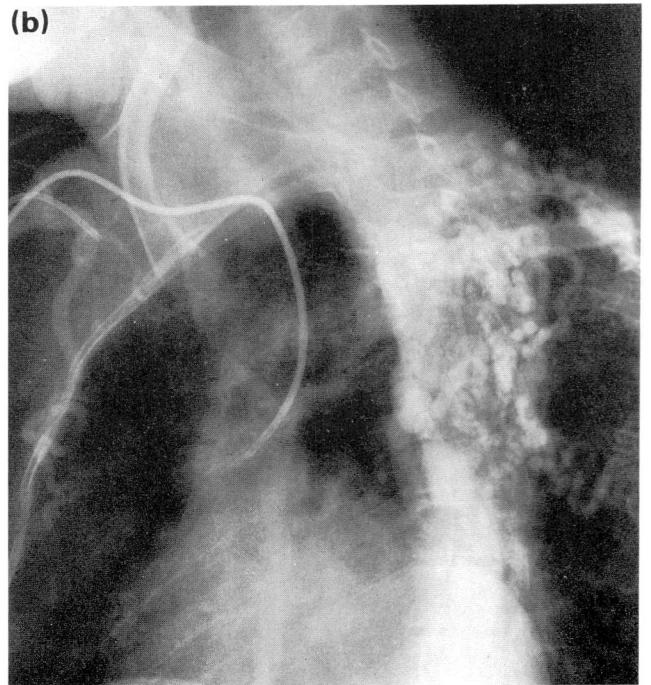

Fig. 20.14 (a and b) Severe coarctation in an older child. An enlarged internal mammary artery is seen providing a collateral channel for blood to reach the lower body (arrow). In a later film (b) a leash of collaterals is seen and there is now some opacification of the descending aorta.

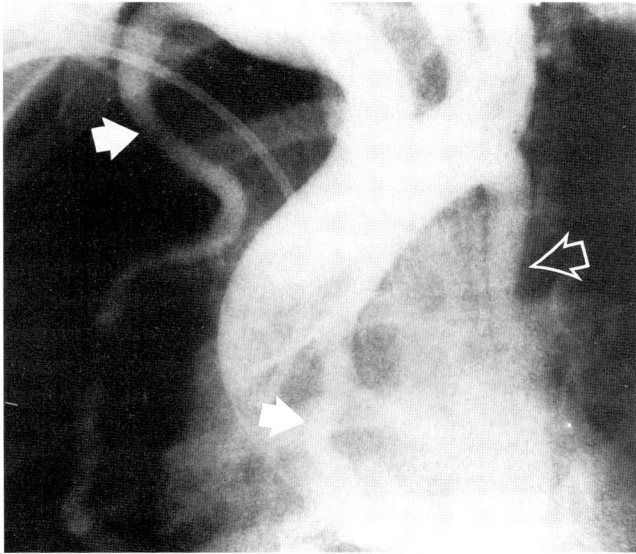

Fig. 20.15 Another example of coarctation (open arrow) with large internal mammary arteries (solid arrows) forming a collateral pathway.

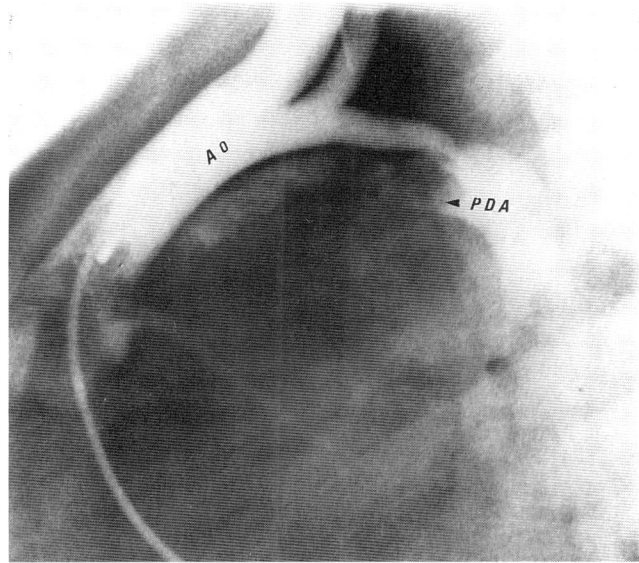

Fig. 20.17 *Isthmal hypoplasia*. Lateral view of an aortogram in a neonate with double inlet left ventricle and ventriculo-arterial discordance. The aorta (Ao) arises anteriorly (from the right ventricle). Isthmal hypoplasia is characteristic of conditions in which, during foetal life, flow is directed away from the aorta and into the pulmonary artery and ductus (PDA). Conversely isthmal hypoplasia is not to be expected in conditions characterised by low pulmonary flow (e.g. the tetralogy of Fallot).

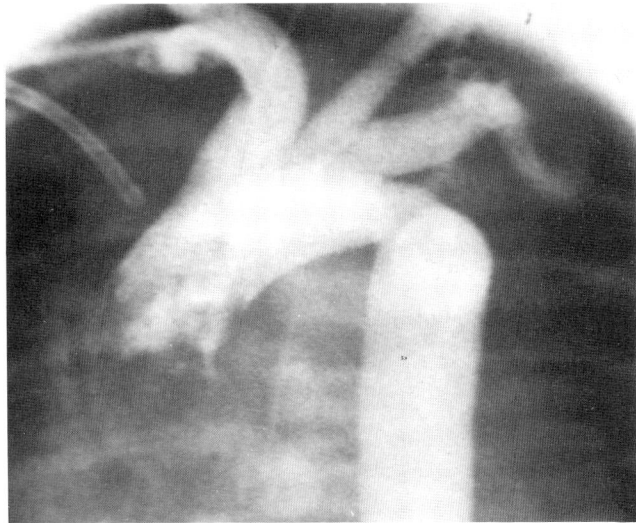

Fig. 20.16 Mild coarctation of the aorta. The appearances are similar to those illustrated in Fig. 20.18.

that coarctation can result from conditions which exaggerate duct flow in relation to aortic flow. Thus coarctation is commonly associated with left-sided obstructive lesions (e.g. Shone syndrome) in which isthmal flow may be expected to be decreased in relation to duct flow. Conversely coarctation is rare in association with right sided obstructive lesions in which pulmonary artery and duct flow is reduced

and aortic and isthmal flow correspondingly increased [7−8]. Isthmal narrowing and localised juxtaductal coarctation can coexist; either may be found in association with other cardiac anomalies but a localised coarctation can be an isolated finding and is the pattern to be expected in older children and adults. Aortography will demonstrate the lesion; a left oblique or left lateral projection are required but on occasion other, angulated, views may be needed. Retrograde catheterisation from the arm avoids the danger of the catheter failing to traverse the coarctation when the approach is from the leg but unless the arterial repair is perfect carries the disadvantage that resulting diminution of right arm pulse pressure makes it impossible to measure upper body pressure postoperatively since the left subclavian is sacrificed in the angioplastic repair. Aberrant right subclavian may be associated with coarctation; the right arm pulses will be reduced and in such cases catheterisation must be from the femoral artery. Aortography (or left ventriculography) may also reveal dilated collateral vessels (Figs 20.14 and 20.15), particularly in the adolescent and adult, and some 'poststenotic' dilatation of the aorta immediately distal to the coarctation.

'Pseudocoarctation' [9] is characterised by elongation and redundancy of the aorta above the coarctation site without a significant gradient. The condition is most likely to be met with in the adult; the aetiology is unknown (Fig. 20.18).

Patent ductus arteriosus (Figs 20.19 to 20.21)

Catheterisation is rarely needed to establish the diagnosis but may be indicated for determining the pulmonary arteriolar resistance. The presence of a patent ductus is established if the catheter passes from the origin of the left pulmonary artery to the descending aorta and can be advanced to below the diaphragm. (In aortopulmonary septal defect it is the *ascending* aorta that will be entered.) The opportunity can be taken to inject contrast medium while withdrawing the catheter from the aorta to the pulmonary artery. Aortography is the conventional method of visualising a patent ductus. A steep left oblique projection with some caudal angulation is ideal. The morphology of a patent ductus is variable; it may be short and fat or it may be long and thin. Aneurysm formation (Fig. 20.20) is seen rarely and may be associated with either a patent or a closed ductus. Calcification can be seen in the ductus in the adult and also occurs in ductus aneurysm. Finally a ductus 'dimple' is commonly seen at the aortic or pulmonary end of a closed ductus (Fig. 20.23).

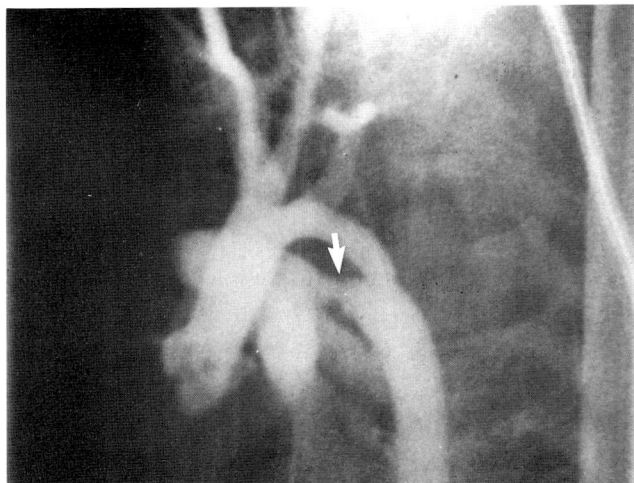

Fig. 20.19 *Aortopulmonary communications*. Patent (persistent) ductus arteriosus (arrow) profiled in a steep left oblique projection. Contrast medium was injected into the aorta and has resulted in opacification of the pulmonary artery and duct.

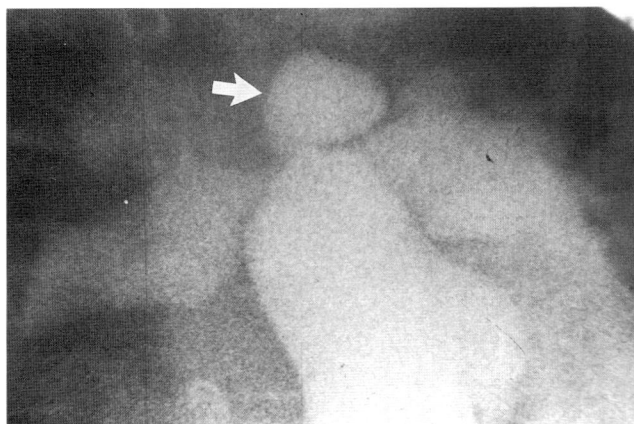

Fig. 20.20 Aneurysms of the ductus occur — in this case at the pulmonary arterial end (arrow).

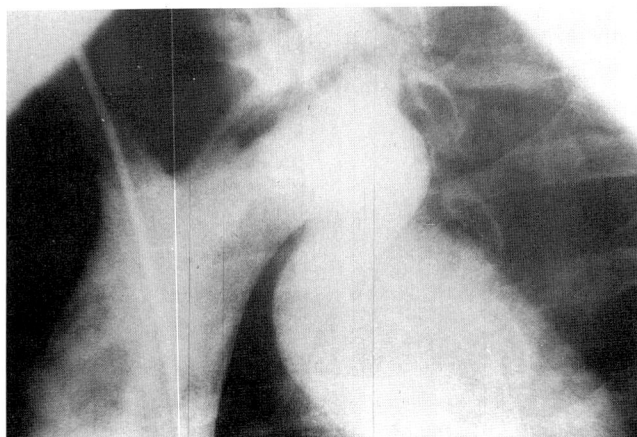

Fig. 20.18 *Pseudocoarctation*. Aortogram in an elderly patient suggesting coarctation. The appearances are due to unfolding and redundancy of the aorta; there was no pressure gradient between ascending and descending aorta.

Aortopulmonary septal defect ('window')

Aortopulmonary 'window' (Figs 20.25 and 20.26) is an uncommon malformation accounting for only 0.5% of cases of congenital heart disease catheterised in our unit [10]. There is a communication between the ascending aorta and pulmonary artery but there are two discrete outflow tracts supporting separate ventriculo-arterial valves and ascending portions of the great arteries. The condition may exist as an isolated anomaly but is frequently associated with

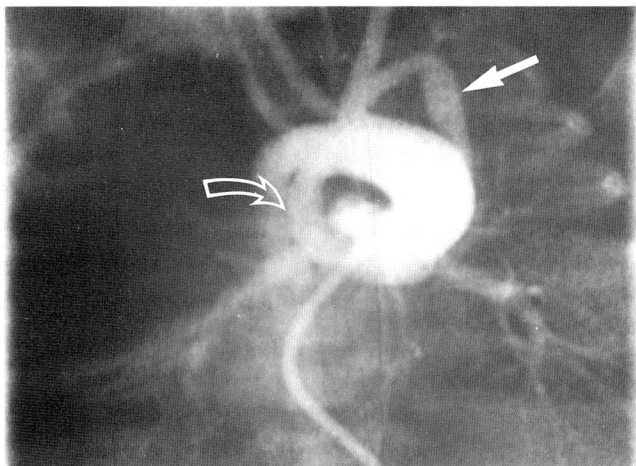

Fig. 20.21 *Aortopulmonary communications.* Right aortic arch with patent *right* duct (open arrow). Bilateral ducti occur but in this example the structure which resembles a left ductus (solid arrow) is a left Blalock shunt.

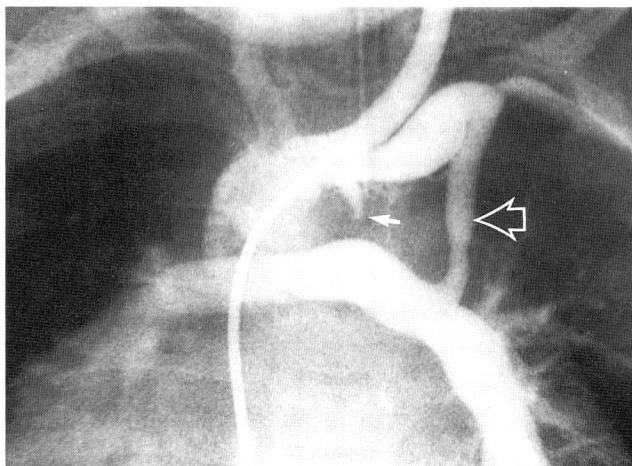

Fig. 20.23 *Aortopulmonary communications.* Another example of a surgical systemic-to-pulmonary shunt (open arrow) in a patient with pulmonary atresia. In this case the shunt is an interposition (Gore—Tex) graft — the left subclavian artery has not been sacrificed (as it is in a classical Blalock shunt) but can be seen continuing towards the left axilla. Also visible is the stump of a closed ductus (small arrow).

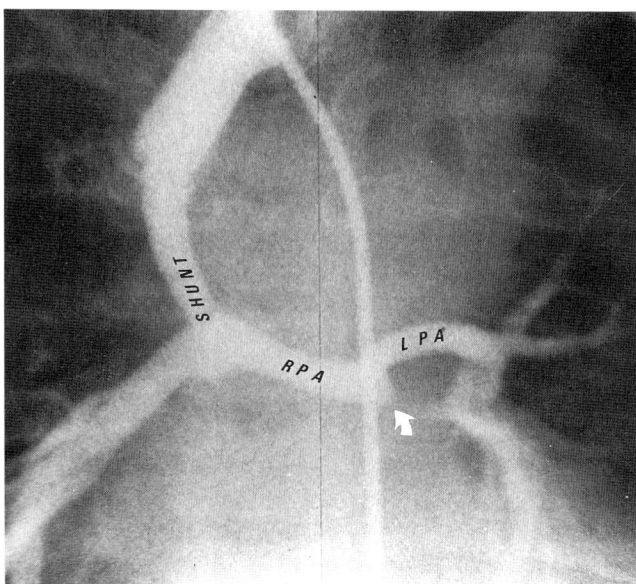

Fig. 20.22 An example of a surgically-created aortopulmonary communication — a right sided Blalock shunt. The pulmonary arteries are very small but the right (RPA) and left (LPA) pulmonary arteries are in continuity. There is pulmonary atresia but the atretic pulmonary trunk (arrow) can be seen indicating potential communication with the ventricular mass.

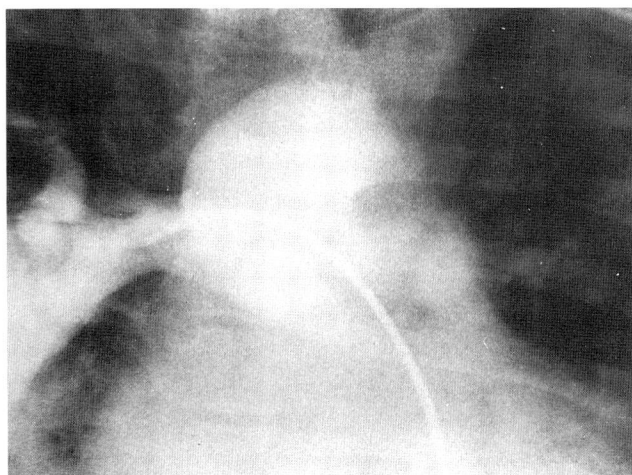

Fig. 20.24 An example of a surgically-created shunt between the ascending aorta and the right pulmonary artery — a Waterston shunt.

other congenital cardiac anomalies including interrupted aortic arch [10—11], ventricular septal defect, anomalous origin of the subclavian, right aortic arch and pulmonary atresia. The associated lesions may determine the clinical presentation in the neonate and the combination of, for example, aortic interruption and aortopulmonary window may produce considerable difficulties in interpretation of the angiogram. Selective aortography is needed to establish the diagnosis.

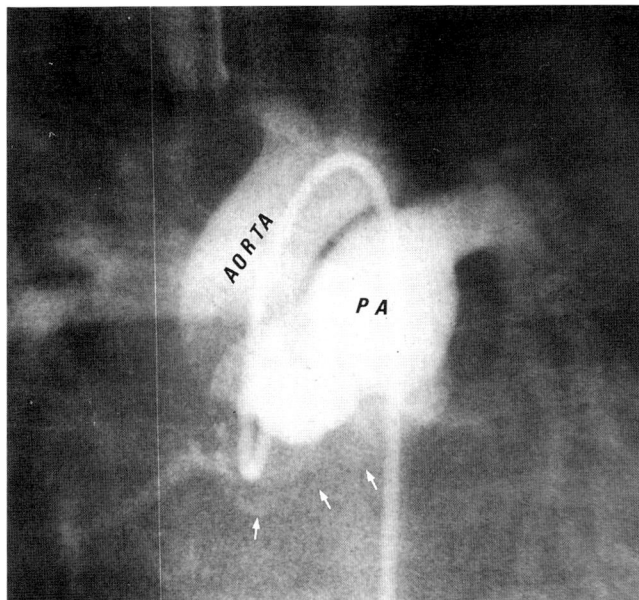

Fig. 20.25 *Aortopulmonary septal defect (window).* This is a rare malformation. The appearances here are similar to persistent truncus arteriosus but the two separate arterial valves can be seen — the aortic valve is indicated by the small arrows.

Truncus arteriosus

Truncus arteriosus communis (Figs 20.27 and 20.28) exists when one great artery arises from the heart and gives origin to the coronary, pulmonary and systemic arteries. There is a single ventriculo-arterial valve which may have two to four cusps (Fig. 20.28); this valve may be incompetent or (rarely) stenotic [12]. Truncus may be classified [13] according to the presence (Type A) or absence (Type B) of a ventricular septal defect and the mode of origin of the pulmonary arteries which may originate from a partially separate main pulmonary artery (Type A1) or directly from the truncus (Type A2). One or other pulmonary artery may be absent (Type A3) with a collateral supply to the other lung. Finally there may be underdevelopment of the aortic arch — hypoplasia, coarctation, atresia or interruption (Type A4). As with aortopulmonary window the association of aortic interruption can provide diagnostic difficulties and aortography is required to demonstrate the anatomy.

Cardiac catheterisation carries a high risk in persistent truncus. A large volume of contrast medium is needed to demonstrate the defect(s) but is poorly tolerated; worsening heart failure and death is not uncommon following angiocardiography in the sick neonate with persistent truncus. Fortunately echocardiography now allows surgical correction without prior catheterisation. If angiography *is* requested the number of injections should be limited — a single injection in the trunk is ideal — and non-ionic contrast medium should be used.

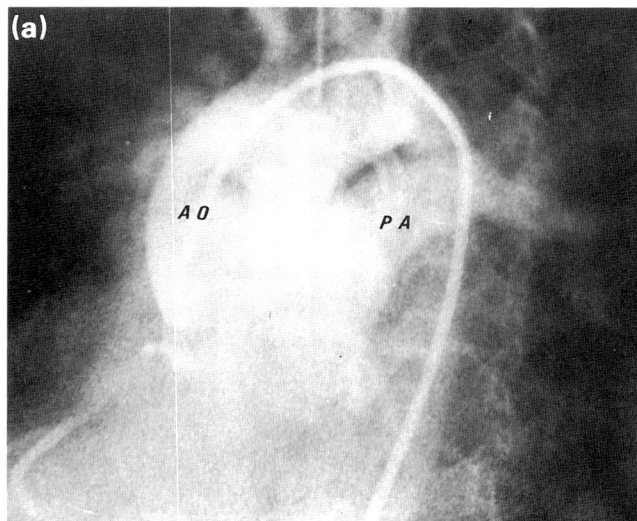

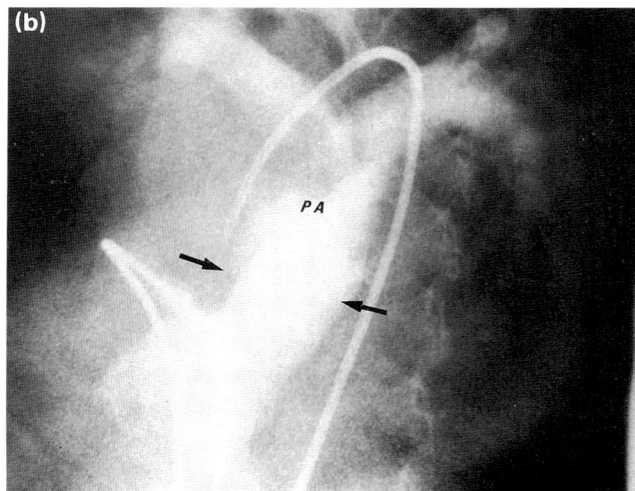

Fig. 20.26 *Aortopulmonary septal defect.* In (a) an aortogram has produced an appearance indistinguishable from persistent truncus arteriosus but a subsequent injection into the right ventricle (b) has opacified a separate pulmonary artery without any opacification of the aorta. The arrows indicate the level of the pulmonary valve.

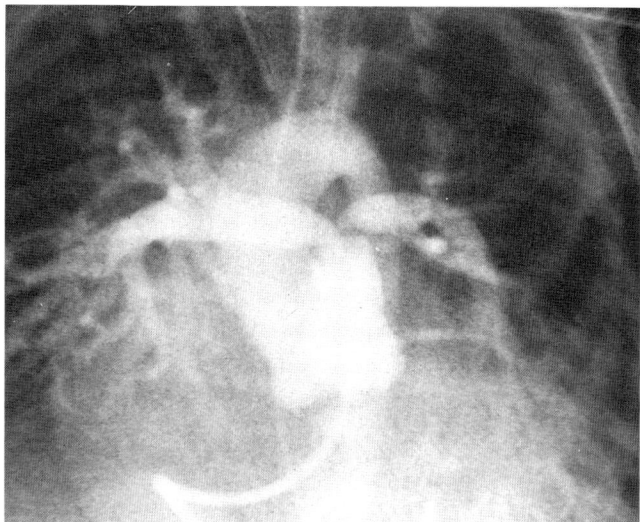

Fig. 20.27 *Persistent truncus arteriosus.* There is a single arterial (truncal) valve and the pulmonary arteries arise from the truncus as a single vessel which then divides into the left and right branches. The origin of the left pulmonary artery is narrowed.

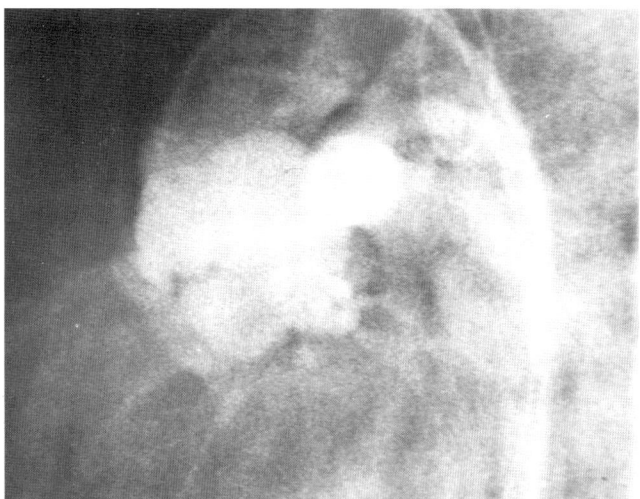

Fig. 20.28 *Persistent truncus arteriosus.* Multiple (? four) valve cusps are seen.

Systemic-to-pulmonary collaterals

Systemic-to-pulmonary collaterals, such as are found in pulmonary atresia with ventricular septal defect, are illustrated in Figs 20.29 to 20.31.

Supravalve aortic stenosis (Figs 20.32 and 20.33)

This lesion is found in association with infantile

hypercalcaemia (Williams syndrome) and may therefore be accompanied by peripheral pulmonary artery stenoses. It may also occur in the rubella syndrome. Most commonly the stenosis takes the form of a sharply localised narrowing at the upper border of the sinuses of Valsalva; on occasion there is a tubular narrowing of the ascending aorta and, rarely, there may be a 'diaphragm' causing a stenosis. The investigation of a child suspected of having Williams syndrome (elfin facies, mental retardation) should include a pulmonary arteriogram *and* an aortogram.

Sinus of Valsalva aneurysms (Figs 20.35 to 20.37)

Aneurysm of the sinus of Valsalva is rare. The right sinus is most commonly involved followed by the non-coronary sinus. Aneurysms of the left sinus of Valsalva are the least common. Patients may present at any age; usually as a result of rupture of the aneurysm into a cardiac chamber. When rupture occurs it is usually into the right ventricle. The aneurysm may bulge into the right ventricular outflow tract and outflow tract gradients from this cause have been reported.

ACQUIRED ABNORMALITIES OF THE THORACIC AORTA

The 'adult cardiologist' is unlikely to encounter any of the conditions described in the preceding section other than coarctation and patent ductus which frequently present in adult life. He will be concerned with:

1 Aortic aneurysm.
2 Aortic dissection.
3 Aortitis.
4 Annulo-aortic ectasia.
5 Aortic rupture.
6 Infective endocarditis and abcess formation.

Aortic aneurysm (Fig. 20.39)

The wall of a 'true aneurysm' includes at least one of the three layers — intima, media and adventitia. A 'false aneurysm' results from extravasation of blood through the aortic wall and is surrounded by adjacent tissues and fibrous tissue. True aneurysms may be associated with many of the conditions to be described in this section but atherosclerosis is by far

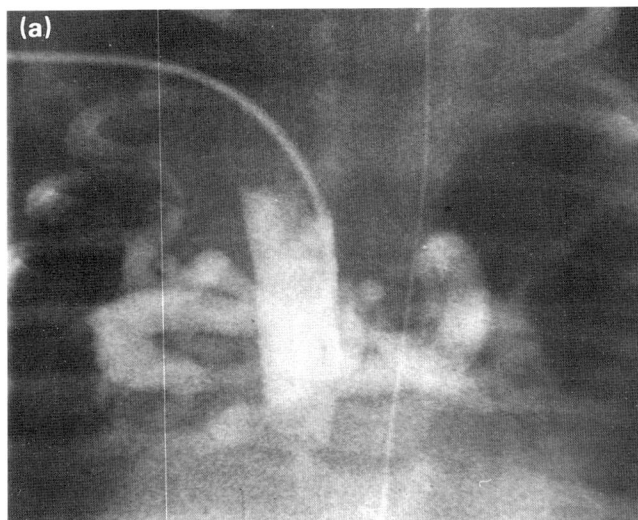

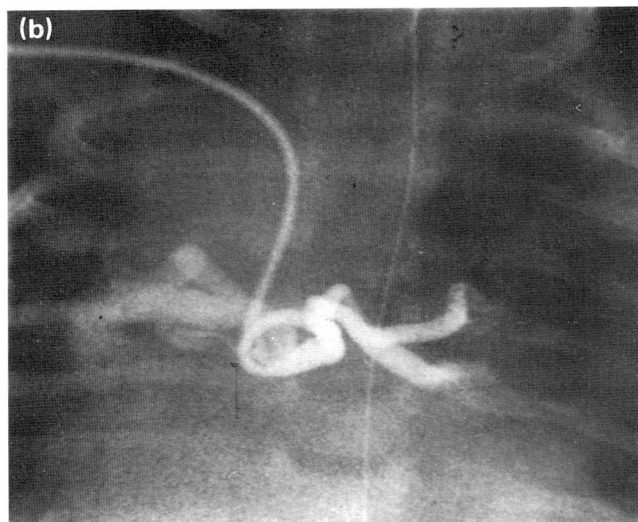

Fig. 20.29 *Aortopulmonary communications.* Pulmonary atresia with ventricular septal defect and pulmonary arterial supply by systemic-to-pulmonary collaterals arising from the descending thoracic aorta. Sometimes called 'pseudotruncus' or 'truncus Type IV' this condition is quite distinct; the single patent arterial valve is a true aortic valve and in many cases a separate, atretic, pulmonary trunk can be traced back to the ventricular mass. In (a) an injection into the descending aorta has demonstrated several, large, systemic-to-pulmonary collateral vessels. Full investigation requires selective injections into each of the collateral vessels as in (b).

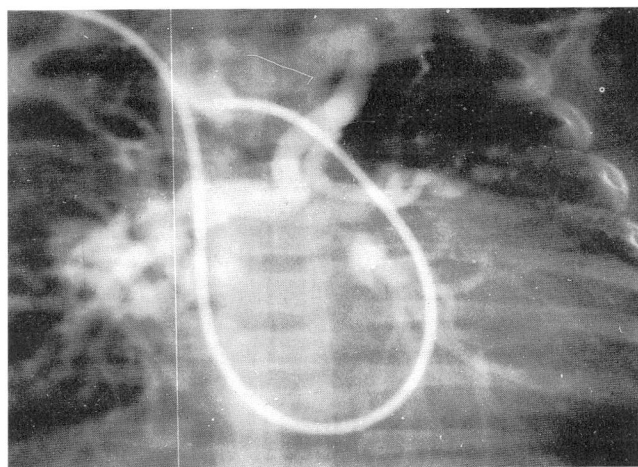

Fig. 20.30 Another example of pulmonary atresia with ventricular septal defect and multifocal pulmonary arterial supply from systemic-to-pulmonary collaterals.

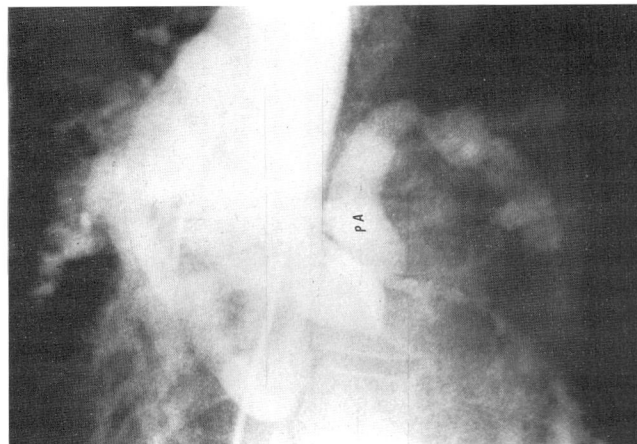

Fig. 20.31 In cases of pulmonary atresia with VSD there may, or may not, be central pulmonary arteries. In this example systemic-to-pulmonary collaterals (not seen) have filled a small pulmonary trunk (PA) which remains densely opacified as there is no 'wash-out' of contrast medium by antegrade flow.

the commonest cause of thoracic aortic aneurysm. Atherosclerotic aneurysms occur most commonly in the abdominal aorta (Fig. 20.40) but about one-third involve the thoracic aorta; of these most occur in the descending aorta followed, in order of frequency, by the arch and ascending aorta. The aneurysms are most often fusiform but may be saccular. Angio-

graphically the associated extensive atheromatous change is likely to cause irregularity of the aortic wall elsewhere. Laminated thrombus may be present within the aneurysm and is detected by increased thickness of the wall between the contrast-filled lumen and the soft tissue shadow of the outer limit of the aneurysm. Generalised dilatation and

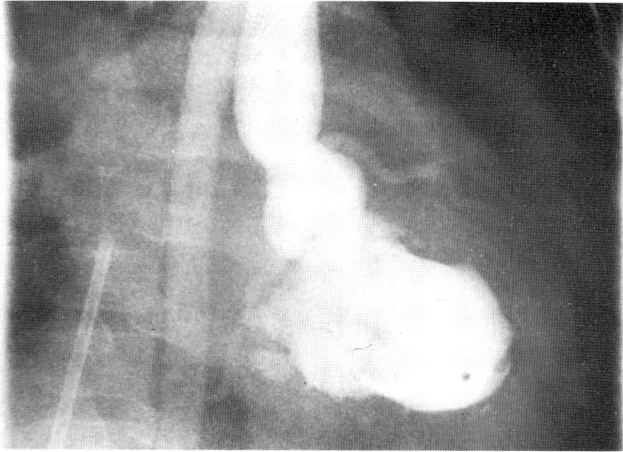

Fig. 20.32 Congenital aortic stenosis may be at subvalve level (see section on the ventricles), at valve level or at supravalve level in the ascending aorta. Mild supravalve aortic stenosis of the 'hour glass' type; waisting immediately above the aortic sinuses.

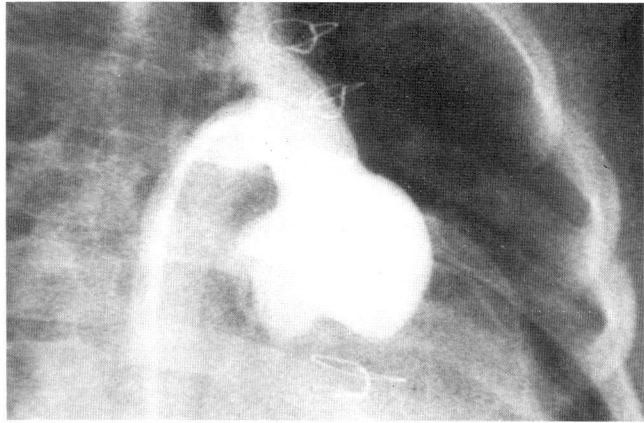

Fig. 20.34 The appearances of supravalve aortic stenosis are mimicked following an arterial 'switch' operation for transposition of the great arteries. The large pulmonary valve and ring are anastomosed to a smaller aorta — hence the appearances illustrated here.

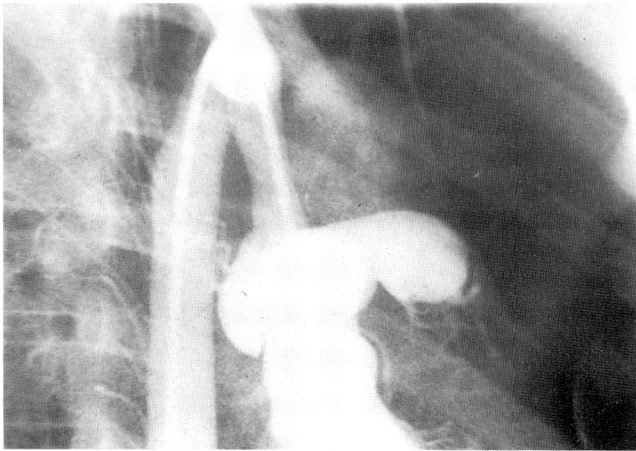

Fig. 20.33 Supravalve aortic stenosis of the tubular type; in this patient there is also gross dilatation of the left sinus of Valsalva.

elongation of the thoracic aorta without localised aneurysm formation ('unfolded aorta') occurs in the elderly; a common reason for aortography is to distinguish an 'unfolded aorta' from a localised aneurysm since both cause widening of the aorta as seen on the plain chest X-ray.

Aortic dissection (Figs 20.41 and 20.42)

Almost all aortic dissections start either at the aortic isthmus at the level of the point of attachment of the ductus ligament or in the ascending aorta just above the sinuses of Valsalva. A widely used classification is that of DeBakey [14]. In this classification Type 1 and Type 2 both originate in the ascending aorta; in Type 1 the dissection involves the ascending aorta, arch and descending aorta while in Type 2 the dissection is confined to the ascending aorta. Type 3 dissections in this classification start in the descending aorta (at the level of the ductus ligament) and extend distally. An alternative classification recognises the fact that management and prognosis depend on whether or not the ascending aorta is involved; dissections are then classified into two types — those that involve the ascending aorta and those that do not.

Dissection involving the ascending aorta may be complicated by aortic regurgitation and/or bleeding into the pericardium with tamponade. Aortic regurgitation may be due to dilatation of the valve ring, to interference with cusp function due to distortion by haematoma or to disruption of the annulus by retrograde extension of the dissection.

Retrograde aortography provides the definitive diagnosis though computerised tomography or magnetic resonance imaging are alternatives. There is no place for non-selective angiography (e.g. pulmonary artery injections) unless digital subtraction is available and shown to be a reliable diagnostic technique. Both the transfemoral and transbrachial approach are used and have their advocates; it is possible that the catheter will enter the false lumen

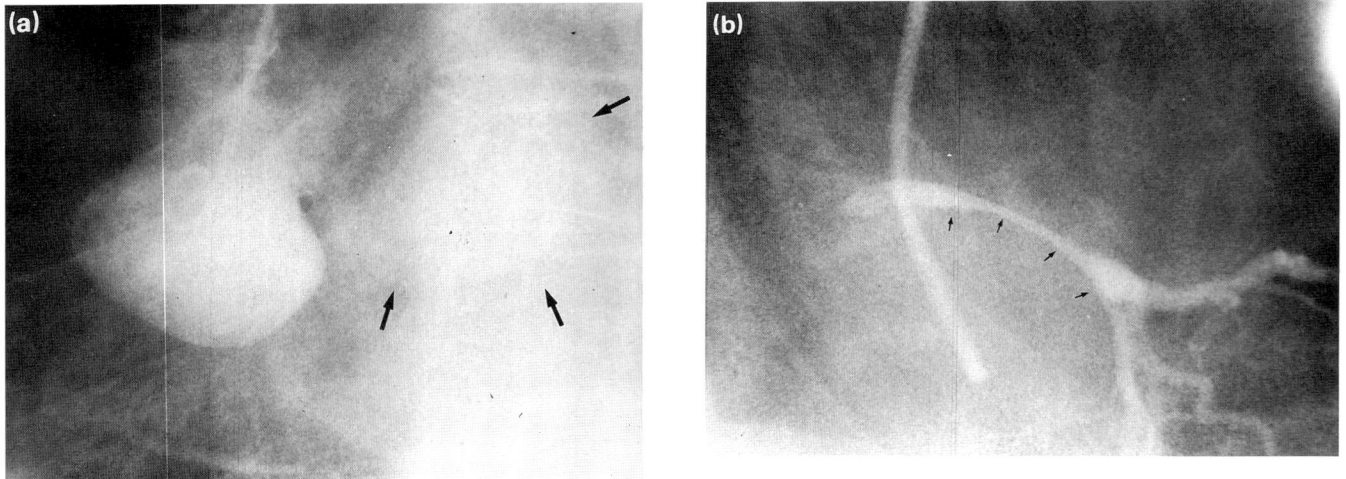

Fig. 20.35 (a) Sinus of the Valsalva aneurysm in an adult. There is gross dilatation of the opacified non-coronary sinus in a patient with Noonan syndrome. There is even more marked enlargement of the left sinus of Valsalva (arrows) though this is only faintly opacified. (b) In the same patient the mainstem left coronary artery is seen to be stretched and elongated as it passes over the aneurysmal left sinus of Valsalva.

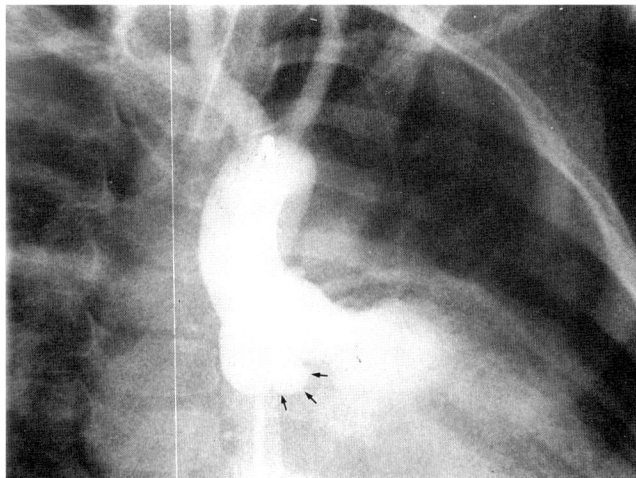

Fig. 20.36 A small sinus of Valsalva aneurysm (arrows). There is also aortic regurgitation which may be due to deformation of the valve cusps.

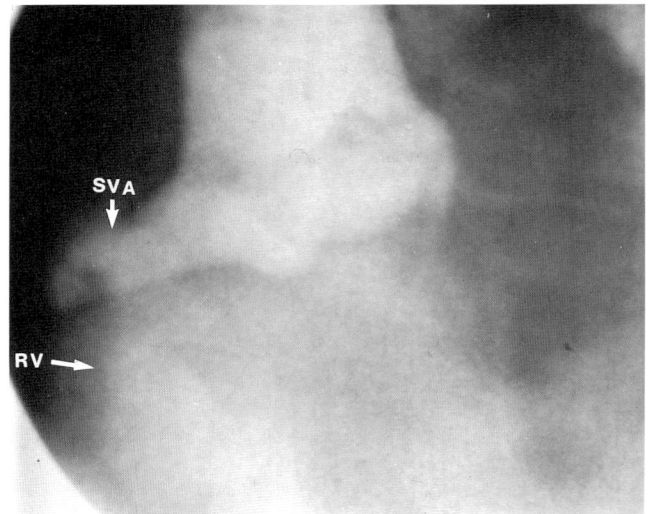

Fig. 20.37 Ruptured sinus of Valsalva aneurysm (SVA). In this case the aneurysm had ruptured into the right ventricle (RV).

which ever approach is used. Unequal volume pulses are a feature of aortic dissection and may be due to compression of the vessel by surrounding haematoma or occlusion of its ostium by an intimal flap. If the transfemoral approach is used entry should be from the side with the better pulse pressure. It is our practice to use the transbrachial approach *unless* the right brachial pulse is diminished in volume as compared with other pulses. A thin-wall angio-

graphic catheter or a pigtail catheter should be used and advanced with caution — never against resistance. Small test injections may be used to check the catheter position before a large volume of contrast is given for definitive angiography. No attempt should be made to cross the aortic valve; it is possible that the catheter is in the false lumen of an ascending aortic dissection and only the absence of coronary artery filling may provide the clue that what appears

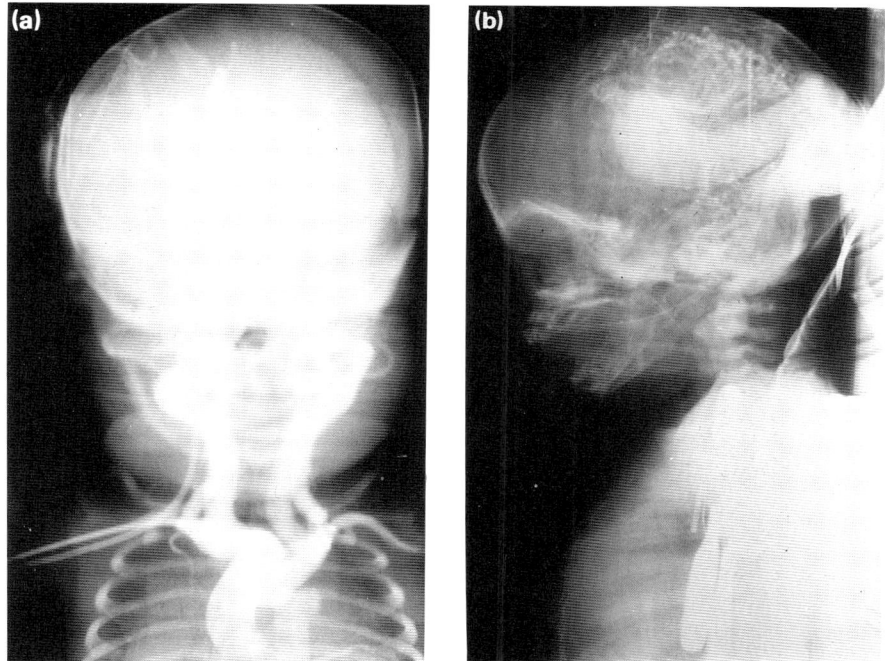

Fig. 20.38 The size (diameter) of a vessel is directly proportional to the flow through it. This is well illustrated by this neonate who presented with congestive heart failure. In (a) an aortogram demonstrates enormous enlargement of the carotid arteries. In (b) the explanation is apparent; there is torrential flow through the carotid arteries due to the presence of a large cerebral arteriovenous fistula. The draining vein is also enormously enlarged due to high flow — leading to one name for this condition: 'vein of Galen aneurysm'.

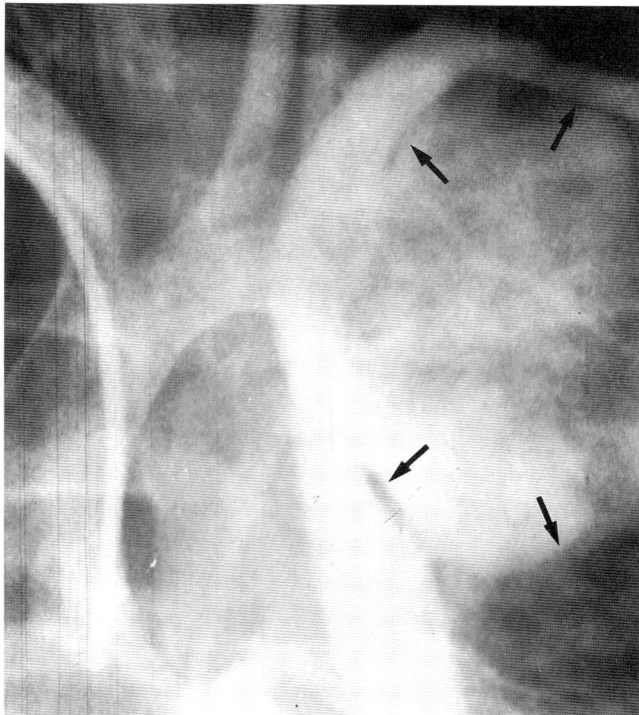

Fig. 20.39 *Aortography — acquired lesions.* A large, saccular, aneurysm of the thoracic aorta (arrows) — possibly a false aneurysm.

to be a dilated ascending aorta is, in fact, the false lumen. Cine angiography will demonstrate one, or more, of the features of aortic dissection. These are: (1) a linear filling defect representing the intimal flap separating the true from the false lumen, (2) contrast medium in the true lumen which is narrowed (compressed) by the false lumen, (3) a variable degree of filling of the false lumen, and (4) a change in calibre of the aorta together with a slight irregularity of its contour at the point of origin of the dissection. It is usually possible to move the table top so as to follow the advancing contrast down the descending aorta (panning) and demonstrate the extent of the dissection and the re-entry point. This may also allow demonstration of occluded aortic branches (renal and mesenteric arteries, etc.). A film of the renal area should follow aortography since an absent nephrogram will suggest renal artery involvement.

Aortitis

Syphillis classically affects the ascending aorta and may result in aneurysm formation and/or aortic regurgitation. Calcification is common resulting in linear shadows outlining the aortic wall. Aortography will reveal irregularities of the wall instead of the normally smooth intima and will define the extent

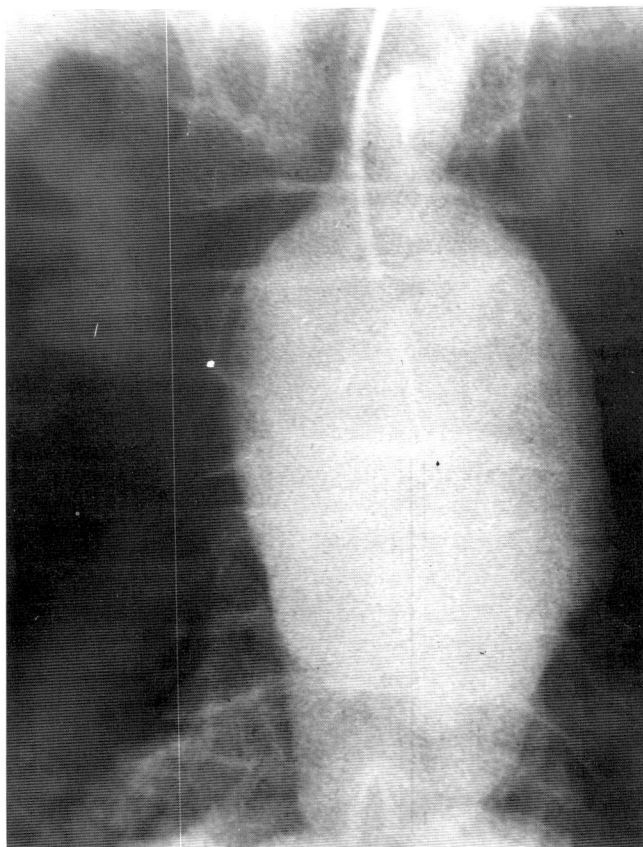

Fig. 20.40 *Abdominal aortic aneurysm.* Although the aneurysm is well seen the injection should have been made in a more proximal site in order to display the renal arteries.

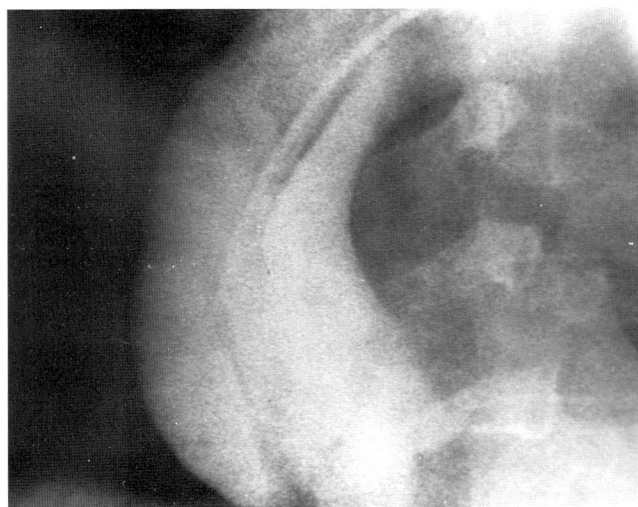

Fig. 20.41 Aortic dissection involving the ascending aorta. A linear filling defect is seen representing the intimal flap which separates the false lumen (on the patient's right) from the true lumen and aortic valve on the left.

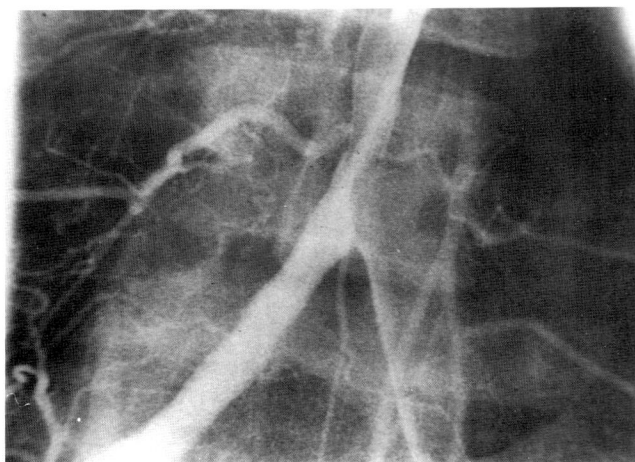

Fig. 20.42 Aortic dissection involving the descending aorta and (left) iliac artery. There is extreme narrowing of the true lumen due to compression by blood in the false lumen.

of an aneurysm if one is present. Although syphilitic aortitis is rarely seen today when it does occur involvement of the coronary ostia is common with resulting ostial stenosis (see Chapter 13). Coronary arteriography is therefore part of the investigation of a patient with suspected syphilitic aortitis.

Takayasu aortitis [15–16] is predominantly a disease of young adult oriental females but can occur in all races and in both sexes. The term 'pulseless disease' describes one form of the disease in which the origins of the aortic arch vessels (subclavian, carotid, innominate) are stenosed or occluded (Figs 20.43 and 20.44b). Typically the vessel is smoothly narrowed for a centimetre or so and then widens to a normal calibre but sharply localised stenoses can occur or the vessel may be narrowed for a considerable distance — as far as the base of the skull. The aortic arch itself may be involved and of irregular

outline. In another form of the disease the descending and/or abdominal aorta are involved (Fig. 20.44a), renal artery stenoses or occlusion are common. Of importance to the cardiologist is the fact that there may be severe stenoses of the proximal coronary arteries producing ostial and left main stem stenosis in young adults (Fig. 20.45). Aneurysm formation can occur in association as can aortic valve involve-

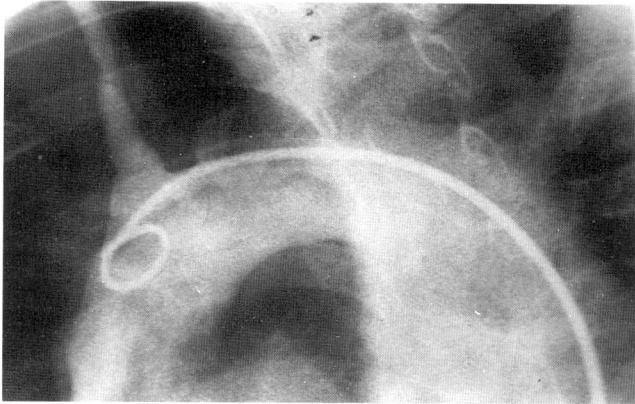

Fig. 20.43 *Aortitis — Takayasu disease*. The aorta in this 20 year old male is irregular and both right and left subclavian as well as the left common carotid arteries are occluded. The only arch vessel seen is the right common carotid and the lumen of this vessel is also irregular. The coronary arteriographic findings in this patient are illustrated in Fig. 20.45.

ment (rarely) with regurgitation. Finally there is often involvement of the pulmonary vasculature resulting in pulmonary hypertension; it is possible that some

cases of so-called 'primary pulmonary hypertension' are, in reality, due to Takayasu disease.

Aortic involvement can occur in giant cell arteritis ('temporal arteritis') and aortitis with aortic regurgitation can complicate ankylosing spondylitis [17], psoriatic arthritis [18], ulcerative colitis and Reiter syndrome. Relapsing polychondritis is a rare disease the features of which commonly include inflammation and destruction of cartilage (most frequently of the pinna of the ear), arthralgia and a raised erythrocyte sedimentation rate. Aortitis occurs in a significant proportion of cases with root dilatation and aortic regurgitation [19]. Death can result from aortic regurgitation or from rupture of an abdominal aortic aneurysm.

Aortic rupture (Fig. 20.46)

Aortic rupture occurs as a result of sudden deceleration — as in a road traffic accident. The patient may have sustained blunt trauma to the front of the chest or may have been held by a seat belt. The ascending aorta may rupture but such

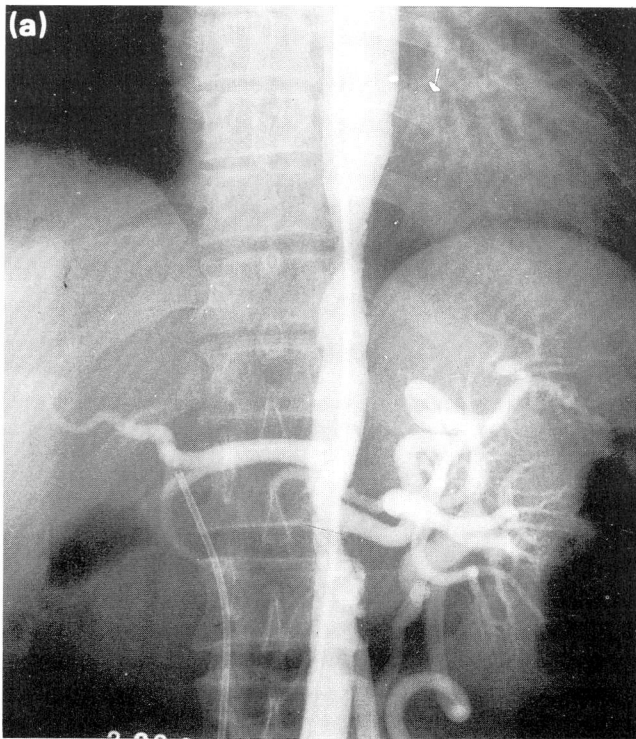

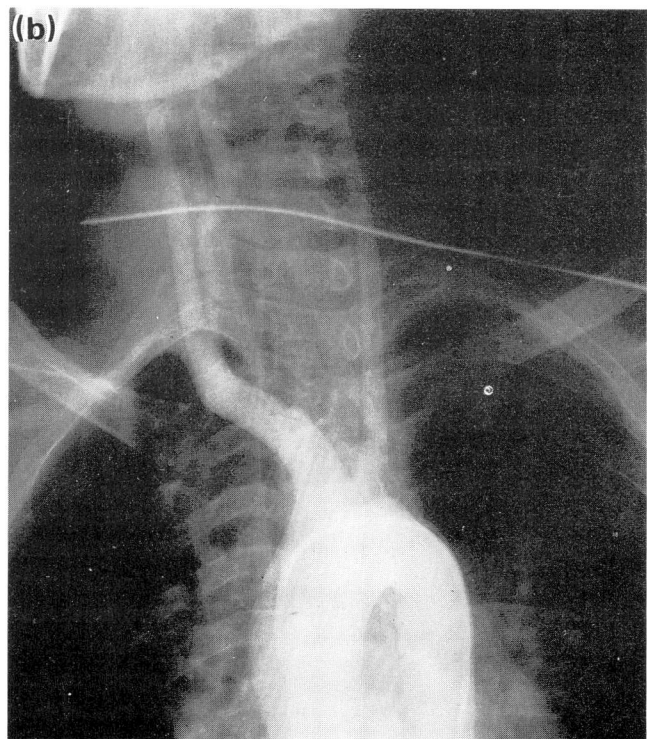

Fig. 20.44 *Aortitis — Takayasu disease*. Involvement of the abdominal aorta (b) and renal arteries in another patient. An ascending aortogram (a) in the same patient reveals occlusion of both subclavian arteries at their origins.

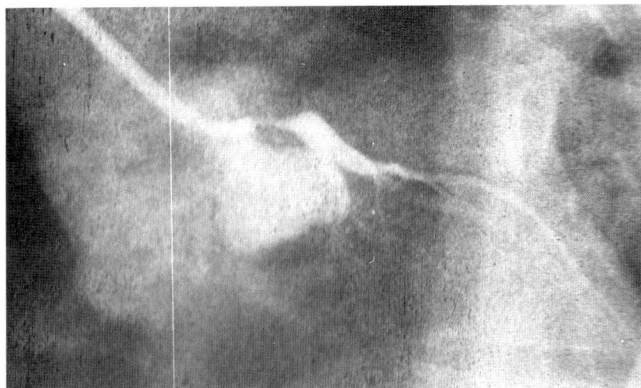

Fig. 20.45 *Aortitis — Takayasu disease.* Severe ostial stenosis of the left coronary artery. There was also right ostial stenosis. The patient presented with angina. The same patient illustrated in Fig. 20.43.

patients are unlikely to survive; the classical site of rupture seen in practice is at the site of attachment of the ductus ligament. Aortography, mandatory whenever the diagnosis is entertained, reveals a change in diameter of the aorta at this site; an intimal flap may produce a linear filling defect and there may be extravasation of contrast medium into sur-

rounding haematoma. Discontinuity may be obvious but the changes, though characteristic, may be subtle. Urgent surgical treatment is needed as the lesion is unstable and rupture and extravasation can occur at any time — even in those few cases who have survived for days or weeks [20].

Annulo-aortic ectasia

The term 'annulo-aortic ectasia' was coined by Ellis *et al.* [21] to encompass cases of aortic regurgitation due to marked dilatation of the aortic valve ring and aorta proximal to the innominate. Although patients with Marfan syndrome provide the best known examples (Fig. 20.47) only about one-third of patients with this condition have other stigmata of Marfan syndrome. A further proportion may be 'formes frustes' while the remainder have some other condition resulting in cystic medial necrosis. The condition is referred to in the chapter on valvular heart disease as it is a cause of aortic regurgitation. Mitral regurgitation, the same process resulting in a 'floppy' mitral valve, is a frequent association. In about half the cases the ascending aorta is 'pear-shaped' with

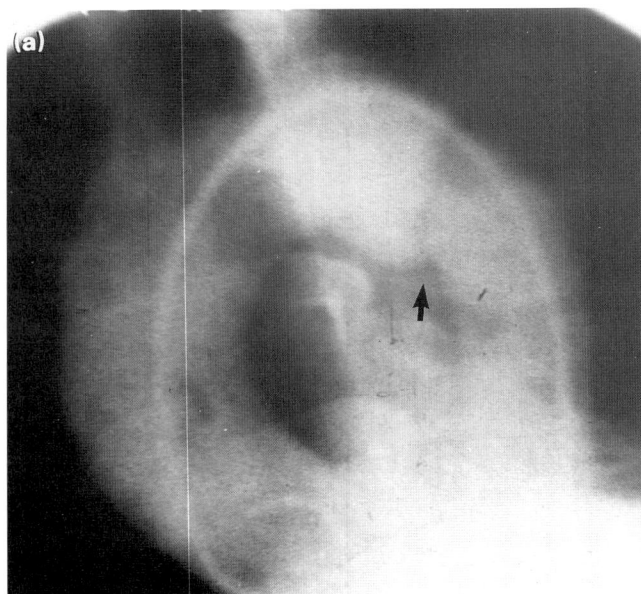

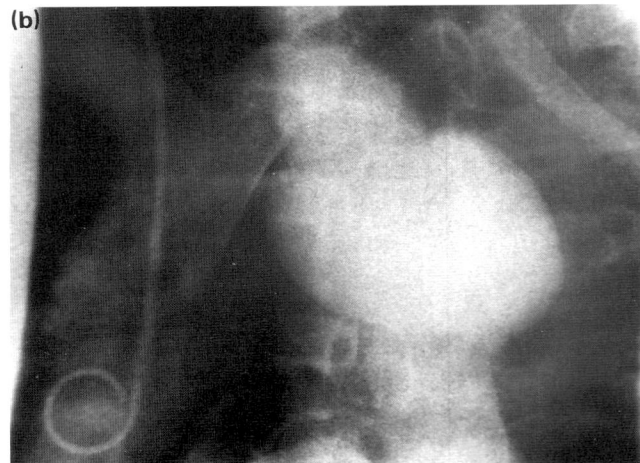

Fig. 20.46 (a) *Aortic rupture.* There is a transverse, linear, translucency at the level of the ductus ligament (arrow) — the characteristic site of rupture in traumatic aortic rupture; due to a road traffic accident in this case. (b) False aneurysm at the site of an aortic rupture which had occurred 2 years previously as a result of a road traffic accident.

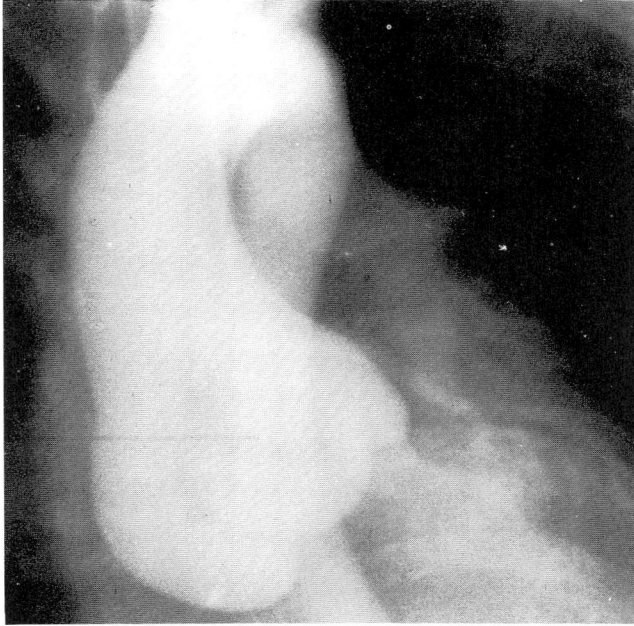

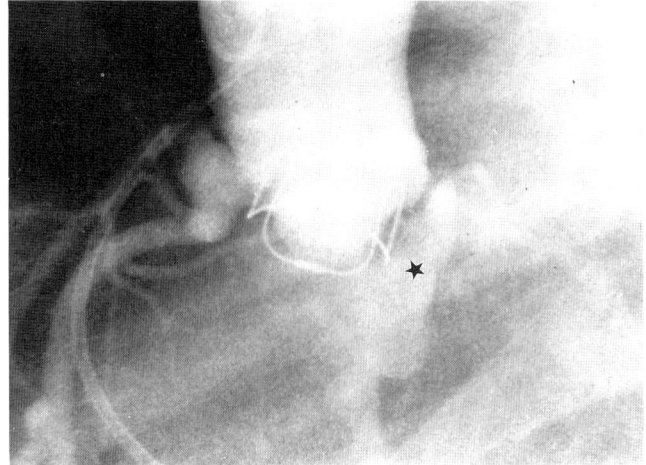

Fig. 20.49 Fistula formation (asterisk) between the aorta and left ventricle following aortic valve replacement (Carpentier—Edwards frame-mounted xenograft).

Fig. 20.47 Annulo-aortic ectasia in Marfan disease. There is obvious dilatation of the aortic root with reduction to a normal calibre before the origin of the head and neck vessels. The aortic valve is competent in this patient since there is no contrast medium visible in the left ventricle. Although probably congenitally determined it is unusual for this condition to become manifest before adulthood.

gross dilatation of the valve ring, aortic sinuses and proximal aorta and abrupt reduction to a normal calibre before the origin of the innominate. Aortic dissection is a frequent complication in those with Marfan syndrome who tend to present at an earlier age — in young adult life. About a quarter of cases exhibit more generalised dilatation of the ascending aorta while, in a small proportion (6%) the dilatation is confined to the aortic sinuses [22]. Rare causes of the condition include the mucopolysaccharidoses — Hunter, Hurler, Morquio and Scheie syndromes [23−24].

Infective endocarditis and aneurysm formation

Although the aorta may be the site of many infections or may be involved by extension of nearby infection the commonest cause that will present to the cardiologist is infective endocarditis related to aortic valve disease or to a prosthetic aortic valve (Figs 20.48 and 20.49). The resulting abcess may extend into the septum and may rupture into another cardiac chamber — the right ventricle for example.

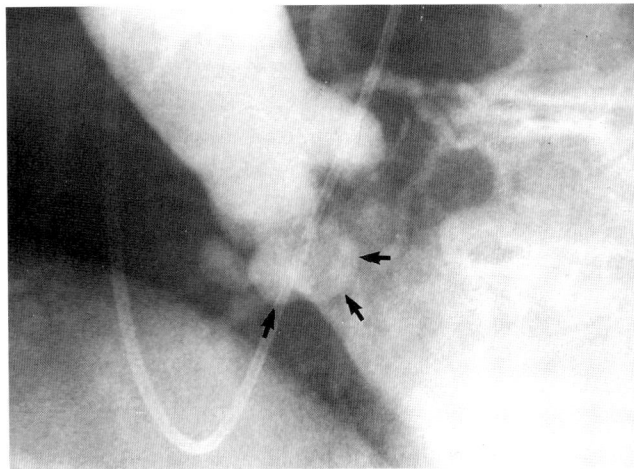

Fig. 20.48 Abcess formation (arrows) in association with infective endocarditis involving a stenotic aortic valve.

REFERENCES

1 Fiddler GI, Partridge JB. Balloon occlusion angiography

in critically ill neonates. *Cathet Cardiovasc Diagn* 1983;**9**:309.

2 Edwards JE. Anomalies of derivatives of aortic arch system. *Med Clin North Am* 1948;**32**:925.

3 Stewart JR, Kincaid OW, Edwards JE. *An atlas of vascular rings and related malformations of the aortic arch system.* Springfield, Charles C Thomas, 1964.

4 Garti IJ, Aygen MM, Vidne B, Levy MJ. Right aortic arch with mirror image branching causing vascular ring. A new classification of the right aortic arch patterns. *Br J Radiol* 1973;**46**:115.

5 Celoria GC, Patton RB. Congenital absence of the aortic arch. *Am Heart J* 1959;**58**:407.

6 Haughton VM, Fellows KE, Rosenbaum AE. The cervical aortic arches. *Pediatr Radiol* 1975;**114**:675.

7 Rudolph AM, Heymann MA, Spitznas U. Haemodynamic considerations in the development of narrowing of the aorta. *Am J Cardiol* 1972;**39**:514.

8 Shinebourne EA, Elseed AM. Relation between fetal flow patterns, coarctation of the aorta, and pulmonary blood flow. *Br Heart J* 1974;**36**:492.

9 Lajos TZ *et al.* Pseudo-coarctation of the aorta. A variant or an entity? *Chest* 1970;**58**:571.

10 Lau KC *et al.* Aorto-pulmonary window. *J Cardiovasc Surg* 1982;**23**:21.

11 Fisher EA, Bubrow IW, Eckner FAO, Hastreiter AR. Aorto-pulmonary septal defect and interrupted aortic arch: a diagnostic challenge. *Am J Cardiol* 1974;**34**:356.

12 Burnell RH, McEnery G, Miller GAH. Truncal valve stenosis. *Br Heart J* 1971;**33**:423.

13 Calder L *et al.* Truncus arteriosus communis. Clinical, angiocardiographic, and pathologic findings in 100 patients. *Am Heart J* 1976;**92**:23.

14 DeBakey ME *et al.* Surgical management of dissecting aneurysms of the aorta. *J Thorac Cardiovasc Surg* 1965;**49**:130.

15 Lupi-Herrera E *et al.* Takayasu's arteritis. Clinical study of 107 cases. *Am Heart J* 1977;**93**:94.

16 Lande A, Bard R, Bole P, Guarnaccia M. Aortic arch syndrome (Takayasu's arteritis). Arteriographic and surgical considerations. *J Cardiovasc Surg* 1978;**19**:507.

17 Bulkley BH, Roberts WC. Ankylosing spondylitis and aortic regurgitation: description of the characteristic cardiovascular lesion from study of eight necropsy patients. *Circulation* 1973;**48**:1014.

18 Muna WF *et al.* Psoriatic arthritis and aortic regurgitation. *JAMA* 1980;**244**:363.

19 Hughes RAC, Berry CL, Seifert M, Lessof MH. Relapsing polychondritis. Three cases with a clinico-pathological study and literature review. *Q J Med* 1972;**41**:363.

20 Bennett DE, Cherry JK. Natural history of traumatic aneurysms of aorta. *Surgery* 1967;**61**:516.

21 Ellis PR, Cooley DA, DeBakey ME. Clinical consideration and surgical treatment of annulo-aortic ectasia. *J Thorac Cardiovasc Surg* 1961;**42**:363.

22 Lemon DK, White CW. Annulo-aortic ectasia. Angiographic, hemodynamic and clinical comparison with aortic valve insufficiency. *Am J Cardiol* 1978;**41**:482.

23 McKusick VA. The genetic mucopolysaccharidoses. *Circulation* 1965;**31**:1.

24 Schieken RM, Kerber RE, Ionasescu VV, Zellweger H. Cardiac manifestations of the mucopolysaccharidoses. *Circulation* 1975;**52**:700.

CHAPTER 21

Management of cardiovascular emergencies in the intensive care unit

Disorders of the circulation are common in the intensive care unit and can be either the cause for admission or a complication occuring in the course of other illness. Multisystem pathology is to be expected and this means that priorities for treatment must be defined and that compromise may be necessary: for example, volume loading will often improve cardiovascular indices in patients with septicaemia but it is likely to do so at the expense of pulmonary function. Rapid change is common too and so the order of clinical priorities alters with time. The combination of multisystem pathology and propensity to sudden change creates a fundamental distinction from the usual practice of the cardiac catheter laboratory. Here, clinical evaluation usually precedes invasive investigation and catheterisation is carried out to confirm the diagnosis, assess severity of disease and its consequences and, in some instances, provide treatment. Haemodynamic investigation in the intensive care unit follows clinical evaluation initially but thereafter the two go hand in hand. This need for catheterisation to fulfil a monitoring role, as distinct from allowing a circumscribed investigation or treatment, influences the choice of catheter and route of access, as does the frequent need to undertake the procedure in unstable patients requiring attention to other systems simultaneously and who are nursed without immediate access to more than limited radiological facilities.

Cardiovascular emergencies in the intensive care unit include resuscitation from cardiac arrest, investigation and treatment of the failing circulation, and the management of dysrhythmias. The first two are discussed in this chapter and dysrhythmias are considered in Chapter 22.

MANAGEMENT OF CARDIAC ARREST

Initial treatment

The nature of intensive care means that the incidence of cardiac arrest is high but the principles of management do not differ from those applying elsewhere. The essential priorities are still maintenance of the Airway, Breathing and Circulation (the 'ABC' of resuscitation). Some distinctions do apply however because immediate recognition, or even recognition of impending arrest, are likely and equipment is easily available. This means that the chances of restoring the heartbeat and achieving survival without neurological damage are higher than when arrest from a comparable cause occurs elsewhere. It may prove possible to terminate the arrest immediately, for example by prompt defibrillation, whereas in other circumstances it would be necessary to start cardiac massage and assist ventilation until the defibrillator is available. An agreed policy by which appropriately trained nursing staff are authorised to use the defibrillator means that treatment can be given with virtually no delay.

Conversely, cardiac arrest in the ICU may be the consequence of failure of the existing apparatus or a complication of treatment, and so the ABC of resuscitation must be combined with an immediate survey of all other aspects of patient management. These include placement and patency of the endotracheal tube, integrity of the ventilator circuit, proper functioning of cardiovascular support equipment, and any other apparatus which could lead to sudden haemodynamic change, such as profound volume loss or air embolism from high-flow perfusion systems. Although many instances of cardiac arrest reflect myocardial instability, often exaggerated by disturbances of body chemistry, temperature or cardiac instrumentation, the most common 'unexpected' events are disorders of ventilation such as respiratory obstruction or hypoxaemia after endotracheal suction or physiotherapy. Tension pneumothorax, abrupt hypovolaemia, cardiac tamponade, pulmonary embolism and coning of the medulla or midbrain are less common.

Restoring the heartbeat

The primary distinction between asystole and ventricular fibrillation is easy to make in the ICU because most patients are monitored continuously. Chronotropic agents such as adrenaline, (epinephrine), isoprenaline (isoproterenol) and occasionally atropine are the immediate choice to control asystole or extreme bradycardia, followed if necessary by electrical pacing. Ionised calcium salts have both inotropic and chronotropic properties and are powerfully stimulant when combined with adrenaline. Extreme stimulation predisposes to myocardial necrosis and so it is wiser, when possible, to maintain the heart rhythm electrically. Sometimes only ECG complexes can be restored with little or no evidence of any forward flow. Sustained cardiac massage may result in improvement but more often this pattern of electromechanical dissociation represents irretrievable myocardial damage. Insertion of pacing wires is also usually ineffective unless additional measures are available to improve pressure and flow. Intra-

thoracic catastrophes such as intrapericardial haemorrhage are more likely to result in asystole than ventricular fibrillation, and resuscitation should not be abandoned without consideration of such possibilities. Emergency thoracotomy and internal cardiac massage are appropriate occasionally and more likely to be followed by success in the ICU where facilities are readily available. However, careful thought should be given to the likely diagnosis and prognosis for each individual before inappropriate and distasteful measures are implemented.

Ventricular fibrillation is treated by external DC defibrillation using the smallest effective shock. High energy defibrillation (200–400 Joules) leads ultimately to a degree of myocardial damage as well as mild skin burns. Antidysrhythmic drug therapy (see Chapter 22) is usually initiated or modified simultaneously, and repeated drug adjustments and repetitive defibrillation may be necessary before a stable rhythm is maintained. Efforts should be made to restore sinus rhythm if this was present before the arrest because loss of atrial systole lowers cardiac output, and this cannot always be tolerated by the acutely ill. During this period of repeated defibrillation and adjustment to drug therapy, cardiac massage should be continued to ensure that flow is maintained to essential tissues. Serial biochemical measurements are needed to adjust chemical variables such as pH and plasma potassium, and sodium bicarbonate is likely to be needed when the arrest is prolonged, even if massage and ventilation were initiated efficiently from the onset. (Fig. 21.1, provides a guide to bicarbonate therapy.)

Aids to calculations in bicarbonate therapy

- A guide to the requirements for bicarbonate to correct acidosis is provided by the measured base excess. The base excess is the number of millimoles of acid or base required to titrate a litre of blood to pH 7.40 at 37 C *while* the P_{aCO_2} is 5.3 kPa (or 40 mmHg); the normal being 0 ± 2.0.
- As the base excess is only affected by non-volatile acids it is a true reflection of the non-respiratory component of an acid-base disturbance.
- The theoretical dose of sodium bicarbonate required to correct acidosis is indicated by the relationship:

$$mmoles\ NaHCO_3 = 0.3 * (body\ weight\ in\ kg) * (base\ excess)$$

- In usual clinical practice, partial correction is attempted with half of the above calculated dose followed by re-evaluation.

Fig. 21.1 Aids to calculations in bicarbonate therapy.

Management after cardiac arrest

No specific measures are required if a transitory rhythm disturbance has been treated by prompt and effective defibrillation, and satisfactory drug therapy to prevent further dysrhythmias has been established. Patients surviving a protracted period of cardiac arrest and resuscitation are likely to need additional treatment to correct new abnormalities, particularly lung injury caused by the inhalation of gastric contents and global ischaemic/hypoxic brain damage. New myocardial damage is possible, induced in part by ischaemia but also by the trauma of cardiac massage or defibrillation, and renal failure is another common sequel of prolonged hypotension. Hepatic and gastrointestinal function often deteriorate too and there is often an increase in serum amylase suggesting pancreatic damage. Hyperglycaemia, hypothermia, acidosis and hyperkalaemia are almost invariable, but are likely to resolve without further treatment provided a satisfactory circulation has been restored.

Management at this stage is influenced by the antecedent pathology, the duration of the arrest, the extent to which new abnormalities are known to have developed — for example, aspiration of gastric contents or the onset of oliguria — and whether or not the haemodynamic status after the arrest is good or parlous. Decisions are likely to be needed in sequence:

1 Is further haemodynamic investigation or treatment necessary?
2 Can spontaneous ventilation be sustained?
3 Can the endotracheal tube be removed if only recently inserted?
4 Are specific measures indicated to treat or prevent complications?

The investigation and management of the failing circulation are considered in more detail on p. 417, and the role of mechanical ventilation in general is described on p. 428. In the specific circumstances of management immediately after cardiac arrest, it is worth noting that the effects of inhaling gastric acid are usually delayed and, if there is any suspicion that aspiration has occured, it is wiser to leave the endotracheal tube in place and continue mechanical ventilation, with sedation if necessary, until it is clear that there is no bronchospasm or progressive hypoxaemia.

Treatment to limit cerebral damage after cardiac arrest is contentious. A number of measures have been advocated, in particular, hypothermia [1, 2] barbiturate coma [3], hyperventilation, and the administration of calcium channel blocking agents [4] or anticonvulsants [5]. Benefit is far easier to demonstrate when treatments are initiated before the ischaemic insult and this alone is likely to limit their role in the management of patients after cardiac arrest.

Haemodynamic side-effects such as hypotension with barbiturates or alkalaemia and hypokalaemia following hyperventilation also curtail their application in these circumstances. Corticosteroids are prescribed most often but there is no evidence that they are of benefit. Their tendency to create or perpetuate hyperglycaemia is almost certainly disadvantageous because the availability of substrate allows the ischaemic brain to continue metabolising anaerobically, so enhancing intracellular acidosis and worsening cerebral damage. Monitoring intracranial pressure improves the outcome of patients with head injury but it is doubtful if comparable benefit can be expected in those suffering an ischaemic insult because the brain is non-compliant rather than exposed to a raised intracranial pressure. If in doubt whether cerebral function is intact after resuscitation from cardiac arrest, it is wise to continue mechanical ventilation to ensure perfect oxygenation and control of the airway. The combination of a head-up tilt and well-maintained systemic blood pressure promotes good cerebral perfusion. Cerebral function should be reassessed at frequent intervals and behavioural patterns at this stage often provide a helpful clue to long-term prognosis. Table 21.1 summarises the features that differentiated patients with the worst prognosis from those most likely to recover following severe ischaemic/hypoxic injury in a large study by Levy et al. [6].

Developments in cardiopulmonary resuscitation

The conventional management of cardiac arrest consists of sternal compression 60–80 times per minute, interrupted briefly while the lungs are inflated. The technique described as 'new' cardiopulmonary resuscitation involves sternal compression for 60% of each cardiac cycle, combined with simultaneous artificial ventilation at an airway pressure of 60–110 cmH$_2$O which is sustained throughout the period of sternal compresion. Systemic blood flow

Table 21.1 Rules that identify patients with good or bad prognosis.

Time post arrest	Clinical sign
Patients with virtually no chance of regaining independence	
Initial examination	No pupillary light reflex
1 day	Motor response no better than flexor and spontaneous eye movements neither orienting nor roving conjugate
3 days	Motor response no better than flexor
1 week	Motor response — not obeying commands and initial spontaneous eye movements neither orienting nor roving conjugate *and* 3-day eye opening *not* spontaneous
Patients with best chance of regaining independence	
Initial examination	Pupillary light reflexes present *and* motor response flexor or extensor *but with* spontaneous eye movements roving conjugate or orienting
1 day	Motor response withdrawal or better and eye opening improved at least two grades
3 days	Motor response withdrawal or better and spontaneous eye movements normal
1 week	Motor response obeying commands
2 weeks	Oculocephalic response normal

and pressure are greater than with the conventional method but new cardiopulmonary resuscitation is more difficult to apply effectively without additional mechanical aids, is associated with a greater risk of visceral damage, and has not been implemented widely. The observed increase in central venous pressure may actually reduce the effective cerebral perfusion pressure [7].

Management in the early postarrest period has also been refined. Enthusiasm for the routine administration of sodium bicarbonate to correct metabolic acidosis has been superceded by the realisation that there are a number of disadvantageous side-effects. These include (1) the volume, osmolar and electrolyte load which are poorly tolerated in the presence of cardiac or renal disease, (2) the production of carbon dioxide in excess of normal metabolism, which requires an increase in alveolar ventilation if homeostasis is to be maintained, and (3) the tendency to develop an intracellular acidosis because carbon dioxide diffuses freely through cell membranes. It remains appropriate to correct the metabolic acidosis of cardiac arrest if resuscitation proves ineffective without, but treatment should be restricted to correc-

tion of the base deficit in the presumptive blood volume in the first instance, with subsequent doses of bicarbonate only if necessary. The mild to moderate acidosis which is apparent after a brief and easily treated cardiac arrest is best left alone: its resolution is a good index of the return of tissue perfusion and normal metabolic activity.

Recognition of the importance of ionised calcium in the regulation of cellular activity, particularly within the myocardium and brain, has led to a reappraisal of the value of calcium salts in the management of cardiac arrest [8]. Bolus injections of calcium salts have been advocated traditionally to restore a coordinated heart beat in patients with asystole, or improve myocardial tone in those with ventricular fibrillation as a prelude to successful defibrillation. Although powerfully inotropic, there is a possibility that this practice increases the chance of myocardial or cerebral injury, and current evidence suggests that early administration of calcium channel blocking agents may provide protection. Until this uncertainty has been resolved, it is probably wise to avoid the use of calcium salts unless other measures have failed.

MANAGEMENT OF THE FAILING CIRCULATION

Assessment and investigations

'Shock' can be defined as failure of the function of vital organs as a result of inadequate perfusion. The common causes are hypovolaemia, myocardial failure, and abnormalities of vascular tone which can include the microcirculation as well as arteries and arterioles. Abnormalities of cellular function ultimately occur in all forms of shock but are apparent much earlier in some circumstances than others, e.g. septicaemia.

The cardinal symptoms and signs are well known: anxiety and restlessness, faintness, pallor and sweating, clouding of consciousness merging into coma and oliguria or anuria. There is systemic hypotension, the heart rate is usually rapid with a pulse of small volume, and the peripheral tissues are cool and often mottled. 'Warm shock' is the term used to describe hypotension associated with vasodilatation and peripheral pulses of good volume.

The simplest haemodynamic indices of severity are systemic arterial pressure, heart rate and the temperature gradient between the peripheral and central tissues (e.g. toe and rectum). End-organ function can be assessed most easily by observation of mental status, the state of the skin, and regular recording of urinary output, preferably with an indwelling catheter. All these measurements can be made with simple apparatus and are virtually non-invasive, but the information available is limited and gives no indication of cause. Even if the aetiology is apparent, e.g. hypovolaemia following trauma in a previously healthy young adult, management of fluid replacement is carried out most accurately if venous filling is monitored by measurements of right atrial (central venous) pressure. If the diagnosis is in doubt, if myocardial, pericardial or pulmonary vascular abnormalities are suspected, and when circulatory failure is so extreme and refractory that each variable has only limited tolerance, more invasive measures are justified so that the filling pressure of both sides of the heart can be followed and changes in cardiac output can be documented. This also allows calculation of other indices of circulatory performance such as systemic and pulmonary vascular resistance, right and left ventricular stroke work, and the relationship between cardiac filling and cardiac performance (see Figs 21.2 and 21.3, and Table 21.2 for a summary of derived cardiovascular indices). This analysis means that there is a progressive spectrum of investigation from simple bedside observations to complex intracardiac manipulation. There is a frequent requirement for invasive monitoring in patients admitted to the intensive care unit but it is not an inevitable necessity, and common sense is needed to select appropriate measures for each patient.

Sphygmomanometry is unsatisfactory as a means of recording arterial pressure when the peripheral pulses are weak and the circulation prone to rapid change. Automated systems which detect peripheral pulses have the advantage of frequent measurement without manual intervention, but most unstable patients are best monitored with an indwelling arterial cannula. This provides beat-to-beat display of the magnitude and waveform of the arterial pulse and permits easy blood sampling, primarily to measure arterial blood gas tensions and pH. The incidence of complications after cannulation of the radial artery with a small (20 or 22 gauge), parallel-sided cannula is low [9]. The dorsalis pedis is an

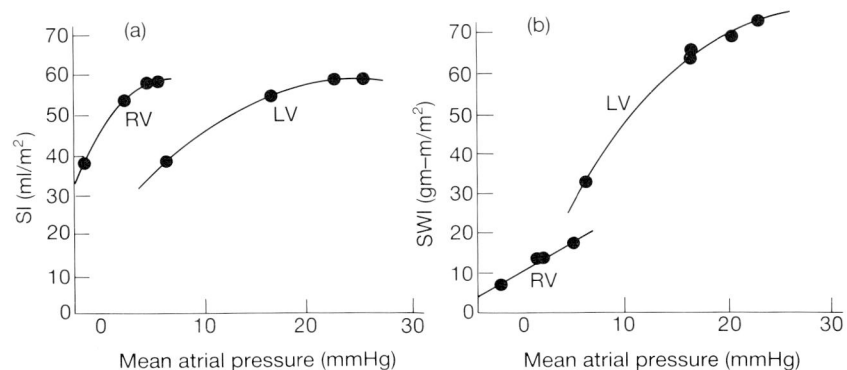

Fig. 21.2 Ventricular function curves for the two sides of the heart. The relation between (a) stroke index (SI) or (b) stroke work index (SWI) and mean atrial pressure in a patient aged 20 suffering from acute glomerulonephritis. Pressure measurements were referred to zero at the sternal angle. RV, right ventricle; LV, left ventricle. (Reproduced from Bradley *et al.* *Cardiovasc Res* 1971;**5**:223, with kind permission of the Editor.)

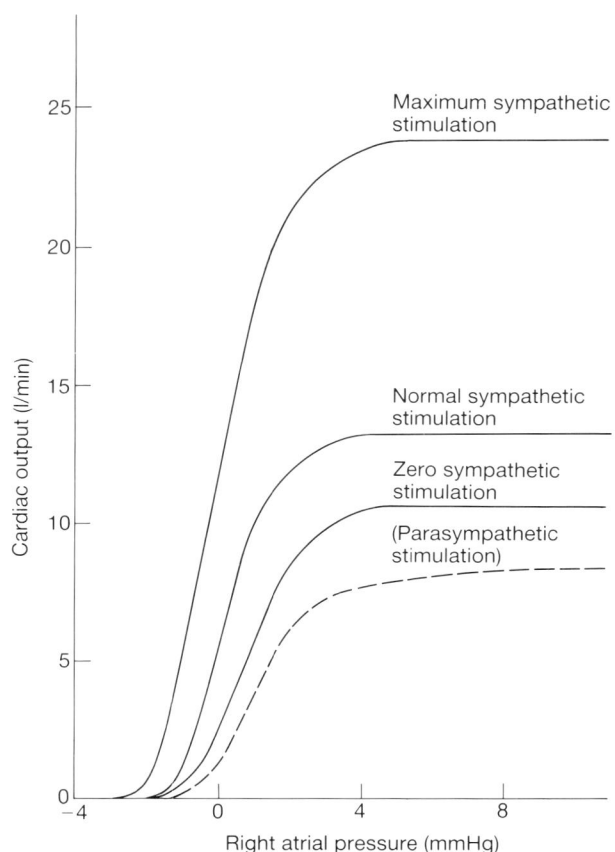

Fig. 21.3 A series of ventricular function curves representing the effects of autonomic stimulation on the heart. (Reproduced from Guyton *et al. Circulatory physiology: cardiac output and its relations.* 1973, with kind permission of WB Saunders)

alternative arterial cannulation site but, even more than the radial artery, may give misleadingly low values for systemic pressure in patients who are vasoconstricted. Cannulation of more proximal vessels (brachial or femoral) is acceptible in the short term but involves a greater risk of distal ischaemia.

Insertion of a central venous catheter is mandatory in a high proportion of patients and only contra-indicated in exceptional circumstances such as gross defects of coagulation. This route of intravenous access provides a reliable means of infusing drugs which are often needed on a continuous basis, and solutions too irritant or hypertonic for administration through peripheral veins. Central venous pressure can be measured too, allowing interpretation of the ease and adequacy of cardiac filling. The internal (occasionally external) jugular and the subclavian veins are the usual routes for central venous access

and either direct cannulation or the Seldinger technique can be used. The right internal jugular vein is probably the most suitable first choice, being easy to locate, in direct line with the superior vena cava and right atrium, and cannulation is associated with a low incidence of complications. Central venous access through the subclavian veins is associated with a much higher incidence of pneumothorax, even in experienced hands, but in practice it is often necessary to use multiple sites in turn. All central venous lines should be inserted with strict attention to sterility because patients requiring intensive care are particularly susceptible to infection and there is a notable incidence of catheter-related sepsis, especially when parenteral nutrients are infused. A subcutaneous tunnel can be fashioned to separate the sites of skin penetration and vascular access and there is some evidence [10] that this decreases the risk of infection. Another useful development has been the introduction of catheters with multiple lumina, which means that separate channels, each 16 or 18 gauge, can be used for vasoactive drug infusions, parenteral nutrition and pressure monitoring.

Catheterisation of the pulmonary artery is necessary if more detailed information about cardiac function and filling is required. A balloon-tipped, flow-guided catheter is chosen most often, sometimes combined with additional channels for on-line oximetry, ventricular pacing or, most commonly, measurement of cardiac output by thermal dilution. The catheter is often surrounded by a sterile sleeve so that it can be manipulated without contamination and it is best inserted through a valved introducer sheath, 1F size larger, usually placed in the right internal jugular or left subclavian vein. Insertion through a cut-down in a peripheral vein is less satisfactory because the valved sheath cannot be used, so preventing subsequent manipulation. A head-down tilt is needed in most patients to minimise the risk of air embolism while the valved sheath is being introduced, but is no longer necessary once the sheath is in place and has been filled with saline. Time in the head-down position should be minimised for conscious patients who find it uncomfortable, and for those with dyspnoea or pulmonary venous engorgement.

The valved sheath, usually 8 or 8.5F, is introduced under local anaesthesia using the Seldinger technique, proceeding from a 22 g 'seeker' venepuncture

Table 21.2 Haemodynamic variables and derived indices.

Variable	Symbol	Formula	Units
Cardiac index	CI	CO/SA	l/min/m^2
Stroke volume	SV	1000*CO/HR	ml
Stroke index	SI	SV/SA	ml/m^2
Systemic vascular resistance	SVR	(MAP − CVP)/CO	Wood units
Pulmonary vascular resistance	PVR	(PAP − LAP)/CO	Wood units
Left ventricular stroke work index	LVSWI	(MAP − LAP)*SI*0.0136	g m/m^2/beat
Right ventricular stroke work index	RVSWI	(PAP − CVP)*SI*0.0136	g m/m^2/beat

Key:
CO = cardiac output (l/min).
SA = surface area (m^2).
HR = heart rate (beats/min).
MAP = mean arterial pressure (mmHg).
PAP = mean pulmonary arterial pressure (mmHg).
LAP = mean left atrial pressure, mmHg (or substitute pulmonary artery 'wedge' pressure or pulmonary arterial diastolic pressure).
CVP = central venous pressure (mmHg) or right atrial pressure.
Note: all vascular pressures referenced to the same point — mid left atrium.

to a thin-walled 18 g needle or 16 g cannula. A double-ended guide wire with a J-tip at one end and a soft, straight tip at the other is useful to ensure easy, unobstructed passage for the wire well beyond the end of the needle or cannula, which is then removed. Next, the vessel dilator is passed through the valve and sheath and threaded over the wire. A small incision is made to open the skin around the wire and, with the guide wire held firmly in place, the dilator and sheath are advanced over it into the vessel. It is important not to let the guide wire advance too because it could perforate the vessel wall [11]. Once the sheath is fully into the vessel, the wire and dilator are discarded and the sheath flushed with saline through the side-channel. The site is then redraped before the pulmonary arterial catheter is inserted.

The balloon is inflated to ensure it fills concentrically and each vascular lumen is flushed with saline.

The distal lumen is used to monitor pressure while the catheter is inserted. The balloon is kept deflated until the catheter tip is beyond the end of the sheath (usually about 20 cm) and then inflated because the balloon is less likely than the unprotected tip to provoke rhythm disturbances during passage through the right ventricle and the outflow tract. The location of the tip is apparent from the dynamic pressure recorded through the distal lumen (Fig. 21.4), and it is usually easy to advance the catheter into the pulmonary artery without any special manipulation. Likely causes of occasional difficulty are severe tricuspid regurgitation, or extreme dilatation of the right atrium or ventricle. Coiling of the catheter in the right ventricle should be avoided to prevent the tip looping through the coil, and it should be withdrawn if the pulmonary artery has not been reached when the outer end has been advanced another 10−15 cm after the right ventricle

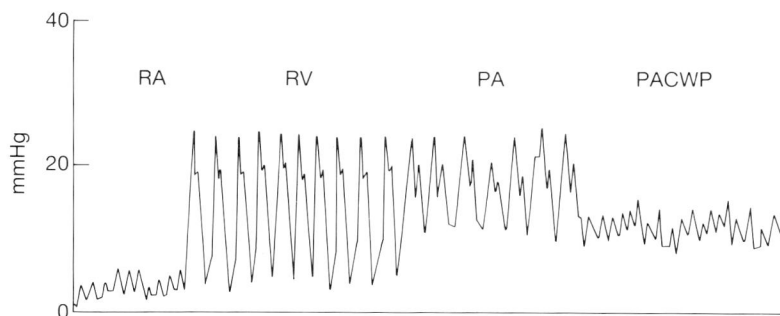

Fig. 21.4 Pressure tracing recorded through a Swan−Ganz catheter traversing the right atrium (RA), right ventricle (RV) and pulmonary artery (PA). The wedge pressure (PACWP) was recorded after the balloon had been inflated.

has been entered. If the catheter with its balloon still inflated is inserted a further 10 cm or so beyond the pulmonary valve, it usually wedges in a branch of the artery and the pulmonary arterial waveform is replaced by that derived indirectly from the left atrium. The balloon should be deflated at this point and the catheter withdrawn a centimetre or two, so that flow in the vessel is not interrupted for more than a few minutes. Provided this sequence is followed, it is unlikely that forward migration of the tip of the catheter after its insertion can lead to unintentional wedging. The catheter can be advanced within its sterile sleeve once more to reach the wedge position and the balloon can be reflated for a few moments when measurements of indirect left atrial pressure are required. There is a close correlation between the end-diastolic pressure in the pulmonary artery and left atrial pressure in patients with a low pulmonary vascular resistance and, once this criterion has been confirmed, it is unnecessary to move the catheter or reflate the balloon at all, but merely display the pulmonary arterial pressure continuously.

Use of balloon-tipped pulmonary arterial catheters can result in pulmonary haemorrhage or infarction and is associated with a definite morbidity and mortality (Table 21.3). The most important requirements for safety are careful and accurate placement of the sheath, insertion of the catheter with the balloon inflated but withdrawal only with the balloon deflated, and avoidance of unintentional wedging with the tip occluding a branch of the pulmonary artery. Presence of abnormally high v waves in the indirect left atrial trace can be confused with the pulmonary arterial waveform and care must be taken

Table 21.3 Causes of morbidity and mortality associated with the use of pulmonary arterial catheters.

Related to insertion:
Trauma (as for all central vascular access)
Air embolism (large valved sheath)
Coiling, kinking, knotting of catheter
Arrhythmia

Related to continued presence:
Infection
Thromboembolism
Pulmonary infarction
Balloon rupture

Related to information gained:
Mesmerism
Misinterpretation

to avoid advancing the catheter even further, or inflating the balloon if the tip is already in the wedged position. Even if these specific hazards are avoided, there is a higher incidence of pulmonary haemorrhage associated with balloon-tipped pulmonary arterial catheterisation in patients with left atrial hypertension and organic mitral incompetence [12]. Pulmonary arterial catheters should not be left in place any longer than necessary and, ideally should be resited if required for more than 36 hours to minimise the risk of infection or thrombosis.

A single-lumen pulmonary arterial catheter permits measurements of pulmonary vascular pressures and intermittent sampling of mixed venous blood. Addition of a separate right atrial lumen and a thermistor near the tip of the distal lumen is the most common modification, allowing measurement of cardiac output by thermal dilution. If a thermistor with a fast response time is used (50 msec), changes in temperature can be followed on a beat to beat basis and can be used to estimate right ventricular ejection fraction with an accuracy comparable to techniques of nuclear cardiology [13]. The frequency with which right ventricular pathology contributes to cardiorespiratory impairment, particularly in patients requiring mechanical ventilation with a sustained, high intrathoracic pressure, emphasises the desirability of investigating both sides of the heart, rather than confining attention solely to left ventricular performance [14]. Computing technology is often used to collate haemodynamic and respiratory data from patients requiring intensive care and, although unnecessary for safe clinical management of the individual, this approach has provided guidelines on pathophysiology, prognosis and the objectives of treatment [15].

A number of other methods of assessment are useful in specific circumstances. Echocardiography is particularly valuable because mobile apparatus can be brought to the bedside and information can be gained quickly. The diagnosis of pericardial effusion, valve defects, unexpected shunts, intracardiac tumours or myocardial dysfunction is often easy but occasional misleading findings are encountered, particularly in patients with a very low cardiac output. The availability of an image intensifier assists placement of the 'difficult' pulmonary arterial catheter or pacing wire and can be used for limited angiographic investigations. Apparatus is available less widely for the detection of myocardial ischaemia using the techniques of nuclear medicine or the measurement of extravascular lung water and pulmonary capillary permeability, but the determination of mechanical and ventilatory indices of pulmonary function is an integral feature of investigation in virtually all patients. Cardiovascular and respiratory pathophysiology are so intimately connected in the acutely ill that it is rarely possible to make a comprehensive diagnosis or initiate a satisfactory treatment policy without considering both systems.

Interpretation of haemodynamic variables

There are two quite separate features which require consideration. One is the nature of the haemodynamic disturbance, the other a need to diagnose the aetiology of the pathophysiological changes which have been identified. Treatment is usually required both to remedy the cause and alleviate the consequences; one without the other is only likely to succeed if the disturbance is minor and self-limiting. The differential diagnosis of the causes of circulatory collapse is beyond the scope of this chapter, the rest of which is confined to consideration of consequences.

It is convenient to divide circulatory disorders into two broad categories, those in which the filling pressure of one or both sides of the heart is elevated, and those in which the converse is true. Right atrial or central venous pressure is a reflection of blood volume, vascular tone (particularly venous tone) and the compliance of the right heart. The pressure at this site is elevated if the blood volume is increased beyond the limits of venous capacitance or the right heart fails to fill easily because of right ventricular failure, tricuspid valve disease or the constraint of a tight pericardium. Right ventricular failure in turn may be an isolated phenomenon or, more commonly, reflects acute or chronic pulmonary vascular disease or the 'back-pressure' effects of left atrial hypertension. Some indication of the diagnosis can be obtained by considering the shape of the right atrial and pulmonary arterial waveforms.

The usual configuration of the right atrial waveform is depicted in Fig. 21.5, and the sustained atrial hypertension and systolic descent (x descent) of a pericardial effusion is contrasted with the postsystolic (y) of constrictive pericarditis in Fig. 21.6. Tricuspid incompetence results in a prominent systolic v wave in the atrial pressure and, if it coexists with a pericar-

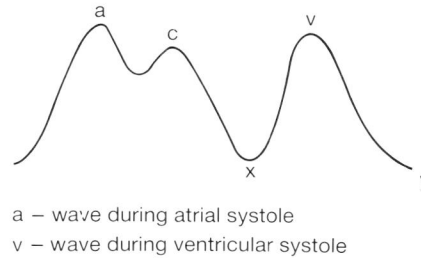

a – wave during atrial systole
v – wave during ventricular systole

Fig. 21.5 Right atrial pressure waveform.

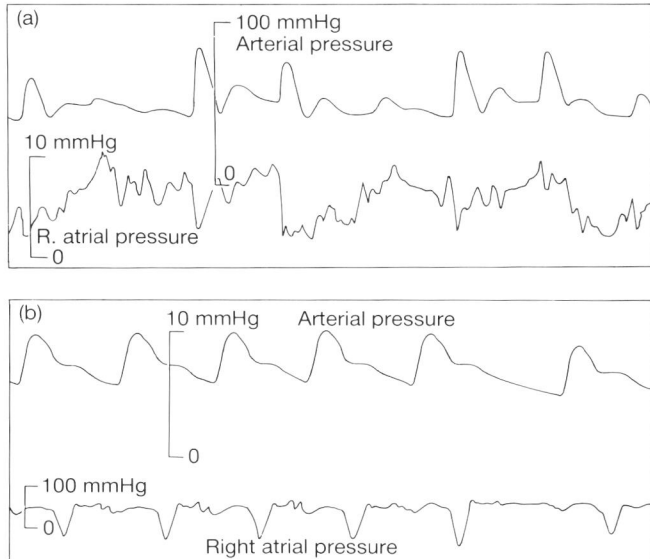

Fig. 21.6 (a) Cardiac tamponade in a male aged 28 years. Systolic descent in the right atrial pressure; pulsus paradoxus is apparent in the arterial blood pressure. The pressure measurements are referred to zero at the sternal angle. (b) Constrictive pericarditis in a male aged 36 years. Postsystolic descent in the right atrial pressure. The pressure measurements are referred to zero at the sternal angle.

dial effusion, both disorders may be missed unless additional investigations are undertaken.

The shape of the pulmonary arterial waveform is also informative, but requires a system with an adequate frequency response. The normal pressure profile is of a fairly sharp systolic upstroke followed by an almost linear fall, interrupted only by a dicrotic notch (Fig. 21.7). A high pulmonary vascular resistance, caused either by obstruction (e.g. pulmonary emboli) or vascular obliteration or spasm (e.g. chronic lung disease), is manifest as an elevated systolic pressure followed by a rapid fall which gives a concave outline to the diastolic phase of the waveform,

Low PVR

Normal

High PVR

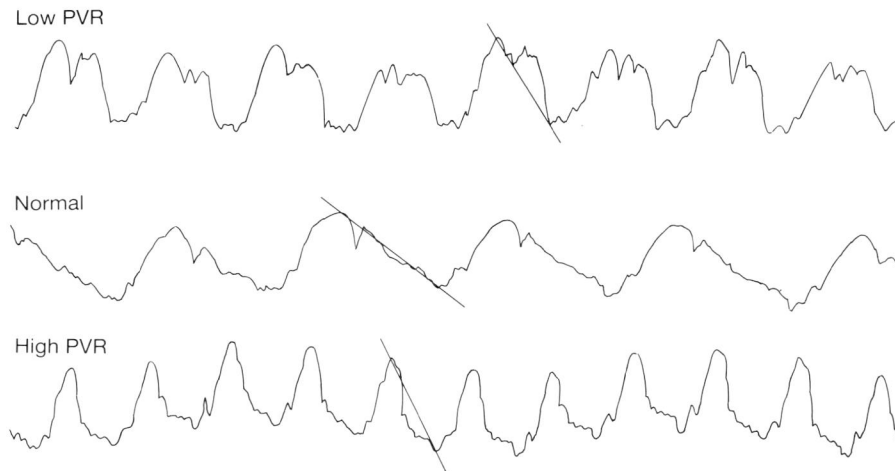

Fig. 21.7 Pulmonary arterial waveforms. For explanation see text.

often with the dicrotic notch barely apparent. Conversely the pulmonary arterial waveform in patients with pulmonary vascular engorgement and left atrial hypertension contains a far larger area under the curve, the dicrotic notch is usually obvious and is followed by a prominent postdicrotic accentuation of pressure which is believed to represent the retrograde transmission of the left atrial v wave. This accentuated postdicrotic wave is also seen when mitral incompetence is only a functional reflection of left ventricular failure.

The magnitude of pulmonary arterial pressure can provide an indication of chronicity because the previously healthy right ventricle can rarely achieve a systolic pressure above approximately 45 mmHg, whereas far higher pressures result when chronic disease is followed by ventricular hypertrophy. This observation should be interpreted with caution however because the pulmonary arterial pressure falls as the cardiac output drops, and a measurement of pulmonary vascular resistance is necessary to confirm the conclusion. Calculation of pulmonary vascular resistance requires a knowledge of mean pulmonary arterial and left atrial pressures as well as cardiac output and it can be difficult to obtain a reliable reading of indirect left atrial pressure from the wedged position of a pulmonary arterial catheter when the resistance of the pulmonary circulation is increased. Indirect left atrial pressure measurements must also be interpreted with caution when high levels of end-expiratory pressure are used during mechanical ventilation. Positive end-expiratory pressure (PEEP) of up to 5 cmH$_2$O is unlikely to

cause confusion, but values above 10 cmH$_2$O will increase the apparent magnitude of the left atrial pressure relative to atmosphere to a degree which depends on the compliance of the lungs. Some authors recommend that PEEP should be withdrawn while haemodynamic measurements are made, but this leads to very rapid changes in the pulmonary circulation which can invalidate the findings, and allows a degree of lung deflation which is usually detrimental and cannot be reversed immediately when PEEP is re-applied. Common sense is usually sufficient to allow adequate interpretation for clinical purposes but direct measurements of intrathoracic pressure are necessary if derived haemodynamic variables are to be calculated with complete accuracy.

Haemodynamic interpretation when the venous pressures are low is usually far easier. The common cause, hypovolaemia, is simple to correct. The only difficulty encountered if volume loss is the sole antecedent event is to recognise the need for ongoing transfusion after the filling pressures have been restored, when the systemic vascular bed dilates as compensatory vasoconstriction wanes. 'Relative hypovolaemia' in which a normal blood volume is inadequate to fill a pathologically dilated vascular bed is more difficult to manage and is seen most often in the sepsis syndrome — circulatory impairment associated with an increased or decreased temperature and white cell count, an identified source of bacterial pathogens or toxins, with or without a positive blood culture. Abnormal vascular permeability as well as abnormal tone is a feature of the condition, and a protein-rich exudate forms around the capillaries of both the systemic and pulmonary vascular beds. The cardiac output is often normal or high, provided filling pressures are maintained, but continued transfusion far in excess of any measured loss leads ultimately to life-threatening pulmonary oedema, often without any increase in left atrial pressure. This therapeutic dilemma is best resolved by the use of pressor agents (discussed later), to increase vascular tone, especially within the systemic veins, so maintaining cardiac filling without overloading the circulation.

The other hazard associated with the correction of hypovolaemia is the presence of marked asymmetry between the performance of the right and left ventricles. The normal relationship between left and right atrial pressure is lost when there is significant ventricular pathology, and the left atrial pressure is often elevated when that on the right is normal or low (Fig. 21.8). Rapid change in the left atrial pressure is common if left ventricular ischaemia is the cause of myocardial dysfunction, and only a modest increase in blood volume, insufficient to alter the right atrial pressure by more than 1 mmHg or so, may suffice to distend the left ventricle and raise the left atrial pressure to levels at which pulmonary oedema results. This underlines the need to monitor the filling pressures on both sides of the heart if serious myocardial dysfunction is suspected in a patient deemed to require transfusion. Once again the effects of respiratory therapy cannot be ignored. Patients with severe pulmonary oedema from any cause — haemodynamic or associated with an increase in pulmonary capillary permeability — require high inflation pressures to secure effective gas exchange during intermittent positive pressure ventilation (IPPV). PEEP is often used as well to increase lung volume and improve arterial oxygenation. Right ventricular integrity is already threatened by the increased pulmonary vascular pressures

associated with pulmonary oedema, and the distortion of the ventricular cavity with marked septal displacement can be demonstrated when high intrathoracic pressures are used as well. This in turn affects both left ventricular filling and performance and it is in these complex circumstances that detailed haemodynamic monitoring has most to offer.

Treatment of the failing circulation

The need to establish an aetiological diagnosis has been mentioned already and specific treatment must be initiated at the same time as attempts are made to correct the haemodynamic disturbance.

The extent to which manipulation of the blood volume can remedy circulatory failure has been outlined in the preceding section. Control of the blood volume combined with attention to non-specific variables such as arterial oxygenation, correction of electrolyte disorders and acid-base status, pain relief and the maintenance of normothermia is all that is required to correct many of the common causes of circulatory collapse. If such measures are unsuccessful, further thought should be given to the cause of the cardiovascular crisis and to the performance of the myocardium. If the signs of inadequate tissue perfusion persist when the filling pressures of the heart are within the normal range, then it is reasonable to assume some impairment of ventricular function. This can be primary, as after myocardial infarction, or secondary to associated pathology such as pulmonary embolism or pericardial effusion. Treatment can only be adjusted once this distinction has been made.

Primary myocardial failure, often ischaemic in origin, is the most common cause of 'cardiogenic shock'. It is mandatory to improve tissue perfusion, including that to the myocardium, but benefit is

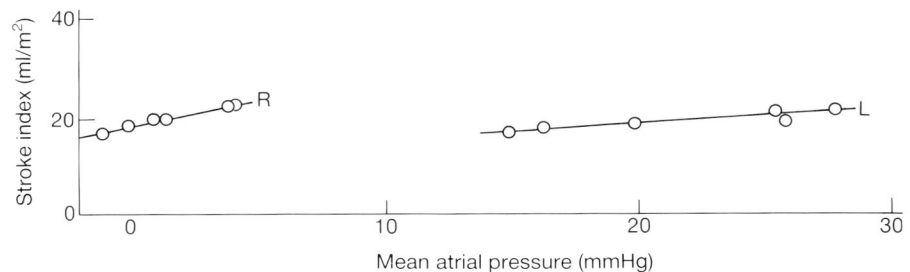

Fig. 21.8 Ventricular function curves recorded from a patient aged 56 years suffering from myocardial infarction.

likely to be transitory if the myocardial oxygen consumption is increased to an extent which outstrips supply. The magnitude of the afterload, heart rate, and the rate of shortening of ventricular muscle fibres govern myocardial oxygen consumption. Oxygen availability depends upon an adequate perfusion pressure (aortic diastolic minus left ventricular diastolic pressure), the duration of diastole, and the ease with which local vascular tone can be adjusted to regulate supply. This last property is eroded by coronary arterial disease, particularly in peripheral vessels, whereas proximal coronary arterial disease is of more importance when considering the head of pressure available to secure myocardial perfusion.

These considerations influence the choice of vasoactive drugs as well as recommendations for other therapy. If the patient is *in extremis* when all the measures described previously have been implemented, there is no alternative to the administration of a powerful inotropic agent such as adrenaline (epinephrine) which also constricts peripheral vessels and so increases the systemic pressure directly. Treatment is often limited by the development of undesirable hypertension, tachycardia or arrhythmia, and agents such as dobutamine or isoprenaline (isoproterenol) may be preferred. The similarities and differences between these agents are listed in Table 21.4 (see also Fig. 21.9).

A drug with predominantly vasopressor properties is chosen occasionally, particularly if there is evidence that a critical perfusion pressure is required for adequate function of the brain, kidneys or even myocardium. Noradrenaline (norepinephrine), metaraminol or phenylephrine can be considered in

Table 21.4 Dose ranges and clinical effects of some commonly used pressor agents.

Agent	Dose range (μ/kg/min)	Chron.	Ino.	Dil.	Constr.
Isoprenaline (isoproterenol)	0.01–0.1	+++	++	++	–
Adrenaline (epinephrine)	0.01–0.1	++	++	+	++
Noradrenaline (norepinephrine)	0.01–0.1	–	+	–	+++
Dopamine	1–20	++	++	++	+++
		(depending on dose used)			
Dobutamine	4–30	–	++	+	–
Salbutamol	0.15–0.4	++	+	++	–
Dopexamine	1–6	+++	?+	++	–

Key: Chron. = chronotropy; Ino. = inotropy; Dil. = vasodilatation; Constr. = vasoconstriction
Note: all doses suggested are meant as a guide only, the actual dose will depend on the individual circumstances.

this context and they are also of value, as an alternative to transfusion (qv), in patients with septicaemia. Raising the systemic arterial resistance in a patient with critical narrowing of one or more coronary arteries is obviously fraught with hazard, and this situation provides the cardinal indication for support by means of aortic counterpulsation, a technique described in more detail below.

Powerful inotropic and vasopressor agents are best avoided unless essential, not only to minimise myocardial oxygen consumption but also because the maintenance of systemic pressure does not guarantee

---

Aids to administered doses of infusion drugs

- Personal computer 'spreadsheet' programmes are eminently suitable for automatically producing a printed array of infusion rates against effective doses, matched for the individual patient's weight and the concentration of the drug solution.
- An alternative is to aim to produce a dilution of drug that results in numerical equivalence (or decimal relationship), between the infusion rate in ml/hour and the dose in mcg/kg/min. One such formula is:

      Drug quantity in mg = 6 * kg (body weight)   (e.g. 6*60 = 360mg)
      made up to   100 ml in appropriate vehicle (e.g. dextrose 5%)
      Then — 5 ml/hour = 5 mcg/kg/min etc

Fig. 21.9 Aids to administered doses of infusion drugs.

appropriate distribution of the cardiac output to essential organs. Renal failure in particular is likely to follow prolonged infusion of vasopressor agents. The susceptibility of the renal vasculature to vasoconstriction and the possibility that coincident mesenteric ischaemia results in the release of a 'myocardial depressant factor', has led to enthusiasm for drugs which influence dopaminergic receptors in the renal cortex and gut to cause selective vasodilatation in these tissue beds. Dopamine in low doses $(2.5-5.0\,\mu g/kg/min)$ is almost exclusively dopaminergic in action whereas higher doses increase myocardial contractility initially and thereafter result in both pulmonary and systemic arterial constriction. Dopexamine may prove a useful alternative because it lacks alpha-adrenergic effects, even at high doses [16].

Drugs which lower vascular tone have assumed increasing importance in recent years, particularly as the need to limit unnecessary myocardial work has been appreciated. The performance of the failing myocardium is influenced far more by changes in afterload than preload. (Fig. 21.10). The normal circulation responds to a reduction in afterload with little or no change in cardiac output but a diminution in contractility. The failing myocardium responds to a reduction in afterload with an increase in cardiac output which is often more than sufficient to offset any fall in systemic perfusion pressure and so does not compromise coronary blood flow. Furthermore, a reduction in preload will diminish intraventricular distension, lower the intraventricular pressure during diastole and so enhance myocardial perfusion.

Drugs which lower vascular tone are useful if the cardiac output is poor and vascular tone high, or if there is pulmonary and systemic venous engorgement with a high venous tone. Infusions of sodium nitroprusside or glyceryl trinitrate are the agents chosen most often to lower vascular resistance, both acting directly but the former primarily on arterial and the latter on venous tone. Other vasodilator drugs are listed in Table 21.5, together with an indication of their mode of action, properties and side-effects. Benefit is often apparent immediately but is not achieved in every case, for example if vasodilatation in healthy vessels deflects blood away from rigid thickened vessels which cannot dilate (the phenomenon of 'vascular steal').

Drug combinations are sometimes helpful, the properties sought being modest inotropic stimulation without any increase in heart rate or propensity to dysrhythmias. The combination of a vasodilator with a diuretic may be sufficient to alleviate pulmonary oedema, especially if the blood volume is greater than normal as a result of chronic fluid retention or inappropriate transfusion. If hypoxaemia or the paucity of renal perfusion render the patient oliguric or anuric, haemofiltration is an effective means of fluid removal. Cannulation of one femoral artery and vein provides a suitable route between patient and filter, and either the systemic pressure or an external pump can be used to maintain flow through it.

There are no drugs at present which selectively lower the pulmonary vascular resistance, and reducing right ventricular afterload in patients with severe pulmonary vascular disease is difficult without lowering the systemic vascular resistance to an unacceptable degree at the same time. Simultaneous infusion of prostacyclin into the pulmonary artery and noradrenaline (norepinephrine) into the left atrium is attractive theoretically, albeit associated with the hazard of systemic embolism. An alternative approach relies on the differing density of vasoactive

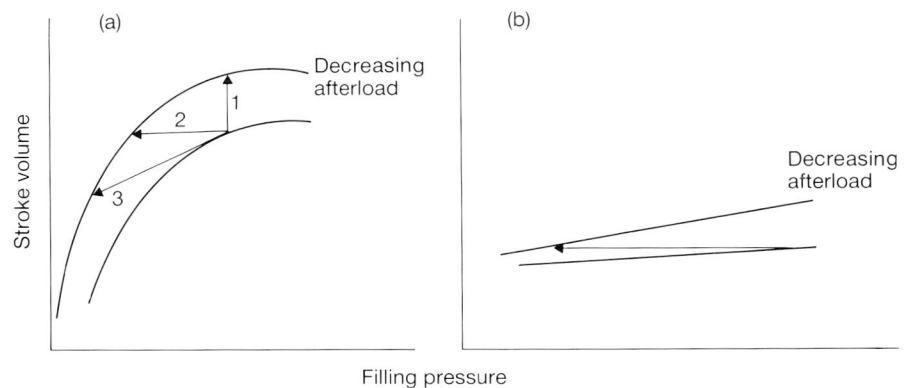

Fig. 21.10 The effect on stroke volume of reducing afterload: (a) when the heart is relatively normal — (1) filling pressure unchanged; (2) moderate fall in filling pressure; (3) profound fall in filling pressure; (b) when heart failure is severe. (Reproduced from Scallan et al. Br J Anaesth 1979;51:649, with kind permission of Macmillan Journals)

Table 21.5 The action and uses of four commonly used vasodilators.

Vasodilator	Dosage	Action	Uses	Problems
Nitroglycerin	Infuse: 0.5– μg/kg/min (no limit) Bolus: 10–20 μg	Mainly venodilator	Reduction of preload (ventricular filling pressure) Treatment of perioperative hypertension Coronary vasodilator Pulmonary vasodilator	Adsorption to polyvinylchloride Risk of reducing cardiac output if filling pressures not elevated
Sodium nitroprusside	Infuse: 0.25–8 μg/kg/ min	Mixed dilator of arterioles and venules (mainly arteriolar)	Treatment of hypertension Reduction of afterload Pulmonary vasodilator	Preparation and toxicity of the agent Sudden hypotension Fall in arterial P_aO_2 Coronary steal?
Phentolamine	Bolus: 1–2.5 mg Duration of action 15–20 min	Mainly arteriolar action. Some increase in venous capacitance. Tachycardia as a reflex or direct β-agonist action	Control of hypertension Control of blood pressure on bypass	Tachycardia
Hydrallazine	Bolus: 5–10 mg Duration of action 10–80 min	Pure direct arteriolar action. No effect venous pressures. Reflex tachycardia	Control of severe vasoconstriction Treatment of postoperative hypertension	Long action after bolus dose Tachycardia

receptor sites in the pulmonary and systemic circulations so that the infusion of glyceryl trinitrate and noradrenaline simultaneously into the right atrium may prove successful.

Intra-aortic counterpulsation (IACP) using an inflatable balloon is intended to mimic some of the haemodynamic advantages which can be achieved with drug therapy. The balloon is inserted either percutaneously or by direct incision into the femoral artery and advanced to the proximal aorta. Systemic anticoagulation is necessary while it is in place. It is inflated with either helium or carbon dioxide in time with each cardiac cycle by triggering the device from the ECG. Both the volume to which the balloon is inflated, and the proportion of cardiac beats which trigger the cycle can be varied according to need. The timing of inflation is of paramount importance: inflated too soon during systole, the balloon offers an insuperable resistance to left ventricular ejection, albeit appearing to support the systolic pressure. Ideally it is inflated to coincide with the dicrotic notch on the systemic arterial waveform so that aortic pressure is sustained by the balloon during diastole, thus enhancing coronary blood flow. The balloon is deflated at the onset of the next ventricular systole,

the consequent reduction in aortic impedence favouring left ventricular ejection. These physiological considerations underline the importance of optimal timing of the cycle of pulsation, but also the harm that can result if synchronisation of balloon inflation with ventricular diastole is not achieved. Vascular damage at the time of insertion or distal ischaemia are other complications of aortic balloon counterpulsation, and the technique should not be employed without good reason. Temporary use of aortic counterpulsation is a means of supporting the circulation and preventing further injury while acute episodes of myocardial damage resolve, e.g. after infarction or postoperatively, and as a prelude to cardiac surgery in patients with unstable angina or an ischaemic ventricular septal defect. The technique is contraindicated if there is more than trivial aortic incompetence and is usually ineffective if the heart rhythm is unstable or the rate is very fast. Severe peripheral vascular disease is a relative contraindication, and only limited benefit can be expected in patients with irretrievable myocardial damage unless there is a prospect of early cardiac transplantation. In these circumstances, other mechanical devices to support the circulation may be preferred.

Although most attention has been given to regulating vascular tone in patients with cardiogenic shock, there are other conditions where similar principles apply. Sudden profound loss of sympathetic tone such as occurs after high spinal cord transection is an indication for vasopressor agents, and a similar situation exists when vasomotor collapse is the result of anaphylaxis. Conversely, vasodilator drugs acting primarily on the peripheral vessels may be of some use in patients with septicaemia if a high cardiac output persists when tissue perfusion is absent or inadequate because of obstruction within the microcirculation. Both salbutamol and dopamine have been used with some success, but neither is of proven benefit and current interest is focussed on opiate agonists and antagonists and prostaglandin derivatives. In spite of the many theoretical advantages, there is little evidence to support the use of large doses of corticosteroids. Table 21.6 provides a simple summary guide to selection of methods of circulatory support.

Table 21.6 Simple guide to the selection of an appropriate method of supporting the failing circulation.

1 *Cardiac output and blood pressure both very low*
  Inotrope: adrenaline (possibly dopamine or isoprenaline)
  If large doses of adrenaline are required, consider the intra-aortic balloon pump
  Once blood pressure rises start vasodilators

2 *Cardiac output and blood pressure low and coronary circulation regarded as critical*
  Aortic counterpulsation (+ inotropes adrenaline or dopamine)

3 *Cardiac output low; blood pressure normal or low; vasoconstriction and oliguria prominent*
  Combined inotrope + vasodilator: adrenaline or dopamine + nitroglycerin or sodium nitroprusside
  For similar effect in one drug consider salbutamol.

4 *Cardiac output low; blood pressures normal or high; venous pressure high*
  Vasodilator: nitroglycerin or sodium nitroprusside

5 *Cardiac output and blood pressure adequate; venous pressures dangerously high*
  Venodilator: nitroglycerin

6 *Cardiac output and blood pressure both normal or high*
  Hypertension prominent: vasodilator — sodium nitroprusside
  Blood pressure normal: myocardial ischaemia present — nitroglycerin: need to limit myocardial oxygen consumption — sodium nitroprusside or nitroglycerin

The cardiorespiratory interface

Dyspnoea is often a feature of shock from any cause and may reflect cerebral ischaemia as in profound hypovolaemia or impending death, or disordered pulmonary function as seen in pulmonary embolic disease or left ventricular failure. There is likely to be an increase in respiratory work in either case, often combined with a very considerable increase in metabolic demand which means that the respiratory muscles require a greater than normal proportion of the cardiac output and available oxygen supply.

If pulmonary function is deranged too, a higher than normal minute ventilation is necessary to achieve normocapnia, and full saturation of arterial blood is unlikely unless the inspired oxygen concentration is increased. Even a physiological intrapulmonary shunt of normal magnitude results in arterial hypoxaemia if the mixed venous blood is markedly desaturated because of a low cardiac output. Tissue oxygenation is impaired even further if there is coincident anaemia or changes in the oxyhaemoglobin dissociation curve which limit oxygen transport.

Patients with mild to moderate circulatory failure should be given oxygen in high concentration by mask. There is little risk of worsening hypercapnia because the presence of a low cardiac output is a vigorous ventilatory stimulant. However, when cardiac failure and the associated disturbances of pulmonary function are sufficiently severe, hypercapnia can develop but must not be misinterpreted as indicating chronic pulmonary disease.

Oxygen by mask is often poorly tolerated by shocked patients because of anxiety and restlessness. Mechanical ventilation secures control of the airway, ensures optimum gas exchange, relieves the work of breathing and, used in conjunction with careful sedation, eliminates the sensation of dyspnoea which is such a potent cause of anxiety, restlessness and increased adrenergic activity. This alone may lead to a reduction in cardiac output, independent of any mechanical consequences of the rise in intrathoracic pressure, but there is an increase rather than a fall in mixed venous oxygen saturation reflecting improved equilibrium between tissue oxygen supply and metabolic requirements.

Intubation is usually carried out using a short-acting anaesthetic agent and a muscle relaxant. Gastric emptying is greatly prolonged by acute illness and the stomach contents are often highly acid which means that the usual precautions to avoid regurgitation and aspiration are necessary. IPPV is started as soon as the tube has been secured, and the residual effects of the same anaesthetic can be used to cover other invasive procedures such as insertion of nasogastric tube or urinary catheter. Most positive pressure ventilators deliver a predetermined tidal volume at an adjustable frequency. (Table 21.7 shows some typical values for ventilator settings in the 'average' 70 kg patient.) The pattern of inspiration can be altered, so influencing the distribution of gas within the lungs as well as the magnitude of the mean intrathoracic pressure. In general, a large tidal volume delivered slowly and followed by a brief end-inspiratory pause (when there is no gas flow into or out of the lungs), is the most effective pattern to secure carbon dioxide clearance (Fig. 21.11). Oxygenation is adjusted by altering the inspired oxygen concentration or, if the lungs are small, by adding a positive end-expiratory pressure to increase the functional residual capacity. Ideally the inspired oxygen concentration should remain below 40% to avoid the risk of pulmonary oxygen toxicity, but this hazard must be set against those of pulmonary barotrauma caused by over-high inflation pressures.

Some of the consequences of IPPV are disadvantageous, in particular innappropriate reduction in arterial carbon dioxide tension which lowers cardiac output in its own right, and impairment of ventricular filling as a result of the increase in mean intrathoracic pressure. If hypovolaemia or a reduction in vascular tone are the cause of circulatory failure, IPPV is likely to impair tissue perfusion even further by lowering cardiac filling and hence output. If myocardial failure is present, and especially if pulmonary oedema has resulted from left atrial hyper-

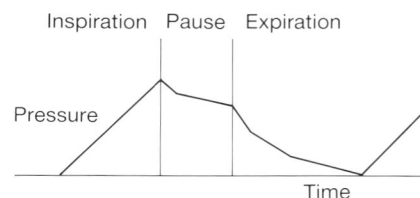

Fig. 21.11 Airway pressure end-inspiratory pause.

tension, mechanical ventilation is therapeutic. Apart from the respiratory benefits enumerated earlier, it displaces blood out of the engorged central vessels, lowers intraventricular distension, enhances coronary perfusion and provides a modest reduction in afterload [17] Qualms that IPPV is detrimental in patients with severe left ventricular failure are unfounded.

Special considerations apply if the pulmonary vascular resistance is very high, or if myocardial function is only moderately impaired. The pressure within the pulmonary circulation in patients with significant pulmonary vascular disease is usually so high that the fairly minor increase associated with IPPV is of little consequence, and is more than outweighed by the advantages of optimising lung volume and hence pulmonary vascular resistance, ensuring adequate gas exchange and eliminating the work of breathing. If pulmonary hypertension of recent onset is associated with profound impairment of pulmonary compliance — a combination seen most often in the adult respiratory distress syndrome (non-cardiogenic pulmonary oedema) — it is necessary to secure the best compromise between respiratory and circulatory function so that tissue oxygen transport, the product of cardiac output and arterial oxygen content, is as high as possible. Increasing the intrathoracic pressure by any of a variety of respiratory manoeuvres may well increase arterial oxygenation but can diminish arterial oxygen transport because the cardiac output falls. Ensuring that tidal ventilation occurs over the most compliant part of the pressure—volume curve of the lung (Fig. 21.12) usually provides the best compromise between arterial oxygenation and cardiac output, and also minimises the risks of damage to oedematous, friable lung caused by excessive airway pressures. It is worth noting in this context that the transmission of airway pressure to the other intrathoracic structures is limited when the lungs are very non-compliant and so it can be both safe and necessary to use high

Table 21.7 'Normal' ventilator settings.

Variable	Symbol	Range	Typically
Tidal volume	V_t	7−10 ml/kg	490−700 ml
Rate	f	12−14	12
Minute volume	MV	100−150 ml/kg	7−10.5 l
O_2 concentration	F_iO_2	0.21−1.0	up to 0.4
Peak pressure	PAP	15−50 cmH$_2$O	15−20 cmH$_2$O
End expiratory pressure	PEEP	2−20 cmH$_2$O	5−10 cmH$_2$O

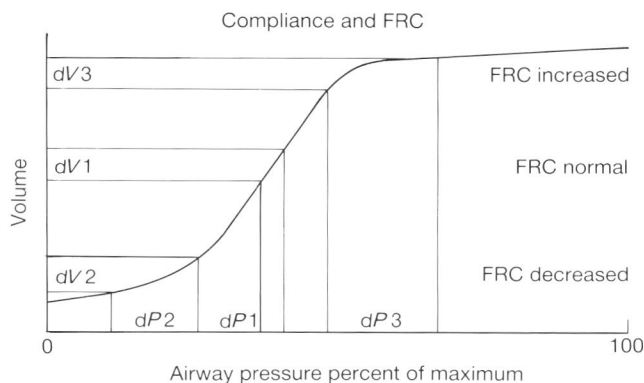

Fig. 21.12 The pressure volume relationship of the lung and chest wall is shown. Equal increments in lung volume ($dV1$, $dV2$ and $dV3$) are plotted against the corresponding pressure change ($dP1$, $dP2$ and $dP3$) required to produce them. Note that in the middle range of lung volume, (with a normal functional residual capacity — FRC), only a small pressure change is required to produce the volume change. At the extremes of the curve, where FRC is low or high, much larger pressure changes are required to produce the same volume change. Clearly ventilation resulting from volume changes over the middle range will be associated with less pressure change and less work.

levels of PEEP, even in the presence of impaired myocardial contractility.

The use of IPPV requires endotracheal intubation, often combined with more sedation than would otherwise be necessary. This has led to some interest in techniques of respiratory support which permit spontaneous ventilation, often without the need for intubation, and usually at a pressure greater than atmospheric. This secures better expansion of the lungs and lessens respiratory work. Although helpful up to a point, there is no evidence that they can replace conventional ventilatory management using IPPV.

Other respiratory measures which are useful in specific circumstances include the administration of bronchodilator drugs or antibiotics, and physical measures to promote sputum clearance. However, the increase in airway resistance which accompanies left ventricular failure responds better to a reduction in pulmonary venous engorgement than to bronchodilators, and endotracheal suction to clear pulmonary oedema is only likely to promote the formation of more oedema. The effort of expectoration is often underestimated, particularly when sputum is copious or viscid, the vital capacity is small and the patient is fatigued. Use of a mini-tracheostomy may prevent sputum retention and subsequent atelectasis. At the other end of the therapeutic spectrum, extracorporeal systems have been used to secure gas exchange when pulmonary function is grossly disorganised. The results are not encouraging [18] and these methods should only be considered if there is a realistic chance of ultimate recovery or a genuine prospect of heart—lung transplantation. The development of exceptional measures for supporting both cardiovascular and respiratory function, combined with techniques for combating failure of other essential systems has introduced new problems. Ethical considerations and the question of financial and human resources are likely to loom large in the intensive care services of the future [19].

REFERENCES

1 Rosomoff HL, Shulman K, Raynor R *et al*. Experimental brain injury and delayed hypothermia. *Surg Gynecol Obstet* 1960;**110**:27.

2 Brader E, Jehle D, Safar P. Protective head cooling during cardiac arrest in dogs. *Ann Emerg Med* 1985;**14**:510 (abs).

3 Abramson NS, Safar P, Detre K *et al*. Brain Resuscitation Clinical Trial (BRCT) I Study Group: randomized clinical study of thiopental loading in comatose cardiac arrest survivors. *N Eng J Med* 1986;**314**:397.

4 Vaagenes P, Cantadore R, Safar P *et al*. Amelioration of brain damage by lidoflazine after prolonged ventricular fibrillation cardiac arrest in dogs. *Crit Care Med* 1984;**12**:846.

5 Cullen JP, Aldrete JA, Jankowsky L *et al*. Protective action of phenytoin in cerebral ischaemia. *Anesth Analg* 1979;**58**:165.

6 Levy DE, Caronna JJ, Singer BH *et al*. Predicting outcome from hypoxic-ischaemic coma. *JAMA* 1985;**253**:1420—6.

7 Bircher N, Safar P. Comparison of standard and 'new' closed-chest CPR and open-chest CPR in dogs. *Crit Care Med* 1981;**9**:384.

8 Dembo DH. Calcium in advanced life support. *Crit Care Med* 1981;**9**:358.

9 Slogoff S, Keats AS, Arlund C. On the safety of radial artery cannulation. *Anesthesiology* 1983;**59**:42—7.

10 Moran KT, McEntee G, Jones B *et al*. To tunnel or not to tunnel catheters for parenteral nutrition. *Ann R Coll Surg Engl* 1987;**69**:235—6.

11 Senderoff E, Lutchman G, Shevde K. Catheter-induced innominate vein perforation: anatomical considerations. *J Cardiothorac Anesth* 1987;**1**:57—8.

12 Shah KB, Rao TLK, Laughlin S *et al*. A review of pulmonary artery catheterization in 6,245 patients. *Anesthesiology* 1984;**61**:271−5.

13 Kay H, Afshan M, Barash PG *et al*. Measurement of ejection fraction by thermal dilution techniques. *J Surg Res* 1983;**34**:337−46.

14 Hines R, Barash P. Intraoperative right ventricular dysfunction detected with a right ventricular ejection fraction catheter. *J Clin Monitoring* 1986;**2**:206−8.

15 Shoemaker WC, Chang P, Czer L *et al*. Cardiorespiratory monitoring in postoperative patients. I: prediction of outcome and severety of illness. *Crit Care Med* 1979;**7**:237−42.

16 Dawson JR, Thompson DS, Signy M *et al*. Acute haemodynamic and metabolic effects of dopexamine, a new dopaminergic agonist, in patients with chronic heart failure. *Br Heart J* 1985;**54**:313−20.

17 Branthwaite MA. Techniques of respiratory support in the management of cardiovascular disease. *Curr Opinion Cardiol* 1987;**1**:702−5.

18 Dorrington KL. Extracorporeal gas exchange in acute respiratory failure. *Br Med J* 1987;**296**:151−29.

19 Jennett B. Inappropriate use of intensive care. *Br Med J* 1984;**289**:1709−11.

CHAPTER 22

Electrophysiology and pacing: techniques of intracardiac electrophysiology — recording, stimulation and treatment

INTRODUCTION

During the last 15 years invasive electrophysiological testing has become the definitive investigation in the majority of arrhythmias. There have been profound advances since earliest recordings identified local atrial and ventricular electrograms, most noticeably the subsequent recording of His bundle activity followed by the introduction of programmed stimulation. These lead the way towards a sophisticated investigation having diagnostic, mechanistic, therapeutic and prognostic implications.

Invasive electrophysiological study has not replaced, but is an adjunct, to surface electrocardiographic interpretation. Surface recordings are limited in their ability to register the complex pattern of depolarisation of the AV conduction system. However this shortcoming did not prevent early pioneers in electrocardiography from applying knowledge of the physiological behaviour of the components of AV conduction to make complex deductions in the mechanisms of most arrhythmias. Electrophysiological study has often achieved little more than confirm these deductions but the test has developed a role in clinical practice by providing accurate diagnoses where surface ECG patterns cannot be precise. For example atrial activity may be difficult to discern on the surface ECG either because of low amplitude or because of rapid QRS complexes, and precise identification by intracardiac studies may be crucial for an accurate diagnosis.

Simple recordings of electrical activity made during an established arrhythmia play a small part in the role of these invasive studies. The use of programmed stimulation allowed the diagnostic role to be extended into the study of paroxysmal arrhythmias by its ability to initiate and terminate many arrhythmias at will. It has also permitted the detailed electrophysiology of the various components of the heart involved in impulse formation and propagation to be studied. This has allowed mechanisms of arrhythmia to be identified and confirmed. Again many of these principles had been proposed before the era of invasive electrophysiological study adding further weight to the doctrine that surface electrocardiography and invasive electrophysiology are complimentary techniques in the approach to patients with arrhythmia. Providing this philosophy is appreciated unnecessary invasive studies on patients will be avoided and maximum benefit obtained when they are necessary.

ELECTROPHYSIOLOGICAL TECHNIQUE

Equipment

In order that the full range of electrophysiological diagnoses can be made the appropriate equipment for undertaking detailed electrophysiological studies must be available. As with other catheterisation procedures electrophysiological studies require a high level of patient safety and, in view of the time these studies may take, require a greater degree of patient comfort than routine angiographic procedures. All electrical equipment should be adequately grounded and checked to ensure that individual leakage currents do not exceed 10 µA. Good quality fluoroscopy is essential for placement of the catheters; for more complex procedures, such as catheter ablation, video tape and freeze-frame facilities are an advantage. As many patients undergoing electro-physiological study also have structural heart disease the capability of undertaking cine-angiography is desirable. Biplane facilities are recommended if endocardial mapping, the detailed study of endo-cardial activation, is to be performed. Full resusci-tation facilities including a reserve defibrillator are essential and in those cases in whom rapid ventricular arrhythmias are likely to occur, requiring prompt cardioversion, the use of adhesive defibrillator pads for the duration of the study is recommended. Regular testing of resuscitative equipment in accordance with local safety regulations is mandatory.

Facilities for recording a full 12—lead ECG must be available. At least three standard ECG leads should be continuously monitored during the study to ensure that axis change and bundle branch block patterns can be detected promptly. A minimum suitable combination would be leads I, AVF and V1 but the addition of a lateral chest lead is desirable. Most centres elect to monitor the electrocardiographic signals on a high quality multichannel oscilloscope capable of displaying the high frequency components of the intracardiac electrograms faithfully. Close and detailed analysis of the traces usually requires hard copy and either an ink jet or photographic recorder are suitable, these being the only recorders capable of displaying, in real time, signals up to 1 kHz. De-tailed analysis of activation patterns may require paper speeds of 200 mm/sec. Storage of signals on magnetic tape provides an optional second medium for the data. However, technological advances in computerised handling, display and storage of these complex signals has now allowed computer con-trolled graphics display systems to be built within reasonable cost limits to replace this hardware.

The catheters used for electrophysiological study are generally constructed from woven Dacron, having small (surface area 12—17 mm^2) ring and tip elec-trodes arranged in pairs (Fig. 22.1). In adults 6F catheters are commonly used and provide adequate torque control and pliability so that they can be manoeuvred to various endocardial sites. Larger catheters provide better torque but their stiffness

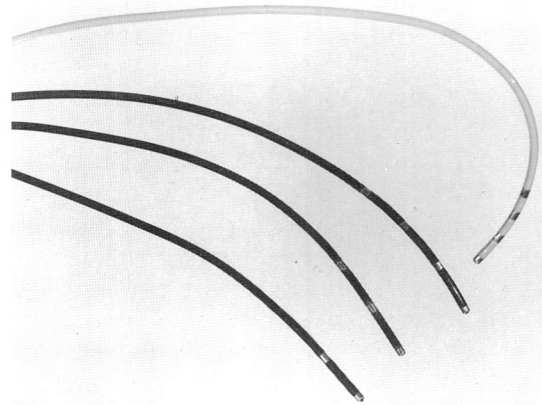

Fig. 22.1 A selection of electrode catheters suitable for electrophysiological study. Bipolar, tripolar and quadripolar arrangements are shown with either 5 mm or 1 cm interpolar spacing.

carries an increased risk of ventricular perforation. Modern technological improvements allow 6F multi-polar catheters to be constructed so that at least two, and often considerably more, bipolar elec-trograms can be obtained from each catheter. With three or four catheters being used routinely it is not unusual for eight bipolar electrograms to be available for analysis. The precise arrangement used will de-pend upon the nature and purpose of the study and the degree of detail required in both clinical and research terms. The number of channels displayed at any one time will be limited by the number of amplifiers and the number of channels on the re-corder. Providing that the display need not be si-multaneous even a relatively modest system can make use of multipolar catheters. However it cannot be recommended that electrophysiological studies are undertaken with a system of less than three surface ECG channels and five intracardiac channels. The amplifiers used for intracardiac signals require filtering of those components of the signals outside the range 40—500 Hz and with continuously variable gain capable of recording signals of 50 µv without any significant mains voltage interference. Each channel should be electrically isolated and should be capable of providing a front-end calibration sig-nal. At present the use of low frequency endocardial recordings or unipolar intracardiac signals has little place in routine electrophysiological investigation.

Bipolar recordings are generally used, the electrodes being 5 or 10 mm apart. This spacing offers sufficiently discrete electrograms for accurate timing and local stimulation. Spacing of 5 mm is recommended for more accurate mapping of activation sequences. For recording the His bundle electrogram a multipolar catheter is recommended so that proximal and distal His bundle activity can be detected.

A stimulator is essential if information beyond simple recording of spontaneous rhythms is to be obtained. It should be capable of delivering up to three premature stimuli synchronised to either paced or spontaneous rhythm as well as rapid continuous pacing over a wide range of heart rates. The device must be capable of delivering constant current stimuli and should preferably have two output channels so that synchronous atrial and ventricular pacing can be performed. The onset of all pacing sequences should be capable of being synchronised to spontaneous rhythm.

Patient selection

Electrophysiological studies are time consuming, expensive and not without potential complications. They should not be undertaken lightly and the goals of the study should be clarified beforehand. Every effort should be made to document spontaneous arrhythmias prior to the investigation especially when the nature of the arrhythmia is not clear from the history, examination and preliminary investigations.

There are few contraindications to electrophysiological study. Obviously radiation poses a risk to women of child-bearing age. Unstable angina and drug toxicity are two other contraindications. It is probably unwise to undertake studies in those with severely depressed left ventricular function.

Vascular complications are infrequent providing careful attention to catheterisation technique is taken. With femoral vein access phlebitis and/or thromboembolism occur in 0.5–1% and heparinisation, which should be routine when catheters are used on the systemic side, should be considered in those thought to be at high risk from venous thrombosis. Endocardial mapping of the left ventricle should be avoided when there is obvious left ventricular thrombus.

All patients should be studied in the fasting state and the majority require premedication, usually with an anxiolytic. Electrophysiological studies take considerably longer than many cardiac catheterisation procedures and may precipitate hypoglycaemia in diabetic and other susceptible patients.

Catheterisation technique

Electrophysiological studies in general require only venous access. Most studies can be performed under local anaesthesia using 0.5 or 1% lignocaine. Care should be taken that none is injected parenterally and preferably no more than 20 ml used. If significant amounts are absorbed the results of the study may be affected. A number of entry sites can be used but the femoral vein is a convenient, large diameter, vessel that can be punctured with ease and little risk. A standard percutaneous technique is used to cannulate the femoral vein. Having identified the course of the femoral artery 1–3 cm below the inguinal crease and instilled local anaesthetic medially one or more small incisions are made over the presumed site of the femoral vein — multiple incisions need be no more than 5 mm apart. The syringe and needle used for local anaesthetic can be used, by advancing with gentle suction, to verify the position of the femoral vein. The subcutaneous tissue below the skin incision should be dilated with forceps. Using the Seldinger or similar technique a guide wire is inserted into the vein. Where more than one catheter is to be used it is easy to insert all the guide wires first. For this reason we soak the guide wires in heparinised saline beforehand. For the majority of patients short guide wires and short dilator sheaths are adequate. Where femoral vein puncture is difficult a number of guide wires can be inserted through a single puncture site using the sheath introduced over the first wire for inserting two or three guide wires. This approach may result in continuous oozing around the sheaths and is not recommended when the venous pressure is high. Multiple (usually no more than three) catheters can be inserted via the femoral vein, this approach offering the optimal route for obtaining the His bundle electrogram.

Catheters can also be advanced to stable positions in the right atrium and the right ventricle, the other two common sites for recording and stimulation. Left atrial and left ventricular activity can be recorded with a catheter in the coronary sinus, a site that can more easily be obtained by a catheter introduced through either subclavian vein. Coronary sinus access can be achieved with a catheter introduced from the femoral vein, although it is less successful; it may occasionally be possible to direct the catheter directly from the IVC across the floor of the right atrium, but the formation of a right atrial loop is usually necessary. If right ventricular pacing and stimulation alone are required, especially if the electrode is to be left *in situ* for a number of days for the purpose of restudy, catheterisation via the subclavian vein may be preferred.

The precise arrangement of electrodes used depends on the nature and goals of the study. Most studies require a His bundle electrogram and a tripolar catheter that allows both proximal and distal His bundle activity to be recorded is recommended. Where atrial stimulation and recording are required a quadripolar catheter is invaluable, one bipole for pacing and the other bipole for sensing. This latter ensures local atrial capture which cannot always be verified by observing surface ECG P-waves. The right atrial appendage offers a stable site for reliable stimulation without the likelihood of producing phrenic nerve stimulation. This site is, however, several centimetres from the sinus node and a position close to the superior vena cava/right atrium

(SVC/RA) junction is essential if direct sinus node recordings are required. A bipolar catheter often suffices for ventricular stimulation as the QRS complexes can be used to ensure ventricular capture. The apex of the right ventricle and the right ventricular outflow tract are the most frequently used sites for ventricular stimulation although the right ventricular inflow tract may be useful in the study of some patients with ventricular tachycardia arising from the right ventricle.

Conduction intervals and principles of stimulation

Electrophysiological investigation rests on two principles — firstly, the intracardiac recording of patterns of activation; and secondly, the response of the various components of the electrical system of the heart to programmed stimulation. In the former, the time for local spread of activation (conduction intervals) as well as the pattern of impulse propagation are examined (Fig. 22.2). By recording the His bundle electrogram AV conduction can be divided into the discrete components that are involved in propagating an impulse from the sinus node to the ventricles The PA interval measures conduction across the right atrium but is of little clinical value. The AH interval indicates AV nodal conduction time and the HV

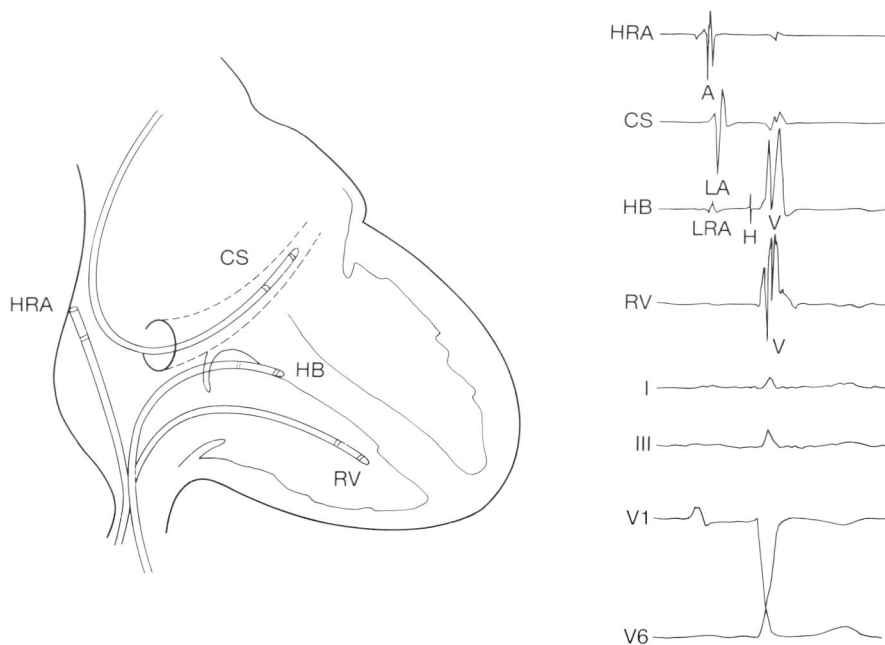

Fig. 22.2 Diagrammatic representation of the heart with electrodes positioned at high right atrium (HRA), adjacent to the His bundle (HB), at the apex of the right ventricle (RV) and in the coronary sinus (CS). Discrete local electrograms from each site are displayed at fast paper speed together with surface leads I, III, VI and V6. The coronary sinus electrogram records left atrial (LA) activity and the His bundle electrogram records low atrial septal activity (LRA), the His bundle potential (H) and upper ventricular septal activity (V).

interval the time for conduction through the His Purkinje system. It is important, for purposes of standardisation, to ensure that a proximal His bundle potential is being recorded; obtained by ensuring that the low right atrial signal is of larger amplitude than the His bundle electrogram. Normal values have been obtained for conduction times through these discrete areas (Table 22.1) [1].

When ventricular depolarisation is normal conduction velocity throughout the fascicular components of the AV conduction system must be similar so that ventricular depolarisation is relatively homogeneous. When there is bundle branch block the HV interval reflects conduction time through the unblocked fascicle(s) with the shortest conduction time — complete or partial disruption of the interrupted fascicle(s) cannot be discriminated. It may however be feasible to identify proximal and distal right bundle branch block based on the interval between the His bundle electrogram and the time of activation of the right ventricular apex [2].

Further observations on the pattern of normal activation are descriptive based on, for example, the spread of anterograde activation across the left atrium after depolarisation of the low right atrium, and activation of the upper ventricular septum and right ventricular outflow tract after activation of the right ventricular apex. The pattern of retrograde atrial depolarisation resulting from conduction over the normal AV node—His bundle axis can also be observed. Low right atrial activity precedes coronary sinus depolarisation, which is then followed by spread of activation across the right atrium simultaneously with spread of activation across the left atrium.

It is important to distinguish conduction of electrical impulses from the property of refractoriness that characterises the response of cardiac tissue to premature stimulation. Although a variety of abnormalities can be identified on the basis of abnormal impulse conduction much of the interpretation during an electrophysiological study rests on the identification of abnormal responses to premature stimulation. Normal values have also been defined for the refractory periods of the various conductive parts of the heart (Table 22.1). Various measurements of refractoriness have been defined and they can be used to characterise the components of the electrical system of the heart in electrophysiological terms. These values can be measured directly in tissues which can be stimulated directly. Alternatively the values can be measured indirectly by examining the ability of areas that cannot be stimulated directly (e.g. the AV node) to propagate impulses generated at a proximal site. Normal myocardial tissue responds differently from AV nodal tissue. Atrial and ventricular myocardium essentially demonstrate the 'all or nothing' phenomenon in which premature stimuli are conducted at the same velocity irrespective of the prematurity of the stimulus. In fact there is a small degree of delay with stimuli very close to the effective refractory period. AV nodal tissue, by contrast, demonstrates decremental conduction, i.e. reduced conduction velocity (increased conduction time) with increasingly premature stimuli over a wide range of intervals.

The distinctive components of refractoriness and conduction are important concepts if mechanisms of arrhythmia, particularly with regard to the influence of programmed stimulation, are to be understood. Similarly the conceptual differences between the mechanism of re-entry and focal automaticity need to be appreciated. While the former can usually be initiated and terminated by premature stimulation, automatic rhythms cannot although they demonstrate overdrive suppression.

Table 22.1 Normal conduction intervals and refractory periods (msec).

	Adults	Children
RA	25—55	20—40
AVN	55—120	40—110
HV	30—55	30—55
Atrial ERP	170—260	160—240
AV nodal ERP	20—440	160—320
Ventricular ERP	180—260	170—220

RA: right atrial; AVN: atrioventricular nodal; HV: His—Purkinje conduction intervals; ERP: effective refractory period.

SINUS NODE FUNCTION

Although surface ECG recordings provide the mainstay of diagnosing sinus node disease electrophysiological study may occasionally be of value. Two measurements of sinus node function have been established; sinus node recovery time and directly or indirectly measured sinoatrial conduction time.

Sinus node recovery time (SNRT)

Cardiac cells demonstrating intrinsic automaticity will be suppressed transiently at the end of a period of overdrive pacing. This phenomenon of overdrive suppression is measurable as the interval between the last externally paced beat and the first spontaneous or return beat from the automatic area [3]. When testing sinus node function, atrial pacing close to the sinus node is performed for at least 30 seconds at a rate just above the intrinsic sinus rate. The interval between the last stimulus and the first atrial depolarisation originating at the high right atrium is taken as the sinus node recovery time. What does this value represent and what are its determinants? The last stimulated atrial depolarisation is conducted across the sino-atrial junction and depolarises the sinus node. Following sinus repolarisation and spontaneous diastolic depolarisation the sinus node discharges and an impulse is conducted back across the sino-atrial junction to depolarise the atria. Therefore besides incorporating sino-atrial conduction time this value is related to the rate and duration of pacing, as well as the underlying intrinsic sinus rate. There are a number of explanations for the variability of the measurements, including the integrity of conduction from the atrium into the sinus node as well as pacemaker shift within the node. In practical terms it is important to repeat the test a number of times and to examine the effect of a range of paced rates. Correction for underlying intrinsic sinus rate can be achieved by subtracting the SNRT from the sinus cycle length and thereby obtaining the corrected SNRT. Values in excess of 525 msec are abnormal (Fig. 22.3). Failure of the last paced beat to be conducted into the sinus node may result in a false negative SNRT; this may however result in a prolonged pause after the first return beat [4]. Such secondary pauses may also indicate significant sinus node disease and a nomogram has been established to allow identification of abnormal pauses [4].

Sino-atrial conduction time (SACT)

Although sinus node dysfunction may result from an inability of the sinus pacemaker cells to generate impulses (disordered automaticity), the perinodal structures may be diseased and prevent the conduction of normally generated impulses from the sinus node into the right atrium. Various methods have therefore been devised for measuring sino-atrial conduction time. Two methods measure SACT indirectly by examining the influence of premature stimulation on atrial response. In the first method the influence of stimuli of increasing prematurity is measured [5]. Atrial premature beats are delivered after every eighth sinus beat and the interval between the last sensed beat and the atrial premature beat compared to the time between the atrial premature stimulus and the next spontaneous sinus beat. These measurements can be normalised by dividing each by the spontaneous sinus cycle length.

The second method uses short (eight beat) episodes of atrial pacing at a rate that just exceeds the intrinsic sinus rate (this rate is assumed not to disturb sinus node automaticity) and measures the interval

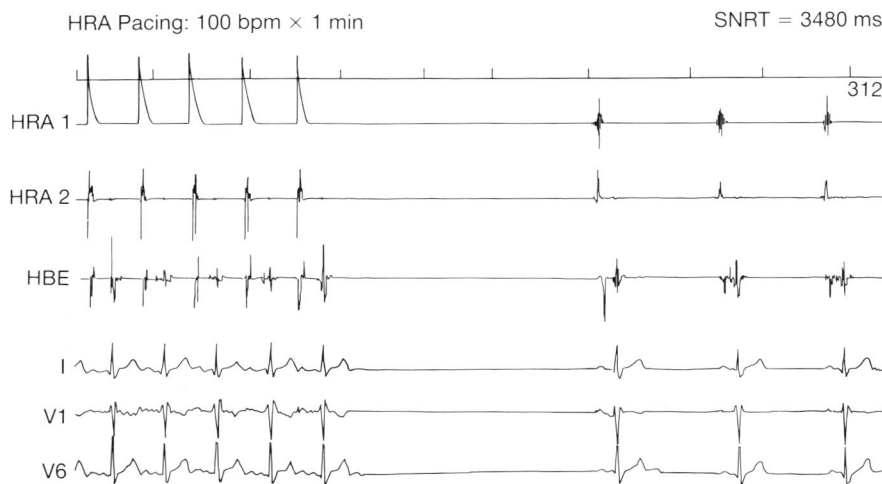

Fig. 22.3 Prolonged sinus node recovery time (SNRT) in a patient with sino-atrial disease following right atrial pacing at 100 bpm for 1 minute (HRA1 and 2 = high right atrial electrograms; HBE = His bundle electrogram; surface ECG leads I, V1 and V6; paper speed 25 mm/second).

between the last paced beat and the first return sinus beat [6]. SACT is the recovery interval minus the mean sinus cycle length. In both techniques SACT measures the combined time an impulse takes to travel into the sinus node and then back to the atrium. The individual unidirectional components cannot be separately identified.

The ability to record sino-atrial activity has provided the first direct measurement of SACT [7]. With an electrode positioned at the high RA/SVC junction low frequency signals have been recorded, preceding atrial activity, and are thought to represent sinus node depolarisation.

There is little agreement between the various methods for assessing sinus node function. This may reflect measurement by the tests of different facets of sino-atrial behaviour and various modifications have been suggested in an attempt either to increase the accuracy of the measurements or to increase the sensitivity of the tests. The recent introduction of a more mathematically derived approach to measurements of sinus node automaticity and sino-atrial conduction [8] may allow these separate facets to be identified more accurately but further experience in a wide variety of patients with sinus node dysfunction will be necessary before it becomes a routine method of assessment. Whether the use of pharmacological adjuncts (e.g. verapamil or disopyramide) that suppress sinus node activity and thereby provoke latent dysfunction will increase the diagnostic sensitivity of these tests remains to be seen.

Clinical electrophysiological testing of patients with suspected sinus node dysfunction lacks the sensitivity and predictive accuracy to make it a reliable test in all patients. However these tests have good specificity and therefore have a role when other tests are normal but there remains a high index of suspicion that there is underlying sinus node disease.

AV CONDUCTION

Despite the inability of surface ECG recordings to reveal individual function of the specific components of the AV conduction system the anatomical location of conduction system disorders can usually be deduced from standard electrocardiographic criteria. Electrophysiological testing therefore has a useful, but limited, role in the assessment of patients with AV conduction disturbances. Its value centres not on making the diagnosis of the degree and type of AV block but on diagnosing the anatomical level of the conduction disturbance and from this allowing prognostic comments to be made concerning the likelihood of progression to higher grade block, for which pacemaker implantation might be indicated.

In the symptomatic individual every effort should be made to obtain ECG documentation during symptomatic episodes rather than relying on electrophysiological testing. When symptoms can be correlated with bradycardia knowledge of the location of AV conduction block is irrelevant. In the asymptomatic individual with resting AV conduction disturbance it was previously felt that precise electrophysiological diagnosis was important. The rationale for this approach was the apparently good prognosis for second degree type I AV block [9], and, therefore, that confirmation by intracardiac study of the proximal nature of the block might remove the need for pacing in the asymptomatic patient. Recent work [10] has however suggested that the prognosis is poor in both forms of second degree block and that in both the prognosis can be improved by pacing. Interestingly the prognosis was uninfluenced by the additional presence of bundle branch block. If these results are confirmed the place of intracardiac study would seem to be limited to those patients with symptomatic first degree AV block in whom ambulatory monitoring cannot reveal higher degrees of AV block. Electrophysiological study would then be used un an attempt to identify resting unsuspected conduction delay in the His—Purkinje system (Fig. 22.4) or to provoke higher degrees of block either by pacing or pharmacologically.

Intraventricular block

A number of studies have examined the role of electrophysiological investigation in patients with fascicular conduction disturbances. These studies have concentrated on patients with bifascicular block and examined and tested the integrity of the remaining fascicle. The HV interval in these patients indicates conduction time in the unblocked fascicle. A number of prospective studies used measurements of the HV interval in patients with bifascicular block to predict those at risk of complete heart block and

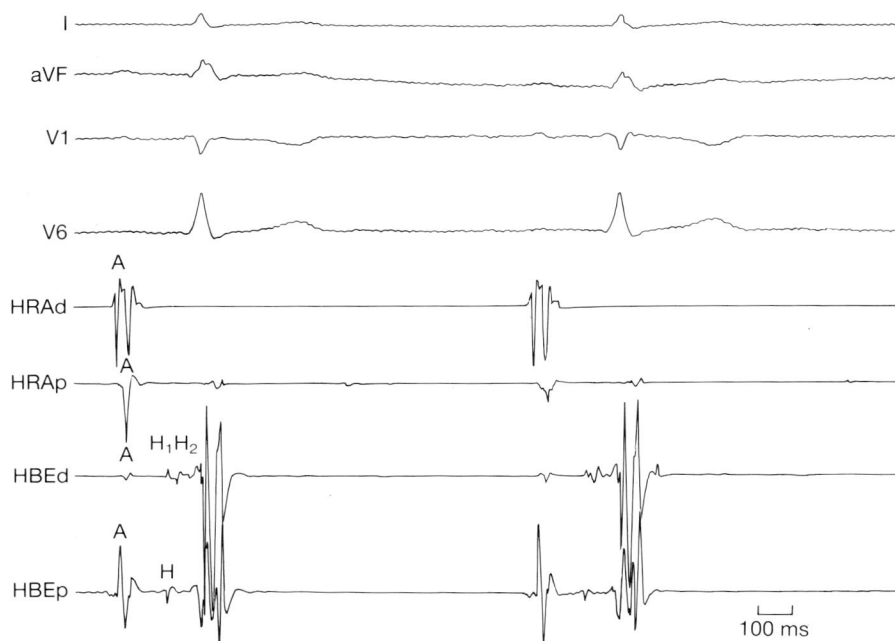

Fig. 22.4 Intrahisian block in a patient with symptomatic first degree AV block. The intracardiac recording shows a split and prolonged His bundle deflection, seen especially on the distal His bundle electrogram (HBEd). Distal and proximal high right atrial and His bundle electrograms are shown together with surface leads I, aVF, V1 and V6.

sudden death [11–13]. Arguably the most important contribution of these studies has been to demonstrate that the prognosis is determined principally by the nature of the underlying cardiac disease rather than the extent of conduction system disease, and that in many sudden death is due to ventricular arrhythmia or myocardial infarction and less frequently to the development of complete heart block. Additionally in almost half the patients examined there was disease at the level of the AV node and not in the remaining intact fascicle. These studies conflict in their conclusion as to the value of the HV interval as an independent predictor of mortality. Furthermore the rate of progression to complete heart block in the asymptomatic patient with bifascicular block is low; in the region of 1% per year. This overall value can, however, be broken down more precisely by knowledge of the HV interval. When there is modest prolongation of the HV interval (55–70 msec) the incidence of progression to second degree AV block or complete heart block is approximately 1% per year. More marked prolongation of the HV interval (70–100 msec) is associated with a 4% per year incidence of high grade AV block and this incidence increases to 8% when the HV interval exceeds 100 msec. There is unfortunately little evidence that pacing improves the prognosis although it may be helpful in the man-

agement of symptoms. Therefore electrophysiological study seems advisable only in those with symptoms, when non-invasive studies have been negative, to clarify abnormal conduction in the remaining fascicle and also to establish (with ventricular stimulation) whether there is inducible sustained ventricular tachycardia [14].

SUPRAVENTRICULAR ARRHYTHMIAS

Atrial flutter and fibrillation

Intracardiac electrophysiological study has little or no part to play in the diagnosis of these arrhythmias. The diagnosis should always be evident on surface electrocardiographic recordings save for the rare case of atrial paralysis in which there may be insufficient electrically active atrial muscle to produce a surface deflection. In such patients an invasive study may demonstrate islands of atrial activity amongst a generally inexcitable atrium.

Paroxysmal supraventricular tachycardia

As with the other arrhythmias referred to in this chapter diagnosis of the precise mechanism of supraventricular tachycardia can usually be obtained from surface ECG recordings [15]. However it was electrophysiological study that confirmed the mechanisms involved in PSVT and allowed surface recordings to be interpreted with more precision than had hitherto been possible [16]. Thus intracardiac electrophysiological study remains the gold standard for diagnosing the precise mechanism of tachycardia thereby allowing antiarrhythmic treatment possibilities to be clarified. For example, in a patient with PSVT the absence of preexcitation on the resting ECG does not exclude the presence of an accessory AV pathway that may be amenable to surgical treatment. The majority of cases of paroxysmal supraventricular tachycardia are associated with re-entry either within the AV node or in association with an accessory pathway. Less frequently re-entry may occur in the region of the sinus node or there may be re-entry or focal activity within atrial myocardium.

An approach to patients with paroxysmal supraventricular tachycardia can be based on whether it is associated with a normal PQRS complex during sinus rhythm or whether there is associated ventricular preexcitation.

PSVT with normal PQRS complex in sinus rhythm

Where the surface ECG is normal and, therefore, does not suggest a mechanism of tachycardia electrophysiological studies are initially directed towards determining whether there is retrograde conduction and its physiological behaviour if present. Re-entry tachycardia associated with either an AV nodal cir-

cuit or in association with an accessory AV pathway requires retrograde conduction from ventricle to atrium and for the pathway to be capable of maintaining 1:1 VA conduction at least to the rate of the tachycardia. Where there is poor retrograde conduction (i.e. retrograde block at rates well below the rate of documented tachycardia) an accessory AV pathway can almost certainly be excluded but AV nodal tachycardia cannot. The retrograde pathway involved in AV nodal re-entry is often richly innervated by the autonomic nervous system and profound changes in retrograde behaviour may occur with sympathetic stimulation. The physiological behaviour of the retrograde pathway in response to incremental pacing or premature stimulation provides the first mechanism for differentiating AV nodal pathways from accessory AV pathways [17]. A retrogradely conducting AV nodal pathway usually demonstrates decremental properties and will activate the low septal right atrium before other atrial sites (Fig. 22.5). Conversely an accessory AV pathway shows fixed retrograde conduction time and may, depending upon it position, activate other atrial sites before the low septal right atrium. Coronary vein mapping (Figs 22.6a and 22.6b) and mapping around the tricuspid valve ring to delineate retrograde atrial activation during sustained tachycardia are essential for confirming an accessory pathway and localising the site. It may be difficult to separate a septal accessory AV pathway participating in a re-entry circuit from AV nodal re-entry, as some AV nodal pathways conduct retrogradely without demonstrating decr-

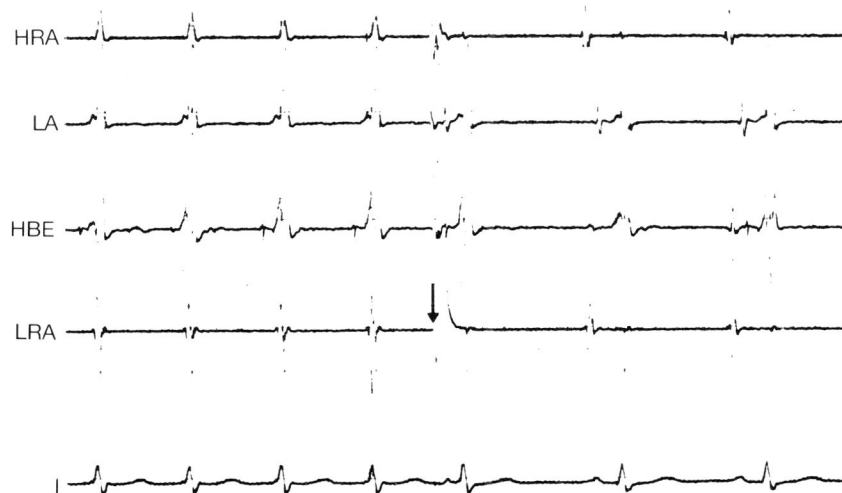

Fig. 22.5 Termination of a sustained supraventricular tachycardia by single premature atrial stimulus (↓) is followed by sinus rhythm with normal PQRS complex. During tachycardia atrial activity occurs coincident with the QRS complex and low septal right atrial activity (LRA) precedes left atrial (LA) and high right atrial activity (HRA).

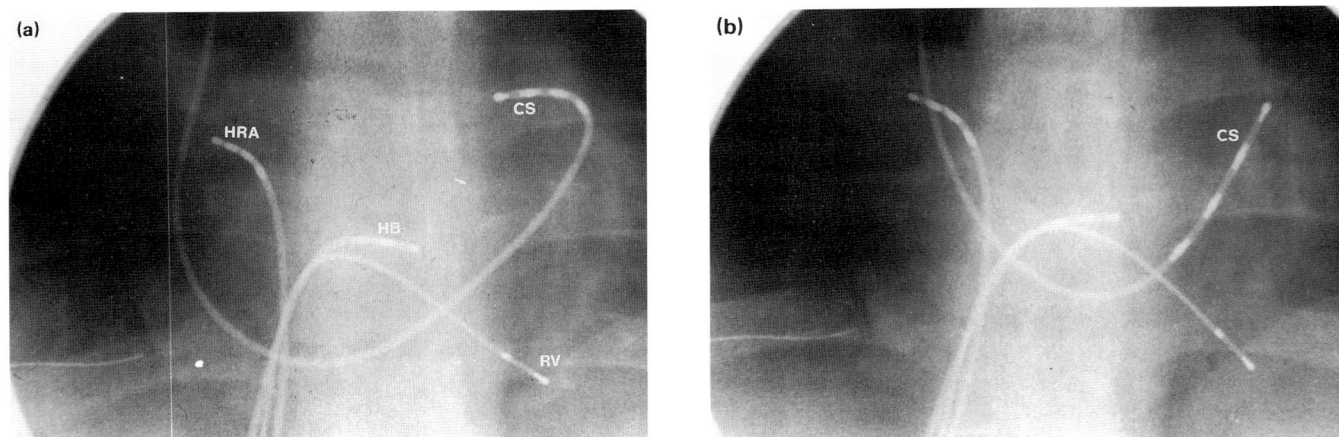

Fig. 22.6 (a and b) X-ray, taken in the AP view, showing the position of the intracardiac electrodes while mapping the coronary vein during electrophysiological study. Three electrodes have been introduced from the right femoral vein and have been positioned at high right atrium (HRA), adjacent to the His bundle (HB) and at the apex of the right ventricle (RV). A catheter introduced from the subclavian vein has been placed in the coronary sinus and advanced as far as possible into the coronary vein (CS) — (a). Recordings are made from the distal site and then the catheter withdrawn proximally to a site where recordings from the middle and proximal extent of the coronary vein are made — (b).

emental properties. Additionally, where there is retrograde conduction over a single AV nodal pathway as well as a left lateral accessory pathway, retrograde conduction may preferentially occur at slow pacing rates over the AV nodal pathway because of its proximity to the site of ventricular pacing when this is right ventricular. Therefore it is always important to examine a wide range of rates and premature intervals in order to achieve decremental conduction in the AV nodal pathway and allow the consistent conduction over the accessory pathway to predominate.

Atrial stimulation (either incremental pacing or atrial premature stimuli) may reveal dual AV nodal pathways with increasing rate or increasing prematurity, the AH interval remaining fixed or prolonging until, at a critical interval or cycle length, this faster conducting pathway becomes refractory. The AH interval suddenly lengthens as a second nodal pathway conducts the atrial impulse. Providing conduction over this second pathway is sufficiently slow the propagating impulse may be able to use the faster pathway in a retrograde direction to re-enter the atrium (to produce an echo beat) and, if the slower pathway has then recovered excitability, AV nodal re-entry tachycardia may ensue. Dual AH pathways and echo beats are both suggestive of a substrate for sustained AV nodal re-entry tachycardia but are probably also present in a percentage of

subjects who never experience PSVT. Therefore manipulation of AV nodal conduction either with catecholamines or drugs, such as verapamil, that slow AV nodal conduction may be necessary to provoke sustained supraventricular tachycardia.

Either ventricular or atrial pacing may induce sustained supraventricular tachycardia and allow the pattern of retrograde conduction to be studied in detail. Diagnosis of the precise mechanism of tachycardia depends upon the timing, location and physiological response of the retrogradely conducting pathway. Sustained tachycardia therefore represents the optimal situation for its study. Where low septal right atrial activation preceeds the onset of the ventricular component of the His bundle electrogram the diagnosis of AV nodal re-entry is not in doubt although it may require ventricular premature stimulation to allow the sequence of atrial activation to be verified (Fig. 22.7). Where septal atrial activation occurs coincident with septal ventricular activation both AV nodal re-entry and a septal accessory AV pathway are diagnostic possibilities. Discrimination may depend upon determining whether the His bundle is part of the re-entry circuit or whether it is a common final pathway for ventricular activation [18]. Ventricular premature stimuli delivered just after anterograde His bundle activation will only advance retrograde atrial activation when there is an accessory AV pathway (Fig. 22.8). Similarly in re-

Fig. 22.7 During sustained narrow QRS tachycardia low right atrial activity on the His bundle electrogram (A) precedes ventricular activation thereby demonstrating AV nodal re-entry tachycardia. A premature ventricular extrastimulus advances ventricular activation and allows the pattern of retrograde atrial depolarisation to be seen more clearly. Proximal and distal His bundle (HBEp and HBEd) and coronary sinus (CSp and CSd) electrograms are shown together with leads I, aVF, V1 and V6.

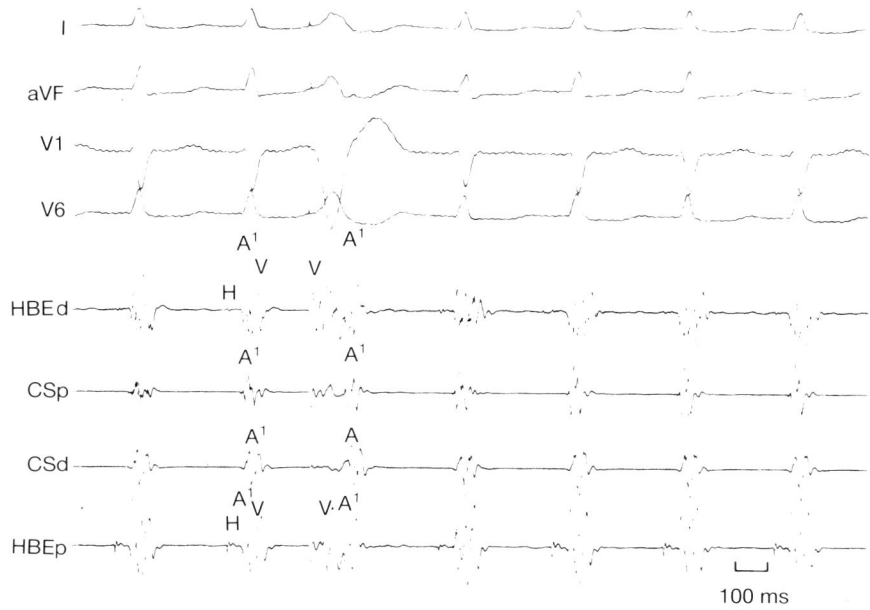

Fig. 22.8 During AV re-entry tachycardia in a patient with Ebstein's anomaly, associated with an right sided accessory AV pathway a late ventricular premature stimulus is delivered with a coupling interval of 380 msec, and causes minimal distortion of the fourth QRS complex. The cycle length of the tachycardia is 385 msec and there is established right bundle branch block — the retrograde VA interval measured on the His bundle electrogram (HBE) is 190 msec. The stimulus is delivered while the His bundle is refractory but results in paradoxically early atrial depolarisation (360 msec) due to the shortened retrograde conduction time (165 msec). Distal and proximal high right atrial (HRA) and low lateral right atrial (LLRA) electrograms are shown with leads I, II, III, V1, V4 and V6.

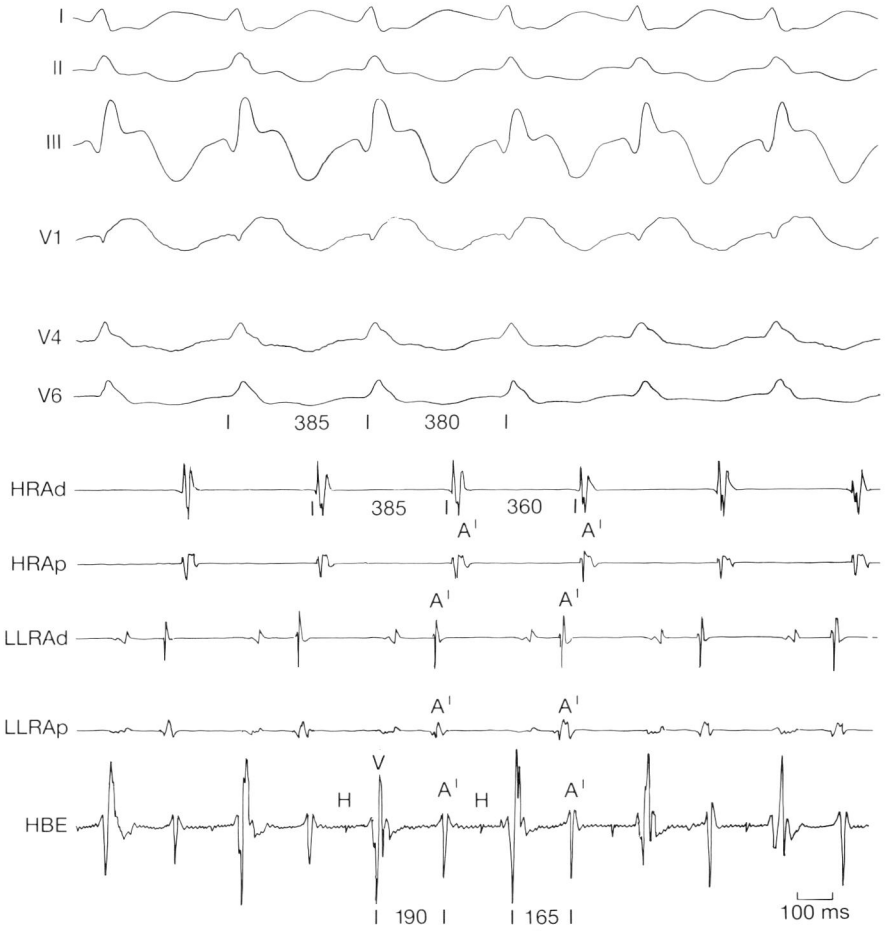

entry circuits involving an accessory AV pathway the bundle branch ipsilateral to the accessory pathway will be involved in the tachycardia circuit. Therefore the influence of bundle branch block on the timing of retrograde atrial activation should be carefully observed [19]. Bundle branch block may occur spontaneously but may also be induced by manipulation of the His bundle catheter against the septum.

Less frequently there may be AV re-entry associated with a posterior septal accessory AV pathway which conducts slowly, shows decremental retrograde conduction and is associated with incessant tachycardia having a long RP' pattern. It may sometimes require electrophysiological study to distinguish this from an atrial tachycardia arising in the septum or coronary sinus [20].

Sinus node re-entry tachycardia is uncommon but may be difficult to differentiate on ECG criteria from an atrial tachycardia arising from the high right atrium.

PSVT in the presence of ventricular preexcitation in sinus rhythm

Various abnormalities of the surface ECG have been recognised as predisposing to PSVT. In each form the ventricles are excited prematurely (pre-

excitation) by an accessory pathway that bypasses the normal AV conduction system. The Wolff—Parkinson—White syndrome is the most common type encountered. Less common forms are the Lown—Ganong—Levine syndrome and those with Mahaim pathways. In each case the pattern of preexcitation results from the presence of a distinct accessory pathway that can be identified anatomically. When tachycardia occurs in such patients it is generally the result of a re-entry circuit being established between the normal AV conduction system and the accessory pathway (Fig. 22.9).

When the mechanism of tachycardia is suggested by the presence of preexcitation on the resting electrocardiogram electrophysiological diagnosis is usually directed towards confirming the participation of an accessory AV pathway in the mechanism of tachycardia. The investigator should bear in mind that multiple mechanisms of tachycardia may be present in patients with preexcitation. Techniques similar to those outlined in the previous section are used to localise and characterise the retrograde pathway during supraventricular tachycardia.

However, it is the risk of sudden death should atrial fibrillation occur that is the prime concern in patients with the Wolff—Parkinson—White syndrome. Atrial fibrillation is more prevalent in patients with the Wolff—Parkinson—White syndrome than in the general population, and more so in those

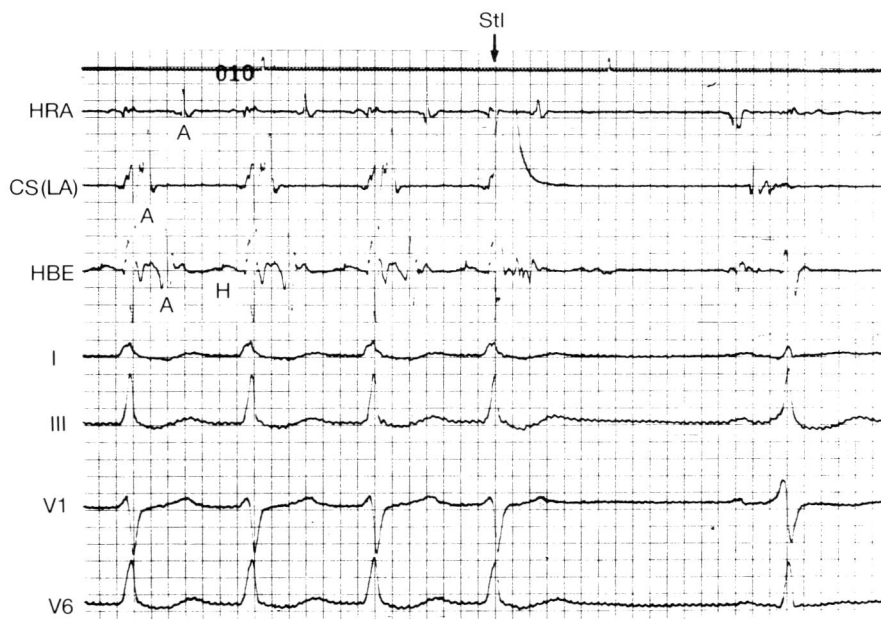

Fig. 22.9 Sustained supraventricular tachycardia in a patient with the Wolff—Parkinson—White syndrome is terminated by a premature atrial stimulus (Stl). During tachycardia the distal left atrium is activated before the low right atrium or high right atrium, indicating a left lateral accessory pathway, and a preexcited QRS complex is evident when sinus rhythm follows termination of tachycardia (paper speed 100 mm/second).

with PSVT. The primary purpose of the study must, therefore, be to establish whether the patient would be at risk should atrial fibrillation occur spontaneously (unless this arrhythmia has been documented previously). Measurement of the anterograde effective refractory period of the accessory pathway and highest rate of 1:1 conduction over the accessory pathway have been shown to correlate with the ventricular rate during atrial fibrillation (Figs 22.10 and 22.11). Induction of atrial fibrillation, however, remains the definitive test but may not always sustain. Assessment of anterograde behaviour requires stimulation at a site as close to the accessory pathway as possible to avoid possible errors due to intra-atrial block or functional properties before the stimulus reaches the accessory pathway. As yet there is no definitive measurement that identifies, prospectively, those at risk. Nor is there a clear consensus of the appropriate therapy for patients with a rapid ventricular response.

Narrow QRS tachycardia with AV dissociation

In unusual cases a narrow QRS complex tachycardia may occur with AV dissociation and it is often impossible to make the diagnosis without recourse to intracardiac study. The tachycardia may be due to AV nodal re-entry without atrial involvement, or may be of His bundle origin either alone or in association with a nodoventricular or fasciculoventricular (Mahaim) pathway. Ectopic tachycardia arising from the His bundle has become well recognised in infants and young children, particularly after corrective surgery for congenital heart defects and especially when surgery involves the ventricular septum. The diagnosis may be difficult to make when there is 1:1 retrograde conduction and electrophysiological study may be of value in ruling out other mechanisms of tachycardia. Despite the difficulty often encountered in treating His bundle tachycardia, it is an important diagnosis to make as

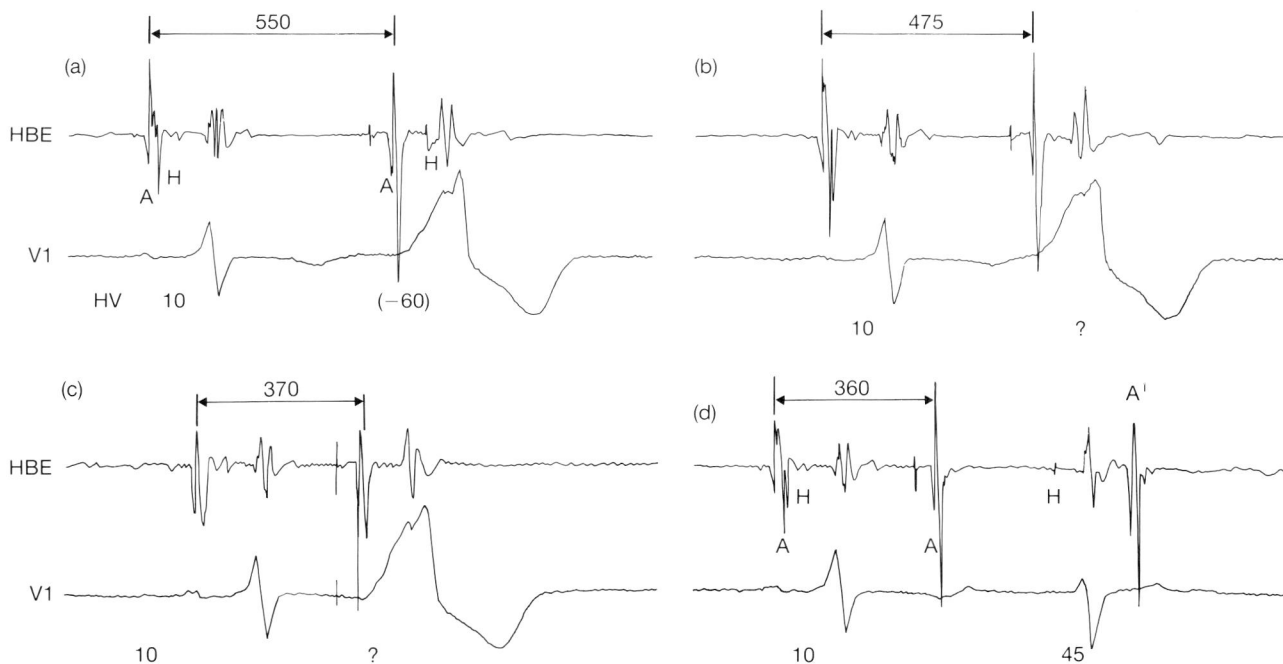

Fig. 22.10 Left atrial stimuli of increasing prematurity are illustrated in a patient with the Wolff–Parkinson–White syndrome. Each panel shows a sinus beat and the QRS complex following the premature stimulus. The HV interval during sinus rhythm is short (10 msec) indicating that the normal AV conduction pathway is being bypassed. Because the premature stimuli are delivered close to the accessory pathway the ventricle is depolarised predominantly via the accessory pathway and thereby producing the widened QRS complex. At an interval of 360 msec (d) the accessory pathway is refractory and conduction occurs via the normal AV conduction system resulting in a normal QRS complex and normal HV interval (45 msec).

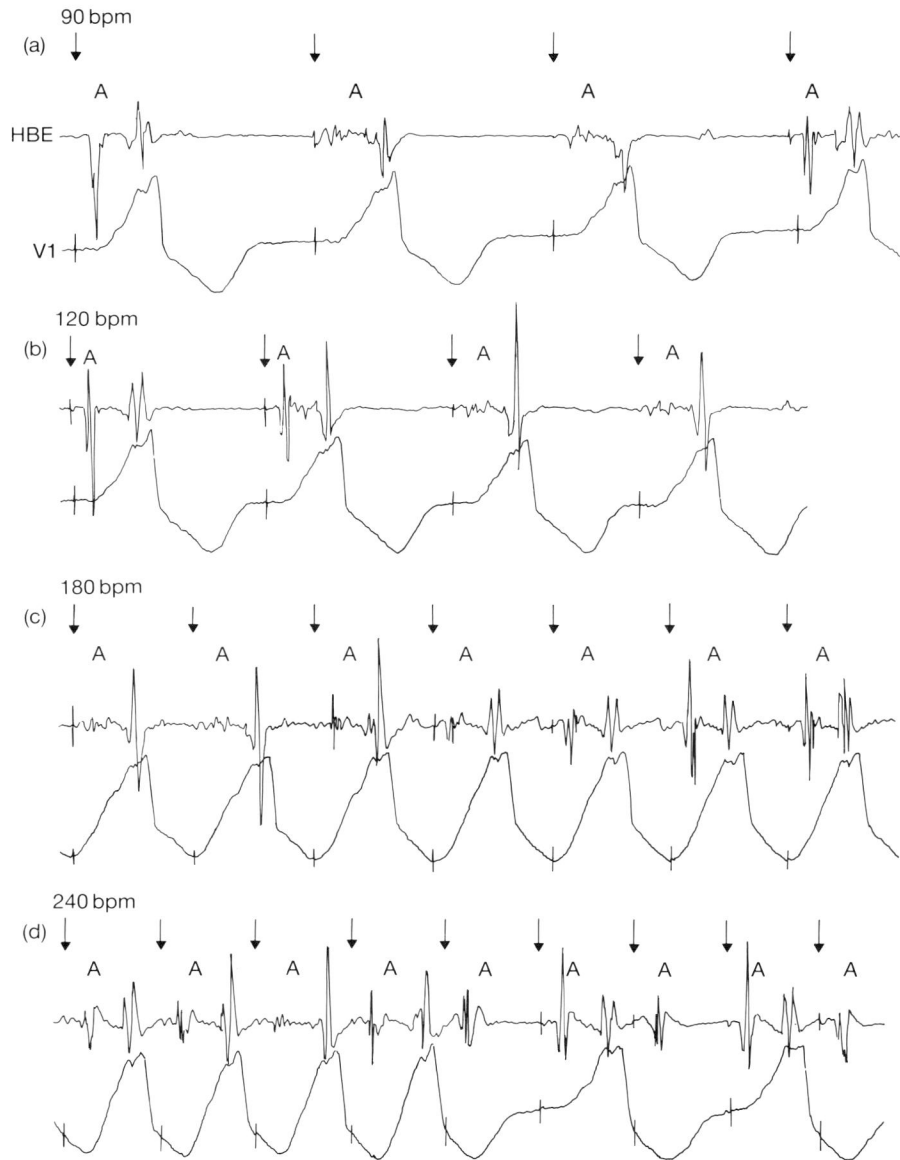

Fig. 22.11 Incremental atrial pacing from the left atrium in a patient with the Wolff–Parkinson–White syndrome and a left sided accessory pathway. 1:1 AV conduction follows increasing rates of atrial pacing (a to c) with a widened QRS complex reflecting predominant AV conduction via the accessory pathway. At a pacing rate of 240 bpm (d) second degree AV block as a result of block in the accessory pathway occurs following the fifth stimulus.

it may be life-threatening. A similar mechanism of tachycardia may occur in adults, usually irregular and catecholamine-sensitive.

WIDE QRS TACHYCARDIA

The ECG features that help to differentiate the possible diagnoses in the presence of a wide QRS tachycardia have received considerable attention and it has been shown that invasive study should rarely

be required in order to establish the diagnosis. However the distinction between VT, SVT with aberration, SVT with anterograde conduction over an accessory AV pathway [21] or tachycardia in association with Mahaim conduction [22] may be impossible when there is 1:1 AV association. There are also cases in which more than one mechanism coexists. The diagnosis of antedromic re-entry tachycardia rests upon the demonstration of an accessory AV pathway used anterogradely and either AV nodal retrograde conduction or another accessory AV pathway used as the retrograde limb. The essential features of Mahaim conduction are decremental anterograde conduction in association with left bundle aberration and shortening HV interval. The Mahaim pathway may be incorporated in the circuit or may be a 'bystander' in the presence of AV nodal or AV re-entry tachycardia.

Ventricular tachycardia

Ventricular tachycardia may occur in a variety of forms that may have mechanistic, prognostic and therapeutic implications. VT can be sustained or non-sustained, monomorphic (uniform) or multi-form (polymorphic). Non-sustained VT is generally defined as lasting more than three beats but terminating spontaneously within 30 seconds. Sustained VT lasts 30 seconds or more or requires immediate termination by pacing or electrical cardioversion. Monoform VT has a consistent QRS morphology while multiform VT has a constantly changing QRS morphology, the interval between the changes being usually no more than a few seconds.

The diagnosis of ventricular tachycardia can be made in most patients from ambulatory or 12-lead ECG recordings during a spontaneous attack. Rarely there may be difficulty in differentiating SVT with aberration from VT. A more frequent indication for invasive study exists when ventricular tachycardia is suspected but spontaneous arrhythmia cannot be documented, and this situation is particularly encountered in patients with syncope of unknown cause. Intracardiac study has therefore been pre-

dominantly used to guide antiarrhythmic therapy although it has also provided supportive evidence for some of the mechanisms of VT. Reproducible initiation of VT with single or double extrastimuli is in favour of re-entry and excludes an automatic mechanism, while rapid pacing is the most effective method for induction of triggered activity (Fig. 22.12). Re-entry is also usually characterised by an inverse relationship between the coupling interval of the extrastimulus that initiates tachycardia and the interval from the extrastimulus to the first beat of tachycardia. Re-entry requires conduction delay and this may be manifest as fractionated electrograms. However, demonstration that such delay is crucial to the mechanism of tachycardia is often difficult as multiple areas of slow conduction may be present, some of them unrelated to the tachycardia.

The diagnostic role of electrophysiological study depends upon the ability to induce clinically relevant ventricular arrhythmia. Ventricular stimulation provides the predominant method for inducing ventricular arrhythmia. Rarely atrial stimulation may induce a form of ventricular tachycardia characterised by a QRS morphology which has a right bundle branch block and left axis deviation configuration. This so-called fascicular tachycardia may involve the left posterior fascicle, and may be the result of triggered automaticity (Fig. 22.13).

A variety of ventricular stimulation protocols have been developed and there is no agreement on what constitutes the ideal protocol. This subject has been reviewed recently [23] and a few generalisations can be given. The sensitivity of the induction protocol is

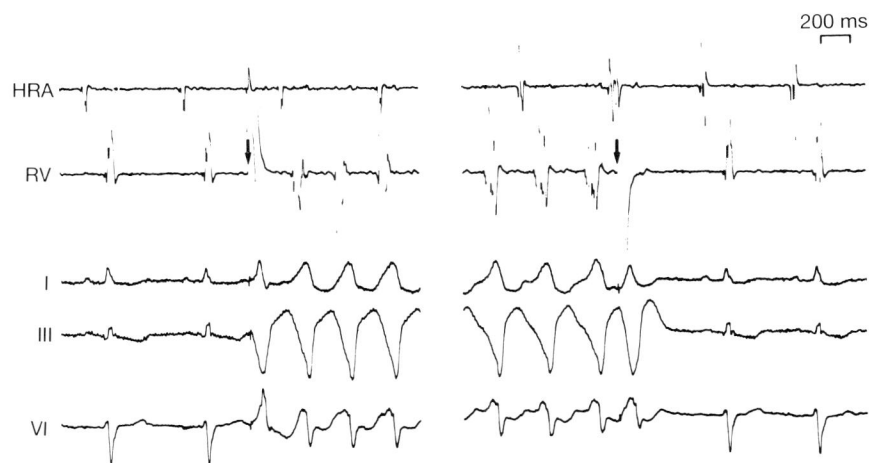

Fig. 22.12 Initiation and termination of sustained ventricular tachycardia by single ventricular premature stimuli. Atrial activity is dissociated both at the onset and termination of the tachycardia.

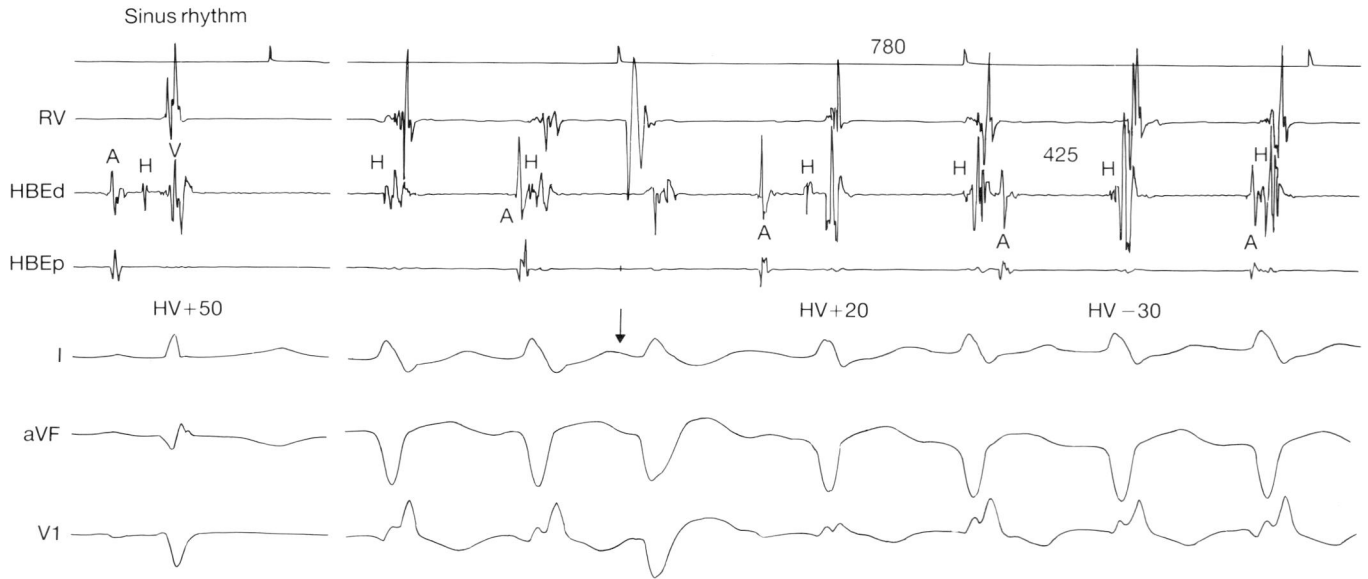

Fig. 22.13 Intracardiac recordings from a patient with fascicular ventricular tachycardia. Normal intracardiac conduction intervals during sinus rhythm are shown in the left hand panel. During sustained tachycardia His bundle depolarisation is evident preceding each septal ventricular deflection on the distal His bundle electrogram (HBEd) but with a negative HV interval (−30 msec). AV dissociation is evident during the tachycardia. Following a ventricular extrastimulus (↓) a fortuitous sinus discharge during the compensatory pause is conducted with fusion and with an intermediate HV interval. Distal and proximal His bundle electrograms (HBEd and HBEp) and right ventricular electrograms (RV) are shown with leads I, aVF and V1 (paper speed 100 mm/second).

increased if (1) more extrastimuli are used, if (2) stimuli are delivered after a train of ventricular paced beats rather than in spontaneous rhythm, and if (3) more than one drive rate is used. Moreover there is an increased yield if there is an abrupt change in rate during the drive, if several sites are stimulated and if stimulus intensity is increased. Using a protocol that includes three extrastimuli at two right ventricular sites and multiple drive cycle lengths VT will remain non-inducible in less than 5% of those with spontaneous VT. When more than two extra-stimuli are used increased sensitivity is balanced by decreased specificity, as non-specific arrhythmias are induced which may be difficult to interpret when no spontaneous arrhythmia has been documented. Therefore in those with syncope of unknown origin it seems appropriate to limit stimulation to two extrastimuli. It would also seem that using two stimuli at multiple sites before introducing a third extrastimulus reduces the incidence of non-specific responses.

However it can be stated that sustained mono-morphic ventricular tachycardia is of clinical significance however it is induced. The induction of either non-sustained or polymorphic ventricular tachycardia or ventricular fibrillation must be interpreted in the light of the aggressiveness of the protocol used.

CATHETER ABLATION

The technique of intracardiac electrophysiological study is of diagnostic value and provides essential information that can be used to select appropriate drug, pacemaker or surgical therapies. Patients with the Wolff—Parkinson—White syndrome undergo electrophysiological testing to demonstrate that an accessory pathway is responsible for the tachycardia. Endocardial electrodes can be placed with such precision that they lie within a few millimetres of the pathway and such localisation is a crucial prerequisite prior to open heart surgical accessory pathway ablation. Similarly in patients with ventricular tachycardia, endocardial mapping is used to locate the 'origin' of the tachycardia (Fig. 22.14).

Catheter ablation has been the logical step that has applied electrophysiological techniques directly to the therapy of various arrhythmias. Intracardiac electrodes used for localising arrhythmias can be used for delivering destructive energies so that the arrhythmia can be abolished. The technique has been used in the treatment of all forms of tachycardia although two areas are of predominant interest.

1 ABLATION OF NORMAL AV CONDUCTION

The technique of catheter ablation was first applied to the treatment of drug resistant supraventricular arrhythmias and clinical experience has been largest in this group [24]. Previously, open heart surgery and destruction of AV conduction by dissection or cryoablation, thereby creating complete heart block, was the only treatment for this group. Catheter ablation can achieve the same end point without the necessity for open heart surgery; the success rates are identical, but the morbidity with catheter ablation lower. The patient is rendered pacemaker-dependent and the technique must be considered an inelegant solution in that it exchanges one arrhythmia for another, albeit that heart block is easier to manage. Catheter ablation of normal AV conduction has been used predominantly for the treatment of resistant atrial fibrillation or atrial flutter and has successfully achieved heart block in approximately two-thirds of patients.

In order to create complete heart block an electrode

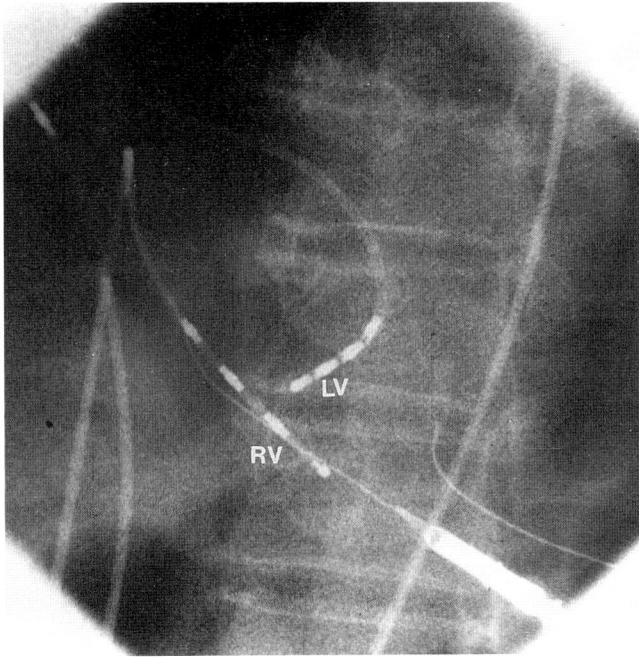

Fig. 22.14 X-ray taken in the LAO projection, during catheter mapping of ventricular tachycardia. This picture was taken after endocardial mapping had identified the earliest site of endocardial activation during ventricular tachycardia. Catheters have been positioned in the right ventricle (RV) and left ventricle (LV) and activation began simultaneously on the septal aspects of the right and left ventricles in this patient with previous anteroseptal myocardial infarction and ventricular tachycardia.

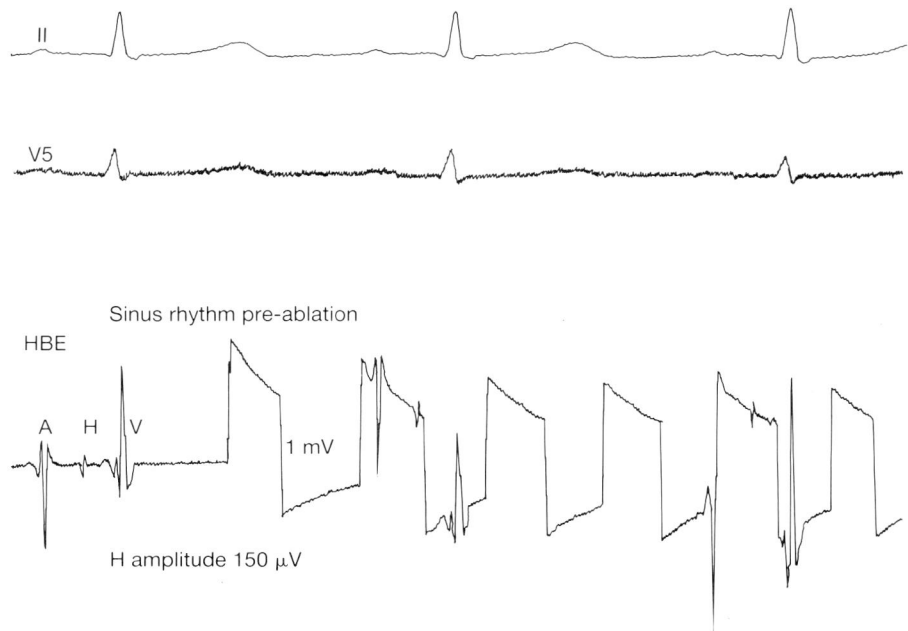

Fig. 22.15 His bundle electrogram together with leads II and V5 recorded before catheter ablation of AV conduction in a patient with paroxysmal atrial fibrillation. The His bundle amplitude is adequate and the large atrial deflection (A) indicates that the catheter is proximal on the AV node-His bundle. 1 mV calibration pulses are seen distorting the His bundle recording.

must be positioned adjacent to the AV node—His bundle — we use a 7F tripolar catheter — and the same technique as described for routine electro-physiological study is used. The best possible His bundle potential should be sought although it has been found that it is not necessarily the amplitude of the His bundle potential that is crucial. It is important to ensure that the catheter is positioned proximally on the AV node—His bundle axis, recog-nised when the low right atrial component of the His bundle electrogram is large (Fig. 22.15). When the electrode is too distal RBBB is produced rather than complete heart block. A right ventricular pacing catheter must be in place for pacing once AV con-duction has been interrupted.

High energy direct current discharges were orig-inally used and most experience has been gained with this form of energy. Discharges of 150—300 J from a standard defibrillator are used. We have de-signed and used a modified DC power source which allowed successful ablation with energies of 2—30 J (Fig. 22.16) [25]. Increasing experience has been gained with radiofrequency energy although the relative merits of the different power sources have not been clarified. One advantage of radiofrequency energy is that unlike DC discharges it does not re-quire general anaesthesia. Whichever power source is used the energy is delivered between the intracar-diac electrode (generally as the cathode) and an in-different large surface area back plate (as the anode). Using a standard defibrillator two or three shocks of 200—300 J are required to create complete heart block. Careful electrocardiographic and haemo-dynamic monitoring is essential as both ventricular arrhythmias and hypotension have occured as immediate complications. Ventricular perforation and tamponade have been described with DC shocks [26].

2 CATHETER ABLATION OF ACCESSORY PATHWAYS AND VENTRICULAR TACHYCARDIA

Surgical techniques for the ablation of the accessory pathway in patients with the Wolff—Parkinson—White syndrome and foci responsible for sustained ventricular tachycardia are well established. Catheter ablation has been used in the treatment of both these conditions using similar techniques to those described above for ablation of normal AV conduc-tion. However, experience has been more limited and in view of the complication rate the procedure for these indications has been limited to relatively few centres. Catheter ablation of accessory pathways using high energy DC shocks has been complicated by rupture of the coronary sinus and fatal tampon-ade, and ablation of ventricular tachycardia compli-cated by fatal hypotension. Despite these rare complications in patients who may have life-threatening arrhythmias further development prom-ises that many of these large groups of patients may be cured of their rhythm disturbances without re-course to open heart surgery or dependence on life-long antiarrhythmic drugs.

TEMPORARY AND PERMANENT PACING

There can be few areas of cardiology that have seen such rapid advances in three decades as that of cardiac pacing. It has benefited from an unpre-cedented advance in electronics. Progress in power source development and integrated technology cir-cuitry has allowed the pulse generator to be a fraction of the size of units implanted 15 years ago (Fig. 22.17). Reliability has reached the stage when gener-ator failure is exceedingly rare. Similarly lead tech-

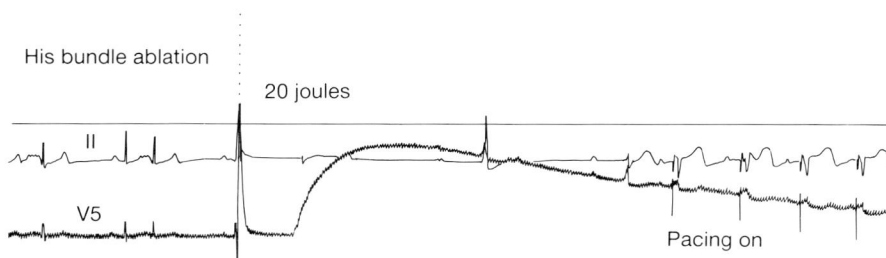

His bundle ablation

20 joules

II

V5

Pacing on

Fig. 22.16 A DC shock of 20 J is delivered synchronous with the QRS complex and between the distal electrode of the His bundle catheter and a back plate resulting in complete heart block. Two escape beats follow before temporary ventricular pacing is established.

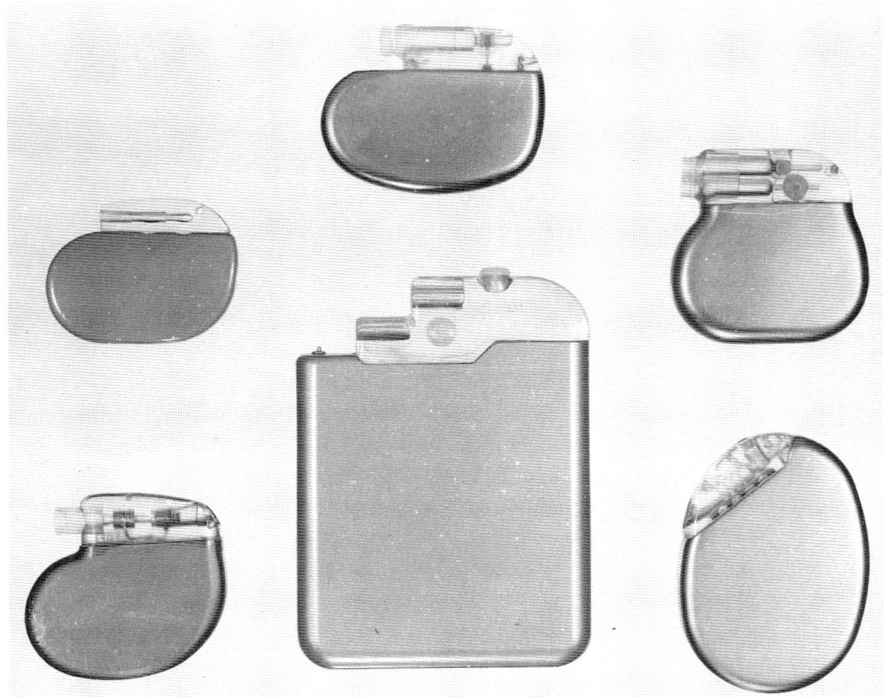

Fig. 22.17 A selection of permanent implantable pulse generators is illustrated. Clockwise from the top is shown a standard multiprogrammable single-chamber pacemaker, a software pacemaker, a dual-chamber pacemaker, an antitachycardia pacemaker and an ultra-small single chamber pacemaker. In the centre is an automatic implantable cardioverter/defibrillator (AICD).

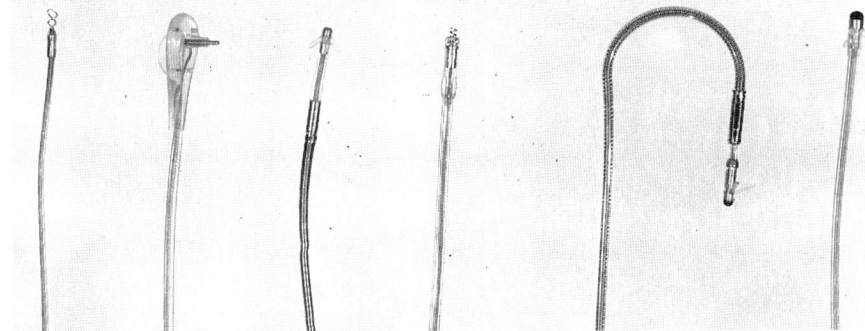

Fig. 22.18 The distal electrodes of a variety of permanent pacing leads are shown. From the left are seen a helical active fixation lead, an epi-myocardial lead, a passive fixation tined bipolar lead, an active fixation 'corkscrew' lead, a passive fixation tined bipolar atrial J-lead and a passive fixation tined carbon tip lead.

nology has allowed the manufacture of leads that will remain functioning for the duration of most pacemaker patients lives (Fig. 22.18).

Not surprisingly, in view of the burgeoning sophistication of pacing units, the choice facing the clinician is often bewildering. Not only are there many devices with similar specifications but in addition, interest in adapting the pacing rate to physiological conditions has produced a multitude of different rate-responsive pacemakers. A conse-

quence of this expansion has been to result in a subspeciality that is poorly understood by many cardiologists and ancillary staff involved in the care of cardiac patients. This has accelerated the need for training and education programmes for those involved in cardiac pacing.

Temporary restoration of the electrical activity of the heart in the setting of acute ventricular standstill or life-threatening bradycardia may be achieved in various ways. Drugs such as atropine, isoprenaline and adrenaline can accelerate or initiate cardiac rhythm. A chest wall thump or direct mechanical stimulation can excite the heart albeit briefly. However electrical stimulation offers the safest and most effective method of re-establishing cardiac contraction either temporarily or permanently. In the acute situation it is possible to pace the ventricles by high voltage chest wall stimulation (27), via pacing needles inserted directly into the myocardium through the chest wall or by oesophageal stimulation. This section will only consider pervenous techniques for cardiac stimulation.

Temporary pacing

BRADYCARDIA

In many circumstances the need for temporary pacing is obvious: generally those patients with arrhythmias producing severe symptoms (dizziness or Stokes—Adams attacks) associated with bradycardia and in whom permanent pacing cannot be immediately undertaken (Table 22.2). In these patients temporary pacing is generally a prelude to imminent permanent pacing and venous access should be gained at some site other than that intended for permanent pacemaker implantation.

In rare instances temporary pacing is warranted as a prophylactic measure because some transient procedure may render a patient at risk from advanced heart block. A well-established indication is when undertaking right heart catheterisation in the presence of left bundle branch block. More frequently patients with conduction system disease undergoing general anaesthesia require temporary pacing, although the indication and requirement are less clear-cut. Patients with atrial fibrillation and underlying sick sinus syndrome who are being car-

Table 22.2 Indication for temporary pacing.

Bradycardia:	Symptomatic heart block
	Prophylactic right heart catheterisation in LBBB
	Risk of heart block during general anaesthesia
	Cardioversion of atrial fibrillation in sick sinus syndrome
Tachycardia:	Paroxysmal supraventricular tachycardia
	Atrial flutter
	Torsade de pointes
	Paroxysmal ventricular tachycardia

dioverted may not have a satisfactory sinus rate after cardioversion and may be more satisfactorily managed by temporary pacing. This not only protects against extreme bradycardia and provides an adequate cardiac output should the rate be slow but also, as the atria are excessively irritable in the presence of pronounced bradycardia, this may help to prevent immediate recurrence of atrial fibrillation.

TACHYCARDIA

There are a variety of tachycardias that can be managed by temporary pacing. Paroxysmal supraventricular tachycardia can almost always be terminated by atrial overdrive pacing and is of particular value when the tachycardia is associated with sinus node disease, a situation in which intravenous drugs might terminate the tachycardia but exacerbate the bradycardia. Atrial flutter can frequently be terminated by rapid atrial pacing, a therapeutic option of particular value immediately after cardiac surgery if temporary atrial pacing wires are attached (Fig. 22.19).

Temporary pacing may be invaluable for the control of life-threatening ventricular arrhythmias. It is the treatment of choice for recurrent episodes of torsade de pointes. Increasing the heart rate, prefer-

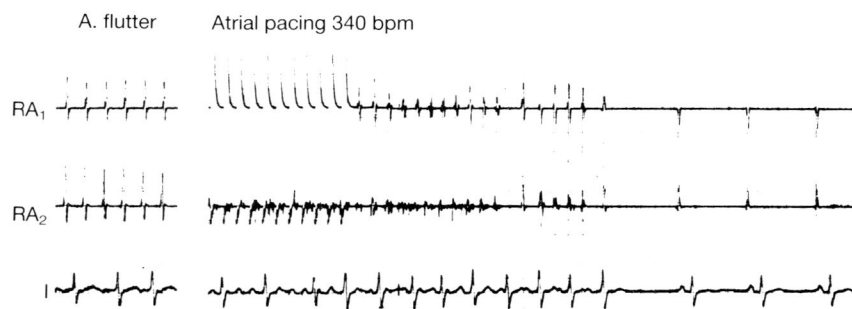

Fig. 22.19 Burst pacing for the termination of atrial flutter. The left hand panel shows atrial flutter with variable AV conduction. Following a period of rapid atrial pacing (340 bpm) atrial activity becomes disorganised but is not supported and sinus rhythm ensues.

ably by atrial pacing but by ventricular pacing if this is not possible, will shorten the QT interval and lower the susceptibility to these unusual arrhythmias which occur in the setting of QT prolongation (Fig. 22.20). Similar modes of preventative pacing also may be useful in the more common monomorphic ventricular tachycardia but if not successful rapid burst overdrive ventricular pacing is usually effective for control of repetitive attacks until some more permanent means of control can be instituted.

EQUIPMENT AND PROCEDURE

Temporary pacing catheters are generally positioned with fluoroscopy although this is not essential. Mobile X-ray machines are preferable so that screening can be performed using a suitable critical care bed.

A selection of temporary pacing catheters should always be available as well as a variety of suitable introducer sets. The satisfactory functioning of the external generator should be checked beforehand.

The route used for venous access depends upon the experience of the operator, the anatomy of the patient, the desired site of pacing, the duration of temporary pacing and the likelihood of imminent permanent pacing. As with other catheterisation procedures full aseptic conditions should be observed.

The infraclavicular approach to the subclavian vein is perhaps the most commonly used site of access. Positioning of the electrodes is relatively straightforward and with the system *in situ* the patient can remain ambulant. In inexperienced hands there is, however, a significant complication rate including pneumothorax, haemothorax, air embolism and trauma to major vessels and nerves. Internal and external jugular veins may be used although both require the patient to be tilted head-down or at least lying

prone if air embolism is to be avoided. Using the forearm veins by cut-down is probably less traumatic to the patient but positioning catheters in the heart by this route can be very difficult. The course the catheter must take is long and may be tortuous, and at a number of sites the vein may be prone to spasm increasing the difficulty of torque control. The femoral vein is the least desirable site for anything but the briefest period of temporary pacing. Ambulation is very difficult and the risk of infection if left for any length of time is high. It is however the preferred site for access to different parts of the right atrium when terminating atrial flutter by overdrive pacing.

The majority of pacing catheters are preshaped and are constructed with adequate torque control. A few specialised catheters, such as some atrial J-shaped leads, also have stylets to aid positioning. Once positioned in a peripheral vein, the catheter should be advanced under fluoroscopic control to the right atrium and from here to the chosen site. For ventricular pacing the apex of the right ventricle is the preferred site and the threshold for pacing should be lower than 1 V.

Temporary pacing electrodes use a bipolar configuration and although the threshold of stimulation will be lower if the distal electrode is used as the cathode, in practice the respective polarity of the connections makes little difference. If the acute pacing threshold is higher than 1 V every effort should be made to reposition the electrode to find a more suitable site. The threshold can be expected to increase appreciably within a few days using temporary pacing catheters and, if not low when inserted, capture may be lost after only a few days, even when the maximum output of the pacing unit is selected. Atrial pacing is most reliably achieved by positioning the electrode tip in the right atrial appendage. When placed in this anterior structure the tip of the catheter will describe a horizontal

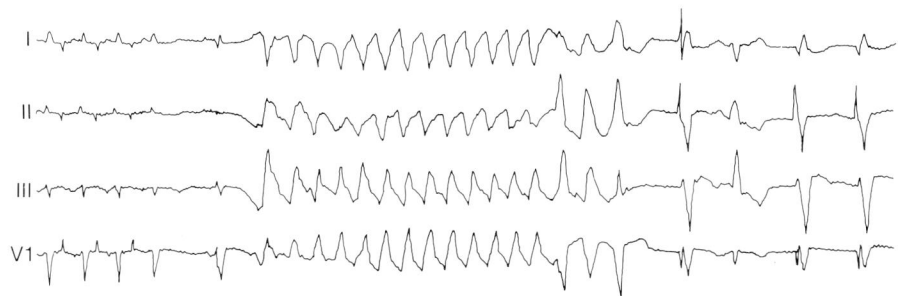

Fig. 22.20 In a patient with episodes of torsade de pointes due to hypokalemia the QT interval is maintained short, and the patient free of arrhythmia, by rapid atrial pacing at 135 bpm, seen in the first four QRS complexes. At this point pacing is discontinued and the first postpacing sinus beat shows massive QT prolongation and the spontaneous appearance of non-sustained polymorphous ventricular tachycardia.

figure-of-eight movement with each cardiac cycle. For reliable atrial pacing in the ambulant patient a J-shaped electrode should be inroduced from a superior vein, using a stylet if available, to straighten the electrode, and withdrawing it once the tip is in the right atrium so that the catheter adopts its J-shape with the tip falling into the appendage. Correctly positioned the acute pacing threshold should be less than 1 V. It is possible to pace the right atrium with standard pacing catheters designed for the ventricle but they usually require the formation of a loop in order to make adequate contact with the atrial wall with the result that they tend to displace easily.

When heart block complicates acute myocardial infarction there may be some benefit from providing optimal haemodynamic support with AV sequential or physiological pacing. Various other conditions have been identified, particularly with regard to permanent pacing, when the atrial contribution to ventricular filling is desirable and these conditions may warrant temporary physiological pacing. Several manufacturers have systems available for temporary dual-chamber pacing. One design consists of a single shaft with a number of proximal electrodes which make contact with the atrial wall when the distal tip lies in the right ventricular apex (Fig. 22.21). Reliable sensing and low stimulation thresholds are, in our experience, rarely maintained for more than a few days. An alternative design consists of a single introducer with two apertures through which separate small diameter atrial and ventricular pacing leads can be positioned individually.

X-ray screening is not essential for positioning temporary pacing leads although it is not recommended that these other techniques should be used except in emergencies when either no fluoroscopy facilities are available or the delay in moving the patient to them would be unacceptable. These techniques also require a degree of familiarity and expertise that can only be gained by experience of placing temporary pacing catheters under fluoroscopic control. They depend upon blindly advancing the catheter via the site of venous access and either using electrogram recording or stimulation to verify that the tip is in the desired location.

When there is spontaneous cardiac activity the catheter can be advanced while monitoring the sensed signal from the pacing electrodes. This can best be performed using an intracardiac amplifier as

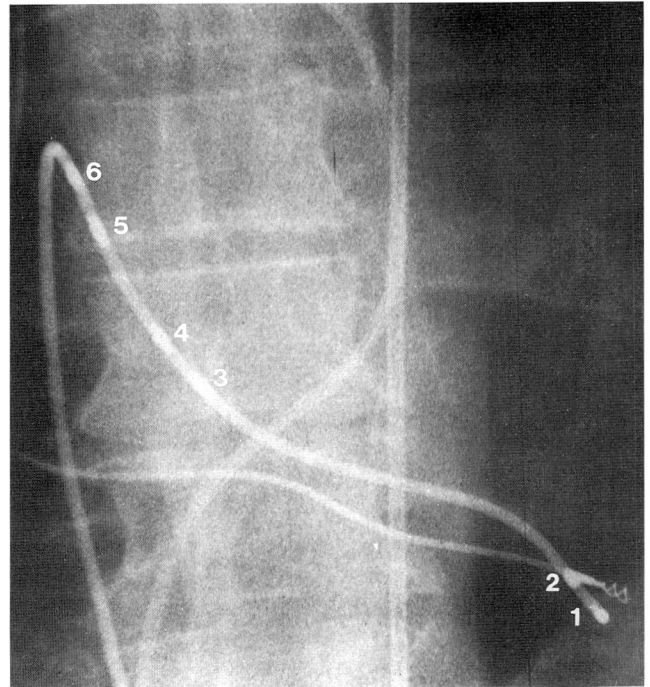

Fig. 22.21 Use of a multipolar electrode catheter for temporary dual-chamber pacing. The tip of the Helifix permanent pacing lead is seen at the apex of the right ventricle. The tip of a temporary hexapolar catheter has also been positioned at the apex of the right ventricle and the distal bipole (electrodes 1 and 2) used for ventricular pacing. When the tip is at the right ventricular apex the proximal 4 electrodes (3–6) are in contact with the atrial wall and can be used for atrial sensing and/or pacing.

used during electrophysiological study. An alternative method is to use a standard, preferably multichannel, ECG machine. As mentioned previously it is imperative that any ECG machines used in this fashion are tested electrically at regular intervals to ensure that it is safe to connect to an intracardiac electrode. The pacing lead can be monitored either in a unipolar or bipolar configuration. In the unipolar mode the distal tip electrode is connected to a V-lead and the appropriate lead recorded. In the bipolar mode the distal electrode is connected to the right-arm cable, the proximal electrode to the left-arm cable and lead-I monitored.

As the catheter is advanced towards the heart the cardiac electrical activity will increase in amplitude, ventricular activity almost always being evident, especially with the unipolar mode of recording. When the electrode(s) are within the right atrium, right atrial activity will be recorded coincident with surface

P waves. Further advancement into the ventricle will result in loss of atrial activity and increased amplitude of the ventricular signal. Once it is felt that the electrode tip has met resistance the electrodes should be connected to a stimulator to ensure an adequate pacing threshold. If not, further manipulation should be performed until a satisfactory threshold is found. Should an atrial component persist while the ventricular component increases, and the pacing threshold remain high it is likely that the catheter has been positioned in the coronary sinus. When a satisfactory electrical position has been obtained it is prudent to obtain a chest X-ray to ensure that the catheter is also in a satisfactory anatomical position. If difficulty is experienced in advancing the catheter tip to the right ventricle a balloon-tipped catheter may be used to float the tip in the venous stream across the tricuspid valve.

This form of 'monitoring-positioning' is only feasible if the intrinsic heart rate is sufficient to support the circulation. When there is an inadequate rate the pacing lead can be positioned while connected to an external pacing unit which has been set to an adequate rate and the maximum output. In this manner cardiac excitation will be seen immediately the electrodes contact ventricular (or atrial) myocardium.

Carefully positioned at the apex of the right ventricle with a low stimulation threshold under careful aseptic conditions and carefully secured a temporary pacing system should continue to function for at least a week. It is essential that the pacing threshold and the adequacy of the batteries in the stimulator are checked daily. One aspect of the system that is frequently overlooked is the pacing lead-external pacemaker connection. A variety of external pacing boxes are available, some carried by the patient, some strapped to the patient's arm and some requiring interconnecting cables, some connecting directly. Whatever the system these connectors must be included in the daily check and if possible the connection between the pacing lead and the pacemakers made such that should the pacing unit fall the connector given way rather than dragging the catheter out of the patient.

Permanent pacing

The indications for insertion of permanent pacemakers have been clarified in a number of recent publications [28]. These resulted from advances in the understanding of those patients who would benefit from pacing but also the suggestion that in some instances pacemakers had been implanted unnecessarily. Intriguingly the rates of pacemaker implantation continue to differ dramatically from one country to another for reasons that are not entirely clear. Further differences in clinical practice are also evident in the decision regarding the type of pacemaker most suited to an individual patient. Although dual-chamber pacing followed shortly after the introduction of single-chamber permanent pacing the units were technically limited and largely fell into disuse. Advances in integrated circuitry have now allowed the generator to contain the necessary technological sophistication that makes dual chamber pacing safe and efficient. Currently, in the UK 12% of pacemakers implanted annually are dual chamber. There remain, however, a considerable number of patients in whom the atria do not provide an adequate signal for rate-responsiveness on exercise. The last 6 years has seen the introduction and expansion of single-chamber pacemakers that are able to increase the pacing rate in response to physical demand and a number of rate-responsive pacemakers are available for clinical use. The rate of use of these types of pacemaker already equals that of dual-chamber pacers and there is little doubt that they will exceed this, possibly accounting for as many as half of all implants.

EQUIPMENT AND PREOPERATIVE DECISIONS

In addition to the screening facilities that are essential to pacemaker implantation, the modern pacing laboratory requires complex and sophisticated technical back-up (Table 22.3).

Pacemaker implantation requires close collaboration between the physician undertaking the operation and the technical staff responsible for making the technical measurements and any necessary

Table 22.3 Equipment for permanent pacing.

ECG monitor
Intracardiac ECG — three channel ECG machine
Pacing system analysers
Selection of pacemakers and leads
Appropriate programmers

adjustment to the pulse generator. In an individual patient this must begin with a decision regarding the type of pacemaker that should ideally be implanted, with the understanding that difficulties during the procedure may make it impossible to implant a more sophisticated unit. Alternative generators and leads should always be available at short notice.

Most pacemaker implants can be performed under local anaesthetic; however, the procedure is uncomfortable and may be frightening to many and all but exceptional cases require modest to heavy sedation. For routine single-chamber pacemaker implants antibiotics are unnecessary. They should be used routinely when there is a risk of endocarditis and probably are of value given intraoperatively when the procedure is prolonged beyond 2 hours.

PROCEDURE

Pacemaker implantation requires the highest possible level of operative sterility. Infection is the single most serious complication and if a pacemaker becomes infected it is all but impossible to eradicate the infection without removal of the pacing system. However, with the progressive and now almost total move from the epicardial to endocardial route for routine pacemaker implantation few institutions can afford a separate fully sterile operating theatre with radiological facilities. Most institutions use a catheterisation laboratory which undertakes routine cardiac catheterisation as well as pacemaker implantation. Every effort must be made to attain sterile conditions. The experience and speed of the operator is probably the most important factor in preventing infection, but awareness by other laboratory staff of the need for sterility as well as undertaking pacemaker implants as the first procedure of the day's list also contribute to lower infection rates.

The subclavian vein is the most common route for venous access and it may be reached by direct puncture or indirectly through the cephalic vein. Few physicians nowadays implant preferentially through the jugular vein as the pacing lead has to bend acutely to traverse downwards and is liable to skin erosion as it lies superficially over the clavicle. The infraclavciular approach allows both the lead and generator to be inserted through a single incision. The cephalic vein lies in the deltopectoral groove

and with experience can be identified and isolated in little more than the time it takes to puncture the subclavian vein. When found, the cephalic vein is suitable for single-lead placement in 80% of cases and for two leads in 50%. Frequently a neurovascular bundle traverses the cephalic vein, its nature obvious from the arterial pulsation, and may rarely require division. The cephalic vein may lie under the lateral edge of pectorals and may not be immediately obvious. When the cephalic vein is seen as a plexus in the deltopectoral grove, it will rarely be satisfactory for lead placement and the direct subclavian approach must be used.

The cephalic vein approach is preferred predominantly because of the lower complication rate (see under temporary pacing) compared to direct puncture. However, when two leads are used the cephalic vein may only be large enough for one and the subclavian route needed for the other. When two leads can be placed in the cephalic vein it may be difficult to manipulate each lead independently especially if they are silicone leads — polyurethane leads are more suitable because their smoother surface allows them to slide against each other. If leads are to be used via the cephalic and subclavian routes it is preferable to puncture the subclavian vein first for fear of lacerating the cephalic lead with the needle. However, if the cephalic lead has been introduced it does aid subclavian puncture as screening the lead will show the location of the vein. Similarly if the cephalic vein cannot be used and difficulty is experienced locating the subclavian vein, injection of contrast into an ipsilateral arm vein will demonstrate its position. Alternatively it will demonstrate that puncture has failed because the vein is thrombosed.

The 'feel' of permanent pacing leads is quite unlike the leads used for temporary pacing. They are soft and impossible to manipulate unaided. A straight stylet is provided which passes through the central channel in the wound-wire conductor to stiffen the lead; the stylet can be shaped to the desired curve in order to help negotiate the tip of the lead through the venous system. A straight stylet is preferable for positioning the tip at the apex of the right ventricle but when straight it may be difficult to negotiate the tip through the tricuspid valve — the straightened lead tends to go into the IVC. If the stylet is withdrawn several inches the lead tip may now curve towards the ventricle as it floats more freely in the blood stream and with further advancing of both wire and stylet may pass across the valve. Clockwise rotation during this manoeuvre may help. If unsuccessful the stylet should be shaped with the largest radius curve possible over the last 5—7.5 cm (2—3 in) to allow the valve to be crossed. A gentle curve will aid passage of the tip down to the right ventricular apex rather than up towards the outflow tract which tends to occur if the curve of the stylet is too severe. Alternatively once across the valve the stylet can be exchanged for a straight version (usually two are supplied). It has often been suggested that the tip of the lead should be advanced to the outflow tract and then pulled back to allow the tip to fall into the apex of the right of the right ventricle. Such manoeuvres are more appropriate to the older type of non-fixation electrode which are now seldom used. Fixation electrodes do not require such precise positioning at the apex as was essential with non-fixation leads, although the apical position adds a further insurance against displacement.

Once the lead tip has reached a satisfactory radiographic position the contact and stability of the lead should be assessed. This is tested mechanically and after the stylet has been withdrawn. The wire should be pulled gently and the restraining effect of the tip lodged in the ventricular myocardium will be felt when it is satisfactorily positioned. Contact with the myocardium is assessed electrically and is measured both in terms of the electrical signal from the heart 'seen' by the electrode and the threshold for myocardial excitation.

The electrogram recorded by the lead must be of adequate amplitude for correct pacemaker sensing. A signal of at least 2 mV is generally required for ventricular sensing and an R wave of at least 5 mV should be obtained at implant. Not only should the amplitude be sufficient but the character of the signal should be 'matched' to the sensing amplifier of the pacemaker. In order to limit sensing of other unwanted signals (e.g. T waves) the amplifier senses signals with a rapid rise time (slew-rate) which should be at least 1 mV/msec. The amplitude can be measured with a pacing systems analyser but the integrity of electrical contact with the myocardium is measured by recording a unipolar electrogram from the tip electrode. When the tip is satisfactorily positioned a contact electrogram will be recorded showing at least 5 mV S-T segment elevation. If there is a marked biphasic pattern to the unipolar elec-

trogram the tip may have perforated the ventricle and should be withdrawn and repositioned.

Electrical contact is also assessed by measuring the pacing threshold. The pacing threshold must be low at implant to ensure that long term ventricular capture within the limited output of the pacing generator can be assured. The threshold will always rise in the first few weeks following implant, will then fall and usually increase again, stabilising at two to three times above the implant value. If the initial value is high the threshold may increase above the output of the generator soon after implant. But equally importantly the pacing rate is designed to fall as the battery capacity runs down towards its end-of-life. This indicates, when the rate falls to a specified value, that the generator requires replacement. However, this rate decline is the response to a decline in the output and if the pacing threshold lies just below the nominal output of the generator ventricular capture will be lost before the warning decline in pacing rate has been reached. This problem has been largely circumvented in modern pacemakers which incorporate threshold measuring circuitry within their programming features so that the chronic threshold can be followed and the output maintained at least 100% above the pacing threshold.

When measuring the threshold with a unipolar lead it is important to use an indifferent electrode (anode) which matches that of the permanent pacemaker. Special metal disks are available that can be placed in the pacemaker pocket. With modern fixation electrodes the pacing threshold should always be below 1.0 V and is usually below 0.5 V when using a stimulus with a pulse width of 0.5 msec. This threshold is dependent on the width of pulse used and may increase sharply at lower pulse widths. As the permanent pacemaker uses pulses of 0.5 msec as the standard setting it should be assured that the pacing threshold is satisfactorily low at much shorter pulse width than the standard setting. We measure the pacing threshold at 0.1, 0.5 and 1.0 msec and ensure that the threshold at the lower pulse width does not exceed twice the value at the other settings. A number of other measurements should be made before accepting the position as satisfactory. Beat to beat stability of electrical contact is reflected in the current drawn with each impulse in a constant voltage pacemaker and any variability should be less than 1 mA, when using an output of 5 V and 0.5 msec.

The tip of a pacing lead placed near the right ventricular apex may lie on the inferior wall adjacent to the diaphragm. In some instance this results in diaphragmatic as well as myocardial stimulation. When this occurs with pulses of 5 V the lead must be repositioned. We also increase the output of the pacemaker system analyser to 10 V to ensure that the diaphragm is not stimulated at this higher output, which is available in some pacemakers and may be used if the chronic threshold rises so that capture is lost at lower outputs.

Once a satisfactory position for the lead tip has been established the course of the lead should be checked radiographically to ensure that it lies satisfactorily in the floor of the right ventricle and in the right atrium. The lead should be seen to 'buckle' slightly against the tricuspid valve and have enough 'slack' in the right atrium such that the tip is not pulled when the patient inspires, coughs or stands up. Alternatively there should not be an excessive length of lead in the atrium that might loop into the IVC or outflow tract and dislodge the tip.

There may be a number of reasons for the apex of the right ventricle being an unsatisfactory position for the lead tip. This area may be infarcted or fibrosed and the threshold for pacing unsatisfactorily high. With fixation electrodes, particularly the active variety, other sites can be used. The septum or outflow tract are the usual alternatives and can be paced satisfactorily. When using an activation fixation electrode it is prudent to wait several minutes if the initial threshold immediately after placement is high, as it often falls to acceptable levels.

Once a satisfactory endocardial position has been established the paced ECG should be recorded, preferably on a multichannel ECG machine. If there is retrograde atrial depolarisation the patient is at considerable risk of symptoms of the pacemaker syndrome and a dual-chamber pacing system should be considered. The QRS morphology of the paced beats should also be scrutinised to ensure that the expected pattern is seen. Unusual patterns, such as a paced QRS showing a RBBB pattern should alert the operator to the possibility that the lead has been placed in the coronary vein or has perforated the right ventricle and is pacing the left ventricle.

When the intravascular part of the lead is satisfactory the lead should be secured as soon as possible after it emerges from the vein. A silicone sleeve is generally provided to protect the lead insulation from the direct pressure of the securing stitch and should always be used with polyurethane leads, which are more susceptible to lead fracture if secured directly. This sleeve should be secured away from the area immediately below the skin incision: its bulk can lead to erosion of the skin; particularly in the individual with little adipose tissue.

Prior to final connection of the full system a check on the pacing generator should be performed. With programmable pacers this can be achieved by using the programmer to verify that it is set to its nominal values, or these changed to selected values. Non-programmable units should be checked by connecting to the pacing systems analyser and ensuring that the unit is producing pulses of the correct amplitude and pulse width.

Dual-chamber pacing

Two leads are generally required for dual-chamber pacing although leads have been produced in which atrial sensing electrodes are mounted proximally on a ventricular lead. When two leads are to be used in a new system both should be inserted into the venous system before positioning. If the cephalic vein is large it may take both leads. Alternatively both can be inserted via the subclavian vein. In the latter case a single puncture, double introducer technique can be used although bleeding from the puncture site and haemothorax have been described.

For the atrium fixation electrodes are essential. When there is an atrial appendage — it has usually been amputated if the patient has had previous cardiopulmonary bypass — a tined J-shaped lead is generally satisfactory. When this site cannot be used an active fixation lead with or without a J-shape will be required. These can usually be positioned at any site on the anterior or lateral atrial wall. The atrial lead should always be positioned after the ventricular lead. When the tip of the atrial lead is in the atrial appendage it has characteristic horizontal figure-of-eight movement on fluoroscopy. This position in the atrial appendage, which is anterior is generally quite obvious on anteroposterior screening, but if in doubt, screening in the RAO projection will confirm the location.

The method of positioning the atrial electrode depends on the type of lead used. With J-shaped leads a straight stylet should be used to straighten the lead and guide the tip of the electrode to the IVC or low atrium. Then whilst withdrawing the lead and at the same time withdrawing the stylet from within the lead the tip will be seen to curl upwards, the lead being rotated if necessary to turn the tip anteriorly towards the appendage. When the tip is caught in the atrial wall the characteristic movement will seen and the J-shape begin to straighten if the lead is retracted further. The straight stylet can then be exchanged for a J-shaped stylet which can be used, with small but firm tugs on the stylet and lead, to embed the lead fully into the atrial wall. If a straight, ventricular-style lead is to be used in the atrium a similar technique using only the J-shaped stylet can be employed.

When in a satisfactory radiographic position the same techniques described for ventricular lead assessment are used although differences in the values obtained will be seen. The amplitude of the electrogram will be smaller but a site producing an electrogram of at least 2 mV should be sought. Similarly the degree of injury current will be less than is seen with the ventricular lead. The pacing threshold is usually higher than with ventricular leads but should always be less than 1 V.

Antitachycardia pacing

Electrophysiological investigation has shown that most paroxysmal supraventricular tachycardias and many cases of ventricular tachycardia can be terminated by premature stimulation. Special pacemakers have been designed that can automatically detect the onset of paroxysmal tachycardia and stimulate the heart until the arrhythmia is terminated. Sophisticated software pacemakers are available for the treatment of supraventricular tachycardia that have a vast array of termination algorithms such that almost all cases of paroxysmal supraventricular tachycardia are amenable. The earliest automatic devices were crude in their ability to distinguish paroxysmal tachycardia from sinus tachycardia and although modern units are more complex this still remains their major deficiency.

As rapid overdrive pacing is the most usual mode of stimulation for terminating paroxysmal supraventricular tachycardia atrial pacing is used exclusively, ventricular pacing having been abandoned. Bipolar pacing leads are essential in order that rate sensing is accurate — a unipolar atrial lead may well sense ventricular in addition to atrial activity and lead to inaccurate rate counting. The atrial appendage is the most satisfactory site but active fixation electrodes allow almost any atrial site to be used. In addition to the electrical measurements described for atrial leads used in dual-chamber pacemakers the sensed electrogram should be examined both in sinus rhythm as well as during tachycardia to ensure that far-field ventricular activity is not recorded.

Although overdrive ventricular pacing will terminate most episodes of sustained monomorphic ventricular tachycardia it is associated with a high incidence of tachycardia acceleration and induction of ventricular fibrillation. Therefore the risk of implantable automatic antitachycardia pacemakers is too high to consider them as a longterm option in most patients. However, such antitachycardia devices may well become incorporated into units that are able to automatically defibrillate the heart. The automatic implantable cardioverter/defibrillator senses the onset of vetricular tachycardia or ventricular fibrillation by analysing the rate and morphology of electrical acitivity sensed by a bipolar sensing lead and two epicardial patches. The patches are also used for delivering one or more shocks (25–38 J) which are capable of converting ventricular tachycardia or ventricular fibrillation [29]. Such devices offer the possibility of improving the prognosis in patients with life-threatening ventricular arrhythmias, an ideal which may not be possible with drugs or surgery.

REFERENCES

1 Josephson ME, Seides SF. *Clinical cardiac electrophysiology. Techniques and interpretations.* Philadelphia, Lea and Febiger, 1979;28.

2 Sung RJ, Tamer DM, Garcia OL *et al.* Analysis of surgically induced right bundle branch block pattern using intracardiac recording techniques. *Circulation* 1976;**54**: 422–6.

3 Mandell W, Hayakawa H, Danzig R, Marcus HS. Evaluation of sinoatrial function in man by overdrive suppression. *Circulation* 1971;**44**:59–65.

4 Benditt DG, Strauss HC, Scheinmann MM *et al.* Analysis of secondary pauses following termination of rapid atrial pacing in man. *Circulation* 1976;**54**:436–40.

5 Strauss HC, Saroff AL, Bigger JT, Giardina EGV. Premature atrial stimulation as a key to the understanding of sinoatrial conduction in man. *Circulation* 1973; **58**:86.

6 Narula OS *et al.* A new method for measurement of sinoatrial conduction time. *Circulation* 1978;**58**:706.

7 Reiffel JA *et al.* The human sinus node electrogram. A transvenous catheter technique and a comparison of directly measured and indirectly estimated sinoatrial conduction time in adults. *Circulation* 1980;**62**:1324.

8 Heddle WF, Jones ME, Tonkin AM. Sinus node sequences after atrial stimulation: similarities of effects of different methods. *Br Heart J* 1985;**54**:568–76.

9 Strasberg B, Amat-y-Leon F, Dhingra RC *et al.* Natural history of chronic second degree atrioventricular nodal block. *Circulation* 1981;**63**:1043–9.

10 Shaw DB, Kekwick CA, Veale D, Gowers J, Whistance T. Survival in second degree atrioventricular block. *Br Heart J* 1985;**53**:587–93.

11 Scheinman MM, Peters RW, Morady F *et al.* Electrophysiologic studies in patients with hundle branch block. PACE 1983;**6**:1157.

12 McAnulty JH, Rahimtoola SH, Murphy E *et al.* Natural history of 'high risk' bundle branch block: final report of a prospective study. *N Engl J Med* 1982;**307**:137.

13 Dhingra RC, Palileo E, Strasberg B *et al.* Significance of the HV interval in 517 patients with chronic bifascicular block. *Circulation* 1981;**64**:1265.

14 Ezri M, Lerman BB, Marchlinski FE *et al.* Electrophysiologic evaluation of syncope in patients with bifascicular block. *Am Heart J* 1983;**106**:693–9.

15 Wu D, Denes P, Amat-y-Leon F *et al.* Clinical, electrocardiographic and electrophysiologic observations in patients with paroxysmal supraventricular tachycardia. *Am J Cardiol* 1978;**41**:1045.

16 Wellens HJJ. Value and limitations of programmed electrical stimulation of the heart in the study and treatment of tachycardias. *Circulation* 1978;**57**:845.

17 Akhtar M, Damato AN, Ruskin JN *et al.* Antegrade and retrograde conduction characteristics in three patterns of paroxysmal atrioventricular junctional reentrant tachycardia. *Am Heart J* 1978;**95**:22.

18 Barold S, Coumel P. Concealed preexcitation. *Am J Cardiol* 1978;**41**:937.

19 Coumel P, Attuel P. Reciprocating tachycardia in overt and latent preexcitation: influence of bundle branch block on the rate of the tachycardia. *Eur Heart J* 1974; **4**:293.

20 Brugada P, Farre J, Green M *et al.* Observations in patients with supraventricular tachycardia having a PR interval shorter than the RP interval. Differentiation between atrial tachycardia and a circus-movement tachycardia using an accessory pathway. *Am Heart J* 1984;**107**:556.

21 Bardy GH, Packer DL, German LD, Gallagher JJ. Preexcited reciprocating tachycardia in patients with Wolff-Parkinson-White syndrome: Incidence and mechanisms. *Circulation* 1981;**70**:377.

22 Gallagher JJ. Variance of preexcitation: update 1984. In: Zipes DP Jalife J, eds. *Cardiac electrophysiology, and arrhythmias.* New York, Grune & Stratton, 1985; 419–33.

23 Mason JW, Anderson KP, Freedman RA. Techniques and criteria in electrophysiologic study of ventricular tachycardia. *Circulation* 1987;**75**(III):125–30.

24 Evans GT, Scheinmann MM, Zipes DP *et al.* The percutaneous cardiac mapping and ablation registry: summary of results. PACE 1987;**10**:1395–99.

25 Rowland E, Cunningham AD, Ahsan A, Rickards AF. Catheter ablation of AV conduction using a new power source. *Br Heart J* (in press).

26 Fisher J, Soo K, Matos J *et al.* Complications of catheter ablation of tachyarrhythmias: occurrence, protection, prevention. *Clin Prog Electrophysiol Pacing* 1985;**3**:292–8.

27 Zoll PM *et al.* External non-invasive temporary cardiac pacing: clinical trials. *Circulation* 1985;**71**:937.

28 American College of Cardiology/American Heart Association Task Force on Assessment of Cardiovascular Procedures (Subcommittee on Pacemaker Implantation). Guidelines for permanent cardiac pacemaker implantation May 1984. *J Am Coll Cardiol* 1984;**4**:434 and *Circulation* 1984;**70**:331A.

29 Mirowski M, Reid PR, Mower MM *et al.* Automatic implantable cardioverter-defibrillator: clinical results. *PACE* 1984;**7**:1345–50.

CHAPTER 23

The role of the catheterisation laboratory in heart and heart—lung transplantation

HEART TRANSPLANTATION

Introduction

Cardiac transplantation is now an accepted treatment for selected patients with end-stage heart disease in whom medical therapy or conventional cardiac surgery has failed or is inappropriate. The majority of patients undergoing cardiac transplantation have severe impairment of myocardial function as a result of coronary artery disease or a dilated cardiomyopathy (Table 23.1).

By 1987, 3623 heart transplant procedures had been reported worldwide to the International Heart Transplant Registry, 1415 of which were undertaken in 1986 [1] (Fig. 23.1). Numerous improvements in the management of the transplant patient have been responsible for the steady increase in patient survival following the procedure. Recipient selection is now the most important determinant of postoperative results; other important factors include the progress in surgical expertise which makes the operation itself relatively straightforward, the routine use of endomyocardial biopsy coupled with other non-invasive techniques to monitor allograft rejection, and the advent of more effective immunosuppressive protocols, particularly the addition of cyclosporine A in 1980.

Actuarial survival for all patients in the Registry

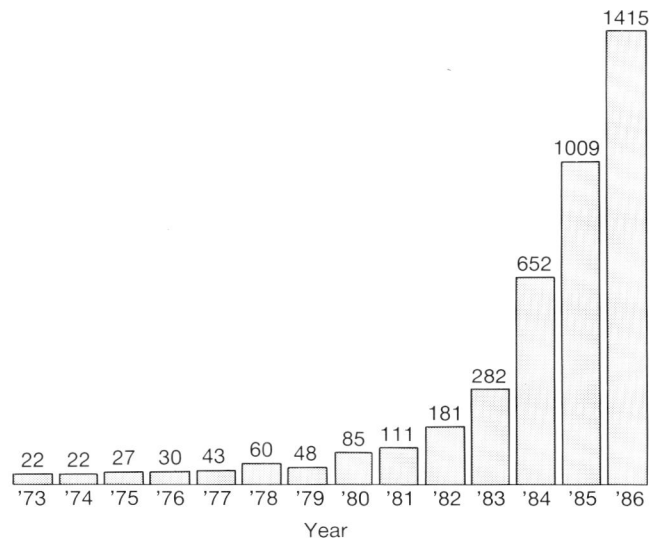

Fig. 23.1 Number of heart transplants worldwide (1973—1986) (redrawn with permission).

Table 23.1 Indications for cardiac transplantation.

Idiopathic dilated cardiomyopathy
Coronary artery disease with poor ventricular function
   (unsuitable for conventional surgery)
Valvular heart disease with poor ventricular function
Myocarditis unresponsive to immunosuppression
Cardiac tumours
Posttraumatic aneurysm

undergoing orthotopic and heterotopic heart transplantation is 76% at 1 year and 71.3% at 5 years which increases to 80.6% and 78.3% respectively for patients treated with cyclosporine [1]. These figures compare favourably with results of other solid organ transplants, for example liver and kidney, and are superior to the survival of many patients with malignant disease treated by surgery or chemotherapy. Early (30-day) mortality following cardiac transplantation has fallen from 16.8% in 1980 to 7.4% in 1986 [1].

With this reduction in early postoperative mortality, attention has turned to the medium and long-term function of the transplanted heart, both from the haemodynamic point of view (at rest and with exercise), and how function in the transplanted heart might be modified by denervation, episodes of rejection, and the immunosuppressive drugs themselves.

HAEMODYNAMICS AT REST

Many factors result in the haemodynamic profile of the transplanted heart differing from that seen in a normal subject. On a background of cardiac denervation must be added the effects of myocardial ischaemia at the time of transplantation, acute and chronic rejection, coronary artery disease, systemic hypertension — all common in transplant recipients together with possible toxicity of the immunosuppressive drugs, for example cyclosporine, on the myocardium.

Reinnervation has never been documented after orthotopic cardiac transplantation in humans [2], such that the donor heart rate does not respond to the Valsalva manoeuvre, amyl nitrate or atropine, and Holter monitoring shows a fixed RR interval without sinus arrhythmia. Adrenergic receptors remain intact however, with a normal haemodynamic response to exogenous catecholamines, β-blockade and the administration of glucagon.

In the first few days after transplantation, graft function is depressed as evidenced by a low cardiac output due mainly to a reduction in stroke volume; this effect is likely to relate to perioperative myocardial ischaemia rather than be due to an immune basis. By the fourth day however resting haemodynamics are essentially normal. Follow-up data from cardiac catheterisation undertaken 1 or more years after transplantation continue to indicate normal or near normal haemodynamics. Resting heart rate is higher than normal (80—100/min) reflecting cardiac denervation, right and left heart filling pressures are normal and cardiac output is in the low normal range [3]; furthermore, the inotropic state of transplant left ventricle as determined by load-independent indices is normal [4].

HAEMODYNAMICS WITH EXERCISE

Despite cardiac denervation, long-term transplant recipients demonstrate an adequate heart rate response to dynamic exercise. The time—rate relationship differs from normal subjects in that the resting heart rate is higher in the transplanted heart, peak heart rate is reached more gradually and the return to the pre-exercise heart rate occurs more slowly [5].

In contrast, the recipient P wave activity from the innervated sinus node accelerates rapidly reaching a peak within 2 minutes of the onset of exercise, with a rapid return to normal after the cessation of exercise. The initial increase in cardiac output associated with exercise is achieved by increased venous return secondary to muscular activity, subsequently cardiac output is further augmented by the increase in contractility and heart rate secondary to the rise in plasma catecholamines [5]. Exercise ejection fraction as determined by radionuclide angiography is normal, and there are some data suggesting that the use of cyclosporine (compared with conventional immunosuppression) favourably affects exercise ejection fraction although this finding has not been universal.

HAEMODYNAMIC CHANGES WITH REJECTION

Impaired haemodynamic function occurs late in the course of rejection and changes in systolic indices or contractility are not useful as a practical method of assessing rejection. The physiological effects of early rejection can be compared with myocardial restriction leading to an increase in venous pressure and a reduction in ventricular compliance. Untreated rejection in animal models results in impaired systolic function and systemic hypotension leading to death. In the long term, the number of rejection episodes does not seem to affect late graft function.

CARDIAC ALLOGRAFT SURVEILLANCE

Once it had been appreciated that graft failure occurred as a result of allograft rejection and that this process could be modified by immunosuppression, numerous investigators have studied methods of identifying rejection so that it might be promptly treated. Whereas episodes of acute rejection were a common cause of death in the early days of cardiac transplantation, recent experience indicates that death is more frequently related to side-effects of the immunosuppressive agents themselves (e.g. opportunistic infection, lymphoma). As a result, attempts have been made to minimise the immunosuppression, making allograft surveillance even more crucial.

Two broad approaches have been used in the assessment of allograft rejection: myocardial structure and function have been analysed either indirectly (e.g. electrocardiography, echocardiography, Doppler) or directly (endomyocardial biopsy); alternatively, immunological monitoring has been applied to the peripheral blood lymphocytes and more recently attention has turned to the identification of lymphocyte subsets within cardiac biopsy specimens.

ENDOMYOCARDIAL BIOPSY

Without a sensitive and specific method for the early detection of episodes of rejection, allograft rejection remained a major cause of mortality in the late 1960s and early 1970s. In view of the rapidly progressive nature of the rejection process in patients treated with conventional immunosuppression (prior to the advent of cyclosporine) and the fact the reduction in the ECG voltage (see below) was delayed 24—48 hours after histological evidence of rejection [6], a more reliable technique was needed.

In 1953, Casten [7] performed percutaneous needle biopsy of the moving heart in closed-chest dogs for the purpose of serial metabolic studies. This technique was applied to humans in 1956 [8], and despite the high complication rate, continued to be used clinically until the early 1970s. In 1962 Sakakibara and Konno from Japan reported a catheter technique for cardiac biopsy via the saphenous vein [9], and in 1972 Caves working in Stanford, using a percutaneous approach, modified the Sakakibara—Konno bioptome for use in cardiac transplant recipients [10]. This was perhaps the most significant advance in cardiac transplantation since the initial reports of Lower and Shumway some 11 years previously [11, 12].

Although endomyocardial biopsy is most frequently used in the diagnosis of rejection episodes in transplant recipients, the technique has been applied to many conditions (Table 23.2). Histological findings on biopsy may be specific and diagnostic (e.g. cardiac amyloidosis, adriamycin cardiotoxicity) or non-specific (e.g. cardiac muscle hypertrophy). Furthermore, serial endomyocardial biopsies are the only reliable method of monitoring the response of acute myocarditis to treatment with immunosuppression. In a series of 700 non-transplant biopsies, a firm conclusion, either by confirmation or exclusion of a clinical diagnosis was achieved in 60% of cases, and in 13% a new and unsuspected diagnosis was made on the basis of histology [13].

Table 23.2 Indications for endomyocardial biopsy.

Diagnosis of specific heart muscle disease
  Amyloid
  Carcinoid
  Eosinophilic heart disease
  Fabry's disease
  Glycogen storage diseases
  Haemochromatosis
  Hypertrophic cardiomyopathy
  Irradiation injury
  Myocarditis (including gaint cell myocarditis)
Monitoring cardiac allograft rejection
Monitoring adriamycin therapy

Procedures

There are three techniques for right ventricular endomyocardial biopsy in general use. The method developed by Caves *et al.* using the Stanford bioptome is the predominant technique used in the USA, whereas in Japan and elsewhere the Sakakibara—Konno technique is widely practiced. In the UK, the King's bioptome adapted from Olympus bronchoscopy forceps has its advocates and is now marketed by Cordis. No large scale comparisons of the three methods have been published, but there are some advantages of the Stanford bioptome, in particular the sample size is significantly larger than that obtained with other instruments and the bioptome can be re-used.

STANFORD BIOPTOME

The Stanford bioptome is 50 cm long and is usually introduced via the internal jugular or subclavian veins (Fig. 23.2). The short length improves ma-

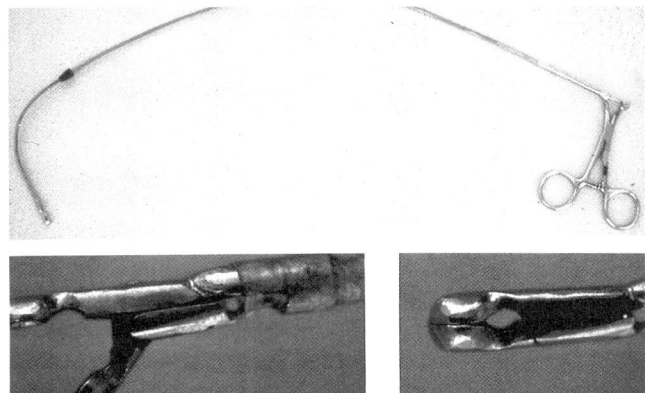

Fig. 23.2 Stanford bioptome.

noeverability and increases the mechanical efficiency of the closing mechanism, but make it unsuitable for the femoral approach. Two hemispherical jaws with an internal diameter of 2.5 mm are attached via a single hinge to a stiff drive wire which pushes the jaws closed and pulls them open via a handle at the operators end. The drive wire courses through a flexible metallic shaft which is covered in non-thrombogenic plastic. The distal end of the bioptome is curved in the same direction as the handle which allows the operator to steer the distal end of the device in a known direction.

An approach using the right internal jugular vein allows direct entry into the right ventricle with minimal manipulation of the bioptome, and without traversing any bends in the vasculature. The right internal jugular vein is entered percutaneously using a Seldinger technique in the standard fashion with the patient lying flat or in the head down (Trendelenburg) position. The head should be turned to the left and local anaesthetic is introduced into the skin 3 cm above the right clavicle between the two heads of the sternocleidomastoid muscle which can usually be identified by visual inspection. Occasionally the muscle is not visible, in which case it can be palpated if the patient lifts his head off the catheter table. After infiltration of the skin, a 21 gauge probe needle is introduced in a caudal direction 30° to the vertical via a small stab incision. With constant suction on a 10 ml syringe, the internal jugular vein is entered 0.65–2.5 cm (0.25–1 in) beneath the skin at which time blood can be drawn freely into the syringe. The needle is left *in situ*, and acts as a guide for the introduction of an 18 gauge thin-walled needle which is also advanced into the vein under constant suction. A short 0.038" diameter guide wire is then introduced through the thin-walled needle, and a 9F valved introducer and sheath is advanced over the wire.

The bioptome is inserted through the valve of the sheath with the jaws closed, and advanced under fluoroscopic control into the lower third of the right atrium with the tip directed to the right. The bioptome is then rotated so that the tip points to the left and passes through the tricuspid valve in the horizontal plane. Subsequent rotation posteromedially brings the tip of the bioptome into contact with the interventricular septum. Proper positioning of the bioptome can be visualised by fluoroscopy when the tip is seen to lie approximately

5 cm (2.5 in) to the left of the vertebral bodies and below the level of the left hemidiaphragm. In addition, ventricular premature beats are often apparent once the ventricle has been entered, and ventricular contraction may be appreciated via transmission through the bioptome to the operators hands. The bioptome is then withdrawn 1 cm (approx. 0.5 in) and the jaws opened; the instrument is then advanced once more with minimal force so that the open jaws lie against the apical portion of the interventricular septum, The jaws are then closed briskly, and the biopsy is removed with gentle traction. Occasionally more traction is required to separate the biopsy from the remaining myocardium, and rarely the biopsy cannot be separated in which case the jaws must be re-opened and an alternative site attempted. Usually between three and six biopsies are obtained and placed in fixative for histological examination by light and electron microscopy. Typically the procedure can be completed within 10–15 minutes, and the jugular approach can be used quite safely on an outpatient basis.

KING'S (CORDIS) BIOPTOME

The King's bioptome is manufactured by Cordis UK Ltd and is available in two lengths, 50 and 104 cm, and two diameters 5.3 and 7F (Fig. 23.3). The principle of right ventricular biopsy with this instrument is similar to that described with the Stanford bioptome. Using the shorter 50 cm bioptome, the right internal jugular vein is identified and entered as described previously. Whereas the curve of the Stanford bioptome can be bent into the desired shape by the operator, undue bending of the shaft of the Cordis bioptome (which is packaged straight), interferes with the opening and closing of the jaw mechanism. To circumvent this problem a long sheath technique is often used in conjuction with the bioptome. Cordis can supply a valved sheath (Fig. 23.4) and introducer set in two lengths (45 and 98 cm) and two sizes (7 and 8F), with either a straight tip or an angled tip. Using an angled tip, the sheath can be directed towards the septum, and the bioptome then advanced through the sheath to remove the biopsy. Alternatively, the 104 cm version of this bioptome can be used to biopsy the right ventricle via the right (or left) femoral vein. The vein is entered using a Seldinger approach (as described in Chapter

(a)

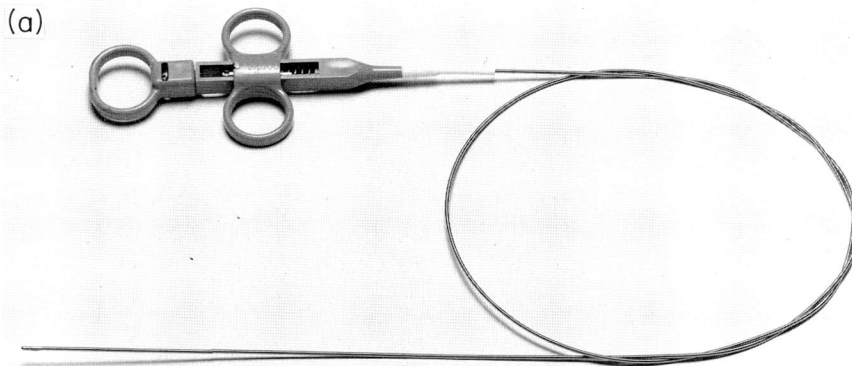

Fig. 23.3 (a) King's (Cordis) bioptome with (b) closed jaws, and (c) open jaws.

(b)

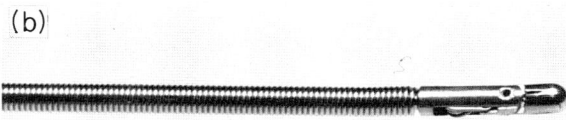

(c)

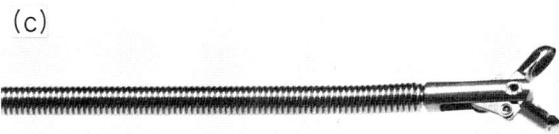

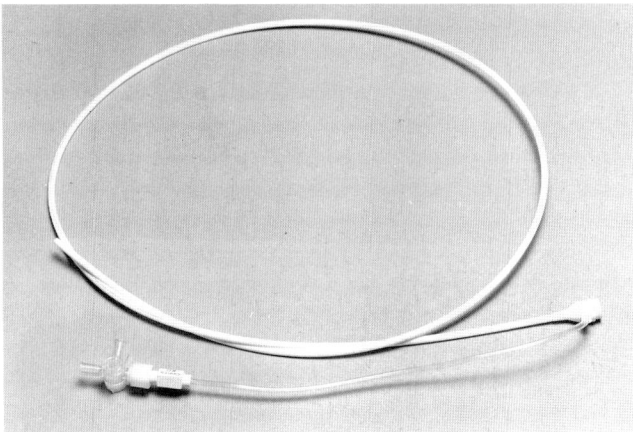

Fig. 23.4 Cordis valved sheath (98 cm).

3) and the long sheath advanced over a 0.038″ diameter guide wire into the right ventricle under fluoroscopic control. Because the sheath itself is made of a rather floppy construction with a tendency to fold, it is best supported with a standard 7 or 8F pigtail catheter which is advanced through the sheath prior to insertion, and then removed once the tip of the sheath is *in situ* so that the bioptome may be introduced in its place. The tip of the pigtail catheter

protrudes through the end of the sheath which prevents the sheath catching on side branches of the inferior vena cava as it is advanced; in addition the pigtail may facilitate making the right angle turn through the tricuspid valve which is necessary when using a femoral approach.

The long (104 cm) version of the Cordis bioptome is also suitable for left ventricular biopsy using the right (or left) femoral approach. The principle of the technique is similar to that described for the right ventricle. The artery is entered using a Seldinger approach, and the sheath and pigtail advanced over a 0.038″ diameter wire retrogradely into the aorta and through the aortic valve into the left ventricle. Arterial pressure can be monitored continuously through the side arm of the long sheath and the usual precautions for flushing the system must be observed, with particular care in relation to the sheath. Using a straight sheath, the bioptome comes to lie naturally on the inferior aspect of the left ventricle which is a suitable area for biopsy (Fig. 23.5). It is possible to advance the sheath along the inferior wall of the ventricle so that biopsies can be obtained from different sites between the apex and mitral valve (Fig. 23.6). The apex itself is best avoided as the myocardium may be thin at that point, and occasionally the bioptome becomes entangled with

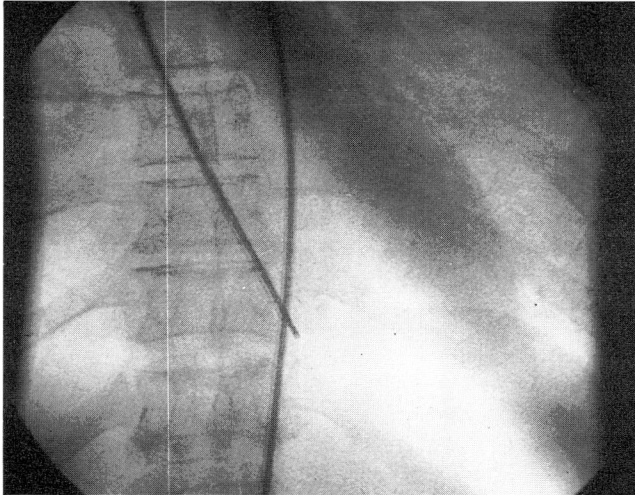

Fig. 23.5 King's (Cordis) bioptome in position for left ventricular biopsy.

the subvalve apparatus (posterolateral papillary muscle and attached chordae) when biopsies are taken close to the mitral valve.

Once the closed bioptome has been withdrawn from the patient, the bioptome is opened and myocardial tissue removed from the jaws with the point of a needle. Samples for histology are placed in 10% phosphate buffered formalin for light microscopy or 2.5% gluteraldehyde for ultrastructural

examination using thin sections or electron microscopy. Tissue processing and paraffin embedding takes 18 to 24 hours, although rapid processors are available which provide permanent sections within 3 to 4 hours. Routine staining includes haematoxylin and eosin to examine myocardial structure, Masson's Trichrome to assess the degree of fibrosis and methyl-green pyronine to aid in the diagnosis of rejection. Alternatively, tissue may be 'snap frozen' in liquid nitrogen for immunofluorescent studies or longterm storage. If other specific disorders are suspected, specialised stains may be required; for example Perl's iron stain for haemochromatosis, Congo red (or polarising light) for the diagnosis of amyloidosis.

Problems with the technique and complications

The small sample size (less than 5 mg of myocardial tissue) obtained using endomyocardial biopsy does not seem to have been a problem in terms of practical patient management; sampling error is reduced to an acceptable level if six or more biopsies are taken from various sites at any one time.

As with many techniques, the complication rate is related to operator experience, and in most large series the complication rate is low. The most serious complication is cardiac perforation resulting in cardiac tamponade. In the days of needle biopsy, tamponade was common, for example Shirey reported

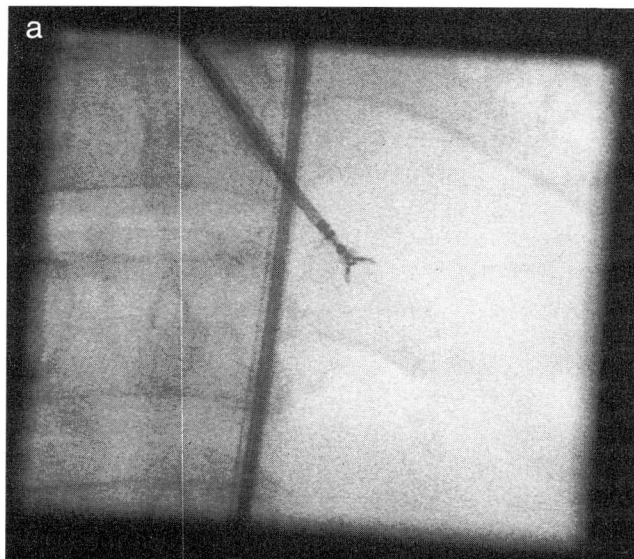

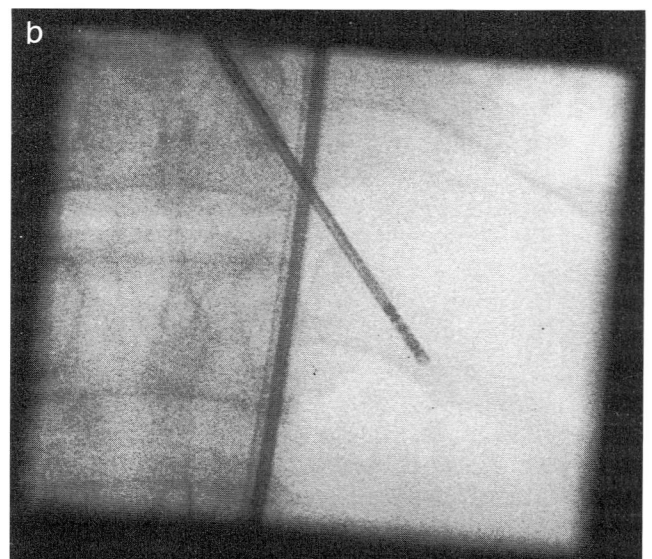

Fig. 23.6 King's (Cordis bioptome) (a) open and (b) closed.

an 8% incidence in a series of 198 patients, half of whom required emergency thoracotomy. In the first 2500 cases in the Stanford series (representing more than 8000 right ventricular biopsies) cardiac tamponade occurred in only four patients (incidence 0.16%) [14]. If care is taken to biopsy the interventricular septum (rather than the ventricular free wall), perforation is very rare. Other occasional complications reported in the literature include transient arrhythmias (e.g. atrial fibrillation) and 'postcardiotomy' syndrome; using the jugular approach, pneumothorax, air embolism, transient right recurrent laryngeal nerve palsy and Horner syndrome have all been described. Systemic thromboembolism appears to be a surprisingly uncommon complication of left ventricular biopsy.

Right or left ventricular biopsy?

There is debate in the literature as to whether it is more appropriate to biopsy the right or left ventricle. In general, the cardiomyopathies can be adequately studied using tissue from either ventricle. Carcinoid heart disease usually affects the right ventricle and radiation changes may be more easily appreciated on the right side. The functional abnormalities in hypertrophic obstructive cardiomyopathy commonly interfere with the left ventricle, although the ultrastructural changes are often diffuse. It has always been assumed that allograft rejection in transplant recipients affects the ventricular mass in a uniform manner; there are however some animal data suggesting that rejection as judged by histology is more marked in the right ventricle for reasons that are unclear [15]. In a routine non-transplant case it is often convenient to biopsy the left ventricle following completion of a diagnostic left and right heart catheter using the femoral approach.

HISTOLOGICAL CHANGES IN TRANSPLANT RECIPIENTS

Routine use of endomyocardial biopsy has allowed the natural history of cardiac allograft rejection to be more fully understood; in particular it was observed that augmentation of the immunosuppression resulted in restoration of the appearance of the myocardium to normal. The histological appearances of acute rejection have been divided by Billingham into four grades of increasing severity (Table 23.3)

Table 23.3 Classification of acute cardiac rejection by endomyocardial biopsy.

Mild rejection
  Early perivascular infiltrate
  Mononuclear cells (lyphocytes) are pyroninophilic
Moderate rejection
  Increased interstitial, perivascular and endocardial infiltrate
  Infiltrate is predominantly mononuclear and pyroninophilic
  Focal myocyte necrosis present
Severe rejection
  Increased inflammatory infiltrate includes neutrophils
  Mononuclear cells are pyroninophilic
  Interstitial haemorrhage and oedema
  Diffuse myocyte necrosis
Resolving rejection
  Decreased or absent infiltrate
  Active fibrosis and scar
  Residual mononuclear cells are non-pyroninophilic
  Residual lipochrome pigment

[16], and this classification is now generally accepted. Early (mild) rejection and focal myocyte necrosis (myocytolysis) can be easily reversed with augmented immunosuppression; indeed, more than 50% of biopsies showing a mild infiltrate resolve spontaneously on maintenance immunosuppression without specific treatment. Formerly, severe rejection was rarely reversible in patients treated with azathioprine, but it can often be reversed effectively in patients treated with cyclosporine. A fine, diffuse interstitial fibrosis can be seen in the myocardium of all patients treated with cyclosporine; the cause of this observation is unclear, but it appears to be a dose related phenomenon.

OTHER METHODS OF MONITORING REJECTION

Numerous other techniques have been used to monitor rejection in an attempt to provide a satisfactory non-invasive alternative to endomyocardial biopsy. At present, changes in cardiac structure as determined by biopsy remain the 'gold standard' against which these other methods are compared. None have been found to be entirely satisfactory, but there is no doubt that they can provide clinically useful information and may permit a reduction in the frequency of biopsy.

Electrocardiography

The value of recording serial electrocardiograms in transplant recipients was first described in dogs by Lower *et al.* in 1965 [17]. Conduction abnormalities, shifts in electrical axis, changes in heart rhythm and atrial and ventricular arrhythmias all accompanied episodes of acute rejection, but the only consistent finding and reliable indicator of acute rejection was a reduction in the amplitude of the R-wave, particularly in standard lead II. They also observed that this reduction in voltage could be reversed following successful treatment with augmented corticosteroids. The actual cause of the reduction in QRS voltage remained unclear, although it was suggested that the myocardial oedema associated with rejection may have been responsible. The same technique was applied to humans and the summated QRS voltage in leads I, II, III, V_1 and V_6 was the index used by most centres, a 15% reduction is summated voltage being taken as significant for rejection. When endomyocardial biopsy was developed and applied to transplant recipients by Caves in 1974, it became clear that the ECG manifestations of acute rejection developed 24–48 hours after histological evidence of rejection was demonstrable by biopsy. Since the advent of cyclosporine, the ECG has lost both sensitivity and specificity in detecting episodes of allograft rejection, possibly because myocardial oedema associated with allograft rejection is less impressive in patients treated with cyclosporine compared with patients treated with conventional immunosuppression.

Echocardiography and Doppler

Ultrasound was first applied to cardiac transplant recipients in 1969 [18], when it was noted that an increase in posterior left ventricular wall thickness and right ventricular dilatation were associated episodes of acute rejection. Similarly, changes in left ventricular mass appear to be related to the biopsy appearance in patients treated with conventional immunosuppression [19].

In patients treated with cyclosporine, haemodynamic compromise as evidenced by impaired systolic function is an uncommon manifestation of allograft rejection. It appears however that changes in diastolic function are related to rejection episodes, and these include a shortening of the isovolumic

relaxation period, premature mitral valve opening and a reduction in the peak rate of posterior left ventricular wall thinning (Fig. 23.7) [20, 21]. Similar results can be demonstrated by Doppler techniques [22].

Radionuclide imaging

Imaging with [201]thallium appears to be unreliable as a method of demonstrating episodes of acute rejection. In one study [23], fixed and reversible defects were demonstrated although their significance was unclear.

McGiffin compared the results of multigated acquisition (MUGA) scanning with endomyocardial biopsy after orthotopic cardiac transplantation and could find no significant relationship between the appearance of the endomyocardial biopsy and the MUGA ejection fraction [24]. Novitsky *et al.* compared MUGA scanning with simultaneous endomyocardial biopsy and found that a reduction in stroke volume and a decrease in end-diastolic volume correlated with acute rejection in the biopsy [25]; care is needed in the interpretation of this study however, because five of the seven patients had received heterotopic transplants and the haemodynamic contribution of the native heart to the circulation may have varied in this subgroup. At least some of the difficulties in the assessment of the radionuclide ventriculogram result from the abnormal plane of the transplanted heart within the chest cavity and the effects of the elevated resting heart rate in transplant recipients [26]. In experimental animal models, [111]indium labelled leucocytes [27] and ^{99m}Tc pyrophosphate [28] have been used with some success.

Immunological techniques

Cytoimmunological monitoring of peripheral blood lymphocytes although time consuming may allow a significant reduction in the frequency of endomyocardial biopsy [29], and *in situ* identification of lymphocyte subpopulations in cardiac biopsies may also be useful in monitoring episodes of acute rejection and predicting outcome [30].

Coronary artery disease in transplant recipients

Clinically significant coronary artery disease has

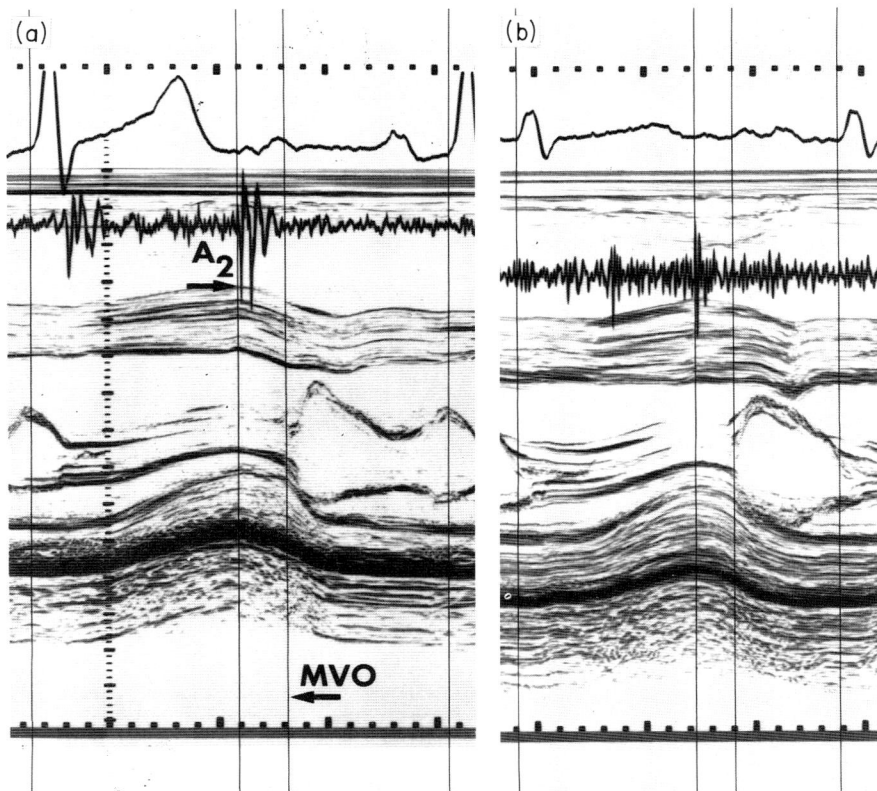

Fig. 23.7 M-mode echocardiogram in (a) a patient with a normal cardiac biopsy — no rejection; and (b) in the same patient during acute rejection with myocyte necrosis. The thickness of the septum and posterior wall has increased in association with a loss of posterior wall thinning in early diastole. During rejection the isovolumic period (aortic closure A_2 to mitral valve opening MVO) shortens.

been documented as early as 13—15 months after orthotopic cardiac transplantation [31, 32]. The pathogenesis of this aggressive form of coronary artery disease in transplant recipients is likely to be related to chronic immune mediated endothelial injury possibly exacerbated by hyperlipidaemia, systemic hypertension, smoking and prolonged graft ischaemia at the time of transplantation. In support of this theory of chronic immune injury, Hess *et al.* have emphasised the importance of cytotoxic B-cell antibodies in this subgroup [33]. The angiographic appearances of this type of coronary disease differ from that seen in a non-transplant population in that there is frequently diffuse tubular narrowing of an entire coronary artery branch, or alternatively close comparison of two sequential arteriograms on the same patient will reveal 'missing' branches. Coronary artery disease of the more usual type is also seen in transplant recipients [34], and coronary angioplasty has been successfully applied to these patients.

Graft atherosclerosis is a significant cause of late morbidity and mortality in transplant recipients due to acute myocardial infarction and sudden death. Denervation of the heart presents an additional problem in that the transplant recipient does not experience angina, and therefore coronary disease is only detected at routine follow-up coronary arteriography. Retransplantation is necessary in the majority of patients with significant coronary disease.

HEART—LUNG TRANSPLANTATION

Introduction

The most common indications for combined heart and lung transplantation remain patients with primary pulmonary hypertension and Eisenmenger syndrome; more recently a number of other groups of patients have proved to be suitable recipients, including patients with parenchymal lung disease, in particular cystic fibrosis (Table 23.4).

Patients undergoing combined heart and lung transplantation fare less well when compared with

Table 23.4 Indications for combined heart and lung transplantation.

Primary pulmonary hypertension
Eisenmenger syndrome
Chronic pulmonary disease
  Chronic bronchitis with Cor pulmonale
  Emphysema (including α_1-antitrypsin deficiency)
Interstitial lung disease
  Fibrosing alveolitis
  Pulmonary fibrosis (including drug reactions)
  Sarcoidosis
Cystic fibrosis
Alveolar proteinosis
Pulmonary venocclusive disease
Left ventricular disease with elevated PVR (>6 Wood units)

heart transplant recipients. Data submitted to the International Heart Transplant Registry reported in 1987 indicate an actuarial 1 year survival of 55.4% and a 5 year survival of 51.9% for all patients [1]. Individual centres however have reported significantly superior results [35].

Poor results achieved with isolated lung transplants in man [36] called for an alternative approach, and although sporadic reports of human heart–lung transplantation [37, 38] appeared after Cooley's initial attempt in 1968 [39], it was not until the heart–lung transplant programme commenced in Stanford in 1981 that the procedure could be regarded as anything other than experimental [40].

Many factors contributed to the successful development of human heart–lung transplantation. Extensive experience had been obtained with simple heart transplantation and the management of opportunistic infection and rejection were largely understood. Long-term survival in primates had been achieved for both auto- and allografts [41] due both to improved operative techniques and the application of new immunosuppressive agents, in particular cyclosporine. Importantly, it was assumed that rejection of the heart and lung would occur *pari passu*, so that rejection of the heart as judged by endomyocardial biopsy would reflect changes in the lung thereby avoiding the need for lung biopsy [42]. Finally, a number of modifications in the technique for removing the heart–lung bloc from the recipient [43] led to a reduction in early postoperative complications especially haemorrhage.

FUNCTION OF THE TRANSPLANTED LUNG

It is clear that long-term survival following combined heart and lung transplantation is critically dependent on satisfactory function of the transplanted lung, and it is the failure of pulmonary rather than cardiac function that is responsible for the less good results following the combined procedure.

Abnormalities of pulmonary haemodynamics, blood gas exchange or respiratory function following heart–lung transplantation may occur as a consequence of cardiopulmonary denervation, recurrent infection, drug toxicity, or pulmonary rejection. Furthermore, the loss of bronchial arterial supply and lymphatic drainage may be important in the early postoperative period.

HAEMODYNAMICS

Preoperative pulmonary hypertension is immediately corrected by combined heart and lung transplantation, and pulmonary artery pressure, pulmonary vascular resistance and cardiac output remain normal in most patients up to 3 years after surgery [44]. Similarly, left ventricular cine angiography has demonstrated normal systolic function with no localised wall motion abnormalities 12 months after transplantation.

CORONARY ARTERIOGRAPHY

Extensive colateral vessels develop from the atrial branches of the left and right coronary arteries in heart–lung transplant recipients. These vessels usually arise proximally from the right coronary artery or left circumflex and feed the mediastinum in the region of the tracheal anastomosis (Fig. 23.8). The presence of this network of collateral vessels is presumed to be fundamental to the lack of complications at the tracheal suture line in combined heart–lung transplant recipients compared with patients undergoing isolated unilateral lung transplantation.

Graft atherosclerosis has also been observed in heart–lung transplant recipients, similar in nature to that seen after simple heart transplantation. Proliferative atherosclerosis not apparent at routine coronary arteriography may be demonstrated histologically (Fig. 23.9), emphasising the difficulty in detecting this abnormality by conventional methods.

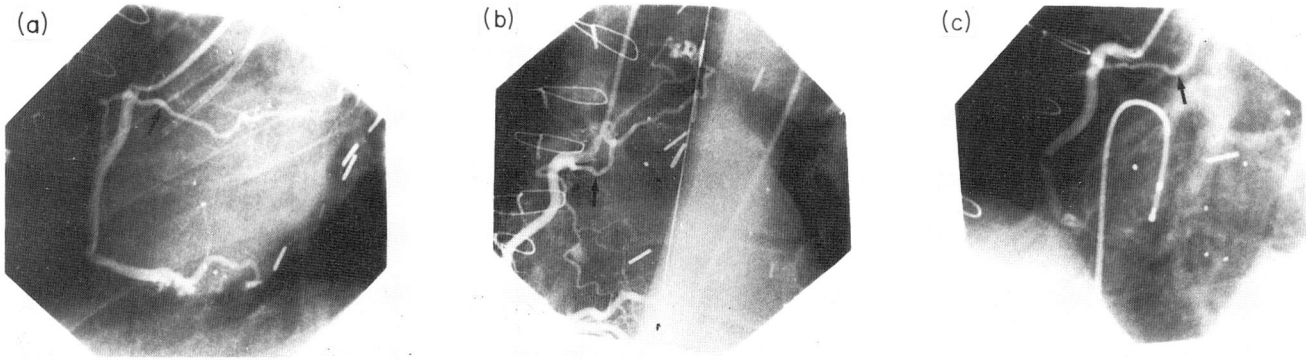

Fig. 23.8 Heart—lung transplant recipient: collateral vessels arising from the right coronary artery 1, 2 and 3 years after transplantation (reproduced with permission).

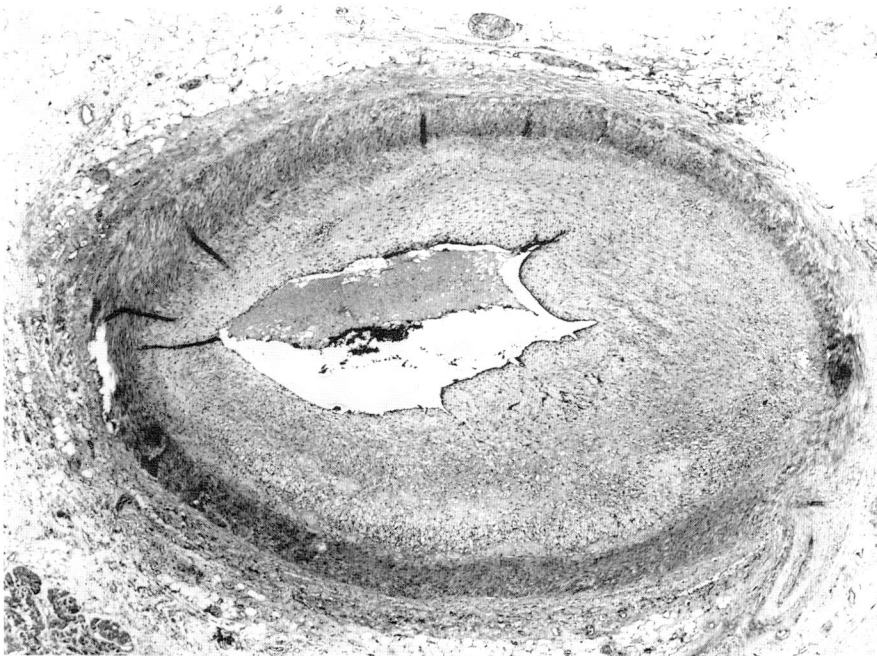

Fig. 23.9 Proliferative coronary atherosclerosis in a heart—lung transplant recipient.

BLOOD GAS EXCHANGE AND RESPIRATORY FUNCTION

Prior to heart—lung transplantation, severe arterial hypoxaemia is associated with a low $P_a\text{CO}_2$; hypoxia is more profound in those patients suffering from Eisenmenger syndrome. Following transplantation, arterial blood gases return to within normal limits, although the alveolar—arterial gradient for oxygen, a sensitive index of the efficiency of gas exchange, is increased in most transplant recipients 1 year after surgery [45]. Of clinical interest is the fact that nail clubbing rapidly regresses in most patients.

In the early postoperative period there is a marked decrease in lung volumes resulting in a moderately severe restrictive ventilatory defect. Reduced flow parameters are related to decreased lung volumes and do not necessarily imply intrinsic airflow obstruction. Abnormalities in lung volumes in the early postoperative period are probably attributable to thoracic surgery together with donor-recipient mismatch (as there is a tendency to transplant smaller lungs into a larger recipient), and are not sufficient to cause breathlessness. In uncomplicated cases, static lung function returns towards normal apart from a minor restrictive defect and mild impairment of gas exchange which improves with time.

Following heart—lung transplantation most patients show a dramatic improvement in symptoms and overall functional capacity. The improvement in objective exercise tolerance is primarily due to favourable changes in the circulatory response to exercise [46]. Ventilation and the ventilatory response to exercise are essentially normal; however the maximum oxygen uptake (Vo_2) is approximately 50% of predicted indicating some degree of circulatory limitation, partially explained by cardiopulmonary denervation and physical deconditioning of the recipients. Long-term follow-up shows further improvement in objective exercise capacity although Vo_2 changes little.

REIMPLANTATION RESPONSE

One of the most difficult aspects of the early postoperative care of the heart—lung transplant recipient is the assessment of the chest radiograph. Within the first 3 weeks after surgery, the radiographic appearance of the lung deteriorates in virtually all patients (Fig. 23.10). This may be alarming, with severe interstitial oedema and large pleural effusions resulting in impaired respiratory mechanics, ventilation—perfusion mismatch and arterial hypoxaemia, sufficient to require reventilation in a proportion of patients. Veith has called this syndrome the 'reimplantation response' [47]; the aetiology appears to be multifactorial, and contributing factors may include denervation of the cardiopulmonary axis, interruption of the lymphatics, surgical trauma and ischaemia. Alternatively, it may be a manifestation of an immune response to blood, blood products or antithymocyte globulin used in the perioperative period. Although rejection must be considered (see below), the syndrome is seen in lung autografts as well as allografts [41]. Daily screening for infection is mandatory because pyogenic or opportunistic infection mistaken for the 'reimplantation response' may prove fatal.

CHANGES ASSOCIATED WITH REJECTION

The assumption that heart and lung rejection was concomitant in heart—lung transplant recipients has

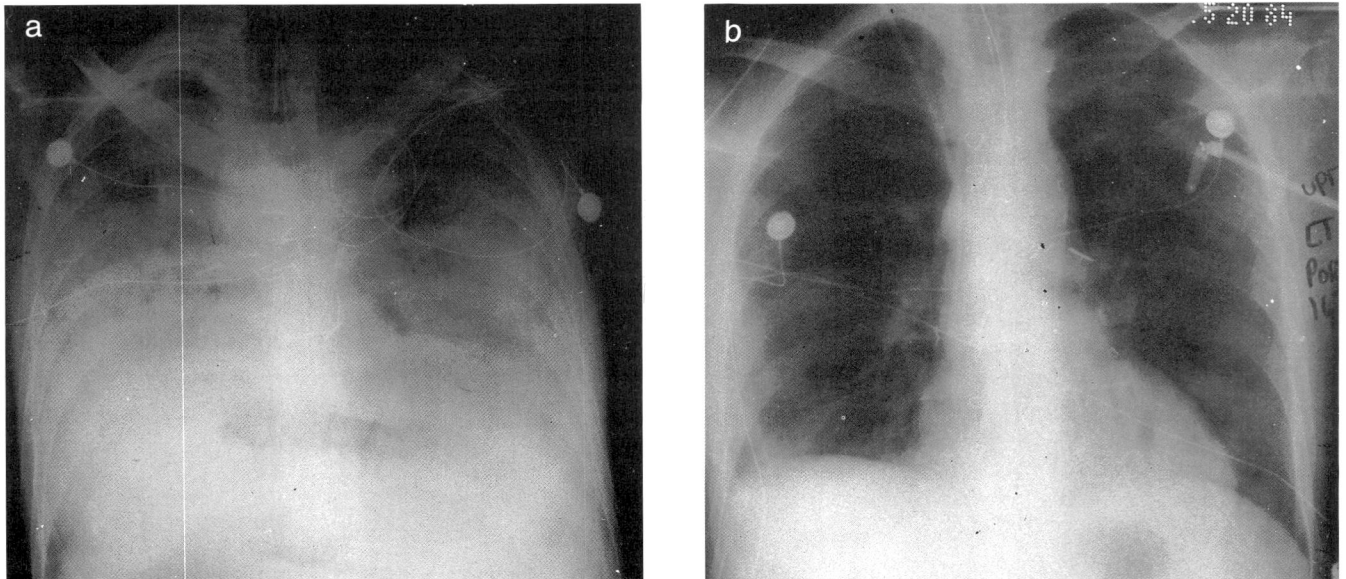

Fig. 23.10 Chest radiographs in a heart—lung transplant recipient showing the reimplantation response (a) with clearing four days later (b).

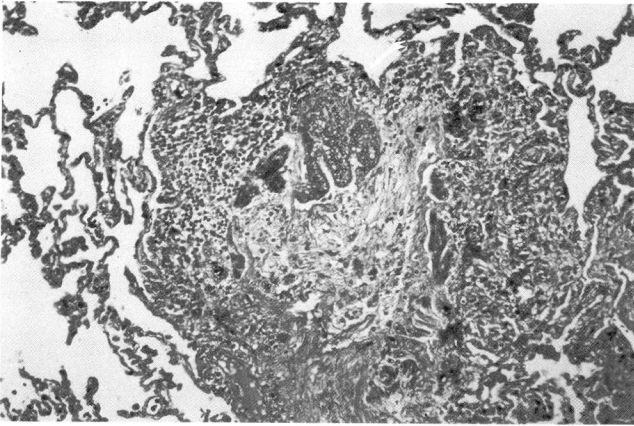

Fig. 23.11 Obliterative bronchiolitis in a heart-lung transplant recipient.

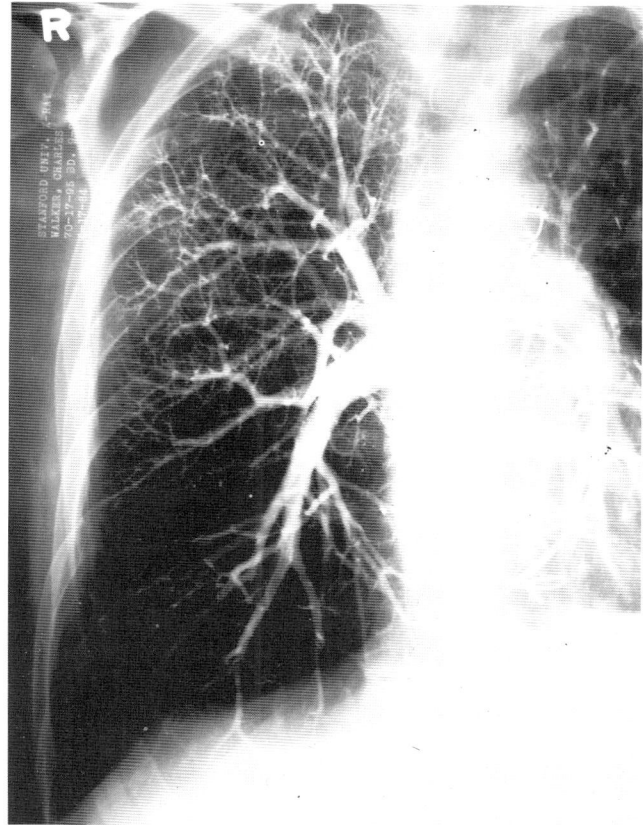

Fig. 23.12 Pulmonary arteriogram in a heart-lung transplant recipient 3 years after surgery showing attenuation of lower lobe pulmonary arteries with loss of fine distal branches.

been shown to be incorrect, firstly in primates [48], and more recently in man [49]. The lung appears to be a more immunogenic organ than the heart, and additionally a more delicate and complex structure, with the result that it is more prone to rejection and the effects of rejection are more devastating and less easily reversible with augmented immunosuppression. Difficulties in management are compounded by the practical problems in obtaining pulmonary material for histology. Repeated open lung biopsy is not feasible, transbronchial biopsy provides small specimens subject to sampling error, and the assessment of cell types from bronchial lavage is unreliable.

Symptoms of rhinitis, postnasal drainage and a cough productive of mucopurulent sputum may be indicative of early pulmonary rejection. Dyspnoea is not a feature until airflow obstruction is advanced. The most sensitive indicators of pulmonary rejection appear to be sequential measurements of the alveolar-arterial oxygen difference, specific airway conductance (S_{GAW}) and the FEF_{25-75}. In advanced cases, open lung biopsy shows evidence of obliterative bronchiolitis (Fig. 23.11) and intimal proliferation in small pulmonary arterioles. The similarity in the appearances of the pulmonary vessels to the coronary arteries suggests that this process has an immune basis and is a manifestation of rejection. Furthermore, recipients in whom abnormal pulmonary vessels have been demonstrated by angiography (Fig. 23.12) or histology all have had additional coronary artery disease.

The exact cause of obliterative bronchiolitis in transplant recipients is a matter of speculation [50]. Abnormalities of mucociliary transport, and inability to clear foreign antigens, chronic infection, pulmonary rejection and cyclosporine toxicity may all be factors important in the development of obliterative bronchiolitis. Once the process is established, the clinical course appears to be rapidly downhill leading to respiratory failure and death, although there are some data suggesting that early aggressive treatment with augmented immunosuppression may be effective [51]. Retransplantation may be necessary if this approach fails.

REFERENCES

1 Kaye MP. The registry of the International Society for Heart Transplantation: Fourth Official Report — 1987. *J Heart Transplant* 1987;**6**:63−7.

2 Schroeder JS. Hemodynamic performance of the human transplanted heart. *Transplant Proc* 1979;**11**:304−8.

3 Schroeder JS, Stinson EB, Dong E, Flamm MD, Shumway NE, Harrison DC. Cardiac transplantation in four patients: hemodynamic function in the immediate postoperative period. *J Thorac Cardiovasc Surg* 1970;**59**:155−64.

4 Dawkins KD. Non-invasive assessment of left ventricular function following cardiac transplantation. MD Thesis, University of London 1984.

5 Savin WM, Schroeder JS, Haskell WL. Response of cardiac transplant recipients to static and dynamic exercise: a review. *J Heart Transplant* 1982;**1**:72−9.

6 Billingham ME, Caves PK, Dong E, Clark DA, Shumway NE. The diagnosis of canine orthotopic cardiac allograft rejection by transvenous endomyocardial biopsy. *Transplant Proc* 1973;**5**:741−3.

7 Casten GG, March JB. Metabolic studies on cardiac tissue obtained by needle biopsy of the intact unanesthetized dog. *Circ Res* 1953;**1**:226−9.

8 Sutton DC, Sutton GC, Kent G. Needle biopsy of the human ventricular myocardium. *Q Bull Northwestern Univ Med School* 1956;**30**:213.

9 Sakakibara S, Konno S. Endomyocardial biopsy. *Jpn Heart J* 1962;**3**:537−543.

10 Caves PK, Stinson EB, Billingham ME, Rider AK, Shumway NE. Diagnosis of human cardiac allograft rejection by serial cardiac biopsy. *J Thorac Cardiovasc Surg* 1973;**66**:461−6.

11 Lower RR, Shumway NE. Studies on orthotopic homotransplantation of the canine heart. *Surg Forum* 1960;**11**:18−19.

12 Lower RR, Stofer RC, Shumway NE. Homovital transplantation of the heart. *J Thorac Cardiovasc Surg* 1961;**41**:196−204.

13 Billingham ME. Some recent advances in human pathology. *Hum Pathol* 1979;**10**:367−86.

14 Mason JW, Billingham ME. In: Yu PN, Goodwin JF (eds.) *Myocardial biopsy. Progress in Cardiology*, Volume 9. Philadelphia, Lea & Febiger, 1980;113−46.

15 Haverich A, Scott WC, Dawkins KD, Billingham ME, Jamieson SW. Asymmetric pattern of rejection following orthotopic cardiac transplantation in primates. *J Heart Transplant* 1984;**3**:280−5.

16 Billingham ME. Diagnosis of cardiac rejection by endomyocardial biopsy. *J Heart Transplant* 1982;**1**:25−30.

17 Lower PR, Dong E, Shumway NE. Long-term survival of cardiac homografts. *Surgery* 1965;**58**:110−19.

18 Schroeder JS, Popp RL, Atinson EB, Dong E, Shumway NE, Harrison DC. Acute rejection following cardiac transplantation: phonocardiographic and ultrasound observations. *Circulation* 1969;**30**:155−64.

19 Sagar KB, Hastillo A, Wolfgang TC, Lower RR, Hess ML. Left ventricular mass by M-mode echocardiography in cardiac transplant patients and acute rejection. *Circulation* 1981;**64**(suppl II):216−20.

20 Dawkins KD, Oldershaw PJ, Billingham ME, Hunt SA, Oyer PE, Jamieson SW et al. Changes in diastolic function as a non-invasive marker of cardiac allograft rejection. *J Heart Transplant* 1984;**3**:286−94.

21 Dawkins KD, Oldershaw PJ, Billingham ME, Hunt SA, Jamieson SW, Oyer PE et al. Non-invasive assessment of cardiac allograft rejection. *Transplant Proc* 1985;**17**:215−17.

22 Valantine HA. Doppler echocardiographic assessment of left ventricular function in cardiac allografts and its application to rejection surveillance. MD Thesis, University of London 1987.

23 McKillop JH, Goris ML. Thallium-201 myocardial imaging in patients with previous cardiac transplantation. *Clin Radiol* 1981;**32**:447−9.

24 McGiffin DC, Karp RB, Logic JR, Tauxe WN, Ceballos R. Results of radionuclide assessment of cardiac function following transplantation of the heart. *Ann Thorac Surg* 1984;**37**:382−6.

25 Novitzky D, Boniaszczuk J, Cooper DK, Isaacs SS, Rose AG, Smith J et al. Prediction of acute cardiac rejection by using radionuclide techniques. *S Afr Med J* 1984;**65**:5−7.

26 Dietz RR, Patton DD, Copeland JG, McNeill GC. Characteristics of the transplanted heart in the radionuclide ventriculogram. *J Heart Transplant* 1986;**5**:113−21.

27 Oluwole S, Wang T, Fawwaz R, Satake K, Nowygrod R, Reemtsma K et al. Use of indium-111-labeled cells in measurement of cellular dynamics of experimental cardiac allograft rejection. *Transplantation* 1981;**31**:51−5.

28 McGregor CGA, Hatz R, Aziz S, Billingham ME, McDougall IR. Technetium-99m pyrophosphate in diagnosis of acute cardiac rejection in the rat with effect of cyclosporine: concise communication. *J Nucl Med* 1984;**25**:870−3.

29 Ertel W, Reichenspurner H, Lersch C, Hammer C, Plahl M, Lehmann M et al. Cytoimmunological monitoring in acute rejection and following viral, bacterial or fungal infection following transplantation. *J Heart Transplant* 1985;**4**:390−4.

30 Kawaguchi A, Goldman MH, Hoshinaga K, Posner M, Page S, Mendez-Picon B et al. Monitoring of lymphocyte subpopulations in cyclosporine- and azathioprine-treated cardiac allograft recipients. *Transplant Proc* 1984;**16**:1542.

31 Hastillo A, Hess ML, Lower RR. Cardiac transplantation; expectations and limitations. *Mod Concepts Cardiovasc Dis* 1981;**50**:13−18.

32 Bieber C, Stinson E, Shumway N. Immunology of

cardiac transplantation. In: Zabriskie JB, Engle MA, Villareal H (eds.) *Clinical immunology of the heart.* New York, John Wiley & Sons, 1981;111—42.

33 Hess ML, Hastillo A, Mohanakumar T, Cowley MJ, Vetrovac G, Szentpetery S *et al.* Accelerated athereosclerosis in cardiac transplantation: role of cytotoxic B-cell antibodies and hyperlipidemia. *Circulation* 1983;**68**: (suppl II):94—101.

34 Shao-Zhou G, Alderman EL, Schroeder JS, Silverman JF, Hunt SA. Accelerated coronary vascular disease in the heart transplant patient: coronary arteriographic findings. *J Am Coll Cardiol* 1988;**12**:334—40.

35 Hutter JA, Despins P, Higgenbottam T, Stewart S, Wallwork J. Heart—lung transplantation: better use of resources. *Am J Med* 1988;**85**:4—11.

36 Veith FJ, Montefusco C, Kamholz SL, Mollenkopf FP. Lung transplantation. *J Heart Transplant* 1983;**2**:155—64.

37 Lillihei CW. In: Wildevuur CRG, Benfield JR. *A review of 23 human lung transplantations by 20 surgeons. Ann Thorac Surg* 1970;**9**:489—515.

38 Barnard CN, Cooper DKC. Clinical transplantation of the heart: a review of 13 years' personal experience. *J R Soc Med* 1981;**74**:670—4.

39 Cooley DA, Bloodwell RD, Hallman GL, Nora JJ, Harrison GM, Leachman RD. Organ transplantation for advanced cardiopulmonary disease. *Ann Thorac Surg* 1969;**8**:30—42.

40 Reitz BA, Wallwork JL, Hunt SA, Pennock JL, Billingham ME, Oyer PE *et al.* Heart—lung transplantation: successful therapy for patients with pulmonary vascular disease. *N Engl J Med* 1982;**306**:557—64.

41 Reitz BA, Burton NA, Jamieson SW, Bieber CP, Pennock JL, Stinson EB *et al.* Heart and lung transplantation: autotransplantation and allotransplantation in primates with extended survival. *J Thorac Cardiovasc Surg* 1980;**80**:360—71.

42 Reitz BA, Gaudiani VA, Hunt SA, Wallwork J, Billingham ME, Oyer PE *et al.* Diagnosis and treatment of allograft rejection in heart—lung transplant recipients. *J Thorac Cardiovasc Surg* 1983;**85**:354—61.

43 Jamieson SW, Reitz BA, Oyer PE, Billingham M, Modry D, Baldwin J *et al.* Combined heart and lung transplantation. *Lancet* 1983;**1**:1130—1.

44 Dawkins KD, Jamieson SW, Hunt SA, Baldwin JC, Burke CM, Billingham ME *et al.* Longterm results, hemodynamics and complications following combined heart and lung transplantation. *Circulation* 1985;**71**:919—26.

45 Theodore J, Jamieson SW, Burke CM, Reitz BA, Stinson EB, Van Kessel A *et al.* Physiologic aspects of human heart—lung transplantation: pulmonary function status of the post-transplanted lung. *Chest* 1984;**86**:349—57.

46 Theodore J, Burke C, Dawkins K, Jamieson SW, Stinson EB, Van Kessel A *et al.* Circulatory versus respiratory limitations to exercise before and after human heart—lung transplantation. *J Am Coll Cardiol* 1984;**3**:509.

47 Siegelman SS, Sinha SB, Veith FJ. Pulmonary reimplantation response. *Ann Surg* 1973;**177**:30—6.

48 Scott WC, Haverich A, Billingham ME, Dawkins KD, Jamieson SW. Lethal lung rejection without significant cardiac rejection in primate heart—lung allotransplants. *J Heart Transplant* 1984;**4**:33—8.

49 McGregor CGA, Jamieson SW, Baldwin JC, Burke CM, Dawkins KD, Stinson EB *et al.* Combined heart—lung transplantation in the treatment of Eisenmenger's syndrome. *J Thorac Cardiovasc Surg* 1985;**90**:623—6.

50 Burke CM, Theodore J, Dawkins KD, Yousem SA, Blank N, Billingham ME *et al.* Post-transplant obliterative bronchiolitis and other late sequelae in human heart—lung transplantation. *Chest* 1984;**86**:824—9.

51 Burke CM, Morris AJR, Dawkins KD, McGregor CGA, Yousem SA, Allen M *et al.* Late airflow obstruction in heart—lung transplant recipients. *J Heart Transplant* 1985;**4**:437—40.

Appendices

Manufacturers and equipment

	Cine film	Cardiac catheters	Catheter-tip manometers	Angioplasty-valvuloplasty	Recording systems	Disposable pressure monitoring	Thermodilution catheters	Oximeters/blood-gas analysers	X-ray equipment	Contrast media	Pacemaker leads (temporary)	Pacemaker leads (permanent)	Pacemakers
Abbott													
ACS													
Agfa Gevaert													
Argon													
American Edwards													
APC													
Biotek													
Biotronic													
Cambridge													
Camino													
Cardiac Recorders													
Cardiologic													
Ciba–Corning													
Cook													
Cordis													
Daig													
ELA													
Elecath													
Gaeltec													
General Electric													
Gould													
Hewlett Packard													
Intermedics													
Kimal													
Kodak													
Mallinckrodt													
Mansfield													
Meadox													
Medtronic													
Medex													
Millar													
Nycomed													
Phillips													
Picker													
PPG/Hellige													
Radiometer													
Schering													
Schneider													
Scimed													
Shiley													
Siemens													
Siemens Pacesetter													
S & W													
Sorin													
S–Pace													
Squibb													
Telectronics													
UMI													
USCI													
Vitatron													
Vygon													
Waters													
Winthrop													

Addresses

The following list of companies supplying equipment, contrast media, etc. used in cardiac catheterisation and pacemaking is inevitably incomplete. Addresses change and companies change their names with bewildering frequency; the list is provided in the hope that it may be of use but no responsibility can be taken for any present — or future — inaccuracies.

Abbott Laboratories
Abbot Critical Care Systems. Abbott Laboratories, North Chicago, Illinois 60064 USA.
UK Agents: Abbott House, Moorbridge Road, Maidenhead, Berkshire, SL6 8JG.

Advanced Cardiovascular Systems, Inc., (ACS)
ACS 1395 Charleston Road, Mountain View, California 94039−7101 USA.
UK Agents: Intervention Ltd., 1 Redman Court, Bell Street, Princes Risborough, Buckinghamshire HP17 OAA.

Agfa Gevaert
UK Agents: 27 Great West Road, Brentford, Middlesex TW8 9AX.

Angiomedics Inc., — see Shiley

Argon Medical Corporation
PO Box 1970, Athens TX 75751 USA.
UK Agents: Polystan (GB) Ltd., 34 Nottingham South and Wilford Industrial Estate, Ruddington Lane, Wilford, Nottingham NG11 7EP.

American Edwards Laboratories, Inc.,
Anasco, Puerto Rico, 00610.
UK Agents: Baxters Health Care Ltd., Wallingford Road, Compton, Nr. Newbury, Berkshire RD16 OQW.

APC Medical
2 Little Ridge, Ridgeway, Welwyn Garden City, Hertfordshire AL7 2BH.

Biotek
Via Dell Arcoveggio 70, 40129 Bologna, Italy.
UK Agents: JPR Ltd., Weirbank, Bray-on-Thames, Maidenhead SL6 2ED.

Biotronic
Biotronic Berlin GmbH, Woermannkehre 1, D-100, Berlin 47, Germany.
UK Agents: Biotronic, 135/137 High Street, Slough SL1 1DN.

Cambridge Medical Equipments
73 Spring Street, Ossining, New York 10562 USA.

UK Agents: Cambridge Medical Equipments Ltd., 50 Clifton Industrial Estate, Cherry Hinton Road, Cambridge CB1 4FJ.

Camino
7550 Trade Street, San Diego, California 92121 USA.
UK Agents: Camino (UK) Ltd., 14 Vincent Road, Selsey, West Sussex PO20 9DH.

Cardiac Recorders Ltd.,
34 Scarborough Road, London N4 4LU.

Cardiologic (CPI)
4100 Hamline Avenue North, St. Paul, Minnesota MN 55112−5798 USA.
UK Agents: Alliance House, Roman Ridge Road, Sheffield S9 1GB.

Ciba−Corning
Medfield MA02052 USA.
UK Agents: Ciba Laboratories, Wimblehurst Road, Horsham, West Sussex RM124AB.

William Cook
PO Box 489, Bloomington, Indiana 47402 USA.
European Agents: William Cook Europe A/S, Sandet 6, DK-4632, Bjaeverskov, Denmark.
UK Agents: William Cook, 9 Glebe Road, Letchworth, Hertfordshire SG6 1DS.

Cordis Corporation
PO Box 370428, Miami, Florida 33137 USA.
European Agents: Cordis Europa, NV Postbus 38, 9300 AA Roden, The Netherlands.
UK Agents: Cordis UK, Cordis House, Syon Gate Way, Brentford, Middlesex TW8 9DD.

Daig Corporation
14901 Minnetonka Industrial Road, Minnetonka 55343 USA.
UK Agents: see Kimal Scientific Products Ltd.

ELA
ELA Medical, 98/100 Rue Maurice−Arnoux, 93120 Montrouge, France.
US Agents: ELA Medical Inc., 37−40 Williston Road, Minnetonka MN 55343.
UK Agents: Lawlite, 4 Barnfield Road, Sevenoaks, Kent TN13 2AY.

ELECATH
Electro-catheter Corporation, 2100 Felder Court, PO Box 1241C, Rahaway, New Jersey 07065 USA.
UK Agents: Franklin Life Support Systems, Cressex Industrial Estate, High Wycombe, Buckinghamshire.

Gaeltec Ltd.,
Dunvegan, Isle of Skye, Scotland IV55 8GU.
US Agents: Medical Measurements Incorporated (MMI), 53 Main Street, Hackensack, New Jersey 07601 USA.

General Electric
GE (General Electric) Medical Systems, PO Box 414, Milwaukee W153201 USA.
UK Agents: IGE (International General Electric) Medical Systems Ltd., Coolidge House, 260 Bath Road, Slough, Berkshire SL1 4ER.

Gould Inc.
Instruments Division, 3631 Perkins Avenue, Cleveland, Ohio 44114 USA.
UK Agents: Gould Medical (and Spectramed Ltd.) Advanced Technology Unit 11, University of Warwick Science Park, Coventry CV4 7E2.

Gould Electronics Ltd.,
Stanford House, Science Park South, Warrington, Cheshire WA3 7BH.
GU Manufacturing Company Ltd., Plympton Street, London NW8 8ABW.

Hewlett Packard
1501 Page Hill Road, Palo Alto, California 94304 USA.
UK Agents: Hewlett Packard Ltd., Medical Group, Harman House, 1 George Street, Uxbridge, Middlesex UB8 1TH.

Intermedics
International Medical Devices, PO Box 617 Freeport, Texas 77541 USA.
UK Agents: 557–579 Harehill Lane, Leeds LS9 6NQ.

Kimal Scientific Products Ltd.,
Unit E, Eskdale Road Industrial Estate, Uxbridge, Middlesex UB8 2RT.

Kodak
Eastman Kodak Company, 343 State Street, Rochester, New York 14650 USA.
UK Agents: Kodak Company Ltd., Box 33, Swallowdale Road, Hemel Hempstead, Hertfordshire.

Lexington Instruments
Waltham, Massachusetts, USA.

Mallinckrodt Inc.,
Post Office Box 5840, St. Louis, Missouri 63134 USA.
UK Agents: Mallinckrodt Diagnostica (UK) Ltd., Building 223 Norwood Crescent, Heathrow Airport, Hounslow, Middlesex TW6 1JH

Mansfield Scientific Inc.,
135 Forbes Boulevard, Mansfield, Massachusetts 02048 USA.
UK Agents: S-Pace Medical Ltd., Lydgate House, Lydgate Lane, Sheffield S10 5FH.

Meadox Surgimed
112 Bauer Drive, Oakland, New Jersey 07436 USA.
European Agents: Meadox Surgimed A/S, Smedeland 5, DK-2600 Glostrup, Denmark.

UK Agents: Meadox Prosthetics Ltd., 11 Wycombe Road, Prestwood, Great Missenden, Buckinghamshire, HP16 ONX.

Medtronic
Medtronic Inc., 6951 Central Avenue NE Minneapolis MN5543Z USA.
UK Agents: Medtronic (UK) Ltd., Marlins House, Marlins Meadow, Watford, Hertfordshire WD1 8RG.

Medex
Medex Inc., 3637 Lacon Road, Hilliard, Ohio 43026 USA.
UK Agents: Medex Medical Inc., 12 Bentwood Road, Carrs Industrial Estate, Haslingden, Rossendale, Lancashire BB4 5HH.

Millar Instruments
PO Box 230227 Houston, Texas 77223 0227 USA.
UK Agents: see Kimal Scientific Products Ltd.

Nycomed AS
Postboks 4220 Torshov N-0401, Oslo 4, Norway.
UK Agents: Nycomed (UK) Ltd., Nycomed House, 2111 Coventry Road, Sheldon, Birmingham B26 3EA.

Phillips Medical Systems
PO Box 10000, 5680 Best, Eindhoven, The Netherlands.
UK Agents: Phillips Medical Systems. Kelvin House, 63/75 Glenthorne Road, Hammersmith, London W4 OLJ.

Picker
595 Miner Road, Cleveland, Ohio 44143 USA.
UK Agents: Picker International Ltd., PO Box No. 2, East Lane, Wembley Middlesex HA9 7PR.

PPG/Hellige
PPG/Hellige GmbH, Heinrich Von Stephan Strasse 4, D7800 Freiburg-im-Breisgau, West Germany.
UK Agents: PPG/Hellige Ltd., Unit 8, Hogwood Lane, Finchampstead, Berkshire RG11 4QW.

Radiometer
Radiometer Copenhagen, 72 Emdrupvej, DK-2400, Copenhagen N.V. Denmark.
UK Agents: V.A. Howe, 12–14 St. Anne's Crescent, London SW18 2LS.

Schering
Schering AG, 1 Berlin 65, Mullerstrasse 170–172.
US Agents: Berlex Laboratories, 300 Fairfield Road, Wayne New Jersey 07470 USA.
UK Agents: Schering Health Care Ltd., The Brow, Burgess Hill, West Susex, RH15 9NE

Schneider Medintag AG
Scharenmoostrasse 115, 8052 Zurich, Switzerland.
US Agents: Schneider–Shiley, 2905 Northwest Boulevard. Minneapolis, Minnesota.

Scimed Life Systems Inc.,
1300 County Road 6, Minneapolis, Minnesota, MN 55441 USA.

UK Agents: Biomedical Systems Ltd., (BMS) Ashley Drive, Bothwell, Strathclyde, Scotland.

Shiley

US Agents: 17600 Gillette Ave., Irvine, California 92714.

UK Agents: Shiley House, 42 Thames Street, Windsor, Berkshire SL4 1PR

Siemens AG

Henkestrasse 127, Postfach 32 60, D-8520 Erlangen, Federal Republic of Germany.

UK Agents: Siemens House. Windmill Road, Sunbury-on-Thames TW16 7HS.

US Agents: Siemens Medical Systems Inc., 186 Wood Avenue South, Iselin, New Jersey 08830.

Siemens/Pacesetter

UK Agents: Siemens House, Windmill Road, Sunbury-on-Thames TW16 7HS.

US Agents: Siemens Medical Systems Inc., 186 Wood Avenue South, Iselin, New Jersey 08830.

Simonsen and Weel (S&W)

Medico Teknik A/S Denmark Hersteduang 8, DK 2620 Albertslund, Denmark.

UK Agents: S&W Ltd., Ruxley Corner, Sidcup, Kent DA14 5BL.

Sorin

Sorin Biomedica 13040 Saluggia (Vercelli), Italy.

UK Agents: Lithmedica Ltd., 48 Mill Road., Cambridge CB1 2AS.

S-Pace

S-Pace Medical Ltd., Lydgate House, Lydgate Lane, Sheffield S10 5FH

Squibb

ER Squibb and sons Inc., Princeton, New Jersey USA.

Telectronics

Telectronics Pty Ltd., 2 Sirius Road, Lane Cove, Sydney, New South Wales 2066 Australia.

US Agents: Telectronics Ltd., 301 West Vogel Avenue, Milwaukee, Wisconsin 53207.

UK Agents: 5 Delta Business Centre, Colindeep Lane, London NW9 6BX.

Universal Medical Instrument Corporation (UMI)

Box 100, Ballston Spa, New York 12020−0100 USA.

USCI (United States Catheter and Instrument)

Division of CR Bard Inc., 1200 Technology Park Drive, PO Box 7025, Billerica, Massachusetts 01821 USA.

UK Agents: USCI International Ltd., Norris House, Burrell Road, Haywards Heath, West Sussex.

Vitatron

Vitatron BV, PO Box 76, 6950 AB, Dieren, The Netherlands.

UK Agents: Vitatron UK, Kings House, 18 Kings Street, Maidenhead, Berkshire SL6 2ED.

Vygon

BP 7−95440 Ecouen, France.

UK Agents: Vygon (UK) Ltd., Bridge Road, Cirencester, Gloucester GL7 1PH.

Waters Inst. Co.,

PO Box 6117, Rochester, Minnesota 55903−6117 USA.

UK Agents: Watco Services, PO Box 86, Basingstoke, Hampshire.

Winthrop Pharmaceuticals

Division of Sterling Drugs Inc., New York 10016 USA.

UK Agents: Sterling Winthrop House, Onslow Street, Guildford, Surrey GU1 4YS.

Address list prepared by Mrs. Sue Jones, Chief Cardiac Technician, The Brompton Hospital, London.

Index